The Oxford Handbook of Cultural
Neuroscience and Global Mental Health

The Oxford Handbook of Criminal
Neuroscience and Global Mental Health

The Oxford Handbook of Cultural Neuroscience and Global Mental Health

Edited by

Joan Y. Chiao, Shu-Chen Li, Robert Turner,

Su Yeon Lee-Tauler, and Beverly A. Pringle

OXFORD
UNIVERSITY PRESS

OXFORD
UNIVERSITY PRESS

Oxford University Press is a department of the University of Oxford. It furthers
the University's objective of excellence in research, scholarship, and education
by publishing worldwide. Oxford is a registered trade mark of Oxford University
Press in the UK and certain other countries.

Published in the United States of America by Oxford University Press
198 Madison Avenue, New York, NY 10016, United States of America.

Library of Congress Cataloging-in-Publication Data
Names: Chiao, Joan Y., editor. | Li, Shu-Chen (Research scientist) editor.
Title: The Oxford handbook of cultural neuroscience and global mental health /
edited by Joan Y. Chiao, Shu-Chen Li, Robert Turner, Su Yeon Lee-Tauler,
Beverly A. Pringle.
Description: New York : Oxford University Press, 2021. |
Series: Oxford library of psychology series | Includes bibliographical references
and index.
Identifiers: LCCN 2020058290 (print) | LCCN 2020058291 (ebook) |
ISBN 9780190057695 (hardback) | ISBN 9780190057718 (epub)
Subjects: LCSH: Neurosciences—Social aspects. | Mental illness—Social
aspects. | Cognition and culture.
Classification: LCC RC343.3 .O94 2021 (print) | LCC RC343.3 (ebook) |
DDC 362.196/8—dc23
LC record available at https://lccn.loc.gov/2020058290
LC ebook record available at https://lccn.loc.gov/2020058291

DOI: 10.1093/oxfordhb/9780190057695.001.0001

9 8 7 6 5 4 3 2 1

Printed by Integrated Books International, United States of America

CONTENTS

PREFACE

Introduction to the Field

Cultural neuroscience and global mental health is an interdisciplinary field of study that integrates theoretical, methodological, and empirical approaches in cultural neuroscience to address grand challenges in global mental health. The study of cultural neuroscience and global mental health addresses how evidence-based research that identifies root causes and risk and preventative factors in global mental health can help to improve and achieve health equity for all people across the world. The goal of discovery and delivery science to find cures, preventions, and interventions for global mental health fulfills one of the human development goals to cure disease and improve health for all. Mental health for all is crucial to the development of security and empowerment across societies and nations. The achievement of health equity for all reflects the total and complete well-being of individuals, societies, and nations and the human capability to live a long and healthy life.

Brief Description of History and Developments of the Field

The history of the field of cultural neuroscience and global mental health builds from the international collaboration of interdisciplinary networks of researchers, practitioners, and policymakers. The growth of the field has been steadily shaped by several major developments. The emergence of cultural neuroscience as a research field traces back to the epistemological understanding of the mutual influences of culture and biology on human health throughout intellectual history. In the 7th century, Isidori of Seville introduced the conceptual notion of human diversity and early conceptualizations of culture in his encyclopedia *Etymologiae*. The epistemology of ancient Western and Eastern philosophical thought, from Locke to Lao Tzu, reflects cultural variation in conceptualizations of the notion of object and the environment. Contemporary notions of cultural influences on mental health build from ancient philosophical thought of culture and human nature and expand into detailed efforts of scientific observation to investigate the influences of culture on the human mind, brain, and behavior. The notion that cures for mental health arise from cultural practices and their underlying neurobiological bases exemplifies the rationale and goal of scientific efforts in cultural neuroscience.

The systematic study of cultural influences on the human brain strengthens the human capability for the achievement of health equity. In 2011, the scientific initiatives of the International Cultural Neuroscience Consortium, an interdisciplinary organization of researchers, led to the coordination of social and financial investment for priority setting in the systematic study of cultural neuroscience. Chief priorities include the expansion of theoretical, methodological, and empirical approaches in cultural neuroscience to address reducing the gap in population health disparities. The development of cultural neuroscience as a research field has steadily grown with targeted capacity-building initiatives that have led to the establishment and achievement of interdisciplinary goals. The advancement of evidence-based research provides a foundation to systematically address issues of culture in health equity and health policy.

The political will and commitment for the achievement of health equity for all has been recognized across all nations through the Sustainable Development Goals program of the United Nations and the World Health Organization Mental Health program. The Movement for Global Mental Health reflects the systematic coordination of collaborative efforts to achieve mental health for all through the societal efforts of researchers, policymakers, and advocates. In 2011, the research agenda and priority setting of the Grand Challenges in Global Mental Health Initiative strengthened the political commitment of nations to the achievement of health equity. Social and financial investment in the research agenda and priorities for global mental health promotes efforts in human development and empowerment for the achievement of health equity for all. Plans of action to achieve health equity and to discover cures for mental health require long-term investment, support, and responsivity of stakeholders to coordinate for integrated research and policy interventions.

Broad Review of the Chapter Contributions

The effective coordination of research and policy stakeholders to support the efforts in discovery and delivery science for the elimination of mental, neurological, and substance abuse (MNS) disorders reflects a chief goal of cultural neuroscience and global mental health. The *Handbook* consists of chapters that provide a detailed and comprehensive review of the main themes and topics in the interdisciplinary field of cultural neuroscience and global mental health. The chapters develop main themes and topics in cultural neuroscience and global mental health that identify root causes and risk and protective factors in mental health across cultural settings. The international authors contribute on themes and topics of research in cultural neuroscience and global mental health from distinct regions across the world. The *Handbook* provides a foundation of research that raises awareness of the global burden in mental health and contributes to international aid and development programs. The development and implementation of mental health policy and practice reflect the culmination of coordinated efforts of researchers, advocates, and policymakers to provide evidence-based research for plans of action that promote mental health for all.

Mission of the Field

Mental health is vital to the development and empowerment of individuals, societies, and nations. The promotion of mental health practices and policies that advance plans of action for the elimination of mental health disorders enhances health equity for all. The achievement of total well-being for all relies on the sustained commitment to practices and policies that ensure human security and empowerment. The strengthening of human capabilities for protection from vulnerabilities, from poverty to armed conflict, and for empowerment, including social and economic equality and independence, expands the range of human freedoms that ensure human fulfillment. The United Nations Sustainable Development Goals plan of action includes the elimination of diseases by 2030 to achieve good health and well-being for all. The goal to eliminate mental health disorders and disease reflects global objectives that are at the core of the development mission. Sustained action and investment toward such goals of the development agenda are necessary for the promotion and, ultimately, the achievement of health equity and equality for all.

Joan Y. Chiao
Shu-Chen Li
Robert Turner
Su Yeon Lee-Tauler
Beverly A. Pringle

ACKNOWLEDGMENTS

The *Oxford Handbook of Cultural Neuroscience and Global Mental Health* represents the second collection of scholarly contributions from the International Cultural Neuroscience Consortium (ICNC) with the International Cultural Neuroscience and Global Mental Health Network (ICNGMHN), organizations of interdisciplinary scholars dedicated to international cooperation and scientific advancement in culture and health. The *Handbook* is intended to provide future generations of scholars with the foundations in cultural neuroscience to address grand challenges in global mental health in the 21st century. The translation of research into practice and policy strengthens the advancement of scientific and technological progress in the cultural neuroscience and global mental health field for the benefit of all.

The volume editors would like to thank Dr. Bill Elwood (National Institute of Mental Health [NIMH]) for his programmatic support of ICNC scholars. We are grateful to Ishmael Amarreh, Pamela Collins, Roberto Delgado, Tamara Lewis-Johnson, Chunling Lu, and Makeda Williams from the annual National Institutes of Health (NIH) Global Mental Health Workshop convened with the NIMH Office for Research on Disparities and Global Mental Health and Grand Challenges Canada for their innovative and dedicated support. We warmly thank Technische Universität Dresden, the Max Planck Institute, the NIMH Office for Research on Disparities and Global Mental Health, and the NIMH Center for Global Mental Health Research for their support. We are grateful to the editors from Oxford University Press for their editorial guidance.

Joan Y. Chiao

Shu-Chen Li

Robert Turner

Su Yeon Lee-Tauler

Beverly A. Pringle

CONTRIBUTORS

Gabriella M. Alvarez
  Department of Psychology and
  Neuroscience
  University of North Carolina
  Chapel Hill
  Chapel Hill, North Carolina
  USA

Diane-Jo Bart-Plange
  Department of Psychology
  University of Virginia
  Charlottesville, Virginia
  USA

Genna M. Bebko
  Department of Psychiatry
  University of Pittsburgh
  Pittsburgh, Pennsylvania
  USA

Caroline Blais
  Department of Psychology
  University of Quebec in Outaouais
  Quebec, Canada
  Canada

Katherine D. Blizinsky
  National Institutes of Health
  Bethesda, Maryland
  USA

Roberto Caldara
  Department of Psychology
  University of Fribourg
  Fribourg, Switzerland
  Switzerland

Yoojin Chae
  Department of Human Development
  & Family Sciences
  Texas Tech University
  Lubbock, Texas
  USA

Joan Y. Chiao
  International Cultural Neuroscience
  Consortium
  Highland Park, Illinois and
  Bethesda, MD
  USA

Morgan Gianola
  Department of Psychology
  University of Miami
  Miami, Florida
  USA

Joshua O. S. Goh
  Graduate Institute of Brain and
  Mind Sciences
  National Taiwan University
  Taipei, Taiwan
  Taiwan

Sharon G. Goto
  Department of Psychological Science
  Pomona College
  Claremont, California
  USA

Sarah Grayzel-Ward
  Department of Psychological Science
  Pomona College
  Claremont, California
  USA

Patricia M. Greenfield
Department of Psychology
University of California Los Angeles
Los Angeles, California
USA

Angela Gutchess
Department of Psychology
Brandeis University
Waltham, Massachusetts
USA

Ryan S. Hampton
Department of Psychology
Arizona State University
Tempe, Arizona
USA

Lasana T. Harris
Department of Experimental
Psychology
University College London
London, United Kingdom
United Kingdom

Hyisung C. Hwang
Department of Psychology
San Francisco State University
San Francisco, California
USA

Tetsuya Iidaka
Brain & Mind Research Center
Nagoya University
Nagoya, Japan
Japan

Lene Arnett Jensen
Department of Psychology
Clark University
Worcester, Massachusetts
USA

Hajin Lee
Department of Psychology
University of Alberta
Edmonton, Alberta
Canada

Su Yeon Lee-Tauler
Uniformed Services University of the
Health Sciences
Bethesda, MD
USA

Richard S. Lewis
Department of Psychological Science
Pomona College
Claremont, California
USA

Shu-Chen Li
Faculty of Psychology
Centre for Tactile Internet with
Human-in-the-Loop
Technische Universität Dresden
Germany

Zhang Li
Department of Psychology
Capitol Normal University
Beijing, China
China

Elizabeth A. Reynolds Losin
Department of Psychology
University of Miami
Miami, Florida
USA

Yoko Mano
National Institute for Physiological
Sciences
Okazaki, Japan
Japan

Takahiko Masuda
Department of Psychology
University of Alberta
Edmonton, Alberta
Canada

David Matsumoto
Department of Psychology
San Francisco State University
San Francisco, California
USA

Nishaat Mukadam
Department of Psychology
Brandeis University
Waltham, Massachusetts
USA

Keely A. Muscatell
Department of Psychology and
Neuroscience
University of North Carolina
Chapel Hill
Chapel Hill, North Carolina
USA

Michael Muthukrishna
Department of Psychological and
Behavioral Science
London School of Economics
London, United Kingdom
United Kingdom

Michio Nomura
Department of Education
Kyoto University
Kyoto, Japan
Japan

Georg Northoff
Institute of Mental Health
Research
University of Ottawa
Ottawa, Canada
Canada

Beverly A. Pringle
National Institute of Health
Bethesda, MD
USA

Jeremy Rappleye
Graduate School of
Education
Kyoto University
Kyoto, Japan
Japan

Matthew J. Russell
Department of Psychology
University of Alberta
Edmonton, Alberta
Canada

Norihiro Sadato
Division of Cerebral Integration
Department of System Neuroscience
National Institute for Physiological
Sciences
Okazaki, Japan
Japan

Emily P. Sands
Department of Experimental
Psychology
University College London
London, United Kingdom
United Kingdom

Kate M. Scott
Department of Psychological Medicine
Dunedin School of Medicine
University of Otago
Dunedin, New Zealand
New Zealand

Dan J. Stein
Department of Psychiatry
University of Cape Town
Cape Town, South Africa
South Africa

Rongxiang Tang
Department of Psychology
Washington University in St. Louis
St. Louis, Missouri
USA

Yi-Yuan Tang
Department of Psychology
Texas Tech University
Lubbock, Texas
USA

Sophie Trawalter
Department of Public Policy and
Psychology
University of Virginia
Charlottesville, Virginia
USA

Ayano Tsuda
Graduate School of
Education
Kyoto University
Kyoto, Japan
Japan

Robert Turner
Max Planck Institute
Leipzig, Germany
Germany
and
University of Nottingham
Nottingham, United Kingdom
United Kingdom

Ryutaro Uchiyama
Centre for Lifelong Learning and
Individualised Cognition
Nanyang Technological
University
Singapore

Michael E. W. Varnum
Department of Psychology
Arizona State University
Tempe, Arizona
USA

Yolanda Vasquez-Salgado
Department of Psychology
California State University
Northridge
Northridge, California
USA

Qi Wang
Department of Human Development
Cornell University
Ithaca, New York
USA

Wanbing Zhang
Department of Psychology
Brandeis University
Waltham, Massachusetts
USA

Xin Zhang
Department of Psychology
Brandeis University
Waltham, Massachusetts
USA

Joan Y. Chiao, Shu-Chen Li, Robert Turner, Su Yeon Lee-Tauler, *and* Beverly A. Pringle

Cultural Neuroscience and Global Mental Health

The goal of the *Oxford Handbook of Cultural Neuroscience and Global Mental Health* is to provide a comprehensive review of evidence-based research in cultural neuroscience to address grand challenges in global mental health. The epidemiology of mental disorders shows geographic variation in the cultural and genetic factors that affect the global prevalence of disease and disorder.

One of the grand challenges in global mental health is to identify biomarkers underlying the etiology of mental, neurological, and substance abuse (MNS) disorders (Collins et al., 2011). MNS disorders make up approximately 13% of the global burden of disease and are an unmet societal burden. The identification of basic cellular and molecular mechanisms of the human brain provides important insights for the discovery of cures for, preventions of, and interventions for MNS disorders.

Research in cultural neuroscience consists of theoretical, methodological, and empirical approaches to the study of cultural influences on neurobiological mechanisms of mental health. The identification of root causes, risk, and preventative factors in MNS disorders builds novel pathways for discovery and delivery science in global mental health. Theoretical approaches in cultural neuroscience build conceptual models and frameworks that provide causal explanations of the mutual influences of cultural and biological systems on the mind, brain, and behavior. Methodological approaches in cultural neuroscience describe complementary tools that allow for the observation of patterns of neural activity during mental function across spatiotemporal scales. Empirical approaches in cultural neuroscience seek to identify the phenotypes and endophenotypes of MNS disorders across cultural settings.

The *Handbook* chapters provide detailed and systematic reviews of themes and topics in cultural neuroscience and global mental health. This setting of the research agenda is a core function of building research capacity in the field. Specific areas for targeted development consist of scientific research initiatives that systematically define problems, develop scientifically evaluated solutions, and share and apply the generation of scientific knowledge in the field. Research priorities in the field illustrate the specific areas of growth and development of new scientific knowledge. The research agenda in the field details the specific priority research areas for the development and implementation of policies and interventions. Specific research areas with an established evidence base across cultures are necessary for the communication of scientific knowledge to become an evidence-based practice in global mental health.

Organization of the Handbook

The *Oxford Handbook of Cultural Neuroscience and Global Mental Health* is a scholarly collection of chapters organized into five parts. The chapters consist of comprehensive reviews on theoretical, methodological, and empirical foundations in cultural neuroscience and global mental health.

Part I introduces theoretical foundations in cultural neuroscience and global mental health. Chapters 1 through 9 introduce fundamental laws and principles that characterize the necessary and sufficient conditions of scientific explanations in cultural neuroscience and global mental health. The chapters explore the theoretical foundations of culture to explain the etiology of mental disorders in global mental health, ascertain the breadth and depth of causal patterns of cultural and neural phenomena in the natural world, and explore the characteristics of cultural and neural systems and their emergent properties.

In Chapter 1, Scott discusses the cross-national prevalence of mental disorders from the World Mental Health Surveys Initiative. The cross-national prevalence of mental disorders varies across distinct factors. Cross-national variation in mental disorders highlights the importance of understanding how culture affects the manifestation and assessment of mental disorders.

In Chapter 2, Uchiyama and Muthukrishna articulate theories of cultural evolutionary neuroscience to explain processes of cultural and genetic adaptation that guide the evolutionary history of the brain. Cultural evolutionary neuroscience theories elaborate the mutual influence of culture and genetic processes on fundamental elements of the brain across the evolutionary timescale. Processes of cultural transmission and cultural change alter pathways of psychological adaptation.

In Chapter 3, Matsumoto and Hwang introduce theoretical frameworks to understand human culture and its relation to psychological processes. Cultural elements consist of a range of psychological processes that regulate behaviors. Understanding the fundamentals of the psychological construction of culture contributes to the investigation of global mental health.

In Chapter 4, Northoff introduces the foundational concepts to the study of culture and neurophilosophy. Northoff characterizes the processes of embrainment to explain how culture is encoded within neuronal activity and enculturation to illustrate how culture is manifested from neuronal activity of the mental functions of affect and cognition.

Northoff articulates how the cultural processes of embrainment and enculturation of the self in neuronal activity are key components of mental health across cultural settings.

In Chapter 5, Chiao, Mano, Li, Bebko, Blizinsky, and Turner review theoretical and methodological approaches to understanding how culture influences neurobiological mechanisms of behavior. Empirical approaches in cultural neuroscience detail programs of research that explain fundamental multilevel mechanisms of culture within the organization of the nervous system. Research in cultural neuroscience aims to identify root causes underlying the etiology of mental disorders.

In Chapter 6, Chiao and Sadato review psychophysiological approaches in cultural neuroscience and global mental health. Cultural processes are instantiated in psychophysiological mechanisms within the central and autonomic nervous system. Spatiotemporal patterns of physiological arousal and electrocortical responses characterize cultural processes in mental constructs.

In Chapter 7, Chiao, Li, and Sadato review cultural and genomic systems that maintain and regulate neurobiological mechanisms of behavior. Cultural processes guide the expression of behavior and genes in the functional activity of neural circuitry. The interaction of genes and environment affects neural and behavioral expression within cultural contexts.

In Chapter 8, Vasquez-Salgado and Greenfield introduce theoretical principles in sociocultural developmental neuroscience. Interdisciplinary work in the field integrates research approaches from sociocultural, developmental, and neuroscience traditions. Sociocultural factors play an important role in shaping neurodevelopmental trajectories.

In Chapter 9, Li discusses the population prospects of an aging population that is undergoing rapid future growth. The growing aging population suggests the importance of preventions and interventions in global mental health that maintain and enhance cognitive functioning and socioemotional well-being. The interaction of the aging brain with cultural resources shows the malleability of brain plasticity through experience and learning.

Part II

Part II provides review on the systematic investigation of the etiology of mental health disorders across cultures. Chapters 10 through 18 detail programs of research for the discovery of root causes and risk and protective factors underlying mental disorders across cultures. The chapters describe the impact of global concerns on societal factors affecting mental health and review programs of research that characterize the role of culture in psychological processes and neurobiological mechanisms of behavior. The chapters provide conceptual models of social and biological factors that affect risk and resilience for mental disorders. Scientific progress and achievement in cultural neuroscience are paramount to the discovery of cures, preventions, and interventions in global mental health.

In Chapter 10, Chiao, Mano, Stein, and Sadato present causal models of cultural influences on mental constructs and neurobiological mechanisms of emotion. Culture affects multilevel mechanisms of emotion. Standard paradigms provide methodological tools for the measurement and observation of patterns of emotion phenomena across cultures.

In Chapter 11, Nomura, Tsuda, and Rappleye discuss the importance of culture as a protective factor in mental health. Culture guides the experience of positive and negative emotion. Cultural factors affecting the experience of positive emotion are beneficial to mental health.

In Chapter 12, Masuda, Lee, and Russell review cultural variation in social cognition. Cultural variation in psychological processes, such as attention, are instantiated within cognitive and neural mechanisms. Understanding cultural variation in fundamental psychological processes in cognitive and neural mechanisms contributes to empirical advances in mental health.

In Chapter 13, Tang and Tang review cultural differences in the representation and processing of numerical cognition. Cultural factors play an important role in guiding the acquisition of numerical cognition. Understanding how culture affects numerical cognition has important implications for mathematical education and mental health.

In Chapter 14, Gutchess, Mukadam, Zhang, and Zhang review cultural influences on memory and aging. Culture shapes the malleability of memory and cognition in healthy aging. Culture affects the modification of risk and protective factors of mental disorders.

In Chapter 15, Goto, Lewis, and Grayzel-Ward review cultural variation in self-construal. Cultural influences on self-construal affect cognition and behavior. Understanding how culture affects self-construal contributes to understanding of preventions and interventions for mental disorders.

In Chapter 16, Blais and Caldara discuss cultural differences in visual perception. Cultural and environmental factors affect visual processing of social cues. The influence of culture on visual and social perception, such as on face and emotion recognition, affect the modification of risk and protective factors of mental health.

In Chapter 17, Gianola and Reynolds Losin review theoretical, methodological, and empirical foundations of cultural learning as processes of imitation. Imitation is a core cognitive process of cultural learning. Multilevel mechanisms of cultural learning contribute to alterations in behavioral, cognitive, and neural systems that contribute to mental disorders.

In Chapter 18, Sands and Harris discuss intergroup theories of dehumanization as a societal factor affecting fundamental cognitive processes. Cultural influences on cognitive processes affect social reasoning in intergroup contexts. Systematic investigation of dehumanization contributes to the modification of risk and protective factors affecting global mental health.

Part III

Part III discusses the societal and environmental influences that affect prevention and early intervention in global mental health. Chapters 19 to 23 provide a systematic review of cultural factors affecting the development and implementation of prevention of and early intervention for mental disorders in global mental health.

In Chapter 19, Varnum and Hampton articulate systematic research programs that investigate patterns of cultural change. Theoretical frameworks in behavioral ecology posit ecological factors that affect causal patterns of cultural change. The neuroscience of cultural change investigates the environmental influences on the structure and function of the brain across cultures.

In Chapter 20, Goh postulates characteristics of neuroplasticity that contribute to neural mechanisms of behavioral acculturation. Processes of behavioral acculturation affect neurocomputation. Investigation of the relation between the dynamics of neuroplasticity and acculturation may provide insight into biomarkers of mental disorders.

In Chapter 21, Chiao, Mano, and Sadato review the translation of evidence-based research in cultural neuroscience into the development and implementation of technological innovations for prevention and early intervention in global mental health. The use of evidence-based cultural neuroscience research in the practice of global mental health requires the transformation of new scientific knowledge into technological innovation for the development of mental health promotion. Evidence-based research in cultural neuroscience informs the design and practical application of technological innovations for prevention and early intervention in global mental health.

In Chapter 22, Chiao, Mano, and Sadato review the mutual influence of cultural and environmental systems. Geographic variations in environmental conditions are a causal influence on the maintenance and regulation of cultural systems. Reciprocally, cultural systems serve as a protective factor in global mental health.

In Chapter 23, Jensen discusses the influence of globalization on human development across cultural contexts. Globalization affects societal exposure to risk and protective factors of mental health across cultures. Systematic research on globalization and its impact on human development across cultures contributes to the development and implementation of prevention of and early intervention for mental disorders in global mental health.

Part IV

Part IV examines strategies for the improvement of treatment and expansion of access to care in global mental health. Chapters 24 and 25 review the societal factors that affect the effectiveness and access to care for MNS disorders across cultural settings.

In Chapter 24, Iidaka provides a systematic analysis of the role of cultural and economic factors that affect the prevalence of mental disorders across nations. Cultural factors contribute to the prevention of and early intervention for mental disorders. Macroeconomic factors affect the effectiveness of interventions for mental disorders within the cultural context.

In Chapter 25, Tang and Tang propose an integrative health model for the development and implementation of prevention of and early intervention for mental disorders in global mental health. Culture affects the development and effectiveness of evidence-based care for mental disorders. The incorporation of cultural factors into the development and implementation of interventions and evidence-based care is an effective strategy for mental health promotion.

Part V

Part V reviews the cultural and socioeconomic factors that affect the prevalence of mental disorders across ethnic groups. Chapters 26 through 29 discuss the contribution of race, ethnicity, stigma, socioeconomic status, as well as social-linguistic and cultural factors on autobiographic memory to variation in the prevalence of health disparities. The chapters discuss research, practice, and policy for the amelioration of mental health disparities across cultural contexts.

In Chapter 26, Chiao and Blizinsky review the cultural factors affecting mental health disparities of racial and ethnic groups. Cultural and genetic variations of ethnic and racial groups contribute to the variation in prevalence of mental disorders. Closing the gap in racial and ethnic disparities in mental health is necessary to achieve health equity.

In Chapter 27, Bart-Plange and Trawalter review the translation of research on stigma into policy that eliminates health disparities and improves health equity. Stigma manifests at multiple levels and contributes to health inequalities. The reduction and elimination of stigma are necessary as a policy solution to reduce social disparities in health.

In Chapter 28, Alvarez and Muscatell review the cultural processes and neural mechanisms that contribute to socioeconomic disparities. Cultural and psychological processes contribute to the perception and subjective experience of socioeconomic status. Mental health promotion strategies that build resilience contribute to the amelioration of socioeconomic health disparities.

In Chapter 29, Chae and Wang review the influences of social-linguistic and other cultural factors, such as family narrative practices and emotional knowledge, on autobiographic memory. The cumulated memory of personal experiences throughout life allows individuals to form clear and distinct representations of themselves. Disturbed or disrupted self-concepts or self-identities are at the core of many mental health issues, including depression and dementia. Cultural differences in mechanisms underlying autobiographic memory thus may moderate relations between self-identity and psychological well-being.

This scholarly collection provides a detailed and in-depth review of themes and topics in cultural neuroscience and global mental health. Addressing grand challenges in global mental health requires a multitude of approaches improving quality of life and reducing the societal burden of mental disorders. Research, practice, and policy in cultural neuroscience and global mental health that build evidence-based approaches to discovery and delivery science provide the necessary foundation for the amelioration of mental disorders across nations.

The advancement of research, practice, and policy in cultural neuroscience and global mental health contributes to the alleviation of the societal and economic burden of mental disorders. Ultimately, through the generation and sharing of novel scientific knowledge, we gain insight into ways that mental health and well-being of individuals, societies, and nations can be achieved.

Reference

Collins, P. Y., Patel, V., Joestl, S. S., March, D., Insel, T. R., Daar, A. S.; Scientific Advisory Board and the Committee of the Grand Challenges on Global Mental Health, Anderson, W., Dhansay, M. A., Phillips, A., Shurin, S., Walport, M., Ewart, W., Savill, S. J., Bordin, I. A., Costello, E. J., Durkin, M., Fairburn, C., Glass, R. I., Hall, W., Huang, Y., Hyman, S. E., Jamison, K., Kaaya, S., Kapur, S., Kleinman, A., Ogunniyi, A., Otero-Ojeda, A., Poo, M. M., Ravindranath, V., Sahakian, B. J., Saxenda, S., Singer, P. A., Stein, D. J. (2011). Grand challenges in global mental health. *Nature, 475*(7354), 27–30.

Cultural Neuroscience and Global Mental Health

PART

1

Cultural
Neuroscience
and Global
Mental Health

The Cross-National Epidemiology of Mental Health Disorders

Kate M. Scott

Abstract

This chapter presents an overview of the recent findings from the World Health Organization World Mental Health Surveys Initiative. Many consistent patterns of association emerge in all countries: mental disorders begin relatively early in the lifespan; they are most prevalent among the young and the socially disadvantaged; they are often highly impairing and frequently comorbid with other disorders; and they are greatly undertreated. These findings have important policy implications indicating the need to prioritize the detection and treatment of mental disorders in young people, to upscale treatment services in low- and middle-income countries in particular, and to coordinate the health policy response with other relevant agencies to reduce the incidence and improve the outcomes of mental disorders among the socially vulnerable. Substantial cross-national variation is also evident, with both prevalence and impairment being lower in low-income countries than in high-income countries. These cross-national patterns are provocative but difficult to interpret given the inability to tease apart the respective contributions of methodological and substantive factors to the cross-national variation observed. A good deal of further research into the ways cultures interact with both the expression and the assessment of mental disorders is required.

Key Words: mental disorders, cross-national, epidemiology, World Mental Health Surveys, World Health Organization

Introduction

Research on the epidemiology of mental disorders initially lagged behind other medical epidemiological research due to a lack of agreement on diagnostic criteria for mental disorders and, connected with that, the absence of a standardized and reliable assessment tool (Kessler, 2000; Stein et al., 2018). These problems were overcome first with the 1980 publication of the *Diagnostic and Statistical Manual of Mental Disorders*, 3rd edition (DSM-III), with clearly operationalized diagnostic criteria, and second with the development the Diagnostic Interview Schedule (DIS; Robins et al., 1981) based on the DSM-III. The DIS was a fully structured research diagnostic interview designed for use by trained nonclinicians and suitable for use in general populations. It was first used in the

Epidemiological Catchment Area study in the United States (Robins et al., 1984), a large, multisite community survey of mental disorders. In a first attempt to learn more about the cross-national epidemiology of selected mental disorders, studies were undertaken with the DIS in a number of different countries (Weissman et al., 1994, 1996).

Initiated by the World Health Organization (WHO) and with support from the US Department of Health and Human Services, work began in the mid-1980s on an expansion of the DIS to incorporate *International Statistical Classification of Diseases* (ICD) criteria and to create a culturally valid translation of the instrument in many different languages. This instrument became known as the WHO Composite International Diagnostic Interview (CIDI; Kessler & Ustun, 2004). The CIDI was first used in the National Comorbidity Survey in the United States and then in a range of other countries under the auspices of the WHO International Consortium in Psychiatric Epidemiology. After a substantial revision of the CIDI in the later 1990s, the WHO launched the World Mental Health (WMH) Surveys Initiative to encourage countries around the world to implement surveys using the revised CIDI (Kessler & Ustun, 2008). Grants from a number of agencies, including the US National Institutes of Health, allowed the creation of a core infrastructure for the WMH surveys. This coordinated approach has provided specialist expertise and oversight of data quality, as well as allowing cost saving for participating countries. Many low- and middle-income countries that had not previously participated in psychiatric epidemiological research due to lack of financial and human resources to undertake such work have been able to conduct large, methodologically rigorous general population surveys and to build capacity in psychiatric epidemiology. The WMH Surveys Initiative now includes over 30 countries and more than 150,000 respondents.

As well as providing data on the prevalence, correlates, and treatment of many mental disorders in a wide range of low-, middle-, and high-income countries, the WMH surveys also provide much-needed data on the degree of functional impairment associated with mental disorders. The first WHO Global Burden of Disease study concluded that mental disorders (especially depression) were among the most disabling health conditions worldwide (Murray & Lopez, 1996), but this conclusion was based in part on estimates by clinical experts of the comparative disability associated with health conditions, rather than on the reports of patients themselves. The WMH surveys were designed to address this limitation (Kessler, 2011) by including a range of measures of disorder-specific and generic disability alongside assessment of the mental disorder symptoms. Disability assessment contributes to the categorization of disorder severity; calculation of the proportion with severe disorders is critical information for mental health service planning.

The WMH surveys have yielded a wealth of data, published in several hundred journal articles and six books. This chapter can provide only a brief overview of the descriptive epidemiology of disorders; due to space limitations, it is not possible to present country-specific estimates for each disorder, so the estimates shown to follow are aggregated across countries and country-income groups (low/lower-middle-income countries;

upper-middle-income countries; high-income countries). Readers interested in country-specific data and more detail on specific disorders are referred to our recent volume (Scott et al., 2018). The WMH surveys website (https://www.hcp.med.harvard.edu/wmh/) provides details on the earlier volumes as well as a chronological listing of articles, many featuring in-depth analytical investigations of a range of hypotheses related to the epidemiology of mental disorders.

Methods

The findings reviewed in this chapter are based on the data from 32 surveys from the following 29 countries: Australia, Belgium, Brazil, Bulgaria, People's Republic of China (PRC; three surveys: Beijing, Shanghai, and Shenzhen), Colombia (two surveys), France, Germany, Iraq, Israel, Italy, Japan, Lebanon, Mexico, Netherlands, New Zealand, Nigeria, Northern Ireland, Peru, Portugal, Poland, Romania, South Africa, Spain, Ukraine, United States, Peru, Portugal, and Poland. A stratified multistage clustered area probability sampling strategy was used to select adult respondents (18+ years) in most WMH countries. Most of the surveys were based on nationally representative household samples, while Colombia, Mexico, and PRC Shenzhen were based on nationally representative household samples in urbanized areas.

An extensive WMH training protocol was developed by the professional survey administration staff at the Survey Research Center (SRC) at the Michigan Institute of Survey Research, with SRC interview supervisors training trainer-supervisors in each WMH country. In most countries, internal subsampling was used to reduce respondent burden by dividing the interview into two parts. All respondents completed Part 1, which included the core diagnostic assessment of most mental disorders. All Part 1 respondents who met lifetime criteria for any mental disorder and a probability sample of respondents without mental disorders were administered Part 2 (at the same interview sitting), which assessed the remaining mental disorders and collected information on physical conditions and covariates. Part 2 respondents were weighted by the inverse of their probability of selection to adjust for differential sampling. Additional weights were used to adjust for differential probabilities of selection within households, to adjust for nonresponse, and to match the samples to population sociodemographic distributions. All survey datasets were cleaned, checked, and analyzed by the Data Coordination Center (DCC) at Harvard University. Translation protocols and measures taken to ensure data accuracy, cross-national consistency, and informed consent are described in detail elsewhere (Kessler & Ustun, 2008; Kessler et al., 2018).

The mental disorders featured in this chapter include *anxiety disorders* (panic disorder, generalized anxiety disorder, specific phobia, social phobia, agoraphobia, posttraumatic stress disorder); *mood disorders* (major depression, bipolar spectrum disorder [bipolar 1 or bipolar II or bipolar subthreshold]); *substance use disorders* (alcohol and drug abuse/dependence); *impulse control disorders* (intermittent explosive disorder, adult attention-deficit-hyperactivity disorder); eating disorders; and some childhood onset disorders (conduct disorder and oppositional defiance disorder). (Readers are referred to Scott et al., 2018, for diagnostic definitions.) In the sections that follow, findings are presented on the lifetime prevalence of these disorders, their average age of onset, the degree of associated functional impairment, and the proportion of those with disorders who sought treatment.

Lifetime Prevalence

Variation Across Disorders

The lifetime prevalence (i.e., the percentage meeting diagnostic criteria at some stage in their lives prior to interview) of specific mental disorders, averaged across all 29 contributing surveys, is shown in the first column of Table 1.1. Major depressive disorder (MDD) is the single most prevalent disorder (10.6%) among those considered here, with intermittent explosive disorder (IED) the least prevalent disorder (0.8%). Other disorders not included in Table 1.1 either because they were not assessed in the WMH surveys (schizophrenia) or due to low case numbers (anorexia) or problems with ascertainment in the CIDI (obsessive compulsive disorder) would also be expected to have low prevalence.

Although MDD is the single most prevalent disorder, anxiety disorders are the most prevalent class of disorders (data not shown). Among the anxiety disorders included here, the most prevalent are the two that usually have early onset (social anxiety disorder and specific phobia at 4.0% and 7.4%, respectively), while agoraphobia is considerably less prevalent (1.2%). The prevalence of adult separation anxiety disorder (SEPAD) is, at 3.1%, perhaps greater than previously understood, falling as it does between generalized anxiety disorder (GAD) at 2.7% and posttraumatic disorder (PTSD) at 3.9%. Alcohol use disorders (AUDs) collectively have one of the higher lifetime estimates shown in Table 1.1 (8.6%), while disruptive behavior disorders and eating disorders are for the most part clustered at the lower end of the prevalence spectrum (from 1.0% for bulimia nervosa to 2.7% for oppositional defiant disorder).

One important interpretation caveat applies to these estimates: because they are based on retrospective data, they are undoubtedly conservative due to recall failure, conscious nondisclosure, and survival bias. One study that illustrates how conservative these prevalence estimates may be compared prospectively assessed lifetime prevalence (the cumulative prevalence obtained from repeated past-year measures of the common mental disorders from age 18 to 32) in a New Zealand birth cohort with the retrospectively assessed lifetime prevalence estimates in the same age group in the New Zealand and American WMH surveys (Moffitt et al., 2010). That study found that the prospective lifetime estimates were approximately double the retrospective lifetime estimates for all the major classes of mental disorders. An even greater discrepancy between lifetime prevalence estimates obtained from retrospective versus prospective methods was observed in long-term follow-up of the Baltimore Epidemiological Catchment Area Study (Takayanagi

Table 1.1. Prevalence, Age of Onset, Impairment, and Treatment Associated With Mental Disorders in the World Mental Health Surveys, All Countries Combined

Type of Mental Disorders	Lifetime Prevalence		Median Age of Onset	Proportion of 12-Month Cases With Severe Role Impairment		Proportion of 12-Month Cases Who Sought Treatment From Health Care Sector[a]	
	%	SE		%	SE	%	SE
Mood Disorders							
Major depressive disorder	10.6	0.1	38	57.0	0.9	38.9	0.7
Bipolar spectrum disorder	1.9	0.1	25	58.5	4.5	54.5	3.8
Anxiety Disorders							
Generalized anxiety disorder	2.7	0.1	38	45.7	1.5	40.0	1.4
Panic disorder	1.7	0.0	32	45.7	1.7	56.0	1.6
Agoraphobia	1.2	0.0	21	41.9	2.0	46.9	1.9
Social anxiety disorder	4.0	0.1	14	37.6	1.0	34.9	0.9
Specific phobia	7.4	0.1	8	18.7	0.6	21.0	0.6
Posttraumatic stress disorder	3.9	0.1	35	49.8	2.1	42.9	1.6
Separation anxiety disorder (adult)	3.1	0.1	27	38.3	2.7	27.7	2.4
Impulse Control Disorders							
Intermittent explosive disorder	0.8	0.0	17	38.9	2.9	25.0	2.6
Conduct disorder	2.3	0.1	13	–	–	23.5	5.3
Oppositional defiant disorder	2.7	0.1	12	41.2	5.3	39.7	5.1
Substance Use Disorders							
Alcohol use disorder	8.6	0.1	23	30.8	2.9	18.0	1.0
Drug use disorder	3.5	0.1	20	45.8	6.8	33.4	2.3
Eating Disorders							
Binge eating disorder	1.8	0.1	24	21.3	3.1	34.0	3.3
Bulimia nervosa	1.0	0.1	21	31.7	4.8	40.7	4.9

[a] Either the specialty mental health sector or the general medical sector.

et al., 2014). Retrospective methods particularly undercount individuals with single, mild episodes (Wells & Horwood, 2004), so the WMH lifetime prevalence estimates are likely to be more representative of the more severe and persistent disorders.

Variation Across Countries as a Function of Country-Level Income

Table 1.2 presents the average lifetime prevalence for each disorder in each of three country income groups: low/lower-middle-income countries, upper-middle-income countries, and high-income countries. These data reveal a consistent pattern in 17 of 18 disorders (SEPAD being the exception) of prevalence being lower in the low/lower-middle-income countries than in the high-income countries. In 15 of 18 disorders prevalence is lowest in the low/lower-middle-income countries, and in 10 of 18 disorders there is a significant positive gradient of increasing prevalence with increasing country income level. This positive association between prevalence of mental disorders and income level of country found in the WMH surveys is consistent with the findings of systematic reviews from the recent Global Burden of Disease (GBD) studies (Baxter et al., 2012; Ferrari, Somerville, et al., 2013; Steel et al., 2014). Nonetheless, it is somewhat counterintuitive because it is opposite in direction to what might be expected based on individual-level inverse associations between socioeconomic status and mental disorder prevalence within countries observed in the WMH data as well as numerous other studies.

Intriguing though it is, this cross-national variation found in the WMH surveys is difficult to interpret because of the unknown role of methodological influences on the differences in prevalence estimates across countries. Although enormous effort went into making the WMH surveys as methodologically consistent as possible (Kessler et al., 2018), differences did occur across surveys in sampling frame, fieldwork quality control, length of the interview, oversampling of population subgroups, use of the two-part interview, degree of clustering and stratification, and obtained response rate. Methodological variation may also have arisen due to the challenge involved in the successful application of the CIDI in cross-cultural research, with a long period of development required to ensure the cultural relevance and cross-cultural equivalence of the constructs and concepts being measured (Ghimire et al., 2013; Harkness et al., 2008; Prince, 2008). Although all WMH surveys adhered in general terms to the WHO translation guidelines for cross-cultural research, it is likely that not all the several steps in this process were followed with equal rigor in every country. A further potential source of variation in prevalence across countries may have come from cross-national variation in the degree to which mental disorders are stigmatized (Gureje et al., 2005; Lasalvia et al., 2013), with flow-on effects on willingness to disclose symptoms (Reavley & Jorm, 2014). In addition to stigma, low-income countries have less of a tradition of health surveys, and this may also inhibit willingness to disclose symptoms to lay interviewers (Gureje et al., 2008).

Although the foregoing section highlights several methodological contenders for the finding of lower prevalence in the lower-income countries, it is worth noting that this

Table 1.2. Lifetime Prevalence of Mental Disorders in the World Mental Health Surveys by Country-Level Income Groups

Type of Mental Disorders	Low-Lower-Middle-Income Countries		Upper-Middle-Income Countries		High-Income Countries		All Countries Combined			
	%	SE	%	SE	%	SE	%	SE	F^a	p
Mood Disorders										
Major depressive disorder	7.1	0.2	9.2	0.3	12.6	0.2	10.6	0.1	259.6	< .001
Bipolar spectrum disorder	1.0	0.1	1.6	0.1	2.5	0.1	1.9	0.1	88.6	< .001
Anxiety Disorders										
Generalized anxiety disorder	1.1	0.1	2.1	0.1	3.7	0.1	2.7	0.1	253.3	< .001
Panic disorder	0.8	0.1	1.1	0.1	2.2	0.1	1.7	0.0	129.9	< .001
Agoraphobia	0.7	0.1	1.5	0.1	1.4	0.1	1.2	0.0	32.3	< .001
Social anxiety disorder	1.6	0.1	2.9	0.1	5.5	0.1	4.0	0.1	387.5	< .001
Specific phobia	5.7	0.2	8.0	0.2	8.1	0.1	7.4	0.1	51.1	< .001
Posttraumatic stress disorder	2.1	0.2	2.3	0.1	5.0	0.1	3.9	0.1	135.8	< .001
Separation anxiety disorder (adult)	3.4	0.3	3.2	0.2	2.9	0.2	3.1	0.1	2.1	0.120
Intermittent explosive disorder	0.6	0.1	0.7	0.1	1.1	0.1	0.8	0.0	19.1	< .001
Impulse Control Disorders										
Conduct disorder	1.5	0.2	1.5	0.1	3.2	0.2	2.3	0.1	21.7	< .001
Oppositional defiant disorder	2.6	0.3	2.1	0.2	3.0	0.2	2.7	0.1	5.3	0.005
Substance Use Disorders										
Alcohol use disorder	5.9	0.2	7.2	0.2	10.4	0.2	8.6	0.1	163.2	< .001
Drug use disorder	0.9	0.1	2.5	0.1	4.8	0.1	3.5	0.1	300.8	< .001
Eating Disorders										
Binge eating disorder	0.8	0.2	3.8	0.3	1.5	0.1	1.8	0.1	38.6	< .001
Bulimia nervosa	0.4	0.1	1.6	0.2	0.9	0.1	1.0	0.1	18.2	< .001

[a] Wald design-corrected test of variation in prevalence across country income groups.

cross-national pattern could also reflect variation in substantive factors. For example, while mental disorders are generally correlated with social disadvantage and stressful exposures within all countries, there may be factors that promote mental health or buffer the effects of these exposures that are more concentrated in lower-income countries or non-Westernized cultures. Such factors might include greater social capital and opportunities for community engagement (Axinn et al., 2015; De Silva et al., 2005; Diener et al., 2010), as well as a greater degree of support from extended family (Daatland et al., 2011; Yeh et al., 2013). Value orientations could also be relevant. For example, in an earlier WMH study it was found that associations between subjective (relative) social status and mental disorders were significantly weaker in the low/lower-middle-income countries than in the higher-income countries (Scott et al., 2014). One interpretation of that finding is that non-Westernized cultures that place less emphasis on individual achievement and status might render their citizens less vulnerable to invidious social comparisons that undermine mental health. In a related vein, some researchers have suggested that the easy access to material things and sense of entitlement that characterize affluent cultures undermine motivation and well-being, thereby creating the conditions for a mismatch between expectations and outcomes that could lead to mental illness (Koplewicz et al., 2009; Luthar et al., 2013).

Before leaving this discussion of possible substantive explanations for the observed cross-national variation in disorder prevalence, it is worth noting the remarkable consistency between the cross-national patterning of mental disorders found in the WMH data and the cross-national patterning of chronic medical conditions such as cardiovascular disease (Lozano et al., 2013). This consistency may be due in part to the well-established bidirectional associations of mental disorders with chronic physical conditions (Prince et al., 2007; Scott et al., 2016), but it may also reflect shared underlying dietary and lifestyle factors that are more prevalent in wealthy countries (Logan & Jacka, 2014; Prescott et al., 2016). In other words, it is conceivable that Western lifestyle may be a contributor to the high rates of both mental disorders and chronic physical conditions in rich countries.

Age of Onset

Although it is clear that the median estimated ages of onset (AOOs) vary considerably across disorders (Table 1.1), it is also the case that for many of the mental disorders under consideration around half of the people who will ever experience the disorder will have first developed it by adolescence or in the first decade of adulthood. There are some notable exceptions to this, with MDD, GAD, and PTSD having median AOOs in the mid- to late 30s. It is also important to note that the dementias and other neurocognitive disorders of aging (not included in the WMH surveys) have much later median AOOs. Nonetheless, these data suggest that most mental disorders typically start within the first decades of life, emphasizing the need for early diagnosis and intervention (Birchwood & Singh, 2013). And in fact, these AOO estimates may be biased upward if older respondents forget disorder episodes occurring earlier in life or if the sample is biased by earlier mortality associated with mental disorders, especially if this is more true for early-onset than later-onset disorders (Walker et al., 2015). As explained in detail elsewhere (Kessler et al., 2018), a series of approaches to minimize recall bias in AOO reports was adopted in the WMH CIDI, and there is some evidence of their success in the absence of the pattern found in previous surveys of AOOs being overrepresented in the 5 years before interview. Nonetheless, it is likely that some recall bias remains in the WMH AOO estimates.

The median AOOs shown in Table 1.1 are averaged across all WMH countries, and it is worth pointing out that they are somewhat higher than those reported in our earlier publications based on high-income WMH countries like the United States (Kessler et al., 2005). They are also somewhat higher than earlier cross-national reports based on WMH surveys (Kessler et al., 2007). This is because the AOO distributions tend to be higher (i.e., with an older median AOO) in lower-income countries, and a greater number of low-income countries are included in these more recent WMH data compared with earlier WMH publications. In addition to the general problem of basing AOO estimates on retrospective data, there are other methodological factors that may have compromised our ability to estimate AOO comparably across countries and so may have contributed to this cross-national variation in AOO estimates. These factors include the possibility of differential early mortality associated with mental disorders across countries, differences in age structure across countries, and cross-national variation in the cognitive representation of time and temporal sequencing (Fuhrman & Boroditsky, 2010; Ghimire et al., 2013).

Functional Impairment

Variation Across Disorders

Role impairment was assessed with a modified version of the Sheehan Disability Scales (SDS; Leon et al., 1997), a widely used self-report measure of condition-specific disability. Our modified version of the SDS consisted of four questions, each asking the respondent to rate on a 0–10 visual analog scale the extent to which a particular disorder interfered with activities in one of four role domains during the month in the past year when the disorder was most severe. The four domains include (a) "your home management, like cleaning, shopping, and taking care of the (house/apartment)"; (b) "your ability to work"; (c) "your social life"; and (d) "your ability to form and maintain close relationships with other people." The 0–10 response options were presented in a visual analog format with the response options of None (0), Mild (1–3), Moderate (4–6), and Severe (7–10). As can be seen from the SDS estimates shown in Table 1.1, most active mental disorders are associated with severe impairment in at least one domain of role functioning in around one-third to one-half of cases. Among the disorders considered here, mood disorders appear to be more impairing than other disorders, with 57% of 12-month MDD cases associated with severe impairment in the worst month of the year. Some qualifications are important to note here. The Sheehan estimate for bipolar disorder is for the bipolar spectrum category and so underestimates the degree of impairment associated with bipolar I or II. Additionally, this relative ranking of impairment is limited by omissions of disorders that are known to be highly impairing such as schizophrenia, dementia, and obsessive compulsive disorder. Nonetheless, our finding that MDD is associated with high impairment is consistent with the recent GBD study that found depression to be the second leading contributor to years lived with disability worldwide (Ferrari, Charlson, et al., 2013).

A comment on assessment methods is in order here in relation to the relatively high degree of impairment associated with depression. As mentioned earlier, basing impairment scores on expert assessment as was done in the first GBD study attracted criticism, but basing it on self-report also has its detractors, particularly in connection with depression. Some researchers have suggested that the high degree of self-reported impairment associated with MDD is because depressed individuals "overreport" disability as a function of the pessimistic outlook that is intrinsic to depression (Morgado et al., 1991). However, a counterpoint to that criticism comes from the ample research showing that depression and other mental disorders can impact motivation, cognition, emotional regulation, and behavior in ways that can be more disabling than the activity limitations associated with physical disabilities (Ormel et al., 2008). These functional limitations, as well as the potentially profound long-term impacts associated with mental disorders, are extensively detailed in an earlier WMH surveys volume (Alonso et al., 2013).

Back to the Sheehan data in Table 1.1: some mental disorders are evidently less impairing than others. Specific phobia is the least impairing of those considered here probably because many individuals with the disorder are able to organize their lives so as to avoid encountering the feared object or situation. Substance use disorders are also associated with lower reported functional impairment, but this might be because minimization or lack of recognition of the deleterious impact of substance use on self or others is a frequent concomitant of these disorders. Reluctance to admit to, or lack of understanding of, the impact of disorder symptoms may also contribute to the relatively low level of reported impairment associated with IED.

Variation Across Countries as a Function of Country-Level Income

An interesting cross-national pattern in the impairment results emerges whereby for 10 of 12 disorders (the two exceptions being binge eating disorder and PTSD), the percent with severe impairment is higher in the high-income countries than in the low/lower-middle-income countries. As discussed earlier in this chapter, there is also a positive gradient of increasing disorder *prevalence* with increasing country income level. The conjunction of these two trends implies that there is a positive association between prevalence and severe impairment across countries. This positive country-level association between prevalence and impairment contrasts with an earlier cross-national WHO study of major depression in primary care patients that found countries with the highest prevalence estimates to report the lowest levels of impairment associated with depression (Simon et al., 2002).

The WMH finding that impairment associated with mental disorders is generally greater in the high-income countries than in the lower-income countries is surprising given the more limited treatment resources (Saxena et al., 2007) and lower treatment uptake for mental disorders (see later) in poorer countries. It is possible that this cross-national pattern is a methodological artifact attributable to the same factors that may have led to lower disorder prevalence in low-income countries. Inconsistent with that suggestion, however, is the fact that the pattern of both lower impairment *and* lower prevalence in the low/lower-middle-income countries is the opposite of what we would expect to see if prevalence estimates were biased downward in low-income countries, or if the CIDI diagnosis thresholds were inappropriately high in low-income countries. This is because a more conservative (higher) diagnostic threshold would normally capture the more severe cases and miss more of the mild cases, resulting in those meeting diagnostic criteria reporting higher rather than lower impairment in the countries where prevalence was underestimated. Yet we find the opposite pattern in the WMH data.

Based on this observation, although we cannot rule out a methodological explanation for this cross-national variation in impairment, it is worth considering a substantive interpretation: that there is genuinely less impairment associated with mental disorders in lower- than in higher-income countries. This could be because mental disorder symptoms interfere less with role demands in lower-income countries, either because of cross-national differences in role or performance expectations or because greater family or community support may help meet role demands among the mentally ill in lower-income countries. There is some indirect evidence in support of this latter suggestion from other WMH data showing that the burden among family caregivers of those with mental health problems is two- to threefold higher in the lower-income countries than in the higher-income countries (Shahly et al., 2013). Moreover, the WMH findings of lower impairment in the lower-income countries is consistent with the findings of earlier cross-national studies that found the course and outcomes associated with schizophrenia to be more benign in developing countries than in developed countries (Harrison et al., 2001; Jablensky et al., 1992). The conclusions drawn from those earlier studies have been disputed (Cohen et al., 2008; Jääskeläinen et al., 2013), and the WMH surveys do not shed any further light on the issue as it relates to schizophrenia. But in relation to other mental disorders, the rather consistent cross-national patterning of impairment seen in the WMH data does suggest that there may be potent cultural modifiers of the disability burden associated with mental disorders. This is an important area for further research as policy initiatives may more easily reduce the impairment associated with disorders than the prevalence of disorders.

Treatment

As shown in Table 1.1, among people who were symptomatic within the 12 months prior to interview, only a minority sought treatment for their mental health problems, ranging from a low of 18% for those with alcohol use disorder to 56% of those with panic disorder. More detailed results presented elsewhere (Evans-Lacko et al., 2018) show that among people with any mental disorders in the prior 12 months, treatment seeking was significantly higher in the wealthier countries, with 33.8% seeking treatment from the health care sector compared with 18.9% in upper-middle-income countries and only 10.8% in low/lower-middle income countries ($F = 249.3$; $p < .001$). In all countries greater disorder severity increased the likelihood of treatment seeking, suggesting some rational allocation of resources. But males, those with less education, and those on lower incomes were less likely to seek treatment, even after taking disorder severity into account. The socioeconomic barriers to access were most pronounced in relation to specialist mental health services (Evans-Lacko et al., 2018). These findings indicate high levels of unmet need, even among those with the most severe disorders. This treatment gap is especially pronounced in the lower-income countries, but even in the high-income countries close to half of those with severe 12-month disorders report no treatment in the prior year (Kessler & Ustun, 2008).

Limitations

As noted in the foregoing, the WMH surveys have several important limitations. They rely on fully structured diagnostic assessments rather than on semistructured diagnostic assessments made by trained clinicians. They rely on retrospective recall of respondents' past experience of disorders, which, together with the possibility of sample survival bias and conscious nondisclosure, means that the lifetime prevalence estimates are conservative. The estimates of AOO are similarly based on respondent recall and thus are likely to be biased to some degree and possibly to vary in degree of bias across countries. Finally, interpretation of the cross-national differences is impeded by the unknown degree of between-surveys methodological variation that may have contributed to the lower estimates of prevalence and impairment in the low-income countries.

Policy Implications

Although there is considerable variation in estimates of prevalence and impairment across countries, from a policy point of view what is most important are the consistent patterns that emerge from the WMH surveys as a whole. These include the findings that mental disorders are common and occur worldwide; that most disorders begin relatively early in the lifespan; that they are most prevalent among the young and the socially disadvantaged; that they are often highly impairing, persistent, and comorbid with other disorders; and that they are greatly undertreated. These central features of the epidemiology of mental disorders underscore the call for health policy and services to place much greater emphasis on the needs of adolescents and young adults with mental disorders given that it is in this age group that most mental disorders first emerge and are most prevalent (Patton et al., 2016). Intervention early in the course of the disorder offers significant potential for long-term social, health, and economic benefits to individuals and societies. This can occur through the reduction of disorder persistence and secondary comorbidity (Kessler

2011), reduced likelihood of lost educational and employment opportunities (Alonso et al., 2013), and delayed development of chronic physical diseases (Scott et al., 2016). That said, knowledge of the public health implications of early intervention for mental disorders is limited because of the lack of focus on this issue in clinical studies.

The WMH surveys make clear that the majority of people with mental disorders are not getting treatment at all and that even fewer are being treated in a timely fashion or in accordance with current evidence of best practices for effective intervention (Thornicroft et al., 2017). This huge treatment gap is especially pronounced among individuals with low socioeconomic status within all countries, and in low/lower-middle-income countries. These findings indicate that for the reduction in prevalence of disorders and prevention of secondary comorbidity, there is much more that could be achieved through better planning and funding of mental health services that are well integrated with primary care (WHO, 2015b) and able to target those most in need (Patel et al., 2016; Thornicroft et al., 2010). The WMH findings also underscore how much more is required in terms of the scaling up and provision of mental disorder treatment services in low- and middle-income countries (Patel et al., 2009; Saxena et al., 2007). The latter is the focus of the WHO Mental Health Gap Action Programme (WHO, 2017).

Addressing this formidable problem will require a much greater investment in mental health service research and delivery than is currently being made by any country in the world, an investment that would help redress the lack of parity in service provision between mental and physical disorders (Wykes et al., 2015). Improved mental health service provision and integration should happen in the context of moving toward universal health coverage (WHO, 2015a). This is a target of the WHO for people in countries at all levels of development to ensure that they receive the quality, essential health services they need without suffering financial hardship. Universal health coverage is a specific component of one of the United Nations' new Sustainable Development Goals (Lu et al., 2015).

Reducing the prevalence and incidence of mental disorders requires a response that extends beyond the responsibilities of the health sector. In all WMH countries, the onset likelihood and current prevalence of mental disorders are highest among the most socially vulnerable: those with less education and low incomes; those who are divorced, separated, or widowed; those who are unemployed or disabled (Scott et al., 2018). These WMH findings replicate much prior research in high-income (Fryers et al., 2003; Wells et al., 2006) and low-income (Lund et al., 2010; Patel & Kleinman, 2003) countries. The direction of causality in the associations between mental disorders and disadvantaged social status is unclear, although evidence exists for both social causation (disadvantaged social status leading to mental disorders) and social selection (mental disorders leading to disadvantaged social status) pathways (J. G. Johnson et al., 1999; Miech et al., 1999; Olesen et al., 2013). Of all the social correlates studied in the WMH surveys, the one that was the most systematically associated with lifetime prevalence of mental disorders was being out of the labor force through unemployment or disability (Scott et al., 2018). In this regard it is relevant to note that most of the WMH surveys were conducted prior to the global financial crisis and that the latter has been associated with substantially increased rates of unemployment (especially among those with existing mental disorders), economic hardship, and associated mental health problems in many affected countries (Evans-Lacko et al., 2013; Karanikolos et al., 2013). The associations of social disadvantage with mental disorders have important policy implications, suggesting that mental disorders and/or their effects on functioning may be amenable to amelioration through a range of social, employment, and welfare policy measures that aim to protect jobs and improve access to financial and housing support (Barr et al., 2015; Karanikolos et al., 2013). This will require a multisectoral strategy where health is embedded in all policies and the health system stewards the other sectors to ensure the mental health and well-being of the population.

Future Directions

Ideally, research that aims to understand the determinants of mental disorders requires a multilevel investigation of a wide range of individual neurobiological and psychological processes together with an equally wide range of social and contextual factors. The few such studies to date have been conducted in high-income countries. When it comes to understanding cross-national variation in rates of disorders, there is the additional need to study how cultural factors, which may vary little within a country, interact with individual factors to contribute to disorder variation across countries. The WMH surveys were optimized to discern consistent within-country correlates and patterns, not to examine hypotheses about cross-national variation. This will be the challenge for future cross-national studies, which could include expanded measurement of relevant attitudes and values thought to vary across countries, as well as individual and community-level indicators of social support and social capital. The WMH findings on cross-national differences in the impairment associated with disorders suggest that we also need a better understanding of cultural variation in the lived experience of those with mental illness, and of the factors that help buffer the impact of the disorder on individuals and families. This kind of research will provide insight into how individuals and families cope in settings where the treatment gap is most pronounced.

But there remains the formidable challenge of understanding how sociocultural factors interact with survey methods. In this respect, to advance the study of cross-national variation in mental disorders, one of the most urgent requirements is for further careful methodological research that can better delineate and thereby help reduce the contribution of methodological variation to cross-national variation in estimates. There is already an active research program devoted to the methodology of comparative cross-national survey design (Harkness et al., 2010; T. Johnson et al., 2018) and the WMH surveys built on some of the accrued insights from this past research. But the challenges in interpretation of the cross-national findings discussed in this chapter highlight the need for extensive further methodological research in certain specific areas. For example, further studies that investigate sociocultural factors that affect willingness to disclose mental health symptoms would be useful, although future surveys are likely to utilize audio computer-assisted self-interviews that can reduce the social effects that may occur with face-to-face interviews. More in-depth studies of the kind conducted in Nepal (Ghimire et al., 2013) that seek to optimize the validation of the translation protocol for diagnostic interviews are needed; these studies can uncover cultural differences in understanding of key concepts that may have a bearing on prevalence estimates. More clinical validation studies in a wider range of countries will be important to test the validity, and cross-national variation in that validity, of lay-administered, fully structured interviews. To further examine the cross-cultural validity of the DSM/ICD classifications themselves, it would be informative to conduct studies within some countries that include both DSM/ICD-based measurement of disorders alongside measures of culture-specific concepts of distress (Kohrt et al., 2014).

Many of the methodological challenges mentioned previously arise because current mental disorder classification systems depend in large part on self-reported symptoms and behaviors. The field of cultural neuroscience that is the subject of this volume has much potential here, both in studying causal processes in mental disorders (Chiao et al., 2017) and in helping to identify biomarkers associated with mental disorders. Figuring out how to implement brain imaging or other psychobiological measures into general population epidemiological studies, especially on a cross-national basis, will be the challenge for the future. The most comprehensive approach to developing an alternative, neurobiologically based way of understanding and classifying mental disorders is the Research Domain Criteria (RDoC; Insel et al., 2010). The RDoC research framework is aimed at facilitating the study of relationships among biological, behavioral, cognitive, and symptomatic measures, and how these vary across developmental and environmental contexts (Clark et al., 2017). The hope is that this research will eventually inform a major revision of current classification systems for mental disorders, but the RDoC framework is still in the early stages and not yet ready for clinical or epidemiological research.

Conclusion

The WMH Surveys Initiative has generated a wealth of epidemiological information on prevalence and sociodemographic patterning of a wide range of DSM-IV disorders in the general populations of a broad range of countries. For most WMH countries these surveys provide the first such descriptive information on the burden of mental disorders in their citizens, and as such they provide an invaluable foundation for health service policy and planning. In all countries surveyed mental disorders begin relatively early in the lifespan; they are most prevalent among the young and the socially disadvantaged; they are often highly impairing and frequently comorbid with other disorders; and they are greatly undertreated. These findings have important policy implications indicating the need to prioritize the detection and treatment of mental disorders in young people, to upscale treatment services in low- and middle-income countries in particular, and to coordinate the health policy response with other relevant agencies to reduce the incidence and improve the outcomes of mental disorders among the socially vulnerable. Substantial cross-national variation is also evident, with both prevalence and impairment being lower in low-income countries than in high-income countries. These cross-national patterns are provocative but difficult to interpret given the inability to tease apart the respective contributions of methodological and substantive factors to the cross-national variation observed. The WMH surveys demonstrate the enormous challenges but rich rewards of cross-national comparative studies of mental disorders in providing an essential foundation for future policy and research in global mental health.

Acknowledgments

Portions of this chapter appeared previously in Scott, K. M., De Jonge, P., Stein, D. J., & Kessler, R. C. (Eds.). (2018). *Mental disorders around the world.* Cambridge University Press.

References

Alonso, J., Chatterji, S., & He, Y. (2013). *The burdens of mental disorders: Global perspectives from the World Mental Health Surveys.* Cambridge University Press.

Axinn, W. G., Ghimire, D. J., Williams, N. E., & Scott, K. M. (2015). Associations between the social organization of communities and psychiatric disorders in rural Asia. *Social Psychiatry and Psychiatric Epidemiology, 50,* 1537–1545.

Barr, B., Kinderman, P., & Whitehead, M. (2015). Trends in mental health inequalities in England during a period of recession, austerity and welfare reform 2004 to 2013. *Social Science & Medicine, 147,* 324–331.

Baxter, A. J., Scott, K. M., Vos, T., & Whiteford, H. A. (2013). Global prevalence of anxiety disorders: A systematic review and meta-regression. *Psychological Medicine, 43,* 897–910.

Birchwood, M., & Singh, S. P. (2013). Mental health services for young people: Matching the service to the need. *British Journal of Psychiatry, 202,* s1–s2.

Chiao, J. Y., Li, S.-C., Turner, R., Lee-Tauler, S. Y., & Pringle, B. A. (2017). Cultural neuroscience and global mental health: Addressing grand challenges. *Culture and Brain, 5,* 4–13.

Psychological Science in the Public Interest, 18, 72–145.

Cohen, A., Patel, V., Thara, R., & Gureje, O. (2008). Questioning an axiom: Better prognosis for schizophrenia in the developing world? *Schizophrenia Bulletin, 34,* 229–244.

Daatland, S. O., Herlofson, K., & Lima, I. A. (2011). Balancing generations: On the strength and character of family norms in the West and East of Europe. *Ageing and Society, 31,* 1159–1179.

De Silva, M. J., McKenzie, K., Harpham, T., & Huttly, S. R. (2005). Social capital and mental illness: A systematic review. *Journal of Epidemiology and Community Health, 59,* 619–627.

Diener, E., Ng, W., Harter, J., & Arora, R. (2010). Wealth and happiness across the world: Material prosperity predicts life evaluation, whereas psychosocial prosperity predicts positive feeling. *Journal of Personality and Social Psychology, 99,* 52.

Evans-Lacko, S., Knapp, M., McCrone, P., Thornicroft, G., & Mojtabai, R. (2013). The mental health consequences of the recession: Economic hardship and employment of people with mental health problems in 27 European countries. *PloS One, 8,* e69792.

Evans-Lacko, S., Tachimori, H., Kovess-Masfety, V., Chatterji, S., & Thornicroft, G. (2018). Service use. In K. M. Scott, P. De Jonge, D. J. Stein, & R. C. Kessler (Eds.), *Mental disorders around the world* (pp. 314–323). Cambridge University Press.

Ferrari, A. J., Charlson, F. J., Norman, R. E., Patten, S. B., Freedman, G., Murray, C. J., Vos, T., & Whiteford, H. A. (2013). Burden of depressive disorders by country, sex, age, and year: Findings from the global burden of disease study 2010. *PLoS Medicine, 10,* e1001547.

Ferrari, A., Somerville, A., Baxter, A., Norman, R., Patten, S., Vos, T., & Whiteford, H. (2013). Global variation in the prevalence and incidence of major depressive disorder: A systematic review of the epidemiological literature. *Psychological Medicine, 43*, 471–481.

Fryers, T., Melzer, D., & Jenkins, R. (2003). Social inequalities and the common mental disorders. *Social Psychiatry and Psychiatric Epidemiology, 38*, 229–237.

Fuhrman, O., & Boroditsky, L. (2010). Cross-cultural differences in mental representations of time: Evidence from an implicit nonlinguistic task. *Cognitive Science, 34*, 1430–1451.

Ghimire, D. J., Chardoul, S., Kessler, R. C., Axinn, W. G., & Adhikari, B. P. (2013). Modifying and validating the Composite International Diagnostic Interview (CIDI) for use in Nepal. *International Journal of Methods in Psychiatric Research, 22*, 71–81.

Gureje, O., Adeyemi, O., Enyidah, N. M. E., Udofia, O., Uwakawe, R., & Wakil, A. (2008). Mental disorders among adult Nigerians: Risks, prevalence and treatment. In R. C. Kessler & T. B. Ustun (Eds.), *The WHO World Mental Health Surveys: Global perspectives on the epidemiology of mental disorders* (pp. 211–237). Cambridge University Press.

Gureje, O., Lasebikan, V. O., Ephraim-Oluwanuga, O., Olley, B. O., & Kola, L. (2005). Community study of knowledge of and attitude to mental illness in Nigeria. *British Journal of Psychiatry, 186*, 436–441.

Harkness, J., Pennell, B., Villar, A., Gebler, N., Aguilar-Gaxiola, S., & Bilgen, I. (2008). Translation procedures and translation assessment in the World Mental Health Survey Initiative. In R. C. Kessler & T. B. Ustun (Eds.), *The WHO World Mental Health Surveys: Global perspectives on the epidemiology of mental disorders* (pp. 91–113). Cambridge University Press.

Harkness, J. A., Braun, M., Edwards, B., Johnson, T. P., Lyberg, L., Mohler, P. P., Pennell, B. E., & Smith, T. W. (2010). *Survey methods in multicultural, multinational, and multiregional contexts.* John Wiley and Sons.

Harrison, G., Hopper, K., Craig, T., Laska, E., Siegel, C., Wanderling, J., Dube, K., Ganev, K., Giel, R., & Der Heiden, W. A. (2001). Recovery from psychotic illness: A 15-and 25-year international follow-up study. *British Journal of Psychiatry, 178*, 506–517.

Insel, T., Cuthbert, B., Garvey, M., Heinssen, R., Pine, D. S., Quinn, K., Sanislow, C., & Wang, P. (2010). *Research domain criteria (RDoC): Toward a new classification framework for research on mental disorders.* American Psychiatric Association.

Jääskeläinen, E., Juola, P., Hirvonen, N., McGrath, J. J., Saha, S., Isohanni, M., Veijola, J., & Miettunen, J. (2013). A systematic review and meta-analysis of recovery in schizophrenia. *Schizophrenia Bulletin, 39*, 1296–1306.

Jablensky, A., Sartorius, N., Ernberg, G., Anker, M., Korten, A., Cooper, J. E., Day, R., & Bertelsen, A. (1992). Schizophrenia: Manifestations, incidence and course in different cultures. A World Health Organization Ten-country Study. *Psychological Medicine,* Monograph Supplement *20*, 1–97.

Johnson, J. G., Cohen, P., Dohrenwend, B. P., Link, B. G., & Brook, J. S. (1999). A longitudinal investigation of social causation and social selection processes involved in the association between socioeconomic status and psychiatric disorders. *Journal of Abnormal Psychology, 108*, 490–499.

Johnson, T., Pennell, B.-E., & Stoop, I. (2018). *Advances in comparative survey methods: Multinational, multiregional and multinational contexts.* John Wiley & Sons.

Karanikolos, M., Mladovsky, P., Cylus, J., Thomson, S., Basu, S., Stuckler, D., Mackenbach, J. P., & McKee, M. (2013). Financial crisis, austerity, and health in Europe. *Lancet, 381*, 1323–1331.

Kessler, R. C. (2000). Psychiatric epidemiology: Selected recent advances and future directions. *Bulletin of the World Health Organization, 78*, 464–471.

Kessler, R. C. (2011). The National Comorbidity Survey (NCS) and its extensions. In M. T. Tsuang, M. Tohen, & P. B. Jones (Eds.), *Textbook of psychiatric epidemiology* (3rd ed.) (pp. 221–242). John Wiley & Sons.

Kessler, R. C., Angermeyer, M., Anthony, J. C., De Graaf, R., Demyttenaere, K., Gasquet, I., De Girolamo, G., Gluzman, S., Gureje, O., Haro, J. M., Kawakami, N., Karam, A., Levinson, D., Medina Mora, M. E., Oakley Browne, M., Posada-Villa, J., Stein, D., Tsang, A., Aguilar-Gaxiola, S., . . . Ustun, T. B. (2007). Lifetime prevalence and age-of-onset distributions of mental disorders in the World Health Organization's World Mental Health Surveys. *World Psychiatry, 6*, 168–176.

Kessler, R. C., Berglund, P., Demler, O., Jin, R., Merikangas, K. R., & Walters, E. E. (2005). Lifetime prevalence and age-of-onset distributions of DSM-IV disorders in the National Comorbidity Survey Replication. *Archives of General Psychiatry, 62*, 593–602.

Kessler, R. C., Heeringa, S. G., Pennell, B., Sampson, N., & Zaslavsky, A. M. (2018). Methods of the World Mental Health Surveys. In K. M. Scott, P. De Jonge, D. J. Stein, & R. C. Kessler (Eds.), *Mental disorders around the world* (pp. 9–40). Cambridge University Press.

Kessler, R. C., & Ustun, B. (2004). The World Mental Health (WMH) Survey Initiative version of the World Health Organization (WHO) Composite International Diagnostic Interview (CIDI). *International Journal of Methods in Psychiatric Research, 13*, 93–121.

Kessler, R. C., & Ustun, T. B. (Eds.). (2008). *The WHO World Mental Health Surveys: Global perspectives on the epidemiology of mental disorders*. Cambridge University Press.

Kohrt, B. A., Rasmussen, A., Kaiser, B. N., Haroz, E. E., Maharjan, S. M., Mutamba, B. B., de Jong, J. T., & Hinton, D. E. (2014). Cultural concepts of distress and psychiatric disorders: Literature review and research recommendations for global mental health epidemiology. *International Journal of Epidemiology, 43*, 365–406.

Koplewicz, H. S., Gurian, A., & Williams, K. (2009). The era of affluence and its discontents. *Journal of the American Academy of Child & Adolescent Psychiatry, 48*, 1053–1055.

Lasalvia, A., Zoppei, S., Van Bortel, T., Bonetto, C., Cristofalo, D., Wahlbeck, K., Bacle, S. V., Van Audenhove, C., Van Weeghel, J., & Reneses, B. (2013). Global pattern of experienced and anticipated discrimination reported by people with major depressive disorder: A cross-sectional survey. *Lancet, 381*, 55–62.

Leon, A. C., Olfson, M., Portera, L., Farber, L., & Sheehan, D. V. (1997). Assessing psychiatric impairment in primary care with the Sheehan Disability Scale. *International Journal of Psychiatry in Medicine, 27*, 93–105.

Logan, A. C., & Jacka, F. N. (2014). Nutritional psychiatry research: An emerging discipline and its intersection with global urbanization, environmental challenges and the evolutionary mismatch. *Journal of Physiological Anthropology, 33*, 22.

Lozano, R., Naghavi, M., Foreman, K., Lim, S., Shibuya, K., Aboyans, V., Abraham, J., Adair, T., Aggarwal, R., & Ahn, S. Y. (2013). Global and regional mortality from 235 causes of death for 20 age groups in 1990 and 2010: A systematic analysis for the Global Burden of Disease Study 2010. *Lancet, 380*, 2095–2128.

Lu, Y., Nakicenovic, N., Visbeck, M., & Stevance, A. (2015). Five priorities for the UN sustainable development goals. *Nature, 520*, 432–433.

Lund, C., Breen, A., Flisher, A. J., Kakuma, R., Corrigall, J., Joska, J. A., Swartz, L., & Patel, V. (2010). Poverty and common mental disorders in low and middle income countries: A systematic review. *Social Science & Medicine, 71*, 517–528.

Luthar, S. S., Barkin, S. H., & Crossman, E. J. (2013). "I can, therefore I must": Fragility in the upper-middle classes. *Development and Psychopathology, 25*, 1529–1549.

Miech, R. A., Caspi, A., Moffitt, T. E., Wright, B. R. E., & Silva, P. A. (1999). Low socioeconomic status and mental disorders: A longitudinal study of selection and causation during young adulthood. *American Journal of Sociology, 104*, 1096–1131.

Moffitt, T., Caspi, A., Taylor, A., Kokaua, J., Milne, B., Polanczyk, G., & Poulton, R. (2010). How common are common mental disorders? Evidence that lifetime prevalence rates are doubled by prospective versus retrospective ascertainment. *Psychological Medicine, 40*, 899.

Morgado, A., Raoux, N., Jourdain, G., Lecrubier, Y., & Widlocher, D. (1991). Over-reporting of maladjustment by depressed subjects. Findings from retesting after recovery. *Social Psychiatry & Psychiatric Epidemiology, 26*, 68–74.

Murray, C. J., & Lopez, A. D. (Eds.). (1996). *The global burden of disease: A comprehensive assessment of mortality and disability from diseases, injuries, and risk factors in 1990 and projected to 2020*. Global Burden of Disease and Injury Series Harvard School of Public Health (on behalf of the World Health Organization).

Olesen, S. C., Butterworth, P., Leach, L. S., Kelaher, M., & Pirkis, J. (2013). Mental health affects future employment as job loss affects mental health: Findings from a longitudinal population study. *BMC Psychiatry, 13*, 144.

Ormel, J., Petukhova, M., Chatterji, S., Aguilar-Gaxiola, S., Alonso, J., Angermeyer, M. C., Bromet, E. J., Burger, H., Demyttenaere, K., de Girolamo, G., Haro, J. M., Huang, I., Karam, E. G., Kawakami, N., Lepine, J. P., Medina Mora, M. E., Posada-Villa, J., Sampson, N., Scott, K. M., . . . Kessler, R. C. (2008). Disability and treatment of specific mental and physical disorders across the world: Results from the WHO World Mental Health Surveys. *British Journal of Psychiatry, 192*, 368–375.

Patel, V., Chisholm, D., Parikh, R., Charlson, F. J., Degenhardt, L., Dua, T., Ferrari, A. J., Hyman, S., Laxminarayan, R., & Levin, C. (2016). Addressing the burden of mental, neurological, and substance use disorders: Key messages from Disease Control Priorities. *Lancet, 387*, 1672–1685.

Patel, V., Goel, D. S., & Desai, R. (2009). Scaling up services for mental and neurological disorders in low-resource settings. *International Health, 1*, 37–44.

Patel, V., & Kleinman, A. (2003). Poverty and common mental disorders in developing countries. *Bulletin of the World Health Organization, 81*, 609–615.

Patton, G. C., Sawyer, S. M., Santelli, J. S., Ross, D. A., Afifi, R., Allen, N. B., Arora, M., Azzopardi, P., Baldwin, W., & Bonell, C. (2016). Our future: A Lancet commission on adolescent health and wellbeing. *Lancet, 387*, 2423–2478.

Prescott, S. L., Millstein, R. A., Katzman, M. A., & Logan, A. C. (2016). Biodiversity, the human microbiome and mental health: Moving toward a new clinical ecology for the 21st century? *International Journal of Biodiversity,*. Article ID 2718275.

Prince, M. (2008). Measurement validity in cross-cultural comparative research. *Epidemiology and Psychiatric Sciences, 17*, 211–220.

Prince, M., Patel, V., Saxena, S., Maj, M., Maselko, J., Phillips, M. R., & Rahman, A. (2007). Global mental health 1: No health without mental health. *Lancet, 370*, 859–877.

Reavley, N. J., & Jorm, A. F. (2014). Willingness to disclose a mental disorder and knowledge of disorders in others: Changes in Australia over 16 years. *Australian & New Zealand Journal of Psychiatry, 48*, 162–168.

Robins, L. N., Helzer, J. E., Croughan, J., & Ratcliff, K. S. (1981). National Institute of Mental Health Diagnostic Interview Schedule: Its history, characteristics, and validity. *Archives of General Psychiatry, 38*, 381–389.

Robins, L. N., Helzer, J. E., Weissman, M. M., Orraschel, H., Gruenberg, E., Burke, J. D. J., & Regier, D. A. (1984). Lifetime prevalence of specific psychiatric disorders in three sites. *Archives of General Psychiatry, 41*, 949–958.

Saxena, S., Thornicroft, G., Knapp, M., & Whiteford, H. (2007). Resources for mental health: Scarcity, inequity, and inefficiency. *Lancet, 370*, 878–889.

Scott, K., Al-Hamzawi, A., Andrade, L., Borges, G., Caldas-de-Almeida, J., Fiestas, F., Gureje, O., Hu, C., Karam, E., Kawakami, N., Lee, S., Levinson, D., Lim, C., Navarro-Mateu, F., Okoliyski, M., Posada-Villa, J., Torres, Y., Williams, D., Zakhozha, V., & Kessler, R (2014). Associations between subjective social status and DSM-IV mental disorders: Results from the World Mental Health Surveys. *JAMA Psychiatry, 71*, 1400–1408.

Scott, K. M., De Jonge, P., Stein, D. J., & Kessler, R. C. (Eds.). (2018). *Mental disorders around the World*. Cambridge University Press.

Scott, K. M., Lim, C., Al-Hamzawi, A., Alonso, J., Bruffaerts, R., Caldas-de-Almeida, J. M., Florescu, S., De Girolamo, G., Hu, C., De Jonge, P., Kawakami, N., Medina-Mora, M. E., Moskalewicz, J., Navarro-Mateu, F., O'Neill, S., Piazza, M., Posada-Villa, J., Torres, Y., & Kessler, R. C. (2016). Association of mental disorders with subsequent chronic physical conditions: World mental health surveys from 17 countries. *JAMA Psychiatry, 73*, 150–158.

Shahly, V., Chatterji, S., Gruber, M., Al-Hamzawi, A., Alonso, J., Andrade, L., Angermeyer, M., Bruffaerts, R., Bunting, B., & Caldas-de-Almeida, J. (2013). Cross-national differences in the prevalence and correlates of burden among older family caregivers in the World Health Organization World Mental Health (WMH) Surveys. *Psychological Medicine, 43*, 865–879.

Simon, G., Goldberg, D., Von Korff, M., & Üstün, T. (2002). Understanding cross-national differences in depression prevalence. *Psychological Medicine, 32*, 585–594.

Steel, Z., Marnane, C., Iranpour, C., Chey, T., Jackson, J. W., Patel, V., & Silove, D. (2014). The global prevalence of common mental disorders: A systematic review and meta-analysis 1980–2013. *International Journal of Epidemiology, 43*, 476–493.

Stein, D. J., De Jonge, P., Kessler, R. C., & Scott, K. M. (2018). The cross-national epidemiology of mental disorders. In K. M. Scott, P. De Jonge, D. J. Stein, & R. C. Kessler (Eds.), *Mental disorders around the world* (pp. 3–8). Cambridge University Press.

Takayanagi, Y., Spira, A. P., Roth, K. B., Gallo, J. J., Eaton, W. W., & Mojtabai, R. (2014). Accuracy of reports of lifetime mental and physical disorders: Results from the Baltimore Epidemiological Catchment Area Study. *JAMA Psychiatry, 71*, 273–280.

Thornicroft, G., Alem, A., Santos, R. A., Barley, E., Drake, R. E., Gregorio, G., Hanlon, C., Ito, H., Latimer, E., & Law, A. (2010). WPA guidance on steps, obstacles and mistakes to avoid in the implementation of community mental health care. *World Psychiatry, 9*, 67–77.

Thornicroft, G., Chatterji, S., Evans-Lacko, S., Gruber, M., Sampson, N., Aguilar-Gaxiola, S., Al-Hamzawi, A., Alonso, J., Andrade, L., & Borges, G. (2017). Undertreatment of people with major depressive disorder in 21 countries. *British Journal of Psychiatry, 210*, 119–124.

Walker, E. R., McGee, R. E., & Druss, B. G. (2015). Mortality in mental disorders and global disease burden implications: A systematic review and meta-analysis. *JAMA Psychiatry, 72*, 334–341.

Weissman, M. M., Bland, R. C., Canino, G. J., Faravelli, C., Greenwald, S., Hwu, H. G., Joyce, P. R., Karam, E. G., Lee, C. K., Lellouch, J., Lepine, J. P., Newman, S. C., Oakley Browne, M. A., Rubio-Stipec, M., Wells, J. E., Wickramaratne, P. J., Wittchen, H. U., & Yeh, E. K. (1996). Cross-national epidemiology of major depression and bipolar disorder. *JAMA, 276*, 293–299.

Weissman, M. M., Bland, R. C., Canino, G. J., & Greenwald, S. (1994). The cross national epidemiology of obsessive compulsive disorder: The Cross National Collaborative Group. *Journal of Clinical Psychiatry, 55*, 5–10.

Wells, J. E., & Horwood, L. J. (2004). How accurate is recall of key symptoms of depression?: A comparison of recall and longitudinal reports. *Psychological Medicine, 34*, 1001–1011.

Wells, J. E., Oakley Browne, M. A., Scott, K. M., McGee, M. A., Baxter, J., & Kokaua, J. (2006). Te Rau Hinengaro: The New Zealand Mental Health Survey (NZMHS): Overview of methods and findings. *Australian and New Zealand Journal of Psychiatry, 40*, 835–844.

World Health Organization (WHO). (2015a). *Tracking universal health coverage: First global monitoring report.*

World Health Organization (WHO). (2015b). *WHO global strategy on people-centred and integrated health services: Interim report.*

World Health Organization (WHO. (2017). *mhGAP training manuals for the mhGAP intervention guide for mental, neurological and substance use disorders in non-specialized health settings-version 2.0 (for field testing).*

Wykes, T., Haro, J. M., Belli, S. R., Obradors-Tarragó, C., Arango, C., Ayuso-Mateos, J. L., Bitter, I., Brunn, M., Chevreul, K., & Demotes-Mainard, J. (2015). Mental health research priorities for Europe. *Lancet Psychiatry, 2*, 1036–1042.

Yeh, K.-H., Yi, C.-C., Tsao, W.-C., & Wan, P.-S. (2013). Filial piety in contemporary Chinese societies: A comparative study of Taiwan, Hong Kong, and China. *International Sociology, 28*, 277–296.

Cultural Evolutionary Neuroscience

Ryutaro Uchiyama *and* Michael Muthukrishna

Abstract

Cultural evolution and cultural neuroscience are complementary approaches to understanding the origins and function of cross-cultural differences in psychology. Cultural evolution, and dual inheritance theory more generally, offers a theoretical framework for understanding cultural transmission and cultural change and how these can change gene frequencies. However, these theories have largely ignored the details of the minds engaging in these processes. Cultural evolutionary models tend to treat the brain as a black box. Cultural neuroscience offers a rich toolkit for examining how cross-cultural psychological differences manifest at a neurological level. However, these tools have largely been used to document differences between populations. Cultural neuroscience tends to ignore why these differences should be expected or how to identify if they are meaningful. This chapter reviews work in each field to carve a pathway for a productive synthesis. This cultural evolutionary neuroscience will benefit both fields and lead to a more complete understanding of human culture.

Key Words: brain evolution, brain development, cultural brain hypothesis, cultural evolution, cultural neuroscience, culture–gene coevolution, dual inheritance, human evolution, life history, social learning

Cultural Neuroscience and Cultural Evolution: An Opportunity for Convergence

Cultural evolution and cultural neuroscience are research programs that cut across traditional disciplinary boundaries and integrate across the biological and social sciences. Both fields try to explain the foundations of human culture, but each draws on different traditions and each relies on different methods, assumptions, and levels of analysis. Although these fields share a common object of inquiry—culture and cultural differences—and although these fields arguably have complementary toolkits, there have been few practical points of contact. In this chapter we hope to sketch out a path toward a productive convergence. To help us understand some of the barriers to this convergence, we'll begin with some history.

Dual inheritance theory and the cultural evolutionary framework began as an attempt to describe how natural selection could lead to a propensity to learn from others rather than by oneself and how this in turn could lead to socially transmitted information—culture—emerging as an independent evolutionary system (for a short introduction to cultural evolution, see Chudek et al., 2015; for a review of the history of dual inheritance theory, see Russell & Muthukrishna, 2018). The approach to answering this question involved developing a series of mathematical models derived from ecology, epidemiology, and population genetics (R. Boyd & Richerson, 1985; Cavalli-Sforza & Feldman, 1981). These seminal models described the evolution of social learning and different social learning strategies, how culture and genes could co-evolve, and the long-run consequences of these transmission and filtering processes. Together these models served as a foundation and convincing case for understanding culture as an evolutionary system, where not only genes, but also socially transmitted information could accumulate adaptations to the environment.

Boyd, Richerson, Cavalli-Sforza, and Feldman offered a productive approach and a revolutionary insight, but just as early population genetics models assumed away the messy details of transmission and molecular genetics, so too did these cultural models assume away the messy details of cultural storage and transmission. Current cultural evolutionary models are "mind blind," often modeling cultural learning as a process akin to contagion. The actual process of cultural transmission involves the selective transfer of information from one brain to another, and just as the messy details of genetics inform and constrain our understanding of genetic evolution (Casillas & Barbadilla, 2017), understanding the architectural and computational particulars of nervous systems should inform and constrain our understanding of cultural evolution.

Cultural neuroscience is a research program that merged methods from cognitive neuroscience with the theoretical and experimental apparatus of cultural psychology (Chiao, 2009; Han et al., 2013; Kitayama & Uskul, 2011). Cultural psychology initially relied on self-report and qualitative description but subsequently cultivated a collection of often ingenious behavioral experimental paradigms, for example, those reviewed in Nisbett and Miyamoto (2005). But techniques such as functional magnetic resonance imaging (fMRI) and event-related potential (ERP) allowed for a cultural *neuroscience* and revealed how those cultural differences manifest at a neurological level. For example, researchers have found cross-cultural differences in neural activity when engaging in psychological processes like self-reflection (Chiao et al., 2009; Ma et al., 2014) and empathy (Cheon et al., 2011). There has also been interesting work done on gene–culture interactions, for example, the effect of an oxytocin receptor gene on social support seeking (Kim et al., 2010), of a serotonin transporter gene on individualist–collectivist cultural values (Chiao & Blizinsky, 2010), and of a dopamine receptor gene on independent–interdependent social orientation (Kitayama et al., 2014): these studies guide us toward a better understanding of the neurogenetic and developmental pathways through which culture makes contact with behavior. As a more conceptual contribution, the advent of cultural neuroscience has highlighted the two-way relationship between culture and brains: the expression of culture in individuals must of course be grounded in an underlying neural substrate, but the neural substrate is also shaped by culture, constituting a system of mutual feedback (Kitayama & Salvador, 2017; see also Lehman et al., 2004). Cultural neuroscience makes clear that investigation of culture is incomplete without investigation of the brain.

Cultural neuroscience is an important step in our scientific understanding of culture, but the conceptual and methodological toolkits inherited from cultural psychology and cognitive neuroscience are limited in their ability to account for aspects of culture that are perhaps fundamental. For example, its change over time. Within the cultural evolutionary framework, cultural change—or more specifically, the ability of cultural practices to adapt to the environment (including the social environment) quicker than genes—is central to both the function and origins of human culture. Measuring cultural traits, neurologically or otherwise, offers only a snapshot of an ongoing adaptive process. As such, any insights gained about current cross-cultural differences are incomplete and sometimes difficult to interpret without a general framework of how these traits evolved and their adaptive function at an individual-level, population-level, and the long-run history of their development (Muthukrishna & Henrich, 2019).

Toward a Cultural Evolutionary Neuroscience

Psychological and behavioral scientists have recently been forced to grapple with the magnitude of psychological differences across societies (Henrich et al., 2010; Muthukrishna et al., 2020; Schulz et al., 2019). Even mental processes often assumed to be universal and hard-wired have been shown to vary cross-culturally. These include low-level visual perception (Nisbett & Miyamoto, 2005), segmentation of continuous sensory experience (Swallow & Wang, 2020), rationality underlying economic decision making (Henrich et al., 2001), internal representation of conceptual categories (Medin & Atran, 2004), and coding of spatial coordinates (Majid et al., 2004). The malleability of the human mind has been vastly underestimated; culture runs deep. This underestimation is in large part due to a systematic sampling bias: the vast majority (96%) of experimental participants are people from Western, educated, industrialized, rich, democratic (WEIRD) countries and most are Americans (68%). Not only is this a narrow slice of human variation, ignoring 88% of the global population, but WEIRD people appear to be extreme on many psychological traits when compared to the full range of global cultural diversity (Henrich et al., 2010b; Muthukrishna et al., 2020; Schulz et al., 2019). This sampling bias, combined with theoretical foundations that assume an invariant human cognitive architecture (e.g., Neisser, 1967; Newell, 1980), has distorted our estimation of the extent to which culture shapes the mind.

Cultural evolutionary theory postulates that our capacity for complex culture has been the primary driver of our extraordinary success as a species (Henrich, 2016). Culture has shaped the ways in which we interact with our environments, and furthermore, through processes like culture–gene coevolution (R. Boyd & Richerson, 1985; Cavalli-Sforza &

Feldman, 1981), it has also shaped our bodies and brains. The genetic evolution of our anatomy and physiology has progressed in tandem with the cultural evolution of our adaptive knowledge, and the trajectory of human brain evolution sits squarely within this intersection of genetic and cultural evolution (Muthukrishna, Doebeli, et al., 2018). Cultural practices such as food sharing (Kaplan et al., 2000), cooking (Wrangham & Carmody, 2010), midwifery (Rosenberg & Trevathan, 2002), and modern medical interventions (Lipschuetz et al., 2015) support our large, costly, difficult-to-birth brains, while reciprocally, our enlarged brains support the storage and transmission of more complex cultural knowledge. This process of *brain–culture* coevolution has allowed human cultural complexity to scale up in dramatic ways, and so cultural transmission is intrinsic to the evolutionary and functional history of our nervous systems (Muthukrishna et al., 2018; Muthukrishna & Henrich, 2016).

Here, we take a step further. Rather than a static picture of brain–culture coevolution that only emphasizes the mutual positive feedback between knowledge and brain size (or brain complexity), we will zoom in on the interaction between two forms of adaptive fluidity: (a) the plasticity of the brain and (b) the intrinsic flexibility of cumulative culture as a dynamical system. Humans appear to have evolved to deal with sharp environmental change in the form of climate fluctuations and their downstream effects (R. Boyd & Richerson, 1985; Ditlevsen et al., 1996; GRIP, 1993; Potts, 1998; Richerson & Boyd, 2000). Given the coincident explosion in human brain size, it is likely that brain plasticity played a key functional role in supporting this kind of ecological resilience (Fiddes et al., 2018; Suzuki et al., 2018). The basic mechanisms of neuroplasticity originate deep in our vertebrate phylogeny (Finlay, 2007; Kirschner & Gerhart, 2005), but the fact that this metabolically expensive organ (Aiello & Wheeler, 1995) expanded at such a rapid rate perhaps suggests that we have exploited these variation-harnessing mechanisms in unusually effective ways. The capacity for cultural variation and for brain plasticity created a doubly flexible system that deals rapidly and effectively with environmental variation.

Culture as a Rapidly Evolvable Neurodevelopmental Regulator

Brain plasticity is usually discussed in the context of reorganization of nervous systems in response to factors like somatic or neurological insult, sensory deficits, training, or socioeconomic deprivation (Kolb & Gibb, 2014), and such conditions are commonly cast as deviations from normal input. Imagine if we were to talk about culture in the same way—as a system that enables populations to "compensate" for nonnormative environmental conditions. This view would hinge upon an illusory reference point; an unhelpful way to think about the organization of culture. To fully appreciate the power of culture, instead of looking for variation around a fixed normative state, we consider the variation that culture enables: for example, the wide range of possible environments that individuals in a society are able to inhabit due to cultural knowledge: we spanned the globe as hunter-gatherers well before the advent of physics, chemistry, or modern medicine. The same holds true for human brains—we should consider the space of possible phenotypes within the constraints of developmental rules. The brain is an adaptive organ not just in the sense of having a good functional fit with a particular environment; more fundamentally, it is adaptive because it is able to support *evolvability*—the ability of a population to respond effectively to environmental change by shifting its phenotypic distribution (Pigliucci, 2008; Wagner & Altenberg, 1996). In other species this is achieved by genomic change and levers around mutation rates. But humans, owing to cumulative culture, are able to adapt in the absence of genotypic change and at a much faster rate (R. Boyd & Richerson, 1985)—a that principle lies at the heart of cultural evolutionary theory. Most species who encountered the range of environments we live in would require considerable genetic change, but we achieved it with very little. For humans, the generation of neural variation and the generation of cultural variation are coupled processes.

Even in the absence of cumulative culture, human brains could still respond effectively to environmental change through standard learning mechanisms: there is evidence across mammalian and avian taxa that brain size explains the ability of species to adapt to new environments (Sol et al., 2005, 2008). In these animals, improvements in brain phenotypes are predominantly driven either genetic adaptation or through direct interaction with the environment. But cumulative culture can, through its own evolutionary dynamics, incrementally improve or sophisticate the neural phenotypes that it produces even while there is no change in the environmental parameters to which the phenotypes are adapted, and at a much faster rate than genetic change. That is, the cultural environment is part of the environment for adaptation. Culturally induced brain phenotypes may exhibit an adaptive match with the non-cultural environment, but this is not because of direct exposure of the learning machinery of the brain to that environment—culture is able to vicariously take the place of environmental stimuli in shaping the nervous system toward a functional match.

For example, there may be some optimal level of risk-seeking in any given environment, which could be tracked either through variation in genes (e.g., neuromodulator genes for serotonin or dopamine; Kuhnen & Chiao, 2009; Kuhnen, Samanez-Larkin, & Knutson, 2013; Riba, Krämer, Heldmann, Richter, & Münte, 2008) or variation in experience (e.g., childhood adversity; Hellemans, Nobrega, & Olmstead, 2005; Lovallo, 2013). In non-cultural species, generation of the latter is dependent upon environmental affordances, and so a shift in the range of experiential variation can come about only through a change in the environment. But cumulative culture, through various channels spanning material artifacts, ritualized action, beliefs, and social norms, is able to furnish a much richer range of possible experience, some of which will be relevant to the programming of the degree of risk-seeking. This diversification would be useful in allowing a population to keep up with environmental change, but it would also be useful for pushing human neurodevelopment into particular regions of phenotypic space that could not be reached by non-cultural environmental input alone. Culture thus confers human populations with enormous flexibility in moving through the space of possible brain phenotypes. We can also expect that the cause-effect relationship between cultural practices and resulting phenotype will often be cryptic: not all cultural practices that influence risk-seeking will be overtly *about* risk, and there are likely to be many indirect, downstream effects of culture that impact neurodevelopment in non-intuitive ways.

These ideas about the role of phenotypic variability and evolvability have been a basic feature of cultural evolutionary theory since its inception (Boyd & Richerson, 1985b), but the discussion has usually been described in terms of the transmission of particular, anthropologically salient skills in domains such as hunting and tool-making. Although the mathematical models are in no way restricted to such examples, the questions asked by researchers in the field have perhaps been unintentionally constrained by this discourse and its origins in anthropology. Here we suggest an extended focus of cultural evolutionary logic from observable behaviors to the organization of the brain.

All aspects of neuroplasticity are raw material on which cultural evolution can potentially act. Given that culture can design specific input regimes for the brain during its development, it has much more flexibility and control in programming the brain than genes do. We can thus expect significant interactions between the structure of neuroplasticity and the particular forms that culture adopts. There is insightful work suggesting for example that the shape of written symbols (Changizi & Shimojo, 2005; Changizi, Zhang, Ye, & Shimojo, 2006; Vinckier et al., 2007), the structure of speech (Giraud & Poeppel, 2012) as well as every other level of language organization (Christiansen & Chater, 2016; Isbilen & Christiansen, 2018), and even the visual statistics of paintings both realist and abstract (Graham & Field, 2007) are all adapted to the intrinsic processing constraints of the nervous system. We believe however that the interaction between the learning gadgetry of the brain and cultural forms is likely to be much more varied and much more extensive. To uncover this mutual feedback, researchers will need to examine variation in cultural products as well as variation in cultural brains.

The focus on WEIRD populations has been a pragmatic choice that has brought us a wealth of preliminary knowledge about the human brain as expressed in one particular (and possibly peculiar) cultural context, but if we want to make sense of human brain function at a more fundamental level, we will need to study the brain across the range of extant cultural variability. This in itself does not give us a dynamic picture of neurophenotypic change in response to cultural evolution, but just as evolutionary biology has made great strides in inferring historical evolutionary trajectories based on the study of extant species, cultural neuroscience (Chiao, 2009; Kitayama & Uskul, 2011) gives us the material we need to interpret contemporary brains within a dynamic, cultural evolutionary framework. Cultural neuroscience is an area of research that looks at cross-cultural differences in neural response. But cultural neuroscience should not just be an additional level of subtlety that serves as a footnote to a "normal" WEIRD neuroscience—to the contrary, the cultural variation is the baseline that needs to be laid down if we are to pursue a science of the human brain that is faithful to its evolutionary history and basic adaptive utility. In the rest of this chapter, we will describe the framework of cultural evolution in more detail as well as discuss how its insights necessitate a conceptual shift in the way in which we view the nature of brain development and the human mind.

An Overview of the Cultural Evolutionary Framework

Cultural Transmission as Evolutionary Inheritance

Let's consider an ability almost synonymous with ecological competence in *Homo sapiens*: control of fire. Darwin (1871) believed that our ancestors' discovery of this skill was "the greatest ever made by man, excepting language." There is evidence that the ability to use fire played a significant role in human evolution; in particular, fire allowed for the cooking of food, and the cooking of food facilitated digestion and thereby contributed to the reallocation of tissue from the gut to the brain, both of which are metabolically costly organs (Aiello & Wheeler, 1995; Navarrete et al., 2011; Wrangham & Carmody, 2010). The control of fire is not a behavior that is typically learned by pure trial and error. Nor is it a genetically encoded behavior. Instead, we learn how to start fires and maintain them by watching or being instructed by other people. It is therefore a problem in which the search through possible solutions is radically narrowed down by social information. This approach to problem solving—*social learning*—exploits the redundancy that exists when multiple agents (both in present and past generations) engage with the same problem: information about the past experiences of other agents can be used as a surrogate for actual exploration through the problem-space. This is not unlike how much better students would do on an exam if they could copy each other's answers.

Social learning has been a significant topic of investigation in both human psychology and animal behavior (Bandura, 1977; Heyes & Galef, 1996; Hoppitt & Laland, 2013; Miller & Dollard, 1945), but it is research conducted within the framework of cultural evolution that has contributed most significantly to our understanding of the deep historical relationship between human ecological success and social learning. Cultural evolution describes how adaptive behaviors can be transmitted down generations not only through genetic inheritance, but also through social learning, and how in humans, extensive use of this second line of inheritance—culture—explains much of our success as a species (R. Boyd & Richerson, 1985; Cavalli-Sforza & Feldman, 1981; Henrich, 2016; Laland, 2018; Mesoudi et al., 2006). Humans employ a rich variety of technologies and other socially acquired skills that are adapted to local ecologies spanning much of the globe. Although social learning has been documented across diverse groups of animals including mammals, birds, fish, reptiles, and insects (Galef & Laland, 2005; Hoppitt & Laland, 2013; Laland & Janik, 2006; Leadbeater & Chittka, 2007; Whiten et al., 2019; Wilkinson et al., 2010), none come as close to humans in the complexity of the information that is transmitted. Humans are the only species with clear evidence of *cumulative culture*: the accumulation of beneficial modifications over the course of iterated social transmission of behaviors to the point where the attained level of complexity would be impossible for any individual to recreate on their own (Dean et al., 2012, 2014; Tennie et al., 2009). Cumulative culture is what has enabled the gradual refinement of numerous tools, techniques, and protocols over the history of our species, as well as the consequent mastery of diverse environments.

We have known for over a half-century how the molecular properties of DNA enable it to function as a genetic code (Crick et al., 1961), but when Darwin initially formulated the theory of evolution by descent with modification, he didn't know about the information-bearing substrate that underlies genetic inheritance nor did he even know about the basic principles of genetic transmission that were being discovered contemporaneously by Mendel. These strands of knowledge would come together in the early 20th century, in what is now known as the Modern Synthesis in evolutionary biology, but the concept of evolution itself was formulated at a level of abstraction that is independent of these biochemical and algorithmic details.

The logic of evolution stripped of its specific manifestations relies on three ingredients: variation in traits, inheritance of these traits between generations, and differential success in the survival of these traits. These criteria sufficiently explained the ubiquity of organisms that are well adapted to their environments, removing reliance on teleological design or foresight. Because of this substrate-independence, the concept of evolution is not intrinsically limited to genetic inheritance. In *The Descent of Man*, Darwin himself postulated that the scope of evolution could be extended to domains of cultural knowledge, in particular that of language, when he wrote about how "the survival or preservation of certain favored words in the struggle for existence is natural selection" (Darwin, 1871).

Despite this initial conceptualization, the study of genetic transmission had been the main driver of evolutionary research throughout much of the 20th century. The Modern Synthesis itself had been constructed on what was virtually an exclusively genetic perspective, a reasonable strategy for the time. This established approach partitions the heritability of traits into genetic and environmental components. But over the years, there has been a gradual accumulation of evidence demonstrating that to fully understand phenotypic change, we need to look at multiple lines of inheritance other than genes and remove the one-way arrow of genes adapting to environments. This includes culture, but also epigenetic modulation of gene expression (Jablonka & Raz, 2009; Richards, 2006); mother-to-offspring transfer of microbiomes during vaginal childbirth, which is reduced in cesarean births (Dominguez-Bello et al., 2016; Ley et al., 2008; Ochman et al., 2010); and inheritance of local environments that are modified through behavior—for example earthworms creating a more moist and richer soil in which subsequent generations can more easily survive (F. J. Odling-Smee et al., 1996; J. Odling-Smee et al., 2013). The theoretical view on evolution that attempts to incorporate all of these inheritance systems under a unitary framework is sometimes known as the "extended evolutionary synthesis" (Laland, 2017; Laland et al., 2015).

Mechanisms of High-Fidelity Cultural Transmission

Genetic transmission relies on a discrete molecular code that carries the information required to regenerate a full organism. In species with sexual reproduction, the genetic information carried by two individuals with complementary reproductive roles is recombined, resulting in offspring whose traits are correlated with both parents. Although cultural transmission also achieves the cross-generational inheritance of behavioral traits, it uses mechanisms that are very different from genetic transmission. One popular way to think about cultural transmission is the copying of information from one brain to another: Richerson and Boyd (2005, p. 61) assert that "culture is (mostly) information stored in human brains, and gets transmitted from brain to brain by way of a variety of social learning processes." But compared to the transmission of genetic information, the brain-to-brain pathway seems riddled with sources of information loss, even in a world of books, videos, and connected computers. Given the enormous complexity of the behaviors that characterize human culture, how do humans transmit behavioral phenotypes through such a noisy channel?

One way in which humans overcome the challenge is through adaptations for causally ignorant social learning. Researchers debate about the degree to which these adaptations are innate or constructed over the course of development (Heyes, 2003) but are generally unified in their recognition that human social learning unfolds at a level of complexity that is unprecedented in the animal kingdom (R. Boyd et al., 2011; Csibra & Gergely, 2011; Mesoudi et al., 2006; Tomasello et al., 2005; Whiten et al., 2009). In particular, humans are thought to be proficient imitators who can perform high-fidelity copying of actions. Human imitation, unlike in chimpanzees, often involves mimicking the specific form of an action, even when the action includes details that are causally irrelevant with respect to the intended effect (Gergely et al., 2002; Horner & Whiten, 2005; Lyons et al., 2007). Although this trait can result in the imitation of ineffective or even maladaptive actions, it also supports the learning of actions whose effects are not immediately obvious. And critically, it doesn't require the learner to know the difference—this gets sifted and filtered over time at a population level through selective learning.

In addition to these adaptations on the part of learners, there is ample evidence that humans are also exceptional in the degree to which they provide guided instruction for the acquisition of behaviors (e.g., slowed-down demonstration or teaching), a practice that is itself adapted to the degree of cultural complexity (we see more and more formalized teaching as cultural complexity increases; Kline, 2015; Muthukrishna & Henrich, 2016). So heavy reliance on both social learning and teaching, at least at high personal cost, appear to be exceptional in humans. Beyond these adaptations of the learning procedure itself, human social organization (Hill et al., 2011; Tomasello et al., 2012; Wilson, 2012) and life history (Gurven et al., 2006; Schniter et al., 2015) also make significant contributions to preparing conditions that are conducive to sophisticated social learning.

Whereas genetic transmission in humans only occurs from parent to child (*vertical transmission*), cultural transmission occurs among individuals within the same generation (*horizontal transmission*), as well as from older nonparents such as teachers (*oblique transmission*) (Cavalli-Sforza & Feldman, 1981). In the early years of life, there is a strong emphasis on vertical transmission of cultural knowledge, as parents are the source of much of the learning that occurs in this period. As development proceeds through childhood and into adolescence, the oblique and horizontal channels become increasingly important, as they offer a greater number and variety of cultural variants from which the learner can choose. Vertical transmission is slow and conservative, as it is constrained to specific relationships as well as to the generational time scale, and is insufficient for cumulative culture (Enquist et al., 2010). Horizontal transmission is unconstrained and can therefore enable the rapid diffusion of knowledge within a population, whereas oblique transmission is expected to be somewhere between these two. Because of these divergent properties, the kinds of knowledge that are transferred down these pathways will also differ.

In the case of vertical transmission, the learner has no choice regarding the model to be learned from, but in horizontal and oblique transmission, the number of available models will scale in proportion to the size of the learner's social network. Although learners benefit from acquiring the most effective cultural variants, it is often difficult to properly evaluate the effectiveness of behaviors, as cause–effect relationships can be ambiguous for a number of reasons, such as long time scales over which effects become manifest or the presence of multiple confounding variables. Due to the ubiquity of this kind of causal opacity (Lyons et al., 2007), learners must rely on various methods for the selection of models, which are collectively referred to as *social learning biases* or *social learning strategies* (Heyes & Pearce, 2015; Laland, 2004; Rendell et al., 2011). There are a large number of social learning strategies that have been proposed as having utility based on either empirical observation or theory (Kendal et al., 2018; Rendell et al., 2011). Two examples of strategies that are thought to be significant in the context of human culture are the *conformist bias* (Henrich & Boyd, 1998; Muthukrishna et al., 2016), in which learners disproportionately tend to adopt behaviors that are observed frequently, and the *prestige bias* (Cheng et al., 2013; Chudek et al., 2012; Henrich & Gil-White, 2001), in which the number of learners already attending to a model is taken to be a cue for the desirability of that model's behaviors. Both of these strategies are expected to be effective ways of selecting adaptive behaviors without having to explicitly evaluate their utility. But this of course involves a trade-off between efficiency and certainty, and sometimes these strategies can result in the propagation of suboptimal or even maladaptive behaviors. One strength of the cultural evolutionary framework is how it can explain the spread of maladaptive behaviors through the lens of evolutionary dynamics.

These cultural evolutionary processes indicate how useful information can spread from brain to brain in an effective manner, but the descriptions fall short of being able to explain how brains become sophisticated enough to carry and transmit this kind of knowledge in the first place. Cultural evolution is only one part of the picture; to understand the role that culture plays in the evolution of organisms, we must, at minimum, understand brains and the coevolutionary dynamic between brains and culture.

The Cultural Brain Hypothesis: How Culture Shaped Our Brains Over Evolutionary History

Just as genetic information is stored in the nucleotide sequences of genomes, cultural information is stored in the neuronal connections of brain tissue (at least until the advent of writing and other forms of distributed cognition). Brains can be scaled in capacity and complexity by evolution, with larger, more complex brains enabling more storage and more sophisticated processing, but with larger energy requirements (Aiello & Wheeler, 1995; Henrich & Boyd, 2008; Kuzawa et al., 2014; Leonard et al., 2003). Humans are an extreme in both brains and energy usage. Our brains tripled in size over the last few million years and are three times as large as chimpanzees, our closest cousins (Bailey & Geary, 2009; Falk, 2012). We also use energy at a faster rate than any other great ape (Pontzer et al., 2016), an achievement we sustain thanks to our efficient extraction of energy from our environment. This efficiency is thanks to culturally acquired food processing techniques, such as cooking, cooperation in food acquisition, parental provisioning, etc., and more recently, the division of labor (Hrdy, 2011; Kaplan et al., 2000; Tomasello et al., 2012; Wrangham & Carmody, 2010). Even our life histories are aligned with this interpersonal transfer of knowledge—we require an extended period of learning to acquire cultural knowledge, whether advanced hunting skills or modern classroom education (Gurven et al., 2006; Koster et al., 2019; Schniter et al., 2015; Schuppli et al., 2012), and indeed, this period may be further extending in developed societies today with longer periods of learning and delayed reproduction (Muthukrishna & Henrich, 2016).

As we can see, there is a complex relationship between sociality, energetic budget, culturally transmitted knowledge, brain size, and life history. In the case of humans, these factors appear to have worked together synergistically, yielding distinct human phenotypes, but the ways in which these variables interact may reflect a more general set of principles that explains evolutionary trajectories across diverse animal taxa. This is the approach taken by the *Cultural Brain Hypothesis* (CBH; Fox et al., 2017; Muthukrishna et al., 2018), which is grounded in theoretical insight from cultural evolutionary theory and empirical observations from the animal behavior literature.

A survey of the literature on primate and human brain evolution reveals a diverse array of explanations for the expansion of brain size that occurred multiple times in primate phylogeny. The most influential such theory over the last two decades has perhaps been the Social Brain Hypothesis (Dunbar, 1992; Dunbar & Shultz, 2007), which claims that primate brains expanded to be able to keep track of interindividual relationships in increasingly large groups; this was later modified to include other aspects of social living. Theories that link primate brain size expansion to various kinds of ecological problem solving have been influential as well (Barton, 1998; DeCasien et al., 2017). A third strand are explanations that attribute primate brain expansion to the ability to learn adaptive behaviors from conspecifics, that is, social learning (Herrmann et al., 2007; Reader et al., 2011; Reader & Laland, 2002; Street et al., 2017; van Schaik & Burkart, 2011; van Schaik et al., 2012). The CBH moves the focus from "social" or "ecological" to "learning" more generally, but also generalizes social and ecological theories.

The CBH formally models the specific causal structure that generates the covarying relationships among variables such as brain size, group size, reliance on social learning, the degree of adaptive knowledge available in the population, and life history profile (Figure 2.1); other theories linking brain evolution to social learning have tended to be more ambiguous about the causal relationships that underlie the covariation. This causal structure builds on other cultural evolutionary theory and is consistent with findings in the empirical literature. Because the CBH is based on a theoretically motivated, process-level model rather than being derived from observations of a particular subset of animal species, it is able to make predictions across the whole space of species traits. For example, it is able to describe how the strength of the relationships between the mentioned variables is expected to vary across the entire gamut of sociality, from the most solitary to the most gregarious species. For example, the CBH predicts that the correlation between brain size and group size should be significantly stronger in species that engage in social learning than in those that do not.

Relatedly, the model presents predictions for the human evolutionary trajectory, with its extreme reliance on cumulative culture, as a special case of the general causal process rather than as something requiring a unique explanation. These predictions are referred to as the Cumulative Cultural Brain Hypothesis (CCBH). In particular, the model predicts two attractors toward which species tend to converge over evolution: one that relies mostly on asocial learning (e.g., trial-and-error learning), but with some amount of social learning usually also taking place, and another that is dominated by social learning. The social learning regime has an extreme that evolves in conditions in which an autocatalytic takeoff occurs through positive feedback between brain size, adaptive knowledge, and sociality—the result being species in which the level of the adaptive knowledge acquired

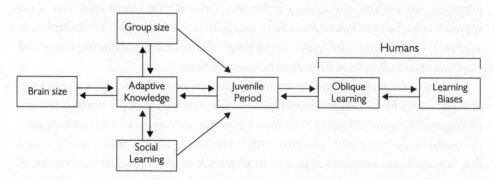

Figure 2.1 Causal relationships predicted by the Cultural Brain Hypothesis (adapted from Muthukrishna et al., 2018).

by individuals greatly exceeds the level that could plausibly be achieved through asocial learning alone. The model operationalizes cumulative cultural evolution (Dean et al., 2012, 2014; Tennie et al., 2009) based on a region where the probability of acquisition through asocial learning is exceedingly unlikely: a human regime.

The CBH gives us a conceptual handle on the kind of dynamics that can explain the covariation among traits such as brain size, length of juvenile period, sociality, and cultural complexity (i.e., level of adaptive knowledge), and does this by making explicit the underlying causal structure. Its explanatory power extends into the case of the human evolutionary trajectory, which exhibits a profound acceleration across all of these variables. However, although the model has many moving parts, its rendition of the brain is representationally minimal: an index of size. We will thus attempt to link the evolutionary dynamics portrayed by the CBH to a more detailed examination of neural architecture and plasticity.

From Large Brains to Networked Minds

Large Brains and the Degrees-of-Freedom Problem

We begin with the principle that as brains become larger, they offer more degrees of freedom in configurability. In mammalian evolution, increased brain size does not result in a linearly corresponding increase in the size of sensory organs—for example, species with vastly different brain sizes have relatively similar eye sizes (Howland et al., 2004). Larger brains do not take in a significantly increased amount of raw data—instead, they provide a greater range of ways in which the same data can be filtered, decomposed, and recombined. Big brains allow more processing and storage options. Roughly the same can be said for action: the difference in brain size between a human and a chimpanzee (a factor of ~3) far outstrips the difference in body size or musculoskeletal organization, but the larger human brain allows for a much wider breadth of options for decision-making and behavior, including various forms of behavioral inhibition (Damasio, 1994; MacLean et al., 2014).

We can therefore say that larger brains enable enhanced control over both sensory processing and action selection, although in actual brain function these two things are deeply intertwined and neither anatomically nor functionally separable (Cisek & Kalaska, 2010; Varela et al., 1991). So large brains not only amplify control options in the sensory and motor domains respectively, but also in their coordination. In the field of cognitive neuroscience, this latter mediational function is referred to as *cognitive control*. The term is roughly synonymous with the older term *executive function*, and Botvinick et al. (2001, p. 624) describe it as "the ability [of a cognitive system] to configure itself for the performance of specific tasks through appropriate adjustments in perceptual selection, response biasing, and the on-line maintenance of contextual information." Cognitive control is a higher-order concept that subsumes component functions such as attention, working memory, error monitoring, inhibitory control, and planning. Cognitive control usually refers to the ability to modulate brain function in real time and in a task-dependent manner, but this kind of adaptive configuration of brain function can also be achieved in part by constraints that stem from processes unfolding over longer time scales, such as brain development and, as we argue, cultural evolution (or more specifically, brain–culture coevolution). The general problem of proliferating control options in large brains demands solutions that span such time scales.

There are at least three characteristics of large brains that make this job easier: One is hierarchy—a hierarchical cortical architecture is able to organize its representations in a combinatorially efficient manner, and owing to fundamental neurodevelopmental constraints, the depth of the cortical processing hierarchy scales systematically with brain size (Charvet et al., 2015; Finlay & Uchiyama, 2015). This is the same computational principle that explains why artificial neural networks become substantially more powerful simply by increasing the number of layers (LeCun et al., 2015). Another characteristic of large brains is the protracted developmental duration that is required to grow them. Brain growth follows a fixed trajectory that is more or less species invariant (Passingham, 1985), and for larger brains, this developmental structure supplies a longer absolute window over which mechanisms of early-life plasticity can be exposed to input from the world. Larger brains therefore undergo more shaping by extrinsic stimuli, or in other words, can learn more. Across all species, this shaping will align with the structure of the ecological environment, but a species with cumulative culture is able to impose additional regimes of shaping that do not exist in the environment per se. Finally, because brain tissue is metabolically expensive, large brains also require greater nutritional provisioning, such as from a calorie-rich environment, availability of food acquisition techniques to be learned, or early provisioning from parents or alloparents. This relationship between large brains and sociality is conducive to the acquisition of adaptive forms of functional configuration via social learning (see Muthukrishna et al., 2018, for a discussion of the two pathways to larger brains).

Brain expansion brings with it a surfeit of processing options, but because it is also accompanied by useful properties like the three properties discussed earlier, there is greater opportunity for converging on adaptive processing options. Culture can play a significant role in this search process, as it is able to change at a much more rapid rate than either genes or the ecological environment. It is also able to support variation in input that would not exist otherwise, which in turn increases phenotypic variability and hence evolvability. Let us examine each of the mentioned concomitants of large brain size in more detail.

Concomitant 1: Large Brains and Deep Hierarchical Abstraction

Larger brains don't just enable an increase in the amount of stored knowledge; they also allow for new ways of representing knowledge. As the neocortex grows larger over evolutionary time, the sizes of early sensory and motor areas expand relatively slowly compared to transmodal association areas that are uncommitted to any particular sensory modality. The largest brains are thus the ones with the greatest proportion of association cortex (Krubitzer, 2009). More association cortex means deeper representational hierarchies, and thus the encoding of increasingly abstract kinds of information, such as complex, context-dependent rules for action or a holistic and variation-tolerant grasp of objects instead of just simple sensory snapshots (DiCarlo et al., 2012). Deeper representational hierarchies also support greater cross-modal integration, so that signals from different sensory systems can be bound together into abstract representations that are independent of particular modalities. For example, speech acquisition in human infants requires the learning of cross-modal associations between visual, auditory, and motor signals.

Human neuroimaging has shown that the lateral frontal cortex and parietal cortex—both patches of association cortex—are organized in a functional hierarchy of the kind described previously, with increasing levels of cognitive abstraction being arranged roughly along a caudal-to-rostral axis (Choi et al., 2018). Increasingly complex tasks (e.g., nesting of conditional rules) recruit cortical areas that correspond to higher levels of the processing hierarchy. Across individuals, a measure of hierarchal organization as estimated by Dynamic Causal Modeling (Friston et al., 2003) not only predicts performance in an explicitly hierarchical cognitive task but also demonstrates a sizable correlation ($r = 0.61$) with a composite intelligence measure that comprises working memory and fluid intelligence (Nee & D'Esposito, 2016). Degree of hierarchical organization may well be an important mediator of the relationship between brain size and intelligence within humans (Gignac & Bates, 2017), as well as across species (MacLean et al., 2014).

In perception too, hierarchical organization is what enables complex forms of object recognition. Deeper levels of the processing hierarchy support abstract representations that are increasingly tolerant to any number of dimensions of variability such as angle of view, within-category variation of exemplars, or sensory modality (DiCarlo et al., 2012). The human visual system is literally able to abstract out the essential features of some target of interest, as illustrated vividly by the discovery of "Jennifer Aniston neurons"—single cells in the medial temporal lobe that respond to a specific individual across various photographic and hand-drawn renditions and even to their printed name, but not to representations of any other individuals (Quiroga et al., 2005). This is precisely the sort of abstraction that is characteristic of a concept or a semantic representation, and in fact it is commonly thought that the anterior temporal lobe, an association area that corresponds to the deepest stage of the ventral visual stream, functions as a hub for the representation of semantic meaning (Chadwick et al., 2016; Patterson et al., 2007).

In general, the more topologically distant a given cortical area is from the primary sensorimotor areas, the more abstract its domain of representation will be. The default-mode network (Raichle, 2015) coincides with the cortical areas that are furthest in this respect (Huntenburg et al., 2018), and not only do these deep association areas display the highest level of cross-modal integration, they also encode the longest temporal windows (e.g., sentences vs. phonemes; Hasson et al., 2015) as well as the most abstract semantic concepts (e.g., "schools" and "lethal" vs. "yellow" and "four"; Huth et al., 2016). In terms of function, this set of areas is known to be most active when dealing with processes such as mind-wandering, mental time-travel (i.e., episodic recollection and thinking about the future), autobiographical memory, narrative comprehension, and social cognition (Spreng et al., 2009). These functions are therefore expected to be the ones that require the most hierarchical depth and hence brain size.

The fact that social cognition, in particular the family of cognitive functions known as "theory of mind," is firmly tied to the network of cortical areas that are at the leading edge of brain expansion is interesting (Schilbach et al., 2008), as it suggests that large brains are useful not only for the social learning of advanced skills but also for understanding the social domain itself. Areas recruited during visual processing of conspecific interactions appear to occupy similar cortical regions (Sliwa & Freiwald, 2017). The fact that these areas encode temporal depth is also significant, as a sophisticated understanding of the behavior of others requires that they be situated within an extended situational context, such as social scripts (e.g., the event structure of "birthday party"; Krueger, Barbey, & Grafman, 2009) or narratives (Nguyen, Vanderwal, & Hasson, 2019; Simony et al., 2016; Zacks, Speer, Swallow, & Maley, 2010). In large-brained species, the behavior of conspecifics is a source of some of the most complex information in the environment (Humphrey, 1976), and it makes sense that the neural representation of the social world will be accommodated by cortical areas that are at the deepest levels of the processing hierarchy. Brain expansion enables a richer representation of the social world.

Concomitant 2: Large Brains and Longer Development

The relationship between brain size and the length of neurodevelopment is highly systematic. For example, the Translating Time model of Finlay and colleagues (Finlay & Darlington, 1995; Workman et al., 2013) is able to use a highly parsimonious but neurodevelopmentally realistic model to predict the nonlinear trajectory of whole brain growth across a variety of mammalian species, along with hundreds of other neurodevelopmental events that span the gamut from the appearance of specific axonal connections to the emergence of walking. For brain growth, the correlation between predicted timing and observed timing is on the order of $r = 0.99$, demonstrating just how systematic brain growth is even when comparing across phylogenetically distant species whose brain masses differ by a factor of ~1000, such as a human versus a mouse (Halley, 2017; Passingham, 1985; Workman et al., 2013). The idea underlying this research is that evolution can create larger brains by temporally stretching the highly structured process of brain development that has been conserved since the ancestor of all extant mammals.

If we look at specific durations, the mouse, for example, reaches 50% of adult brain mass around 26 days postconception or 7 days postpartum (Gottlieb et al., 1977), while humans reach the same milestone around 350 days postconception or 2.5 months after birth (Dekaban & Sadowsky, 1978). We are using 50% brain mass as an arbitrary reference point, but any such reference point can be highly informative precisely because of the systematic and predictable nature of mammalian brain development: if we know the timing of some particular developmental event, we know with a significant degree of accuracy the developmental state of the nervous system as a whole. When the mouse is at its 50% mark, everything else going on in its cranium—the onset and offset of neurogenesis in particular cortical layers, the establishment of dopaminergic axons from the midbrain to the neocortex, or the completion of myelination in the hippocampus—is at roughly the same state as it is in the brain of a human infant who is also achieving the 50% milestone (Workman et al., 2013).

Now consider the interval between 50% and 80% adult brain mass: the mouse progresses through this segment of the neurodevelopmental process (along with every other event that is in sync with it) in a span of just 5 days (Gottlieb et al., 1977), while the human takes about 16 months to go through it (Dekaban & Sadowsky, 1978). The two species are undergoing roughly the same degree of intrinsic brain development within this interval, but for the human infant, the processes of brain development are exposed to more than a year of external stimuli, while the baby mouse only gets a few days. Although it is true that the time scale of an organism's physiological and ontogenetic processes scale down systematically with body size (West et al., 2001), there is simply no way to close the gap in the amount of learning that can occur between the mouse and the human, both within this particular interval and across brain development as a whole. So increasing brain size does not only increase processing power, it also allows more knowledge and skills to be loaded into it during its development, whether this be through trial-and-error or social learning.

In fact, there is likely more to the story than just a longer window of opportunity for learning. The brain itself is of course undergoing considerable organizational changes over development, and this appears to create a learning gradient that unfolds over time, in which early learning is characterized by a broader space of hypotheses about the structure of the world and hence greater flexibility in learning. As maturation progresses, the brain acquires stronger prior hypotheses about what to expect, and information processing becomes more efficient, but also more rigid, consistent with evidence from learning (Gopnik et al., 2017; Lucas et al., 2014).

Making a similar proposal, but with greater neurodevelopmental specificity, Chrysikou and colleagues (Chrysikou et al., 2014; Thompson-Schill et al., 2009) hypothesize that the extended development of the prefrontal cortex and the resulting deficiency of prefrontal function in children (Diamond, 2013) is not a deficit per se, but rather a functional design feature that affords certain learning advantages that are critical in early years. For instance, in language acquisition, children are better at learning irregular verbs and irregular plurals than adults are, and this is attributed to the tendency for children to reiterate utterances that they have actually heard, compared to adults, who tend to search for underlying rules (J. K. Boyd & Goldberg, 2012). This tendency would give children an advantage in learning conventions in general, linguistic or otherwise, because in this domain, veridical reproduction (overimitation) often matters more than finding efficient representations (Lyons et al., 2007).

Reduced prefrontal control early in life may thus confer an advantage in the effective execution of conformity. Paradoxically, it may also confer an advantage for innovation as well (Chrysikou et al., 2014). Older children are more susceptible to "functional fixedness" effects than are younger children, meaning that once they have a concept of what a given tool is for, they have more difficulty coming up with alternative uses for it (Defeyter & German, 2003). There appears to be a marked shift in this tendency between the ages of 5 to 7 years, a period during which prefrontal development is beginning to accelerate (Kanemura et al., 2003). There is also evidence that links prefrontal activity to inhibited performance when adults are asked to come up with novel uses for tools (Chrysikou et al., 2013; Chrysikou & Thompson-Schill, 2011). More generally, artistic creativity may be tied to a reduction of prefrontal control, whether in visual art or jazz improvisation (Chrysikou et al., 2014). These advantages of reduced prefrontal function or *hypofrontality* necessarily accompany the early phase of brain development in a species like ours, in which the mammalian neurodevelopmental program is lengthened to generate a large brain. In other words, large brains, which in the case of humans are also cultural brains, get these advantages "for free" in evolutionary terms—specific selection is not required. And it is not difficult to see why a mutually beneficial relationship between cultural learning and early hypofrontality is plausible. These findings are important to building a more complete picture of human evolution. They inform our understanding of the raw material that natural selection can work with, mapping out the adjacent possible and guiding us in inferring necessary selection pressures and probable adaptations. And although they echo similar dynamics between variation creation and transmission fidelity at a population level (Muthukrishna & Henrich, 2016), at an individual level, they are thus far missing from dual inheritance theory and cultural evolution.

Concomitant 3: Large Brains and Sociality

Brain tissue is expensive, and a large, complex brain needs to pay its energy bills. For humans, at least in early life, provisioning comes from nutritional subsidies offered well beyond nursing and often beyond mothers and even close kin (Hrdy, 2011). Such provisioning requires stable nutritional surpluses, made possible by effective methods for calorie acquisition from cumulative cultural knowledge. The transfer of food resources from the competent to the incompetent appears to be a human universal, and individuals may not attain a production surplus until late into their teens or beyond, meaning that humans go through a long period of dependence during which they acquire the skills needed to produce at a surplus for the next generation (Kaplan et al., 2000). In contrast, chimpanzee juveniles are forced to look after themselves immediately after weaning.

When we evaluate the timing of weaning in relation to the stage of brain maturation across species, we discover that human infants are actually weaned at a noticeably earlier point in the mammalian neurodevelopmental schedule than our closest primate relatives (Finlay & Uchiyama, 2020; Hawkes & Finlay, 2018), and this is also reflected in the timing of weaning being earlier than expected on the basis of brain size: Figure 2.2 (weaning) shows that human weaning occurs much earlier than would expected for a non-human ape with our brain size, and earlier even than would be expected for other primates (i.e., monkeys and prosimians). The box plot displays the range in the timing of weaning across small-scale societies as observed in ethnographic records (Sellen, 2001), revealing substantial variation in human weaning: half of these societies lie below the lower boundary of the 95% prediction interval for apes, and about 1 out of 6 lie below the lower boundary for other primates. These data suggest that in humans, the timing of weaning is determined by both genetic and cultural selection.

Early weaning is tied to a shorter period between births, and hence higher reproductive output. It is striking that the hunter-gatherer interbirth interval of 3 to 4 years is shorter than the 4 to 5 year interval of chimpanzees and gorillas (Robson & Wood, 2008) despite humans being more delayed than the great apes in other aspects of life history, and this is even more remarkable once we take the relationship between brain size and life history into account. Early weaning is possible thanks to the care given by not just mothers but also others (Hrdy, 2011). This high level of sociality also ensures access to a broad assortment of conspecifics at an early stage of life, which may have helped in the evolution of selective social learning biases that extend cultural learning beyond parents and close kin (Muthukrishna et al., 2018; Muthukrishna & Henrich, 2016). The energetic demands of our large brains may thus link us not only to social structures that are able to supply the requisite calories, but also to cultural networks that transfer adaptive information as well.

Another exceptional feature of human life history is our long lifespans (Figure 2.2 reproductive lifespan and maximum longevity). The puzzle of human longevity, including the postmenopausal years, has been a topic of much discussion in the anthropological literature (Hawkes, 2003; Kaplan et al., 2000a), but here we suggest that this feature too may be partly explained by genes adapting to the requirements of cultural learning. In particular, an ever-expanding corpus of skills and knowledge may select for longer lifespans over which more of this cultural knowledge can be acquired and refined and a longer period for it to be exploited or passed on to the next generation (Information Grandmother Hypothesis). Even in relatively simple societies that rely on hunting and 'slash-and-burn' agriculture, competence in foraging skill can peak as late as the 50s (Gurven, Kaplan, & Gutierrez, 2006b; Schniter, Gurven, Kaplan, Wilcox, & Hooper, 2015b), and this may just be a manifestation of a more general positive relationship between social complexity and the late peaking of foraging skill that is observed across mammalian species (Isler & van Schaik, 2009). Accumulation of knowledge may also explain postmenopausal life in other highly social species such as killer whales (Brent et al., 2015). In contrast to traits

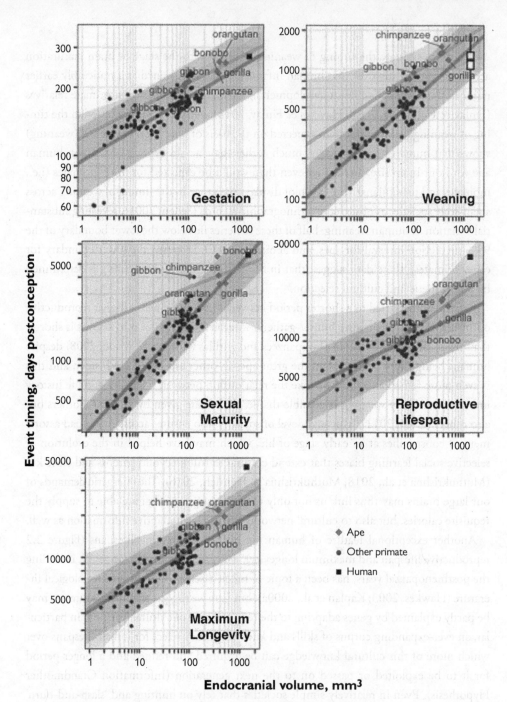

Figure 2.2. Scatterplots displaying the relationships between brain size (endocranial volume) and timing of life history events among primates, for gestation, weaning, sexual maturity, reproductive lifespan, and maximum longevity. Event timings are given in postconception days rather than postnatal days because the former is tightly coupled with the species-invariant state of brain maturation, whereas the latter is not (Workman et al, 2013). Light and dark lines are OLS regression lines for non-human apes and other primates (i.e., monkeys and prosimians) respectively. 95% prediction intervals for each model are shown as bands around the lines. Humans are plotted, but not included in the computation of the models. The box plot in the panel for weaning displays the cross-cultural variation in the timing of human weaning across the ethnographic record, based on Sellen (2001). All plotted data are from Street, Navarrete, Reader & Laland (2017) except for the human endocranial volume of 1349 cm³, which is the average value across 122 ethnic groups from Beals, Smith and Dodd (1984) and the distribution of human weaning.

such as weaning and lifespan, birth and sexual maturity appear to occur in humans at roughly the timing that would be expected for both apes and non-apes (Figure 2.2 gestation and sexual maturity), suggesting differential selection pressures across different facets of life history.

We have reviewed three traits that covary with brain size: deep hierarchies, long development, and high sociality. When brains expand over evolution, this suite of traits gets pulled upward, in some parts as expected, and in other parts deviating from expectations and therefore probably requiring trait-specific genetic, cultural, or culture–gene coevolutionary selection. A cultural evolutionary neuroscience approach thus informs cultural evolution and informs neuroscience.

When cultural knowledge, brain size, and access to the number of brains (i.e., population size) enter a positive feedback loop, as predicted by the CCBH (Muthukrishna et al., 2018), these concomitants of brain expansion play a role in moving information processing from simply the cranial-bound brain to the collective brains bound in a social network, which can in turn empower each individual brain via cultural learning (Muthukrishna & Henrich, 2016).

Cumulative Culture and the Rise of the Collective Brain

Humans are thought to be the only species for which we have evidence of cumulative culture (Dean et al., 2012, 2014; Tennie et al., 2009), and the Cultural Brain Hypothesis (Muthukrishna et al., 2018) models this evolutionary trajectory as the crossing of a threshold in which the individuals that make up a species begin to learn more adaptive knowledge from social learning than they would be able to discover by themselves (CCBH). Once this threshold has been crossed, traits like sociality, brain size, length of juvenile period, and cultural complexity enter a positive feedback loop and shoot upward rapidly. Note that in a scenario like this one (which captures various anomalies of human evolution), large brains can be maintained only because they can come into the world with the expectation that they will be fed with energy and information that is effective enough to be able to pay for their high metabolic cost. In such a species, groups grow in such a way that the collective information-processing capacity eclipses the intrinsic capabilities of the neural hardware itself, and individual brains become informationally and metabolically dependent on others in their societies. The processing power of the group is determined by factors such as the number of individuals that constitute the group, the topology of connections between individuals, and the effectiveness of strategies for selecting what to learn and who to learn from (Derex et al., 2013; Derex & Boyd, 2016; Goldstone & Theiner, 2017; Henrich, 2004; Muthukrishna et al. 2013; Muthukrishna & Henrich, 2016). But inference of the adaptive value of any given behavior or belief is inherently noisy and opaque, as we saw in the discussion on social learning strategies, and so there is always a selection pressure for better search strategies. Former CEO of Google Eric Schmidt unknowingly echoed these insights about the coevolutionary dynamics of culture in 1993 when he quite presciently predicted that "when the network runs as fast as the computer backplane, the computer will hollow out and distribute itself around the network, and profits in the industry will migrate toward the providers of 'sort' and 'search' capabilities" (Gilder, 2013, p. 319). We can say that Schmidt's vision concisely captures what has been happening to the relationship between hardware, software, and networks in recent years—so too in brains, culture, and sociality.

The evolution of human brain *size* is fairly well known even among nonscientists, and discussions of brain evolution often revolve around this manifestly visible characteristic. But according to the perspective that we are outlining here, a focus on size, or for that matter any property of individual brains, is insufficient for explaining human brain evolution. Our social systems, our bodies of culturally accumulated knowledge, our social learning strategies, and even our life histories have all evolved together with our brains, and we need to think of all these factors as an integrated system. To not do so is as misguided as trying to understand the advances in computing solely through understanding advances in hardware specifications.

Muthukrishna and Henrich (2016) refer to this distributed information-processing system as a *collective brain*, nomenclature that emphasizes the information-processing capacities of the network itself. They argue that collective brains are underpinned in particular by our *norm psychology* (Chudek & Henrich, 2011) and *ethnic psychology* (McElreath et al., 2003). Norm psychology refers to the suite of abilities that allow us to infer what the shared behavioral standards of the group are, adhere to them appropriately, and enforce them when flouted. Ethnic psychology refers to the mental abilities that allow us to figure out to which groups we belong. In combination, our norm and ethnic psychology allow us to understand the norms of these groups and to whom these norms apply. Once we have a norm psychology and an ethnic psychology, societies are able to generate complex structures in their networks, for example, through marriage rules that have consequences for the shape of networks beyond immediate kin (e.g., through in-law relationships) and thus for the parameters of the collective brain. Societies also vary on how open they are to outgroup members (e.g., whether exogamous marriage is allowed or to whom; Chapais, 2013; Hill et al., 2011), how tolerant they are to norm deviations (e.g., tightness–looseness; Gelfand et al., 2011), and the amount of migration (Powell et al., 2009). Each of these traits, and no doubt many more, modulate information flow in the collective brain. And since these collective brains in turn change their constituent individual brains, we complete the circle and find ourselves needing not just a neuroscience approach, but a cultural neuroscience approach to cultural evolution and a cultural evolutionary approach to cultural neuroscience.

Much of cultural neuroscience has focused on mapping cross-cultural differences at the level of the brain (just as cultural psychology has mainly focused on mapping cross-cultural differences in psychology). A more systematic approach to cultural evolutionary neuroscience requires an understanding of the sources of those cross-cultural differences (e.g., Schulz et al., 2019) and how they manifest neurologically as well as perhaps genetically, such as via a Baldwinian process (Crispo, 2016) where repeated cultural learning eventually selects for genes that make that learning more effective or more efficient.

Caveats and Conclusions

Cultural neuroscience has revealed variations in human brains, especially between East Asians and Western people, who appear to differ even in core aspects of psychology, such as visuo-spatial judgment (Goh et al., 2013), arithmetic (Tang et al., 2006), and empathy (Cheon et al., 2011). But variations in the neural systems underlying common tasks are present even within a population, because our brains are as variable as we are. For example, Noppeney and colleagues (Noppeney, Penny, et al., 2006; Noppeney, Price, et al., 2006) examined intersubject variability in fMRI activity while participants underwent semantic judgment tasks, within a conventional UK participant sample. Such variability is usually discarded when data is averaged across participants, but Noppeney et al. used analyses that allow detection of differences in the neural systems being recruited for the same task. Across two different experiments, they found overlapping but distinguishable clusters of participants, with each participant cluster corresponding to a different activation profile and suggesting the use of a distinct strategy—for example, semantic discrimination being supported by stimulus-dependent ("bottom-up") versus task-dependent ("top-down") mechanisms (Noppeney, Price, et al., 2006). In this case these differences in neural activation did not predict differences in performance.

The general notion that multiple neural systems can interchangeably implement a common function is an example of what is known as *degeneracy*, defined by Edelman and Gally (2001) as "the ability of elements that are structurally different to perform the same function or yield the same output," or in other words, a many-to-one structure–function mapping (Edelman & Gally, 2001; Price & Friston, 2002; Tononi et al., 1999). The extent of degeneracy in the genetic code is striking: in *Caenorhabditis elegans*, 89% of single-copy (i.e., nonduplicated) genes can be knocked down without any detectable phenotypic effect (Conant & Wagner, 2004). Across levels of biological organization from genes to multiply realizable muscular control of movement, degeneracy is taken to be a key factor in supporting robustness and evolvability, as it enables the generation of phenotypic variation without any immediate consequence for adaptive function and thereby supports the exploration of phenotypic space (Ancel & Fontana, 2000; Edelman & Gally, 2001; Whitacre & Bender, 2010). Although the extent of degeneracy in the brain is not currently known, it has been argued that the rapid recovery of function following focal cortical damage is possible only because neural degeneracy is prevalent (Noppeney et al., 2004). Thus, caution is required when we find cross-cultural differences in neural activity, as they may not necessarily correspond to differences in function. Gordon et al. (2015) found individual differences in the topology of resting state functional connectivity but warn that such whole-brain architectural differences may not necessarily be predictive of cognitive performance and may instead reflect degeneracy. Cultural psychologists have illuminated an impressive collection of cross-cultural psychological differences, but the general strategy of mapping these performance differences onto neural activation differences requires caution, and we should be wary of false positives. In principle, explanations for such behavior-brain mapping are constrained by cultural psychological constructs, such as when greater activation of theory-of-mind-related areas of the brain in East Asians is attributed to their "collectivism" (Han & Ma, 2014), but there is ambiguity in the specific predictions that can be derived from such constructs, and their effectiveness as theoretical constraints for making sense of high-dimensional neuroimaging data is not self-evident.

There are also cases in which an apparent absence of performance difference masks some interesting underlying neurocognitive differences. Comparing patients with Williams Syndrome, a developmental disorder characterized by intellectual impairment in some domains but intact ability in others, with healthy controls, Karmiloff-Smith and colleagues found that the two groups achieve matched performance on some tasks using different cognitive strategies. For example, children with the disorder rely comparatively more on verbal abilities than on visuo-spatial abilities when counting (Ansari et al., 2003), and adult patients were found to use "featural" as opposed to "configural" processing in face perception tasks (Karmiloff-Smith, et al., 2004). Although the example is of a clinical population, studies such as these hint at what we should also be looking for cross-culturally, namely, covert variation in neurodevelopmental trajectories.

In other cases, cross-cultural and within-population differences in neural activation do affect overt performance, such as in the neural response to threat (Coan et al., 2006, 2017), or are likely to have performance implications, such as the relationship between age and brain structure (LeWinn et al., 2017), reading and writing (Bolger et al., 2005; Kobayashi et al., 2007; Tan et al., 2005), collectivism–individualism (Triandis et al., 1988), or tightness–looseness (Gelfand et al., 2011).

These caveats further reinforce the need to understand the origins and function of cross-cultural differences. Disentangling the question of when neurological differences do and do not matter requires the theoretical tools of cultural evolution and the empirical tools of cultural neuroscience. Without cultural neuroscience, cultural evolution remains mind blind. Without cultural evolution, cultural neuroscience continues collecting cross-cultural differences. The confluence of these fields, a cultural evolutionary neuroscience, will give us a more complete understanding of our species.

References

Aiello, L. C., & Wheeler, P. (1995). The expensive-tissue hypothesis: The brain and the digestive system in human and primate evolution. *Current Anthropology*, *36*(2), 199–221. https://doi.org/10.1086/204350

Ancel, L. W., & Fontana, W. (2000). Plasticity, evolvability, and modularity in RNA. *Journal of Experimental Zoology*, *288*(3), 242–283. https://doi.org/10.1002/1097-010X(20001015)288:3<242::AID-JEZ5>3.0.CO;2-O

Ansari, D., Donlan, C., Thomas, M. S. C., Ewing, S. A., Peen, T., & Karmiloff-Smith, A. (2003). What makes counting count? Verbal and visuo-spatial contributions to typical and atypical number development. *Journal of Experimental Child Psychology*, *85*(1), 50–62. https://doi.org/10.1016/S0022-0965(03)00026-2

Bailey, D. H., & Geary, D. C. (2009). Hominid brain evolution: Testing climatic, ecological, and social competition models. *Human Nature*, *20*(1), 67–79. https://doi.org/10.1007/s12110-008-9054-0

Bandura, A. (1977). *Social learning theory*. Prentice Hall.

Barton, R. A. (1998). Visual specialization and brain evolution in primates. *Proceedings of the Royal Society of London. Series B: Biological Sciences, 265*(1409), 1933–1937. https://doi.org/10.1098/rspb.1998.0523

Beals, K. L., Smith, C. L., & Dodd, S. M. (1984). Brain Size, Cranial Morphology, Climate, and Time Machines. *Current Anthropology, 25*(3), 301–318. https://doi.org/10.1086/203138

Bolger, D. J., Perfetti, C. A., & Schneider, W. (2005). Cross-cultural effect on the brain revisited: Universal structures plus writing system variation. *Human Brain Mapping, 25*(1), 92–104. https://doi.org/10.1002/hbm.20124

Botvinick, M. M., Carter, C. S., Braver, T. S., Barch, D. M., & Cohen, J. D. (2001). Conflict monitoring and cognitive control. *Psychological Review, 108*(3), 624–652.

Boyd, J. K., & Goldberg, A. E. (2012). Young children fail to fully generalize a novel argument structure construction when exposed to the same input as older learners. *Journal of Child Language, 39*(3), 457–481. https://doi.org/10.1017/S0305000911000079

Boyd, R., & Richerson, P. J. (1985). *Culture and the evolutionary process*. University of Chicago Press.

Boyd, R., Richerson, P. J., & Henrich, J. (2011). The cultural niche: Why social learning is essential for human adaptation. *Proceedings of the National Academy of Sciences, 108*(Supplement_2), 10918–10925. https://doi.org/10.1073/pnas.1100290108

Brent, L. J. N., Franks, D. W., Foster, E. A., Balcomb, K. C., Cant, M. A., & Croft, D. P. (2015). Ecological Knowledge, Leadership, and the Evolution of Menopause in Killer Whales. *Current Biology, 25*(6), 746–750. https://doi.org/10.1016/j.cub.2015.01.037

Casillas, S., & Barbadilla, A. (2017). Molecular population genetics. *Genetics, 205*(3), 1003–1035. https://doi.org/10/f9zkvj

Cavalli-Sforza, L. L., & Feldman, M. W. (1981). *Cultural transmission and evolution: A quantitative approach*. Princeton University Press.

Chadwick, M. J., Anjum, R. S., Kumaran, D., Schacter, D. L., Spiers, H. J., & Hassabis, D. (2016). Semantic representations in the temporal pole predict false memories. *Proceedings of the National Academy of Sciences, 113*(36), 10180–10185. https://doi.org/10.1073/pnas.1610686113

Changizi, M. A., & Shimojo, S. (2005). Character complexity and redundancy in writing systems over human history. *Proceedings of the Royal Society B: Biological Sciences, 272*(1560), 267–275. https://doi.org/10.1098/rspb.2004.2942

Changizi, M. A., Zhang, Q., Ye, H., & Shimojo, S. (2006). The Structures of Letters and Symbols throughout Human History Are Selected to Match Those Found in Objects in Natural Scenes. *The American Naturalist, 167*(5), E117–E139. https://doi.org/10.1086/502806

Chapais, B. (2013). Monogamy, strongly bonded groups, and the evolution of human social structure. *Evolutionary Anthropology: Issues, News, and Reviews, 22*(2), 52–65. https://doi.org/10.1002/evan.21345

Charvet, C. J., Cahalane, D. J., & Finlay, B. L. (2015). Systematic, cross-cortex variation in neuron numbers in rodents and primates. *Cerebral Cortex, 25*(1), 147–160. https://doi.org/10.1093/cercor/bht214

Cheng, J. T., Tracy, J. L., Foulsham, T., Kingstone, A., & Henrich, J. (2013). Two ways to the top: Evidence that dominance and prestige are distinct yet viable avenues to social rank and influence. *Journal of Personality and Social Psychology, 104*(1), 103–125. https://doi.org/10.1037/a0030398

Cheon, B. K., Im, D., Harada, T., Kim, J.-S., Mathur, V. A., Scimeca, J. M., Parrish, T. B., Park, H. W., & Chiao, J. Y. (2011). Cultural influences on neural basis of intergroup empathy. *NeuroImage, 57*(2), 642–650. https://doi.org/10.1016/j.neuroimage.2011.04.031

Chiao, J. Y. (2009). Cultural neuroscience: A once and future discipline. *Progress in brain research, 178*, 287-304. https://doi.org/10.1016/S0079-6123(09)17821-4

Chiao, J. Y., & Blizinsky, K. D. (2010). Culture–gene coevolution of individualism–collectivism and the serotonin transporter gene. *Proceedings of the Royal Society B: Biological Sciences, 277*(1681), 529–537. https://doi.org/10.1098/rspb.2009.1650

Chiao, J. Y., Harada, T., Komeda, H., Li, Z., Mano, Y., Saito, D., . . . Iidaka, T. (2009). Neural basis of individualistic and collectivistic views of self. *Human Brain Mapping, 30*(9), 2813–2820. https://doi.org/10.1002/hbm.20707

Choi, E. Y., Drayna, G. K., & Badre, D. (2018). Evidence for a functional hierarchy of association networks. *Journal of Cognitive Neuroscience, 30*(5), 722–736. https://doi.org/10.1162/jocn_a_01229

Christiansen, M. H., & Chater, N. (2016). The Now-or-Never bottleneck: A fundamental constraint on language. *Behavioral and Brain Sciences, 39*, e62. https://doi.org/10.1017/S0140525X1500031X

Chrysikou, E. G., Hamilton, R. H., Coslett, H. B., Datta, A., Bikson, M., & Thompson-Schill, S. L. (2013). Noninvasive transcranial direct current stimulation over the left prefrontal cortex facilitates cognitive flexibility in tool use. *Cognitive Neuroscience, 4*(2), 81–89. https://doi.org/10.1080/17588928.2013.768221

Chrysikou, E. G., & Thompson-Schill, S. L. (2011). Dissociable brain states linked to common and creative object use. *Human Brain Mapping, 32*(4), 665–675. https://doi.org/10.1002/hbm.21056

Chrysikou, E. G., Weber, M. J., & Thompson-Schill, S. L. (2014). A matched filter hypothesis for cognitive control. *Neuropsychologia, 62*, 341–355. https://doi.org/10.1016/j.neuropsychologia.2013.10.021

Chudek, M., Heller, S., Birch, S., & Henrich, J. (2012). Prestige-biased cultural learning: Bystander's differential attention to potential models influences children's learning. *Evolution and Human Behavior, 33*(1), 46–56. https://doi.org/10.1016/j.evolhumbehav.2011.05.005

Chudek, M., & Henrich, J. (2011). Culture–gene coevolution, norm-psychology and the emergence of human prosociality. *Trends in Cognitive Sciences, 15*(5), 218–226. https://doi.org/10.1016/j.tics.2011.03.003

Chudek, M., Muthukrishna, M., & Henrich, J. (2015). Cultural Evolution. In D. M. Buss (Ed.), *The Handbook of Evolutionary Psychology* (2nd ed.). John Wiley and Sons.

Cisek, P., & Kalaska, J. F. (2010). Neural mechanisms for interacting with a world full of action choices. *Annual Review of Neuroscience, 33*(1), 269–298. https://doi.org/10.1146/annurev.neuro.051508.135409

Coan, J. A., Beckes, L., Gonzalez, M. Z., Maresh, E. L., Brown, C. L., & Hasselmo, K. (2017). Relationship status and perceived support in the social regulation of neural responses to threat. *Social Cognitive and Affective Neuroscience, 12*(10), 1574–1583. https://doi.org/10/gb2xqj

Coan, J. A., Schaefer, H. S., & Davidson, R. J. (2006). Lending a hand: Social regulation of the neural response to threat. *Psychological Science, 17*(12), 1032–1039. https://doi.org/10.1111/j.1467-9280.2006.01832.x

Conant, G. C., & Wagner, A. (2004). Duplicate genes and robustness to transient gene knock-downs in *Caenorhabditis elegans*. *Proceedings of the Royal Society of London. Series B: Biological Sciences, 271*(1534), 89–96. https://doi.org/10.1098/rspb.2003.2560

Crick, F., Barnett, L., Brenner, S., & Watts-Tobin, R. (1961). General nature of the genetic code for proteins. *Nature, 192*(4809), 1227–1232.

Crispo, E. (2007). Baldwin effect and genetic assimilation: Revisiting two mechanisms of evolutionary change mediated by phenotypic plasticity. *Evolution, 61*(11), 2469–2479. https://doi.org/10.1111/j.1558-5646.2007.00203.x

Csibra, G., & Gergely, G. (2011). Natural pedagogy as evolutionary adaptation. *Philosophical Transactions of the Royal Society B: Biological Sciences, 366*(1567), 1149–1157. https://doi.org/10.1098/rstb.2010.0319

Damasio, A. R. (1994). *Descartes' error: Emotion, reason, and the human brain.* G. P. Putnam. https://search.library.wisc.edu/catalog/999764511802121

Darwin, C. (1871). *The descent of man, and selection in relation to sex.* John Murray.

Dean, L. G., Kendal, R. L., Schapiro, S. J., Thierry, B., & Laland, K. N. (2012). Identification of the social and cognitive processes underlying human cumulative culture. *Science, 335*(6072), 1114–1118. https://doi.org/10.1126/science.1213969

Dean, L. G., Vale, G. L., Laland, K. N., Flynn, E., & Kendal, R. L. (2014). Human cumulative culture: A comparative perspective. *Biological Reviews, 89*(2), 284–301. https://doi.org/10.1111/brv.12053

DeCasien, A. R., Williams, S. A., & Higham, J. P. (2017). Primate brain size is predicted by diet but not sociality. *Nature Ecology & Evolution, 1*(5). https://doi.org/10.1038/s41559-017-0112

Defeyter, M. A., & German, T. P. (2003). Acquiring an understanding of design: Evidence from children's insight problem solving. *Cognition, 89*(2), 133–155. https://doi.org/10.1016/S0010-0277(03)00098-2

Dekaban, A. S., & Sadowsky, D. (1978). Changes in brain weights during the span of human life: Relation of brain weights to body heights and body weights. *Annals of Neurology, 4*(4), 345–356. https://doi.org/10.1002/ana.410040410

Derex, M., Beugin, M.-P., Godelle, B., & Raymond, M. (2013). Experimental evidence for the influence of group size on cultural complexity. *Nature, 503*(7476), 389–391. https://doi.org/10.1038/nature12774

Derex, M., & Boyd, R. (2016). Partial connectivity increases cultural accumulation within groups. *Proceedings of the National Academy of Sciences, 113*(11), 2982–2987. https://doi.org/10.1073/pnas.1518798113

Diamond, A. (2013). Executive functions. *Annual Review of Psychology, 64*(1), 135–168. https://doi.org/10.1146/annurev-psych-113011-143750

DiCarlo, J. J., Zoccolan, D., & Rust, N. C. (2012). How does the brain solve visual object recognition? *Neuron, 73*(3), 415–434. https://doi.org/10.1016/j.neuron.2012.01.010

Ditlevsen, P. D., Svensmark, H., & Johnsen, S. (1996). Contrasting atmospheric and climate dynamics of the last-glacial and Holocene periods. *Nature, 379,* 810–812.

Dominguez-Bello, M. G., De Jesus-Laboy, K. M., Shen, N., Cox, L. M., Amir, A., Gonzalez, A., . . . Clemente, J. C. (2016). Partial restoration of the microbiota of cesarean-born infants via vaginal microbial transfer. *Nature Medicine, 22*(3), 250–253. https://doi.org/10.1038/nm.4039

Dunbar, R. I., & Shultz, S. (2007). Understanding primate brain evolution. *Philosophical Transactions of the Royal Society B: Biological Sciences, 362*(1480), 649–658. https://doi.org/10.1098/rstb.2006.2001

Dunbar, R. I. M. (1992). Neocortex size as a constraint on group size in primates. *Journal of Human Evolution, 22*(6), 469–493. https://doi.org/10.1016/0047-2484(92)90081-J

Edelman, G. M., & Gally, J. A. (2001). Degeneracy and complexity in biological systems. *Proceedings of the National Academy of Sciences, 98*(24), 13763–13768. https://doi.org/10.1073/pnas.231499798

Enquist, M., Strimling, P., Eriksson, K., Laland, K. N., & Sjostrand, J. (2010). One cultural parent makes no culture. *Animal Behaviour, 79*(6), 1353–1362. https://doi.org/10.1016/j.anbehav.2010.03.009

Falk, D. (2012). *Hominin paleoneurology. Where are we now? Progress in brain research* (Vol. 195). Elsevier B.V. https://doi.org/10.1016/B978-0-444-53860-4.00012-X

Fiddes, I. T., Lodewijk, G. A., Mooring, M., Bosworth, C. M., Ewing, A. D., Mantalas, G. L., . . . Haussler, D. (2018). Human-specific NOTCH2NL genes affect Notch signaling and cortical neurogenesis. *Cell, 173*(6), 1356–1369.e22. https://doi.org/10.1016/j.cell.2018.03.051

Finlay, B., & Darlington, R. (1995). Linked regularities in the development and evolution of mammalian brains. *Science, 268*(5217), 1578–1584. https://doi.org/10.1126/science.7777856

Finlay, B. L. (2007). Endless minds most beautiful. *Developmental Science, 10*(1), 30–34. https://doi.org/10.1111/j.1467-7687.2007.00560.x

Finlay, B. L., & Uchiyama, R. (2015). Developmental mechanisms channeling cortical evolution. *Trends in Neurosciences, 38*(2), 69–76. https://doi.org/10.1016/j.tins.2014.11.004

Finlay, B. L., & Uchiyama, R. (2020). The timing of brain maturation, early experience and the human social niche. In *Evolutionary Neuroscience* (2nd ed.). Academic Press. https://doi.org/10.1016/B978-0-12-820584-6.00034-9

Fox, K. C. R., Muthukrishna, M., & Shultz, S. (2017). The social and cultural roots of whale and dolphin brains. *Nature Ecology & Evolution, 1.*https://doi.org/10.1038/s41559-017-0336-y

Friston, K. J., Harrison, L., & Penny, W. (2003). Dynamic causal modelling. *NeuroImage, 19*(4), 1273–1302. https://doi.org/10.1016/S1053-8119(03)00202-7

Galef, B. G., & Laland, K. N. (2005). Social learning in animals: Empirical studies and theoretical models. *Bioscience, 55*(6), 489–499. https://doi.org/doi:10.1641/0006-3568(2005)055[0489:SLIAES]2.0.CO;2

Gelfand, M. J., Raver, J. L., Nishii, L., Leslie, L. M., Lun, J., Lim, B. C., . . . Othman, R. (2011). Differences between tight and loose cultures: A 33-nation study. *Science, New Series, 332*(6033), 1100–1104.

Gergely, G., Bekkering, H., & Kiraly, I. (2002). Rational imitation in preverbal infants. *Nature, 415*(6873), 755–756. https://doi.org/10.1038/415755a

Gignac, G. E., & Bates, T. C. (2017). Brain volume and intelligence: The moderating role of intelligence measurement quality. *Intelligence, 64,* 18–29. https://doi.org/10.1016/j.intell.2017.06.004

Gilder, G. (2013). *Knowledge and power: The information theory of capitalism and how it is revolutionizing our world.* Regnery Publishing.

Giraud, A.-L., & Poeppel, D. (2012). Cortical oscillations and speech processing: emerging computational principles and operations. *Nature Neuroscience, 15*(4), 511–517. https://doi.org/10.1038/nn.3063

Goh, J. O. S., Hebrank, A. C., Sutton, B. P., Chee, M. W. L., Sim, S. K. Y., & Park, D. C. (2013). Culture-related differences in default network activity during visuo-spatial judgments. *Social Cognitive and Affective Neuroscience, 8*(2), 134–142. https://doi.org/10.1093/scan/nsr077

Goldstone, R. L., & Theiner, G. (2017). The multiple, interacting levels of cognitive systems (MILCS) perspective on group cognition. *Philosophical Psychology, 30*(3), 338–372. https://doi.org/10.1080/09515089.2017.1295635

Gopnik, A., O'Grady, S., Lucas, C. G., Griffiths, T. L., Wente, A., Bridgers, S., . . . Dahl, R. E. (2017). Changes in cognitive flexibility and hypothesis search across human life history from childhood to adolescence to adulthood. *Proceedings of the National Academy of Sciences, 114*(30), 7892–7899. https://doi.org/10.1073/pnas.1700811114

Gordon, E. M., Laumann, T. O., Adeyemo, B., & Petersen, S. E. (2015). Individual variability of the system-level organization of the human brain. *Cerebral Cortex, 27*(1), 386–399. https://doi.org/10.1093/cercor/bhv239

Gottlieb, A., Keydar, I., & Epstein, H. T. (1977). Rodent brain growth stages: An analytical review. *Biological Neonate, 32*, 166–176.

Graham, D. J., & Field, D. J. (2007). Statistical regularities of art images and natural scenes: Spectra, sparseness and nonlinearities. *Spatial Vision, 21*(1–2), 149–164.

GRIP (Greenland Ice-core Project Members). (1993). Climate instability during the last interglacial period recorded in the GRIP ice core. *Nature, 364*, 203–207.

Gurven, M., Kaplan, H., & Gutierrez, M. (2006). How long does it take to become a proficient hunter? Implications for the evolution of extended development and long life span. *Journal of Human Evolution, 51*(5), 454–470. https://doi.org/10.1016/j.jhevol.2006.05.003

Halley, A. C. (2017). Minimal variation in eutherian brain growth rates during fetal neurogenesis. *Proceedings of the Royal Society B: Biological Sciences, 284*(1854), 20170219. https://doi.org/10.1098/rspb.2017.0219

Han, S., & Ma, Y. (2014). Cultural differences in human brain activity: A quantitative meta-analysis. *NeuroImage, 99*, 293–300. https://doi.org/10.1016/j.neuroimage.2014.05.062

Han, S., Northoff, G., Vogeley, K., Wexler, B. E., Kitayama, S., & Varnum, M. E. W. (2013). A cultural neuroscience approach to the biosocial nature of the human brain. *Annual Review of Psychology, 64*(1), 335–359. https://doi.org/10/f4k2cm

Hasson, U., Chen, J., & Honey, C. J. (2015). Hierarchical process memory: Memory as an integral component of information processing. *Trends in Cognitive Sciences, 19*(6), 304–313. https://doi.org/10.1016/j.tics.2015.04.006

Hawkes, K. (2003). Grandmothers and the evolution of human longevity. *American Journal of Human Biology, 15*(3), 380–400. https://doi.org/10.1002/ajhb.10156

Hawkes, K., & Finlay, B. L. (2018). Mammalian brain development and our grandmothering life history. *Physiology & Behavior, 193*, 55–68. https://doi.org/10.1016/j.physbeh.2018.01.013

Hellemans, K. G. C., Nobrega, J. N., & Olmstead, M. C. (2005). Early environmental experience alters baseline and ethanol-induced cognitive impulsivity: relationship to forebrain 5-HT1A receptor binding. *Behavioural Brain Research, 159*(2), 207–220. https://doi.org/10.1016/j.bbr.2004.10.018

Henrich, J. (2004). Demography and Cultural Evolution: How Adaptive Cultural Processes can Produce Maladaptive Losses: The Tasmanian Case. *American Antiquity, 69*(2), 197–214. https://doi.org/10.2307/4128416

Henrich, J. (2016). *The secret of our success: How culture is driving human evolution, domesticating our species, and making us smarter*. Princeton University Press.

Henrich, J., & Boyd, R. (1998). The evolution of conformist transmission and the emergence of between-group differences. *Evolution and Human Behavior, 19*(4), 215–241. https://doi.org/10.1016/S1090-5138(98)00018-X

Henrich, J., & Boyd, R. (2008). Division of labor, economic specialization, and the evolution of social stratification. *Current Anthropology, 49*(4), 715–724. https://doi.org/10.1086/587889

Henrich, J., Boyd, R., Bowles, S., Camerer, C., Fehr, E., Gintis, H., & McElreath, R. (2001). In search of homo economicus: Behavioral experiments in 15 small-scale societies. *American Economic Review, 91*(2), 73–78.

Henrich, J., & Gil-White, F. J. (2001). The evolution of prestige: Freely conferred deference as a mechanism for enhancing the benefits of cultural transmission. *Evolution and Human Behavior: Official Journal of the Human Behavior and Evolution Society, 22*(3), 165–196.

Henrich, J., Heine, S. J., & Norenzayan, A. (2010). The weirdest people in the world? *Behavioral and Brain Sciences, 33*(2–3), 61–83. https://doi.org/10.1017/S0140525X0999152X

Herrmann, E., Call, J., Hernandez-Lloreda, M. V., Hare, B., & Tomasello, M. (2007). Humans have evolved specialised skills of social cognition: The cultural intelligence hypothesis. *Science, 317*(5843), 1360–1366. https://doi.org/10.1126/science.1146282

Heyes, C. (2003). Four routes of cognitive evolution. *Psychological Review, 110*(4), 713–727. https://doi.org/10.1037/0033-295X.110.4.713

Heyes, C., & Pearce, J. M. (2015). Not-so-social learning strategies. *Proceedings of the Royal Society B: Biological Sciences, 282*, 20141709. http://dx.doi.org/10.1098/rspb.2014.1709

Heyes, C. M., & Galef, B. G. (1996). *Social learning in animals: The roots of culture*. Academic Press.

Heyes, C., & Pearce, J. M. (2015). Not-so-social learning strategies. *Proceedings of the Royal Society B: Biological Sciences, 282*, 20141709.

Hill, K. R., Walker, R. S., Božičević, M., Eder, J., Headland, T., Hewlett, B., . . . Wood, B. (2011). Co-residence patterns in hunter-gatherer societies show unique human social structure. *Science, 331*, 1286–1289. https://doi.org/10.1126/science.1199071

Hoppitt, W., & Laland, K. N. (2013). *Social learning: An introduction to mechanisms, methods, and models.* Princeton University Press.

Horner, V., & Whiten, A. (2005). Causal knowledge and imitation/emulation switching in chimpanzees (Pan troglodytes) and children (Homo sapiens). *Animal Cognition, 8*(3), 164–181. https://doi.org/10.1007/s10071-004-0239-6

Howland, H. C., Merola, S., & Basarab, J. R. (2004). The allometry and scaling of the size of vertebrate eyes. *Vision Research, 44*(17), 2043–2065. https://doi.org/10.1016/j.visres.2004.03.023

Hrdy, S. B. (2011). *Mothers and others: The evolutionary origins of mutual understanding.* Harvard University Press.

Humphrey, N. K. (1976). The social function of intellect. In P. Bateson & R. Hinde (Eds.), *Growing points in ethology.* Cambridge University Press.

Huntenburg, J. M., Bazin, P.-L., & Margulies, D. S. (2018). Large-scale gradients in human cortical organization. *Trends in Cognitive Sciences, 22*(1), 21–31. https://doi.org/10.1016/j.tics.2017.11.002

Huth, A. G., de Heer, W. A., Griffiths, T. L., Theunissen, F. E., & Gallant, J. L. (2016). Natural speech reveals the semantic maps that tile human cerebral cortex. *Nature, 532*(7600), 453–458. https://doi.org/10.1038/nature17637

Isbilen, E. S., & Christiansen, M. H. (2018). Chunk-Based Memory Constraints on the Cultural Evolution of Language. *Topics in Cognitive Science.* https://doi.org/10.1111/tops.12376

Isler, K., & van Schaik, C. P. (2009). The Expensive Brain: A framework for explaining evolutionary changes in brain size. *Journal of Human Evolution, 57*(4), 392–400. https://doi.org/10.1016/j.jhevol.2009.04.009

Jablonka, E., & Raz, G. (2009). Transgenerational epigenetic inheritance: Prevalence, mechanisms, and implications for the study of heredity and evolution. *Quarterly Review of Biology, 84*(2), 131–176. https://doi.org/10.1086/598822

Kanemura, H., Aihara, M., Aoki, S., Araki, T., & Nakazawa, S. (2003). Development of the prefrontal lobe in infants and children: A three-dimensional magnetic resonance volumetric study. *Brain and Development, 25*(3), 195–199. https://doi.org/10.1016/S0387-7604(02)00214-0

Kaplan, H., Hill, K., Lancaster, J., & Hurtado, M. (2000). A theory of human life history evolution: Diet, intelligence, and longevity. *Evolutionary Anthropology, 9*(4), 156–185. https://doi.org/10.1002/1520-6505(2000)9:4<156::AID-EVAN5>3.3.CO;2-Z

Karmiloff-Smith, A., Thomas, M., Annaz, D., Humphreys, K., Ewing, S., Brace, N., . . . Campbell, R. (2004). Exploring the Williams syndrome face-processing debate: the importance of building developmental trajectories. *Journal of Child Psychology and Psychiatry, 45*(7), 1258–1274. https://doi.org/10.1111/j.1469-7610.2004.00322.x

Kendal, R. L., Boogert, N. J., Rendell, L., Laland, K. N., Webster, M., & Jones, P. L. (2018). Social Learning Strategies: Bridge-Building between Fields. *Trends in Cognitive Sciences, 22*(7), 651–665. https://doi.org/10.1016/j.tics.2018.04.003

Kim, H. S., Sherman, D. K., Sasaki, J. Y., Xu, J., Chu, T. Q., Ryu, C., . . . Taylor, S. E. (2010). Culture, distress, and oxytocin receptor polymorphism (OXTR) interact to influence emotional support seeking. *Proceedings of the National Academy of Sciences, 107*(36), 15717–15721. https://doi.org/10.1073/pnas.1010830107

Kirschner, M., & Gerhart, J. C. (2005). *The plausibility of life: Resolving Darwin's dilemma.* Yale University Press.

Kitayama, S., King, A., Yoon, C., Tompson, S., Huff, S., & Liberzon, I. (2014). The dopamine D4 receptor gene (*DRD4*) moderates cultural difference in independent versus interdependent social orientation. *Psychological Science, 25*(6), 1169–1177. https://doi.org/10.1177/0956797614528338

Kitayama, S., & Salvador, C. E. (2017). Culture embrained: Going beyond the nature-nurture dichotomy. *Perspectives on Psychological Science, 12*(5), 841–854. https://doi.org/10.1177/1745691617707317

Kitayama, S., & Uskul, A. K. (2011). Culture, mind, and the brain: Current evidence and future directions. *Annual Review of Psychology, 62*(1), 419–449. https://doi.org/10.1146/annurev-psych-120709-145357

Kline, M. A. (2015). How to learn about teaching: An evolutionary framework for the study of teaching behavior in humans and other animals. *Behavioral and Brain Sciences, 38*, e31. https://doi.org/10.1017/S0140525X14000090

Kobayashi, C., Glover, G. H., & Temple, E. (2007). Cultural and linguistic effects on neural bases of "Theory of Mind" in American and Japanese children. *Brain Research, 1164*(1), 95–107. https://doi.org/10.1016/j.brainres.2007.06.022

Kolb, B., & Gibb, R. (2014). Searching for the principles of brain plasticity and behavior. *Cortex, 58*, 251–260. https://doi.org/10.1016/j.cortex.2013.11.012

Koster, J., McElreath, R., Hill, K., Yu, D., Shepard, G., van Vliet, N., . . . Ross, C. (2019). The life history of human foraging: Cross-cultural and individual variation. *BioRxiv.* https://doi.org/10/gfwvhn

Krubitzer, L. (2009). In search of a unifying theory of complex brain evolution. *Annals of the New York Academy of Sciences, 1156*(1), 44–67. https://doi.org/10.1111/j.1749-6632.2009.04421.x

Krueger, F., Barbey, A. K., & Grafman, J. (2009). The medial prefrontal cortex mediates social event knowledge. *Trends in Cognitive Sciences, 13*(3), 103–109. https://doi.org/10.1016/j.tics.2008.12.005

Kuhnen, C. M., & Chiao, J. Y. (2009). Genetic Determinants of Financial Risk Taking. *PLoS ONE, 4*(2), e4362. https://doi.org/10.1371/journal.pone.0004362

Kuhnen, C. M., Samanez-Larkin, G. R., & Knutson, B. (2013). Serotonergic Genotypes, Neuroticism, and Financial Choices. *PLoS ONE, 8*(1), e54632. https://doi.org/10.1371/journal.pone.0054632

Kuzawa, C. W., Chugani, H. T., Grossman, L. I., Lipovich, L., Muzik, O., Hof, P. R., . . . Lange, N. (2014). Metabolic costs and evolutionary implications of human brain development. *Proceedings of the National Academy of Sciences, 111*(36), 13010–13015. https://doi.org/10.1073/pnas.1323099111

Laland, K. N. (2004). Social learning strategies. *Animal Learning & Behavior, 32*(1), 4–14. https://doi.org/10.3758/BF03196002

Laland, K. N. (2017). *Darwin's unfinished symphony: How culture made the human mind.* Princeton University Press.

Laland, K. N., & Janik, V. M. (2006). The animal cultures debate. *Trends in Ecology and Evolution, 21*(10), 542–547. https://doi.org/10.1016/j.tree.2006.06.005

Laland, K. N., Uller, T., Feldman, M. W., Sterelny, K., Müller, G. B., Moczek, A., . . . Odling-Smee, J. (2015). The extended evolutionary synthesis: Its structure, assumptions and predictions. *Proceedings of the Royal Society B. Biological Sciences, 282*(1813), 20151019. https://doi.org/10.1098/rspb.2015.1019

Leadbeater, E., & Chittka, L. (2007). Social learning in insects—From miniature brains to consensus building. *Current Biology, 17*(16), 703–713. https://doi.org/10.1016/j.cub.2007.06.012

LeCun, Y., Bengio, Y., & Hinton, G. (2015). Deep learning. *Nature, 521*(7553), 436–444. https://doi.org/10.1038/nature14539

Lehman, D. R., Chiu, C., & Schaller, M. (2004). Psychology and culture. *Annual Review of Psychology, 55*(1), 689–714. https://doi.org/10.1146/annurev.psych.55.090902.141927

Leonard, W. R., Robertson, M. L., Snodgrass, J. J., & Kuzawa, C. W. (2003). Metabolic correlates of hominid brain evolution. *Comparative Biochemistry and Physiology—A Molecular and Integrative Physiology, 136*(1), 5–15. https://doi.org/10.1016/S1095-6433(03)00132-6

LeWinn, K. Z., Sheridan, M. A., Keyes, K. M., Hamilton, A., & McLaughlin, K. A. (2017). Sample composition alters associations between age and brain structure. *Nature Communications, 8*(1). https://doi.org/10.1038/s41467-017-00908-7

Ley, R. E., Lozupone, C. A., Hamady, M., Knight, R., & Gordon, J. I. (2008). Worlds within worlds: Evolution of the vertebrate gut microbiota. *Nature Reviews Microbiology, 6*(10), 776–788. https://doi.org/10.1038/nrmicro1978

Lipschuetz, M., Cohen, S. M., Ein-Mor, E., Sapir, H., Hochner-Celnikier, D., Porat, S., . . . Yagel, S. (2015). A large head circumference is more strongly associated with unplanned cesarean or instrumental delivery and neonatal complications than high birthweight. *American Journal of Obstetrics and Gynecology, 213*(6), 833.e1–833.e12. https://doi.org/10.1016/j.ajog.2015.07.045

Lovallo, W. R. (2013). Early life adversity reduces stress reactivity and enhances impulsive behavior: Implications for health behaviors. *International Journal of Psychophysiology, 90*(1), 8–16. https://doi.org/10.1016/j.ijpsycho.2012.10.006

Lucas, C. G., Bridgers, S., Griffiths, T. L., & Gopnik, A. (2014). When children are better (or at least more open-minded) learners than adults: Developmental differences in learning the forms of causal relationships. *Cognition, 131*(2), 284–299. https://doi.org/10.1016/j.cognition.2013.12.010

Lyons, D. E., Young, A. G., & Keil, F. C. (2007). The hidden structure of overimitation. *Proceedings of the National Academy of Sciences of the United States of America, 104*(50), 19751–19756. https://doi.org/10.1073/pnas.0704452104

Ma, Y., Bang, D., Wang, C., Allen, M., Frith, C., Roepstorff, A., & Han, S. (2014). Sociocultural patterning of neural activity during self-reflection. *Social Cognitive and Affective Neuroscience, 9*(1), 73–80. https://doi.org/10.1093/scan/nss103

MacLean, E. L., Hare, B., Nunn, C. L., Addessi, E., Amici, F., Anderson, R. C., . . . Zhao, Y. (2014). The evolution of self-control. *Proceedings of the National Academy of Sciences, 111*(20), E2140–E2148. https://doi.org/10.1073/pnas.1323533111

Majid, A., Bowerman, M., Kita, S., Haun, D. B. M., & Levinson, S. C. (2004). Can language restructure cognition? The case for space. *Trends in Cognitive Sciences*, *8*(3), 108–114. https://doi.org/10.1016/j.tics.2004.01.003

McElreath, R., Boyd, R., & Richerson, P. J. (2003). Shared norms and the evolution of ethnic markers. *Current Anthropology*, *44*(1), 122–130. https://doi.org/10.1086/345689

Medin, D. L., & Atran, S. (2004). The native mind: Biological categorization and reasoning in development and across cultures. *Psychological Review*, *111*(4), 960–983. https://doi.org/10.1037/0033-295X.111.4.960

Mesoudi, A., Whiten, A., & Laland, K. A. (2006). Towards a unified science of cultural evolution. *Behavioral and Brain Sciences*, *29*, 323–383.

Miller, N. E., & Dollard, J. (1945). *Social learning and imitation*. Routledge.

Muthukrishna, M., Bell, A. V., Henrich, J., Curtin, C. M., Gedranovich, A., McInerney, J., & Thue, B. (2020). Beyond Western, educated, industrial, rich, and democratic (WEIRD) psychology: Measuring and mapping scales of cultural and psychological distance. *Psychological Science*, *31*(6), 678–701. https://journals.sagepub.com/doi/full/10.1177/0956797620916782

Muthukrishna, M., Doebeli, M., Chudek, M., & Henrich, J. (2018). The cultural brain hypothesis: How culture drives brain expansion, sociality, and life history. *PLOS Computational Biology*, *14*(11), e1006504. https://doi.org/10.1371/journal.pcbi.1006504

Muthukrishna, M., & Henrich, J. (2016). Innovation in the collective brain. *Philosophical Transactions of the Royal Society of London. Series B, Biological Sciences*, *371*(1690), 137–148. https://doi.org/10.1098/rstb.2015.0192

Muthukrishna, M., & Henrich, J. (2019). A problem in theory. *Nature Human Behaviour*, *3*(3), 221–229.

Muthukrishna, M., Morgan, T. J. H., & Henrich, J. (2016). The when and who of social learning and conformist transmission. *Evolution and Human Behavior*, *37*(1), 10–20.

Muthukrishna, M., Shulman, B. W., Vasilescu, V., & Henrich, J. (2013). Sociality influences cultural complexity. *Proceedings of the Royal Society B: Biological Sciences*, *281*(1774), 20132511–20132511. https://doi.org/10.1098/rspb.2013.2511

Navarrete, A., van Schaik, C. P., & Isler, K. (2011). Energetics and the evolution of human brain size. *Nature*, *480*(7375), 91–93. https://doi.org/10/bz4zj4

Nee, D. E., & D'Esposito, M. (2016). The hierarchical organization of the lateral prefrontal cortex. *ELife*, *5*. https://doi.org/10.7554/eLife.12112

Neisser, U. (1967). *Cognitive psychology*. Meredith. https://books.google.co.uk/books?hl=en&lr=&id=oyGcBQAAQBAJ

Newell, A. (1980). Physical symbol systems. *Cognitive Science*, *4*(2), 135–183. https://doi.org/10.1016/S0364-0213(80)80015-2

Nguyen, M., Vanderwal, T., & Hasson, U. (2019). Shared understanding of narratives is correlated with shared neural responses. *NeuroImage*, *184*, 161–170. https://doi.org/10.1016/j.neuroimage.2018.09.010

Nisbett, R. E., & Miyamoto, Y. (2005). The influence of culture: Holistic versus analytic perception. *Trends in Cognitive Sciences*, *9*(10), 467–473. https://doi.org/10.1016/j.tics.2005.08.004

Noppeney, U., Friston, K. J., & Price, C. J. (2004). Degenerate neuronal systems sustaining cognitive functions. *Journal of Anatomy*, *205*(6), 433–442. https://doi.org/10.1111/j.0021-8782.2004.00343.x

Noppeney, U., Penny, W. D., Price, C. J., Flandin, G., & Friston, K. J. (2006). Identification of degenerate neuronal systems based on intersubject variability. *NeuroImage*, *30*(3), 885–890. https://doi.org/10.1016/j.neuroimage.2005.10.010

Noppeney, U., Price, C. J., Penny, W. D., & Friston, K. J. (2006). Two distinct neural mechanisms for category-selective responses. *Cerebral Cortex*, *16*(3), 437–445. https://doi.org/10.1093/cercor/bhi123

Ochman, H., Worobey, M., Kuo, C. H., Ndjango, J. B. N., Peeters, M., Hahn, B. H., & Hugenholtz, P. (2010). Evolutionary relationships of wild hominids recapitulated by gut microbial communities. *PLoS Biology*, *8*(11), 3–10. https://doi.org/10.1371/journal.pbio.1000546

Odling-Smee, F. J., Laland, K. N., & Feldman, M. W. (1996). Niche construction. *American Naturalist*, *147*(4), 641–648. https://doi.org/10.1086/285870

Odling-Smee, J., Erwin, D., Palkovacs, E. P., Feldman, M. W., & Laland, K. N. (2013). Niche construction theory: A practical guide for ecologists. *Quarterly Review of Biology*, *88*(1), 3–28.

Passingham, R. E. (1985). Rates of brain development in mammals including man. *Brain, Behavior and Evolution*, *26*, 167–175.

Patterson, K., Nestor, P. J., & Rogers, T. T. (2007). Where do you know what you know? The representation of semantic knowledge in the human brain. *Nature Reviews Neuroscience, 8*(12), 976–987. https://doi.org/10.1038/nrn2277

Pigliucci, M. (2008). Is evolvability evolvable? *Nature Reviews Genetics, 9*(1), 75–82. https://doi.org/10.1038/nrg2278

Pontzer, H., Brown, M. H., Raichlen, D. A., Dunsworth, H., Hare, B., Walker, K., . . . Ross, S. R. (2016). Metabolic acceleration and the evolution of human brain size and life history. *Nature, 533*, 390–392. https://doi.org/10.1038/nature17654

Potts, R. (1998). Variability selection in hominid evolution. *Evolutionary Anthropology: Issues, News, and Reviews, 7*(3), 81–96.

Powell, A., Shennan, S., & Thomas, M. G. (2009). Late Pleistocene demography and the appearance of modern human behavior. *Science (New York, N.Y.), 324*(5932), 1298–1301. https://doi.org/10.1126/science.1170165

Price, C. J., & Friston, K. J. (2002). Degeneracy and cognitive anatomy. *Trends in Cognitive Sciences, 6*(10), 416–421. https://doi.org/10.1016/S1364-6613(02)01976-9

Quiroga, R. Q., Reddy, L., Kreiman, G., Koch, C., & Fried, I. (2005). Invariant visual representation by single neurons in the human brain. *Nature, 435*(7045), 1102–1107. https://doi.org/10.1038/nature03687

Raichle, M. E. (2015). The brain's default mode network. *Annual Review of Neuroscience, 38*(1), 433–447. https://doi.org/10.1146/annurev-neuro-071013-014030

Reader, S. M., Hager, Y., & Laland, K. N. (2011). The evolution of primate general and cultural intelligence. *Philosophical Transactions of the Royal Society B: Biological Sciences, 366*(1567), 1017–1027. https://doi.org/10.1098/rstb.2010.0342

Reader, S. M., & Laland, K. N. (2002). Social intelligence, innovation, and enhanced brain size in primates. *Proceedings of the National Academy of Sciences, 99*(7), 4436–4441. https://doi.org/10.1073/pnas.062041299

Rendell, L., Fogarty, L., Hoppitt, W. J. E., Morgan, T. J. H., Webster, M. M., & Laland, K. N. (2011). Cognitive culture: Theoretical and empirical insights into social learning strategies. *Trends in Cognitive Sciences, 15*(2), 68–76. https://doi.org/10.1016/j.tics.2010.12.002

Riba, J., Krämer, U. M., Heldmann, M., Richter, S., & Münte, T. F. (2008). Dopamine Agonist Increases Risk Taking but Blunts Reward-Related Brain Activity. *PLoS ONE, 3*(6), e2479. https://doi.org/10.1371/journal.pone.0002479

Richards, E. J. (2006). Inherited epigenetic variation—Revisiting soft inheritance. *Nature Reviews Genetics, 7*(5), 395–401. https://doi.org/10.1038/nrg1834

Richerson, P. J., & Boyd, R. (2000). Climate, culture, and the evolution of cognition. In C. Heyes & L. Huber (Eds.), *Evolution of cognition* (pp. 329–346). MIT Press.

Richerson, P. J., & Boyd, R. (2005). *Not by genes alone: How culture transformed human evolution*. University of Chicago Press.

Robson, S. L., & Wood, B. (2008). Hominin life history: Reconstruction and evolution. *Journal of Anatomy, 212*(4), 394–425. https://doi.org/10.1111/j.1469-7580.2008.00867.x

Rosenberg, K., & Trevathan, W. (2002). Birth, obstetrics and human evolution. *BJOG: An International Journal of Obstetrics and Gynaecology, 109*(11), 1199–1206. https://doi.org/10.1046/j.1471-0528.2002.00010.x

Russell, C. J. S., & Muthukrishna, M. (2018). Dual inheritance theory. In T. K. Shackelford & V. A. Weekes-Shackelford (Eds.), *Encyclopedia of evolutionary psychological science* (pp. 1–7). Springer International Publishing. https://doi.org/10.1007/978-3-319-16999-6_1381-1

Schilbach, L., Eickhoff, S. B., Rotarska-Jagiela, A., Fink, G. R., & Vogeley, K. (2008). Minds at rest? Social cognition as the default mode of cognizing and its putative relationship to the "default system" of the brain. *Consciousness and Cognition, 17*(2), 457–467. https://doi.org/10.1016/j.concog.2008.03.013

Schniter, E., Gurven, M., Kaplan, H. S., Wilcox, N. T., & Hooper, P. L. (2015). Skill ontogeny among Tsimane forager-horticulturalists. *American Journal of Physical Anthropology, 158*(1), 3–18. https://doi.org/10.1002/ajpa.22757

Schulz, J. F., Bahrami-Rad, D., Beauchamp, J. P., & Henrich, J. (2019). The Church, intensive kinship, and global psychological variation. *Science, 366*(6466), eaau5141. https://doi.org/10.1126/science.aau5141

Schuppli, C., Isler, K., & Van Schaik, C. P. (2012). How to explain the unusually late age at skill competence among humans. *Journal of Human Evolution, 63*(6), 843–850. https://doi.org/10.1016/j.jhevol.2012.08.009

Sellen, D. W. (2001). Comparison of Infant Feeding Patterns Reported for Nonindustrial Populations with Current Recommendations. *The Journal of Nutrition*, *131*(10), 2707–2715. https://doi.org/10.1093/jn/131.10.2707

Simony, E., Honey, C. J., Chen, J., Lositsky, O., Yeshurun, Y., Wiesel, A., & Hasson, U. (2016). Dynamic reconfiguration of the default mode network during narrative comprehension. *Nature Communications*, *7*(1). https://doi.org/10.1038/ncomms12141

Sliwa, J., & Freiwald, W. A. (2017). A dedicated network for social interaction processing in the primate brain. *Science*, *356*(6339), 745–749. https://doi.org/10.1126/science.aam6383Sol, D., Bacher, S., Reader, S. M., & Lefebvre, L. (2008). Brain size predicts the success of mammal species introduced into novel environments. *American Naturalist*, *172*(S1), S63–S71. https://doi.org/10.1086/588304

Sol, D., Duncan, R. P., Blackburn, T. M., Cassey, P., & Lefebvre, L. (2005). Big brains, enhanced cognition, and response of birds to novel environments. *Proceedings of the National Academy of Sciences*, *102*(15), 5460–5465. https://doi.org/10.1073/pnas.0408145102

Spreng, R. N., Mar, R. A., & Kim, A. S. N. (2009). The common neural basis of autobiographical memory, prospection, navigation, theory of mind, and the default mode: A quantitative meta-analysis. *Journal of Cognitive Neuroscience*, *21*(3), 489–510. https://doi.org/10.1162/jocn.2008.21029

Street, S. E., Navarrete, A. F., Reader, S. M., & Laland, K. N. (2017). Coevolution of cultural intelligence, extended life history, sociality, and brain size in primates. *Proceedings of the National Academy of Sciences*, *114*(30), 7908–7914. https://doi.org/10.1073/pnas.1620734114

Suzuki, I. K., Gacquer, D., Van Heurck, R., Kumar, D., Wojno, M., Bilheu, A., . . . Vanderhaeghen, P. (2018). Human-specific NOTCH2NL genes expand cortical neurogenesis through Delta/Notch regulation. *Cell*, *173*(6), 1370–1384.e16. https://doi.org/10/gdkxhr

Swallow, K. M., & Wang, Q. (2020). Culture influences how people divide continuous sensory experience into events. *Cognition*, *205*, 104450. https://doi.org/10.1016/j.cognition.2020.104450

Tan, L. H., Laird, A. R., Li, K., & Fox, P. T. (2005). Neuroanatomical correlates of phonological processing of Chinese characters and alphabetic words: A meta-analysis. *Human Brain Mapping*, *25*(1), 83–91. https://doi.org/10.1002/hbm.20134

Tang, Y., Zhang, W., Chen, K., Feng, S., Ji, Y., Shen, J., . . . Liu, Y. (2006). Arithmetic processing in the brain shaped by cultures. *Proceedings of the National Academy of Sciences*, *103*(28), 10775–10780. https://doi.org/10.1073/pnas.0604416103

Tennie, C., Call, J., & Tomasello, M. (2009). Ratcheting up the ratchet: On the evolution of cumulative culture. *Philosophical Transactions of the Royal Society B: Biological Sciences*, *364*(1528), 2405–2415. https://doi.org/10.1098/rstb.2009.0052

Thompson-Schill, S. L., Ramscar, M., & Chrysikou, E. G. (2009). Cognition without control: When a little frontal lobe goes a long way. *Current Directions in Psychological Science*, *18*(5), 259–263.

Tomasello, M., Carpenter, M., Call, J., Behne, T., & Moll, H. (2005). Understanding and sharing intentions: The origins of cultural cognition. *Behavioral and Brain Sciences*, *28*(05), 675–735. https://doi.org/10.1017/S0140525X05000129

Tomasello, M., Melis, A. P., Tennie, C., Wyman, E., & Herrmann, E. (2012). Two key steps in the evolution of human cooperation. *Current Anthropology*, *53*(6), 673–692. https://doi.org/10.1086/668207

Tononi, G., Sporns, O., & Edelman, G. M. (1999). Measures of degeneracy and redundancy in biological networks. *Proceedings of the National Academy of Sciences*, *96*(6), 3257–3262. https://doi.org/10.1073/pnas.96.6.3257

Triandis, H. C., Bontempo, R., Villareal, M. J., Asai, M., & Lucca, N. (1988). Individualism and collectivism: Cross-cultural perspectives on self-ingroup relationships. *Journal of Personality and Social Psychology*, *54*(2), 323–338. https://doi.org/10.1037/0022-3514.54.2.323

van Schaik, C. P., & Burkart, J. M. (2011). Social learning and evolution: The cultural intelligence hypothesis. *Philosophical Transactions of the Royal Society B: Biological Sciences*, *366*(1567), 1008–1016. https://doi.org/10.1098/rstb.2010.0304

van Schaik, C. P., Isler, K., & Burkart, J. M. (2012). Explaining brain size variation: From social to cultural brain. *Trends in Cognitive Sciences*, *16*(5), 277–284. https://doi.org/10.1016/j.tics.2012.04.004

Varela, F. J., Thompson, E., & Rosch, E. (1991). *The embodied mind: Cognitive science and human experience.* MIT Press.

Vinckier, F., Dehaene, S., Jobert, A., Dubus, J. P., Sigman, M., & Cohen, L. (2007). Hierarchical Coding of Letter Strings in the Ventral Stream: Dissecting the Inner Organization of the Visual Word-Form System. *Neuron*, *55*(1), 143–156. https://doi.org/10.1016/j.neuron.2007.05.031

Wagner, G. P., & Altenberg, L. (1996). Complex adaptations and the evolution of evolvability. *Evolution*, *50*(3), 967–976. https://doi.org/10.1111/j.1558-5646.1996.tb02339.x

West, G. B., Brown, J. H., & Enquist, B. J. (2001). A general model for ontogenetic growth. *Nature*, *413*(6856), 628–631. https://doi.org/10.1038/35098076

Whitacre, J., & Bender, A. (2010). Degeneracy: A design principle for achieving robustness and evolvability. *Journal of Theoretical Biology*, *263*(1), 143–153. https://doi.org/10.1016/j.jtbi.2009.11.008

Whiten, A. (2019). Cultural Evolution in Animals. *Annual Review of Ecology, Evolution, and Systematics*, *50*(1), 27–48. https://doi.org/10.1146/annurev-ecolsys-110218-025040

Whiten, A., McGuigan, N., Marshall-Pescini, S., & Hopper, L. M. (2009). Emulation, imitation, over-imitation and the scope of culture for child and chimpanzee. *Philosophical Transactions of the Royal Society B: Biological Sciences*, *364*(1528), 2417–2428. https://doi.org/10.1098/rstb.2009.0069

Wilkinson, A., Kuenstner, K., Mueller, J., & Huber, L. (2010). Social learning in a non-social reptile (Geochelone carbonaria). *Biology Letters*, *6*(5), 614–616. https://doi.org/10.1098/rsbl.2010.0092

Wilson, E. O. (2012). *The social conquest of earth*. Liveright Publishing Corp.

Workman, A. D., Charvet, C. J., Clancy, B., Darlington, R. B., & Finlay, B. L. (2013). Modeling transformations of neurodevelopmental sequences across mammalian species. *Journal of Neuroscience*, *33*(17), 7368–7383. https://doi.org/10.1523/JNEUROSCI.5746-12.2013

Wrangham, R., & Carmody, R. (2010). Human adaptation to the control of fire. *Evolutionary Anthropology*, *19*(5), 187–199. https://doi.org/10.1002/evan.20275

Zacks, J. M., Speer, N. K., Swallow, K. M., & Maley, C. J. (2010). The brain's cutting-room floor: segmentation of narrative cinema. *Frontiers in Human Neuroscience*, *4*. https://doi.org/10.3389/fnhum.2010.00168

Culture and Psychology

David Matsumoto *and* Hyisung C. Hwang

Abstract

This chapter introduces readers to a basic model and framework with which to understand how human cultures influence, and are influenced by, psychological processes and behaviors. It provides a working definition of culture; describes the factors that influence the creation, maintenance, evolution, and function of human cultures; distinguishes them from nonhuman cultures; and introduces the subjective elements of human culture on the level of attitudes, values, beliefs, opinions, worldviews, and norms, all of which regulate behavior. The chapter discusses the relation of these elements of culture to psychological processes and social behaviors and introduces the mediating role of context. It also describes universality and culture specifics in psychological processes and behaviors leveraging the concepts of etics and emics. The chapter understands cultures as solutions to the problems of groups' needs to adapt to their contexts and environments in order to survive. Hopefully this very basic framework of the relation between culture and psychological processes provides a basis for understanding the relation between culture and mental health, locally and globally.

Key Words: culture, psychology, context, elements of culture, attitudes, values, beliefs, worldviews, norms, social behavior

Introduction

In this chapter, we introduce readers to culture and its relation to psychological processes and behavior. We discuss factors that influence the evolution, maintenance, evolution, and function of cultures, and distinguish between human and nonhuman cultures. We describe how human cultures manifest themselves on the level of individuals' psychological processes—in attitudes, values, beliefs, opinions, worldviews, norms, and behavior. We then provide readers with a framework with which to understand how human cultures influence, and are influenced by, psychological processes and social behaviors, with context playing an important mediating role. We describe how cultures are solutions to the problem of groups' needs to adapt to their contexts, addressing their members' social motives and biological needs. As adaptational responses to the environment, cultures help to select behaviors, attitudes, values, opinions, and norms that optimize the tapping of resources to meet survival needs. Through this analysis, we hope to convey that cultures play major roles with regard to understanding global mental health, including how to understand, assess, and treat various mental illnesses. We begin first with a discussion of a working definition of culture.

What Is Culture?

A Working Definition

Scholars have attempted to define culture for well over a century, and most definitions of culture focus on the concept of shared ways of living of a group. For example, culture has been defined as all capabilities and habits learned as members of a society (Tylor, 1865); social heredity (Linton, 1936); patterns of and for behavior acquired and transmitted by symbols, constituting the distinct achievements of human groups, including their embodiments in artifacts (Kroeber & Kluckhohn, 1952/1963); the totality of equivalent and complementary learned meanings maintained by a human population or by identifiable segments of a population and transmitted from one generation to the next (Rohner, 1984); a descriptive term that captures not only rules and meanings but also behaviors (Jahoda, 1984); personality (Pelto & Pelto, 1975); shared symbol systems transcending individuals (Geertz, 1975); the shared way of life of a group of people (Berry et al., 1992); and an information-based system that allows people to live together and satisfy their needs (Baumeister, 2005).

Definitions of culture that focus on the concept of shared ways of living, however, encompass all living beings, as all need to adapt to their contexts to meet basic needs and survive. Many animals are social, and in animal societies there are clear hierarchical and distributive social networks. Many animals invent and use tools (Whiten et al., 2005) and communicate with each other. Thus, many social animals have some form of culture (Boesch, 2003; McGrew, 2004).

We make a distinction between human and nonhuman cultures and define human cultures as *unique meaning and information systems shared by groups and transmitted across generations; these meaning and information systems allow groups not only to meet basic needs for survival but also to improve ways in meeting those needs, pursue happiness and well-being, and derive meaning from life* (Matsumoto & Juang, 2016). Our definition of human cultures is slightly different than most traditional definitions of culture but better describes human cultures because of our focus on human cultures as meaning and information systems.

As beings with very complex cognitive abilities, humans are uniquely positioned not only to create meaning and information but also to organize that created meaning and information into systems. Although nonhuman animals certainly have many complex cognitive skills, they lack many of the cognitive abilities of humans and even of human infants (Tomasello, 1999; Tomasello & Herrmann, 2010; Warneken & Tomasello, 2006). Thus, while nonhuman animals have some form of culture, mostly revolving around shared behavioral patterns, human cultures are able to leverage the fact that humans can create meaning and information systems because of their complex cognitive abilities; culture becomes represented in such systems.

Like nonhuman cultures, the meaning and information systems of human cultures exist first to enable humans to meet basic needs of survival. They provide guidelines on how to meet others, procreate and produce offspring, put food on the table, provide shelter from the elements, and care for our daily biological essential needs, all of which are necessary for survival. But human cultures as meaning and information systems also allow people to adapt to their environments to address their social needs and motives by allowing for complex social networks and relationships and enhancing the meaning of normal, daily activities. They allow humans to pursue happiness; to be creative in music, art, and drama; to seek recreation; and to engage in sports and organize competition, whether in the local community Little League or the Olympic Games. They allow humans to search the sea and space; to create mathematics, as well as an educational system; and to go to the moon. Human cultures allow humans to create research laboratories on Antarctica and send probes to Mars, Jupiter, and beyond. Unfortunately, human cultures also allow people to have wars, create weapons of mass destruction, and recruit and train terrorists.

Human cultures do this by creating and maintaining complex social systems, institutionalizing and improving cultural practices, creating beliefs about the world, and communicating meaning systems to other humans and subsequent generations. These characteristics of human cultures differentiate human from nonhuman cultures and enable human cultures to be unique in several ways. Human cultures are cumulative; knowledge, tools, technology, and know-how accumulate over time and continue to improve (Dean et al., 2012; also see later discussion about racheting).

The ability to be cumulative allows human cultures to differ from animal cultures in three ways: *complexity*, *differentiation*, and *institutionalization*. For example, not only do humans make tools, but also humans make tools to make tools and then automate the process of making tools and mass-distribute tools around the world for global consumption. Because humans have complex social cognition, language, shared intentionality, and ratcheting (more later), human social and cultural life is much more complex than that of other animals. Humans are members of multiple groups, each having its own purpose, hierarchy, and networking system, and most humans weave in and out of multiple groups daily (see the related concept of relational mobility: Schug et al., 2010). Much of human cumulative culture is based on uniquely human cognitive skills, such as teaching and learning through verbal instruction, imitation, and prosociality (Dean et al., 2012). Humans have evolved to have unique human cultures, and human cultures ensure a great diversity in life. Increased diversity greatly aids in survival (but comes with some risks; see later). (See also Chapter 2 by Uchiyama and Muthukrishna, this volume, for a different perspective on cultural evolution.)

Factors That Influence the Evolution and Maintenance of Cultures

Deviation from temperate climate. At its core, the culture of any group evolves as a set of adaptations to the environment in which that group exists; thus, environments matter. One core component of environments that influences cultures is climate, and more importantly, *deviation from temperate climate* (van de Vliert, 2009). Humans need to regulate their body temperatures and have an easier time doing so in temperate climates around 22°C. Much colder or hotter climates produce harsher thermoregulatory demands, requiring individuals to do more to adjust and adapt. Harsher climates create greater risks of food shortage and food spoilage, stricter diets, and more health problems. Infectious and parasitic diseases tend to be more frequent in hotter climates (Matsumoto & Fletcher, 1996). Demanding climates require special clothing, housing, and working arrangements; special organizations for the production, transportation, trade, and storage of food; and special care and cure facilities. People in hotter climates tend to organize their daily activities more around shelter, shade, and temperature changes that occur during the day. Thus, more demanding cold or hot climates arouse a chain of needs shared by all inhabitants of an area (van de Vliert, 2009). Geographic latitude-related climato-economic pressures have fairly consistent relations with cultural individualism, political democracy, corruption, aggression, trust, and creativity (Van de Vliert & Kong, 2019).

Resources. Another ecological factor that influences cultures is *resources*. Natural resources are related to the amount of *arable land*—the amount of land on which food can grow and water is available to sustain the individuals in that area. Environments with abundant natural resources and arable land create different ways of living compared to areas with fewer natural resources and readily available food and water. Also, the type of food produced is linked to psychological and cultural differences. Within China, for example, people who live in regions with a history of farming rice are generally more interdependent on others around them; people who live in regions with a history of farming wheat are generally more independent of others around them (Talhelm et al., 2014).

In modern human history, money and affluence have become important resources in influencing cultures. Money is a human cultural product, not a natural resource. Abundant money and affluence can help buffer the consequences of a lack of resources or harsh climates (van de Vliert, 2009). People and groups with more money can afford (literally) to be less reliant on many cultural guidelines to meet basic social and biological needs. People and groups with less money have fewer choices.

Other factors. There are other ecological factors that influence culture, such as *population density*—the ratio of the number of people that live in an area to the size of that area. The combination of population density and resources produces different types of social pressures, which, in turn, create different types of adaptations and adjustments. *Global changes in climate across history* have affected the evolution of humans (Behrensmeyer, 2006), as has the *incidence and prevalence of infectious diseases* in different regions of the world (Murray & Schaller, 2010; Murray et al., 2011; Schaller & Murray, 2008). Unless we consider the very beginnings of human life, most human groups live in a region with a *previous culture*, which will have had an impact on the kind of culture they have now. And environments differ in the amount of *contact they allow with other cultures* through geographical proximity and accessibility. All these factors are likely to influence a group's adaptations and hence their cultures.

The Evolved Human Mind

Many of the factors described previously (with the exception of money, which is a uniquely human cultural product) influence the creation and maintenance of human and nonhuman cultures because all animals need to adapt to their environment to survive. What makes human cultures unique is the evolved human mind, which allows for more advanced and uniquely human adaptations. Humans come to the world with specific needs and motives and with uniquely human abilities and capabilities that provide them with tools to adapt and survive in a uniquely human fashion.

Needs and motives. Humans have basic needs that are ultimately initially related to reproductive success (Boyer, 2000; Buss, 2001). These include physical needs (the need to eat, drink, sleep, deal with waste, and reproduce) as well as safety and security needs (the need for hygiene, shelter, and warmth). These needs are universal to all humans. Basic needs are associated with social motives (Hogan, 1982; Sheldon, 2004), which include the motives to achieve and affiliate with others for social engagement and self-esteem. Over history, people had to have solved a host of distinct social problems to adapt and achieve reproductive success. These social problems included negotiating complex status hierarchies, forming successful work and social groups, attracting mates, fighting off potential rivals for food and sexual partners, giving birth and raising children, and battling nature (Buss, 1988, 1991, 2001). Humans have these needs in their current, everyday lives as well. All individuals and groups have a universal problem of how to adapt to their environments to address these needs; these adaptations are specific to each group because the contexts in which each group exists are different.

Language and complex cognition. Humans bring to the world a *universal psychological toolkit*. This is a term we use to refer to the many abilities and aptitudes with which nature and evolution endowed humans to help them address their basic needs and social motives and ultimately adapt and survive. These tools emerged with the evolution of the human brain and are important parts of the human mind.

Language is one of the tools in the toolkit. Humans, unlike other animals, have the unique ability to symbolize their physical and metaphysical world (Premack, 2004), to create sounds representing those symbols (morphemes), to create rules connecting those symbols to meaning (syntax and grammar), and to put all these together in sentences. Since the use of papyrus to develop paper, humans developed writing systems (another manner of symbolizing the world) so those oral expressions can be reduced to words on paper. This book (and all books) is a uniquely human product.

Another tool in our toolkit involves a host of complex cognitive abilities that allow for complex social cognition, memory, hypothetical reasoning, problem solving, and planning (which, as we mentioned earlier, is the basis for the creation of the meaning and information systems that compose human cultures). For instance, one of the most important thinking abilities that humans have unlike other animals is the ability to believe that other people, in addition to ourselves, are intentional agents—that they have wishes, desires, and intentions to act and behave. This ability produces interesting social dynamics because humans not only know of their own intentions and that others have intentions but also know that others know that they have intentions. Thus, we have causal beliefs (known as *attributions*) and *morality*, which are uniquely human products rooted in this uniquely human complex cognitive ability. This ability apparently turns on in humans around 9 months of age (Tomasello, 1999), which is a critical time of development of many cognitive abilities.

Moreover, humans have the cognitive ability to share their intentions with others. One of the major functions of language is to allow us to *communicate shared intentionality* (Matsumoto & Hwang, 2016; Tomasello & Herrmann, 2010). One of the functions of nonverbal communication is also to share intentions with others, and some types of nonverbal communication are uniquely human (because they map uniquely human cognitive abilities and language; see Cartmill & Goldin-Meadow, 2016). Shared intentionality may be at the heart of social coordination, which allows for the creation of human culture (Fiske, 2000).

Another important ability that humans have that animals do not is the ability to continually build upon improvements, known as the *ratchet effect* (Tomasello et al., 1993, 2005). When humans create something that is effective, it usually evolves to a next generation in which it is even better. This is true for computers, cars, music players, and, unfortunately, weapons. Like a ratchet, an improvement never goes backward; it only goes forward and continues to improve on itself. Because of specialized sociocognitive skills, which include teaching through verbal instructions, imitation, and prosociality, humans can achieve higher-level solutions when solving problems. Other animals do not possess these skills, which prevents them from achieving a cumulative culture that ratchets up (Dean et al., 2012). Human cultures are constantly ratcheting up.

Our cognitive skills also include memory, and because we have memory, we can create histories, and because we can create histories, we have traditions, customs, and heritage (Balter, 2010; Liu & Paez, 2019; Wang & Senzaki, 2019). Our cognitive skills also include the ability to think hypothetically and about the future. This allows us not only to plan things but also to worry about the uncertainty of the future, both of which form the basis of important cultural practices.

Emotions. Humans are also equipped with the ability to have emotions. Emotions are rapid, information-processing systems that aid individuals in reacting to events that require immediate action and have important consequences to one's welfare with minimal cognitive processing (Matsumoto & Hwang, 2019). They are part of an archaic, biologically innate system that is regulated and elaborated on in very unique, complex ways by humans. While some emotions are shared with nonhuman animals, humans have many different types and complexities of emotions, such as self-conscious emotions like pride, shame, guilt, or embarrassment, and moral emotions such as outrage or indignation (which speaks to the complexity of human cultures).

Personality traits. Finally, humans come to the world with personality traits. Humans around the world share a core set of traits that give them predispositions to adapt to their environments, solve social problems, and address their basic needs (Allik & Realo, 2019). Many cultures of the world are associated with differences in mean levels of several personality traits (McCrae et al., 1998, 2005). Questions concerning the origin of the relation between cultures and personality traits raise interesting possibilities. Although it is possible that cultures shaped the average personalities of its members, it is also possible that groups of individuals with certain kinds of personalities and temperaments banded together in certain geographic regions because it was beneficial for their adaptation to the environment, and thus influenced culture (a process of reverse causation: Hofstede & McCrae, 2004; McCrae et al., 2000).

In short, the universal psychological toolkits allow humans to adapt to their environments in order to meet their needs. To be sure, individual differences exist in how much of these toolkits each person has or how they are used. Nevertheless, humans come to the world pre-equipped with an evolved, naturally selected set of abilities and aptitudes that allows them to adapt, survive, and create cultures.

The Function of Cultures

An understanding of the function of cultures begins with an acknowledgment that humans are social animals and have always lived in groups. Group life is, in fact, an adaptation to the environment as humans, like other nonhuman animals, learned many hundreds of thousands of years ago that living in groups was better than living alone. Groups increase our chances for survival because they increase efficiency through division of labor. Division of labor allows groups to accomplish more than any one individual can, which is functional and adaptive for all the members of the group as it increases survival rates. Living in groups also increases safety and security.

A risk to group life is that there is potential for social conflict and chaos because of individual differences. Because of those differences, groups can become inefficient, reducing the probability for survival. And if groups are uncoordinated and individuals do not adapt to their environments with some degree of harmony with others, conflict and disorganization can occur, which can lead to social chaos. Some individuals and groups may even work to subvert, disrupt, or corrupt a larger group.

The function of human cultures, therefore, is to increase social order and coordination while reducing social chaos so that groups can adapt to their environments in order to meet human needs not only to survive but also to flourish. Human cultures achieve this function by creating rules and systems of living, thinking, and being. These become the meaning and information system of a group, which is their culture. Human cultures provide guidelines and roadmaps on what to do, how to think, and what to feel. Those guidelines are passed from one generation to the next so that future generations don't have to keep reinventing the wheel. Moreover, humans are equipped with universal psychological toolkits that allow for advanced, complex cognition and communication, and human cultures leverage these toolkits to increase complexity, differentiation, and institutionalization of the meaning and information systems and thus the ways of living, thinking, and being. These ways become the contents of a group's culture, and cultures help explain and describe those ways (Figure 3.1).

The Contents of Culture

The concept of "culture" is an abstract metaphor and its contents are represented by objective and subjective elements (Kroeber & Kluckhohn, 1952/1963; Triandis, 1972). The latter include all those parts of a culture that do not survive people as physical artifacts and include psychological processes such as attitudes, values, beliefs, and behaviors. The subjective elements of culture represent the meaning and information system aspects of culture. They exist symbolically in the human-made aspects of our environment, reflecting

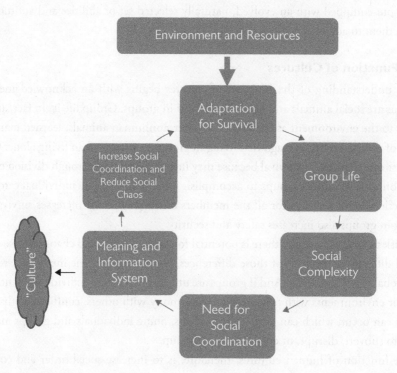

Figure 3.1. A functional perspective of culture.

culture, and they exist as mental representations in humans' minds (see Douglas, 1997, and Verweij et al., 2015, for writings that have had a major influence on thinking about culture and symbols). To follow we briefly describe the major components of the subjective elements of culture as represented in psychology.

Values. Values are guiding principles that refer to desirable goals that motivate behavior. They define the moral, political, social, economic, esthetic, or spiritual ethics of a person or group of people. Values can exist on two levels—personal and cultural. Personal values represent transitional desirable goals that serve as guiding principles in individuals' lives. Cultural values are shared, abstract ideas about what a social collectivity views as good, right, and desirable.

Scientists have suggested several ways in which cultures differ from one another on their values. The most well-known approach to understanding cultural values in psychology comes from work by Hofstede (1980, 2001). He studied work-related values around the world and reported data from 72 countries involving the responses of more than 117,000 employees of a multinational business organization, spanning over 20 different languages and seven occupational levels to 63 work-related values items (Hofstede, 1980, 2001). Using ecological-level factor analyses, Hofstede discerned five culture-level value dimensions:

- *Individualism Versus Collectivism.* This bipolar dimension refers to the degree to which cultures encourage, on one hand, the tendency for people to look after themselves and their immediate family only, or, on the other hand, for people to belong to ingroups that are supposed to look after their members in exchange for loyalty.
- *Power Distance.* This dimension refers to the degree to which cultures encourage less powerful members of groups to accept that power is distributed unequally.
- *Uncertainty Avoidance.* This dimension refers to the degree to which people feel threatened by the unknown or ambiguous situations and have developed beliefs, institutions, or rituals to avoid them.
- *Masculinity Versus Femininity.* This bipolar dimension is characterized on one pole by success, money, and things, and on the other pole by caring for others and quality of life. It refers to the distribution of emotional roles between males and females.
- *Long- Versus Short-Term Orientation.* This bipolar dimension refers to the degree to which cultures encourage delayed gratification of material, social, and emotional needs among its members.

Another major approach to understanding cultural values in psychology comes from the work of Schwartz, who has identified seven cultural values that are universal (Schwartz & Ros, 1995): embeddedness, hierarchy, mastery, intellectual autonomy, affective autonomy, egalitarianism, and harmony. Other approaches to cultural values also exist (House et al., 2003; Smith et al., 1996; Trompenaars & Hampden-Turner, 1998). Of the various cultural values dimensions that have been considered, individualism versus collectivism has by far received the greatest attention in cross-cultural research. It has been used to both predict and explain many differences across cultures, especially in many aspects of thinking and emotions (Oyserman & Lee, 2008; Schimmack et al., 2005; Triandis, 2001), as well as in research on culture and mental health (Griner & Smith, 2006; Huang & Zane, 2019; Leong & Lau, 2001; Tanaka-Matsumi, 2019).

Attitudes. Attitudes are relatively stable evaluations of things occurring in ongoing thoughts about those things or stored in memory. Cultures facilitate attitudes concerning actions and behaviors. Some attitudes generate cultural filters, which serve as the basis of stereotypes and prejudice. Cultures also foster attitudes that are not tied to specific kinds of actions, such as believing that democracy is the best form of government.

Beliefs. Beliefs are propositions regarded as true, and different cultures foster different belief systems. Cultural beliefs are known as *social axioms* (Bond et al., 2004; Leung et al., 2002). These are general beliefs and premises about oneself, the social and physical environment, and the spiritual world. They are assertions about the relationship between two or more entities or concepts; people endorse and use them to guide their behavior in daily living, such as "belief in a religion helps one understand the meaning of life."

On the individual level, five major types of social axioms exist (Leung et al., 2002); on the cultural level, two social axioms dimensions exist (Bond et al., 2004): dynamic externality, which represents an outward-oriented, simplistic grappling with external forces that are construed to include fate and a supreme being, and societal cynicism, which represents a predominantly cognitive apprehension or pessimism of the world confronting people. Culturally facilitated beliefs can impact many aspects of mental health, including beliefs about the causes and origins of mental health issues, beliefs about healers, and beliefs about treatment regimens (Marsella, 1982; Marsella & Yamada, 2000).

One of the major ways by which cultures are reflected in beliefs is through religions. Religions are organized systems of social practices, usually linked closely with beliefs, and are perhaps one of the most important subjective elements of culture (Saroglou, 2011, 2019). They tie together attitudes, values, beliefs, worldviews, and norms and provide guidelines and legitimations for living. At an abstract level, religions are similar in the sense that they serve a specific need—to help people manage themselves and their behaviors with others to avoid social chaos and provide social coordination. They also fulfill a widely shared desire among humans to want to believe in something to promote psychological stability and well-being. But religions achieve these higher-order goals in different ways. As a set of beliefs, religion also can have a major influence on health and mental health (Koenig & Larson, 2001; Levin & Chatters, 1998; Seybold & Hill, 2001).

Worldviews. These are culturally specific belief systems that contain attitudes, beliefs, opinions, and values about the world. They are assumptions people have about their physical and social realities (Koltko-Rivera, 2004). An important component of our worldviews is how we think about our self, which is known as self-concept. Undoubtedly the most influential perspective about cultural self-concepts in psychology has been the independent versus interdependent self-construal distinction (Markus & Kitayama, 1991). Although this perspective has led to much cross-cultural research over the past two-plus decades, recent studies have continually reported evidence challenging that distinction (Matsumoto, 1999; Oyserman et al., 2002; Takano & Osaka, 1999). Also, it has been recognized for millennia that behaviors and cultural worldviews are not necessarily related to each other; a belief about something may not correspond with actual behaviors (Matsumoto, 2006). Today most psychologists agree that the self-concept is multifaceted and accessed differently by people and facilitated to different degrees by national-ethnic cultures (Vignoles et al., 2016).

Norms. Norms are generally accepted standards of behavior for any cultural group. They dictate behaviors that a culture has defined as appropriate in a given situation. All cultures give guidelines about how people are expected to behave through norms. Norms also exist for describing the behaviors of people of other cultures (Shteynberg et al., 2009) as well as for controlling one's expressive behavior when emotional (Matsumoto et al., 2005, 2008). Norms are also related to social rituals and etiquette.

Norms can arise as the unintended consequence of people's efforts to coordinate with each other locally on small scales. Global norms can emerge from small-scale, local interactions even though people have no idea about the larger population or that they are coordinating on a larger, global scale (Centola & Baronchelli, 2015). Thus, large institutions or organizations are not necessary for the development of norms.

An important dimension of cultural variability with respect to norms involves a concept known as *tightness versus looseness* (Pelto, 1968). Tightness–looseness has two key components: the strength of social norms, or how clear and pervasive norms are within societies, and the strength of sanctioning, or how much tolerance there is for deviance from norms within societies. This dimension appears to be part of a loosely integrated system that incorporates ecological and historical components, such as population density, resource availability, history of conflict, and disease, with the strength of everyday recurring situations in facilitating mental processes and behaviors (Gelfand et al., 2011). Interestingly, recent work has suggested that cultural values of tightness–looseness likely coevolved with the serotonin transporter gene (SLC6A4) in the production of moral behavior (Chiao et al., 2013).

The Relation Between Culture, Psychological Processes, and Behavior

Cultures Ascribe Meaning to Situational Contexts

Culture influences thought and action through a rich, constant, and consistent interaction between situational contexts and individual difference factors. Cultures exert their influences on individuals primarily through situational contexts because cultures provide meanings to social contexts. These meanings, via norms and their associated attitudes, values, beliefs, and worldviews, inspire actions that are socially acceptable and desirable within each culture.

Individuals begin the process of learning about their culture, and more specifically, the rules and norms of appropriate behavior in specific situations and contexts, through a process known as *enculturation*. The enculturation process gradually shapes and molds individuals' ways of thinking, including how individuals perceive their worlds, think about the reasons underlying their and others' actions, have and express emotions, and interact with others in specific contexts. As individuals become enculturated, they learn specific behaviors and patterns of activities appropriate and inappropriate for their culture in specific situational contexts. Thus, much of the subjective elements of culture are learned. Much of this learning is unconscious, acquired through a probabilistic internalization of consistent features of lived experience.

At the same time, much of our behaviors and mental processes are influenced by individual factors, which include intention, personality, and biological factors, because humans come to the world with individual differences in personality, temperament, reactivity, and sensitivity. Thus, thought and action are the products of the interaction between two major forces—culture and individual differences. The relative contribution of these depends on contexts: in some contexts, the press of culture weighs relatively more heavily on individuals; in others, the push of individual factors may outweigh culture and context (Figure 3.2).

The relation between culture, psychological processes, and behaviors is not static or uni-directional. It is dynamic and interrelated; it feeds back on and reinforces itself. Cultures evolve over time as the creativity, attitudes, beliefs, values, worldviews, and behaviors of its members change and the environments within which groups exist are changed by them, all the while undergoing other natural changes. Technological developments bring about changes in ways of living that in turn affect culture. Changes in the environment, such as in climate, can bring about changes in ways of living, which will bring about changes in

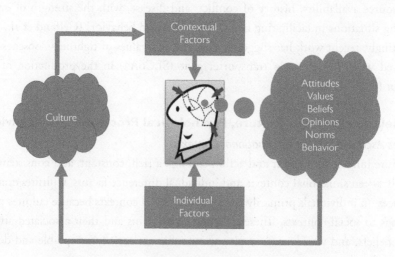

Figure 3.2. The association between culture and psychological processes and behavior.

culture. Changes in affluence of a region, culture, or even individuals bring about changes in ways of living and thus changes in culture. Longitudinal research on changes in culture and cultural products attest to the dynamic, changing nature of culture (Allen et al., 2007; Cai et al., 2019; Matsumoto et al., 1996; Rosenmann & Kurman, 2019). (See also Chapter 19 by Varnum and Hampton, this volume, on cultural change.)

Universals and Culture Specifics: Etics and Emics

Because all humans have the same basic needs and tasks—find food, water, and mates; dispose of waste; build living quarters with shelter and security; raise offspring; conduct the tasks of daily life—some degree of cross-cultural universality in mental processes and even behaviors is expected and reasonable. At the same time, because all human cultures exist in their own specific, unique environment, differences in the ways by which humans achieve these tasks and meet their needs (i.e., adapt) are also expected. In anthropology, folklore studies, and the social and behavioral sciences, the terms *emic* and *etic* refer to two kinds of field research and viewpoints: *emic,* from within the social group (from the perspective of the subject), and *etic,* from outside (from the perspective of the observer). *Etics* is intended to refer to those processes that are consistent across cultures, candidates as universal psychological processes. *Emics* refers typically to participants' characterizations of their life experience, which often differ across cultures, and to culture-specific processes. These terms originated in the study of language (Pike, 1954), with *phonetics* referring to aspects of language that are common across cultures and *phonemes* referring to aspects of language that are specific to a particular culture and language. These linguistic concepts were then borrowed to describe universal versus culturally relative aspects of behavior (Berry, 1969; see also Lonner, 1980, and Norenzayan & Heine, 2005, for more discussion on universal psychological processes).

The concepts of emics and etics are related to an understanding of the relation between culture and mental health in several ways. For example, there have long been accounts of culture-specific (i.e., emic) psychological syndromes, such as *amok, zar, baksbat, susto, latah,* or *koro* (see brief descriptions in Matsumoto & Juang, 2016). At the same time, for decades researchers have been searching for cross-culturally applicable indicators and symptomatology (i.e., etic) of various major psychological disorders such as schizophrenia, depression, and anxiety disorders (see Tanaka-Matsumi, 2019, for a review).

Because cultures aid humans in finding ways to meet their basic needs but at the same time exist in different, sometimes very unique environments, human cultures are very flexible. Sometimes culture is a multiplier, enhancing certain behaviors. Sometimes culture is a creator, empowering novel activities not seen elsewhere. Sometimes culture is an enabler, facilitating and encouraging behaviors. Sometimes culture is a suppresser, discouraging behaviors (Matsumoto & Juang, 2016). And individuals in every culture find their own ways, producing many individual differences within cultures.

Conclusion

Cultures are products of the evolved human mind's response to specific environments in which groups live and the resources available to them. Cultures emerge from the interaction among universal biological needs and functions, universal social problems associated with those needs, the complex cognitive abilities afforded, and the resources available in the environments in which humans live. Cultures are solutions to the problem of groups' needs to adapt to their contexts to address their members' social motives and biological needs. As adaptational responses to the environment, cultures help groups to select behaviors, attitudes, values, opinions, norms, and behaviors that may optimize the tapping of resources to meet survival needs. Out of all the myriad behaviors possible in the human repertoire, cultures help to focus people's behaviors and attention on a few limited alternatives to maximize their effectiveness, given their resources and their environment.

The very basic framework of the relation between culture and psychology described previously provides a basis for understanding the relation between culture and mental health, locally and globally (see also Chapter 1 by Scott, this volume, on cross-national epidemiology of mental disorders). While cultures can of course be similar or different in the incidence rates of mental disorders, cultures also differ in the attitudes, values, beliefs, opinions, and norms concerning the etiology of mental disorders, treatments and treatment methodologies, and mental health caregivers and professionals. Moreover, while national cultures certainly exist, cultural groups also exist within nations, the fact of which leads to interesting questions concerning mental health disparities among various ethnic groups as well as immigrant groups, in the United States and elsewhere. Understanding similarities and differences among and across various cultural groups begins with a basic understanding of the contents and function of culture and their relation to psychological processes, which we have hopefully provided earlier.

To be sure, despite the wealth of knowledge we have about culture and psychology, there is still much we don't know, especially concerning the specific links between culture, context, norms, and neuroscience. Cultures infuse contexts with rich, deep, and sophisticated meanings, all of which are encoded in the human mind. Although we have explicated some of the psychological encoding of those cultural contents at an abstract level in this chapter, the field still does not have a good idea of exactly what those meanings are or how to explicate context along meaningful and measurable dimensions for research. The field has yet to tackle questions concerning the underlying neuropsychological encoding of cultural content or context or how cultural content and context interact with individual neuropsychological structures and substrates individuals come to the world with. The underlying neuropsychology undoubtedly plays a role in influencing and being influenced by mental health. Future research hopefully will endeavor to elucidate these very basic but complex links as they have wide-ranging implications to many aspects of human social life and mental health.

Because of the nature of the relation between culture and psychology, cultures play major roles with regard to understanding global mental health, including how to understand, assess, and treat various mental illnesses. Elucidating etic and emic aspects of mental illnesses and other psychiatric syndromes has been a major focus of cross-cultural research (Tanaka-Matsumi, 2019), as has their treatment (Huang & Zane, 2019). All approaches can be informed by a basic understanding of culture and psychology, which hopefully this chapter has provided.

References

Allen, M. W., Ng, S. H., Ikeda, K. I., Jawan, J. A., Sufi, A. H., Wilson, M., & Yang, K.-S. (2007). Two decades of change in cultural values and economic development in eight East Asian and Pacific Island nations. *Journal of Cross-Cultural Psychology, 38*(3), 247–269. doi:10.1177/0022022107300273

Allik, J., & Realo, A. (2019). Culture and personality. In D. Matsumoto & H. C. Hwang (Eds.), *Oxford handbook of culture and psychology* (pp. 401–430). Oxford University Press.

Balter, M. (2010). Did working memory spark creative culture? *Science, 328,* 160–163. doi:10.1126/science.328.5975.160

Baumeister, R. F. (2005). *The cultural animal: Human nature, meaning, and social life.* Oxford University Press.

Behrensmeyer, A. K. (2006). Climate change and human evolution. *Science, 311,* 476–478. doi:10.1126/science.1116051

Berry, J. W. (1969). On cross-cultural comparability. *International Journal of Psychology, 4,* 119–128. doi:10.1080/00207596908247261

Berry, J. W., Poortinga, Y. H., Segall, M. H., & Dasen, P. R. (1992). *Cross-cultural psychology: Research and applications.* Cambridge University Press.

Boesch, C. (2003). Is culture a golden barrier between human and chimpanzee? *Evolutionary Anthropology, 12,* 82–91. doi:10.1002/evan.10106

Bond, M. H., Leung, K., Au, A., Tong, K. K., Reimel de Carrasquel, S., Murakami, F., Yamaguchi, S., Bierbrauer, G., Singelis, T., Broer, M., Boen, F., Lambert, S. M., Ferreira, M. C., Noels, K. A., van Bavel, J., Safdar, S., Zhang, J., Chen, L., Solcova, I., . . . Lewis, J. R. (2004). Culture-level dimensions of social axioms and their correlates across 41 cultures. *Journal of Cross-Cultural Psychology, 35,* 548–570. doi:10.1177/0022022104268388

Boyer, P. (2000). Evolutionary psychology and cultural transmission. *American Behavioral Scientist, 43*(6), 987–1000. doi:10.1177/00027640021955711

Buss, D. M. (1988). The evolution of human intrasexual competition: Tactics of mate attraction. *Journal of Personality & Social Psychology, 54*(4), 616–628. doi:10.1037/0022-3514.54.4.616

Buss, D. M. (1991). Evolutionary personality psychology. *Annual Review of Psychology, 42,* 459–491. doi:10.1146/annurev.ps.42.020191.002331

Buss, D. M. (2001). Human nature and culture: An evolutionary psychological perspective. *Journal of Personality, 69*(6), 955–978. doi:10.1111/1467-6494.696171

Cai, H., Huang, J., & Jing, Y. (2019). Living in a changing world: The change of culture and psychology. In D. Matsumoto & H. C. Hwang (Eds.), *Oxford handbook of culture and psychology* (pp. 786–810). Oxford University Press.

Cartmill, E. A., & Goldin-Meadow, S. (2016). Gesture. In D. Matsumoto, H. C. Hwang, & M. G. Frank (Eds.), *APA handbook of nonverbal communication* (pp. 307–333). American Psychological Association.

Centola, D., & Baronchelli, A. (2015). The spontaneous emergence of conventions: An experimental study of cultural evolution. *Proceedings of the National Academy of Sciences, 112*(7), 1989–1994. doi:10.1073/pnas.1418838112

Chiao, J. Y., Cheon, B. K., Pornpattananangkul, N., Mrazek, A. J., & Blizinsky, K. D. (2013). Cultural neuroscience: Progress and promise. *Psychological Inquiry, 24*(1), 1–19. doi:10.1080/1047840X.2013.752715

Dean, L. G., Kendal, R. L., Schapiro, S. J., Thierry, B., & Laland, K. N. (2012). Identification of the social and cognitive processes underlying human cumulative culture. *Science, 335,* 1114–1118. doi:10.1126/science.1213969

Douglas, M. (1997). *Natural symbols.* Routledge.

Fiske, A. P. (2000). Complementarity theory: Why human social capacities evolved to require cultural complements. *Personality and Social Psychology Review, 4*(1), 76–94. doi:10.1207/S15327957PSPR0401_7

Geertz, C. (1975). From the natives' point of view: On the nature of anthropological understanding. *American Scientist, 63,* 47–53.

Gelfand, M. J., Raver, J. L., Nishii, L., Leslie, L. M., Lun, J., Lim, B. C., . . . Yamaguchi, S. (2011). Differences between tight and loose cultures: A 33-nation study. *Science, 332,* 1100–1104. doi:10.1126/science.1197754

Griner, D., & Smith, T. B. (2006). Culturally adapted mental health intervention: A meta-analytic review. *Psychotherapy: Theory, Research, Practice, Training, 43*(4), 531–548. doi:10.1037/0033-3204.43.4.531

Hofstede, G. H. (1980). *Culture's consequences: International differences in work-related values.* Sage Publications.

Hofstede, G. H. (2001). *Culture's consequences: Comparing values, behaviors, institutions and organizations across nations* (2nd ed.). Sage Publications.

Hofstede, G. H., & McCrae, R. R. (2004). Personality and culture revisited: Linking traits and dimensions of culture. *Cross-Cultural Research, 38*(1), 52–88. doi:10.1177/1069397103259443

Hogan, R. (1982). A socioanalytic theory of personality. In M. Page (Ed.), *Nebraska symposium on motivation* (Vol. 30, pp. 55–89). University of Nebraska Press.

House, R. J., Hanges, P. J., Javidan, M., Dorfman, P., & Gupta, V. (2003). *GLOBE, cultures, leadership, and organizations: GLOBE study of 62 societies.* Sage.

Huang, C. Y., & Zane, N. (2019). Culture and psychological interventions. In D. Matsumoto & H. C. Hwang (Eds.), *Oxford handbook of culture and psychology* (pp. 468–508). Oxford University Press.

Jahoda, G. (1984). Do we need a concept of culture? *Journal of Cross-Cultural Psychology, 15*(2), 139–151. doi:10.1177/0022002184015002003

Koenig, H. G., & Larson, D. B. (2001). Religion and mental health: Evidence for an association. *International Review of Psychiatry, 13*(2), 67–78. doi:10.1080/09540260124661

Koltko-Rivera, M. E. (2004). The psychology of worldviews. *Review of General Psychology, 8*(1), 3–58. doi:10.1037/1089-2680.8.1.3

Kroeber, A. L., & Kluckhohn, C. (1952/1963). *Culture: A critical review of concepts and definitions.* Harvard University.

Leong, F. T. L., & Lau, A. S. L. (2001). Barriers to providing effective mental health services to Asian Americans. *Mental Health Services Research, 3*(4), 201–214. doi:10.1023/a:1013177014788

Leung, K., Bond, M. H., de Carrasquel, S. R., Muñoz, C., Hernández, M., Murakami, F., . . . Singelis, T. M. (2002). Social axioms: The search for universal dimensions of general beliefs about how the world functions. *Journal of Cross-Cultural Psychology, 33*(3), 286–302. doi:10.1177/0022022102033003005

Levin, J. S., & Chatters, L. M. (1998). Research on religion and mental health: An overview of empirical findings and theoretical issues. In H. G. Koenig (Ed.), *Handbook of religion and mental health* (pp. 33–50). Academic Press.

Linton, R. (1936). *The study of man: An introduction.* Appleton.

Liu, J. H., & Paez, D. (2019). Social representations of history as common ground for processes of intergroup relations and the content of social identities. In D. Matsumoto & H. C. Hwang (Eds.), *Oxford handbook of culture and psychology* (pp. 586–614). Oxford University Press.

Lonner, W. J. (1980). The search for psychological universals. In J. W. Berry, Y. H. Poortinga, & J. Pandey (Eds.), *Handbook of cross-cultural psychology, Vol. 1: Theory and method* (pp. 43–83). Allyn and Bacon.

Markus, H. R., & Kitayama, S. (1991). Culture and the self: Implications for cognition, emotion, and motivation. *Psychological Review, 98*(2), 224–253. doi:10.1037/0033-295X.98.2.224

Marsella, A. J. (1982). Culture and mental health: An overview. In A. J. Marsella & G. M. White (Eds.), *Cultural conceptions of mental health and therapy* (pp. 359–388). Springer Netherlands.

Marsella, A. J., & Yamada, A. M. (2000). Chapter 1—Culture and mental health: An introduction and overview of foundations, concepts, and issues. In I. Cuéllar & F. A. Paniagua (Eds.), *Handbook of multicultural mental health* (pp. 3–24). Academic Press.

Matsumoto, D. (1999). Culture and self: An empirical assessment of Markus and Kitayama's theory of independent and interdependent self-construals. *Asian Journal of Social Psychology, 2,* 289–310. doi:10.1111/1467-839X.00042

Matsumoto, D. (2006). Culture and cultural worldviews: Do verbal descriptions of culture reflect anything other than verbal descriptions of culture? *Culture and Psychology, 12*(1), 33–62. doi:10.1177/1354067X06061592

Matsumoto, D., & Fletcher, D. (1996). Cross-national differences in disease rates as accounted for by meaningful psychological dimensions of cultural variability. *Journal of Gender, Culture, and Health, 1,* 71–82.

Matsumoto, D., & Hwang, H. C. (2016). The cultural bases of nonverbal communication. In D. Matsumoto, H. C. Hwang, & M. G. Frank (Eds.), *APA handbook of nonverbal communication* (pp. 77–101). American Psychological Association.

Matsumoto, D., & Hwang, H. C. (2019). Culture and emotion: Integrating biological universality with cultural specificity. In D. Matsumoto & H. C. Hwang (Eds.), *Oxford handbook of culture and psychology* (pp. 361–400). Oxford University Press.

Matsumoto, D., & Juang, L. P. (2016). *Culture and psychology* (6th ed.). Cengage.

Matsumoto, D., Kudoh, T., & Takeuchi, S. (1996). Changing patterns of individualism and collectivism in the United States and Japan. *Culture and Psychology, 2,* 77–107. doi:10.1177/1354067X9621005

Matsumoto, D., Yoo, S. H., Fontaine, J. R. J., Anguas-Wong, A. M., Arriola, M., Ataca, B., . . . Grossi, E. (2008). Mapping expressive differences around the world: The relationship between emotional display rules and Individualism v. Collectivism. *Journal of Cross-Cultural Psychology, 39*(1), 55–74. doi:10.1177/0022022107311854

Matsumoto, D., Yoo, S. H., Hirayama, S., & Petrova, G. (2005). Validation of an individual-level measure of display rules: The Display Rule Assessment Inventory (DRAI). *Emotion, 5*(1), 23–40. doi:10.1037/1528-3542.5.1.23

McCrae, R. R., Costa, P. T., del Pilar, G. H., Rolland, J.-P., & Parker, W. D. (1998). Cross-cultural assessment of the five-factor model: The revised NEO Personality Inventory. *Journal of Cross-Cultural Psychology, 29*(1), 171–188. doi:10.1177/0022022198291009

McCrae, R. R., Costa, P. T., Ostendorf, F., Angleitner, A., Hrebickova, M., Avia, M. D., . . . Smith, P. B. (2000). Nature over nurture: Temperament, personality, and life span development. *Journal of Personality and Social Psychology, 78*(1), 173–186. doi:10.1037/0022-3514.78.1.173

McCrae, R. R., Terracciano, A., Leibovich, N. B., Schmidt, V., Shakespeare-Finch, J., Neubauer, A., . . . Munyae, M. (2005). Personality profiles of cultures: Aggregate personality traits. *Journal of Personality and Social Psychology, 89*(3), 407–425. doi:10.1037/0022-3514.89.3.407

McGrew, W. C. (2004). *The cultured chimpanzee: Reflections on cultural primatology.* Cambridge University Press.

Murray, D. R., & Schaller, M. (2010). Historical prevalence of infectious diseases within 230 geopolitical regions: A tool for investigating origins of culture. *Journal of Cross-Cultural Psychology, 41*(1), 99–108. doi:10.1177/0022022109349510

Murray, D. R., Trudeau, R., & Schaller, M. (2011). On the origins of cultural differences in conformity: Four tests of the pathogen prevalence hypothesis. *Personality and Social Psychology Bulletin, 37*(3), 318–329.

Norenzayan, A., & Heine, S. J. (2005). Psychological universals: What are they and how can we know? *Psychological Bulletin, 131*(5), 763–784. doi:10.1037/0033-2909.131.5.763

Oyserman, D., Coon, H. M., & Kemmelmeier, M. (2002). Rethinking individualism and collectivism: Evaluation of theoretical assumptions and meta-analyses. *Psychological Bulletin, 128*(1), 3–72. doi:10.1037/0033-2909.128.1.3

Oyserman, D., & Lee, S. W. S. (2008). Does culture influence what and how we think? Effects of priming individualism and collectivism. *Journal of Personality and Social Psychology, 134*(2), 311–342.

Pelto, P. J. (1968). The differences between "tight" and "loose" societies. *Transaction,* 37–40. doi:10.1007/BF03180447

Pelto, P. J., & Pelto, G. H. (1975). Intra-cultural diversity: Some theoretical issues. *American Ethnologist, 2,* 1–18. doi:10.1525/ae.1975.2.1.02a00010

Pike, K. L. (1954). *Language in relation to a unified theory of the structure of human behavior.* Summer Institute of Linguistics.

Premack, D. (2004). Is language the key to human intelligence? *Science, 303,* 318–320. doi:10.1126/science.1093993

Rohner, R. P. (1984). Toward a conception of culture for cross-cultural psychology. *Journal of Cross-Cultural Psychology, 15,* 111–138. doi:10.1177/0022002184015002002

Rosenmann, A., & Kurman, J. (2019). The culturally situated self. In D. Matsumoto & H. C. Hwang (Eds.), *Oxford handbook of culture and psychology* (pp. 538–585). Oxford University Press.

Saroglou, V. (2011). Believing, bonding, behaving, and belonging: The big four religious dimensions and cultural variation. *Journal of Cross-Cultural Psychology, 42*(8), 1320–1340. doi:10.1177/0022022111412267

Saroglou, V. (2019). Religion and related morality across cultures. In D. Matsumoto & H. C. Hwang (Eds.), *Oxford handbook of culture and psychology* (pp. 724–785). Oxford University Press.

Schaller, M., & Murray, D. R. (2008). Pathogens, personality, and culture: Disease prevalence predicts world-wide variability in sociosexuality, extraversion, and openness to experience. *Journal of Personality and Social Psychology, 95*(1), 212–221. doi:10.1037/0022-3514.95.1.212

Schimmack, U., Oishi, S., & Diener, E. (2005). Individualism: A valid and important dimension of cultural differences between nations. *Personality and Social Psychology Review, 9*(1), 17–31. doi:10.1207/s15327957pspr0901_2

Schug, J., Yuki, M., & Maddux, W. (2010). Relational mobility explains between- and within-culture differences in self-disclosure to close friends. *Psychological Science, 21*(10), 1471–1478. doi:10.1177/0956797610382786

Schwartz, S. H., & Ros, M. (1995). Values in the west: A theoretical and empirical challenge to the individualism-collectivism cultural dimension. *World Psychology, 1,* 91–122.

Seybold, K. S., & Hill, P. C. (2001). The role of religion and spirituality in mental and physical health. *Current Directions in Psychological Science, 10*(1), 21–24. doi:10.1111/1467-8721.00106

Sheldon, K. M. (2004). *The psychology of optimal being: An integrated, multi-level perspective.* Erlbaum.

Shteynberg, G., Gelfand, M. J., & Kim, K. (2009). Peering into the "Magnum Mysterium" of culture: The explanatory power of descriptive norms. *Journal of Cross-Cultural Psychology, 40*(1), 46–69. doi:10.1177/0022022108326196

Smith, P. B., Dugan, S., & Trompenaars, F. (1996). National culture and the values of organizational employees: A dimensional analysis across 43 nations. *Journal of Cross-Cultural Psychology, 27*(2), 231–264. doi:10.1177/0022022196272006

Takano, Y., & Osaka, E. (1999). An supported common view: Comparing Japan and the U.S. on individualism/collectivism. *Asian Journal of Social Psychology, 2*(3), 311–341. doi:10.1111/1467-839X.00043

Talhelm, T., Zhang, X., Oishi, S., Shimin, C., Duan, D., Lan, X., & KItayama, S. (2014). Large-scale psychological differences within China explained by rice versus wheat agriculture. *Science, 344,* 603–608. doi:10.1126/science.1246850

Tanaka-Matsumi, J. (2019). Abnormal psychology and culture. In D. Matsumoto & H. C. Hwang (Eds.), *Oxford handbook of culture and psychology* (pp. 431–467). Oxford University Press.

Tomasello, M. (1999). *The cultural origins of human cognition.* Harvard University Press.

Tomasello, M., Carpenter, M., Call, J., Behne, T., & Moll, H. (2005). Understanding and sharing intentions: The origins of cultural cognition. *Behavioral & Brain Sciences, 28,* 675–735. doi:10.1017/S0140525X05000129

Tomasello, M., & Herrmann, E. (2010). Ape and human cognition: What's the difference? *Current Directions in Psychological Science, 19*(1), 3–8. doi:10.1177/0963721409359300

Tomasello, M., Kruger, A. C., & Ratner, H. H. (1993). Cultural learning. *Behavioural and Brain Sciences, 16,* 495–552. doi:10.1017/S0140525X0003123X

Triandis, H. C. (1972). *The analysis of subjective culture.* Wiley.

Triandis, H. C. (2001). Individualism and collectivism: Past, present, and future. In D. Matsumoto (Ed.), *Handbook of culture and psychology* (pp. 35–50). Oxford University Press.

Trompenaars, A., & Hampden-Turner, C. (1998). *Riding the waves of culture: understanding cultural diversity in global business* (2nd ed.). McGraw Hill.

Tylor, E. B. (1865). *Researches into the early history of mankind and development of civilisation.* John Murray.

Van de Vliert, E. (2009). *Climate, affluence, and culture.* Cambridge University Press.

Van de Vliert, E., & Kong, D. T. (2019). Cold, heat, warmth, and culture. In D. Matsumoto & H. C. Hwang (Eds.), *Oxford handbook of culture and psychology* (2nd ed.) (pp. 93–122). Oxford University Press.

Verweij, M., Senior, T., Domínguez, D. J., & Turner, R. (2015). Emotion, rationality, and decision-making: How to link affective and social neuroscience with social theory. *Frontiers in Neuroscience, 9*(332). doi:10.3389/fnins.2015.00332

Vignoles, V. L., Owe, E., Becker, M., Smith, P. B., Easterbrook, M. J., Brown, R., . . . Bond, M. H. (2016). Beyond the 'east–west' dichotomy: Global variation in cultural models of selfhood. *Journal of Experimental Psychology: General, 145*(8), 966–1000. doi:10.1037/xge0000175

Wang, Q., & Senzaki, S. (2019). Culture and cognition. In D. Matsumoto & H. C. Hwang (Eds.), *Oxford handbook of culture and psychology* (pp. 318–360). Oxford University Press.

Warneken, F., & Tomasello, M. (2006). Altruistic helping in human infants and young chimpanzees. *Science, 311,* 1301–1303. doi:10.1126/science.1121448

Whiten, A., Horner, V., & De Waal, F. B. M. (2005). Conformity to cultural norms of tool use in chimpanzees. *Nature, 437*(7059), 737–740. doi:10.1038/nature04047

Embrainment and Enculturation: Culture, Brain, and Self

Georg Northoff

Abstract

Embrainment and enculturation are central concepts in cultural neuroscience, but their mechanisms remain unclear. Embrainment describes how cultural contexts are encoded into the brain's neuronal activity, whereas enculturation means that neuronal activity is impacted by cultural contexts as manifested in the brain's affective and cognitive functions. This chapter takes the self as a paradigmatic example of embrainment and enculturation. It discusses different concepts of self and shows the neuronal correlates of self, which highlight spatiotemporal, scale-free (i.e., across different spatial and temporal scales operating in a self-similar way), and stochastic mechanisms. That very same spatiotemporal, scale-free, and stochastic encoding is manifested on the mental level in human selves, which, therefore, are relational and spatiotemporal. The chapter concludes that embrainment and enculturation reflect two distinct aspects of one and the same underlying process, that is, self-related processing as manifested in the self as relational self. Moreover, as human selves provide the basis of mental health, the here-described mechanisms of embrainment and enculturation of self are central for global mental health as people with their self and the underlying brain's spontaneous activity move across different cultures.

Key Words: embrainment, enculturation, self, cortical midline structure, scale-free properties, spatiotemporal features

Introduction

Cultural neuroscience has demonstrated that culture permeates our affective and cognitive functions as well as their underlying neuronal mechanisms in the brain (Han & Northoff, 2008, 2009; see also Chiao et al., "Cultural Neuroscience," in this volume). Even our self (i.e., sense of self or self-consciousness) is strongly dependent upon the respective cultural context. Markus and Kitayama (1991, 2003) distinguished two different styles or types of self: an independent self that is more focused on itself and less on its respective social context and thus presupposes a more individualistic cultural view (see also Masumoto and Hwang, "Culture and Psychology"; Goto, "Culture and Self-Construal"; and Wang, "Culture and Autobiographical Memory," this volume), and an interdependent self that is less focused on itself and emphasizes more its social relation and context and thus presupposes a more collectivistic view. Following Markus and Kitayama (1991), the independent self is predominant in the Western world, while the interdependent self dominates more in the Far Eastern part of the world. Most interestingly, recent brain imaging studies demonstrated neural differences between independent and interdependent selves (see Han & Ma, 2016; Han & Northoff, 2009; see also Goto, "Culture and Self-Construal" as well as Wang, "Culture and Autobiographical Memory," this volume).

These findings on the self and many other findings in cultural neuroscience raise the question about the mechanisms by which culture comes into the brain. Specifically, we are asking about the mechanisms by which the brain's neuronal activity and the associated self can encode cultural context and are shaped by them. This is the question about what has been described as "embrainment" and "enculturation" or, more or less synonymously, "culture–brain nexus," "neuroculture interaction," or "encultured brain" (Northoff, 2016). Briefly, embrainment describes that cultural contexts are encoded into the brain's neuronal activity such that the latter is shaped by the former—one can thus speak of "embrainment of culture." Enculturation describes that our affective and cognitive functions, including their underlying neural correlates, are adopted to the respective cultural context and thus encultured—one can thus speak of "enculturation" of the brain.

The main aim in this chapter is to understand some of the mechanisms underlying embrainment and enculturation. For that, I take the self as a paradigmatic example appropriate to reveal the mechanisms underlying embrainment and enculturation. The first part will focus on recent concepts of self, which will be complemented in the second part by showing recent empirical (neuroscientific) findings on self. The third part will address the mechanisms of embrainment and enculturation, while the fourth part will focus on the implications of these mechanisms for mental features like the self. The main thesis is that, as based on empirical data, I consider embrainment and enculturation as two distinct aspects of one and the same underlying neuroecological process, that is, self-related processing as manifested in the self as relational self.

Concept of Self

Is the Self a Mental Substance or Property?

What is the self? What must it look like to presuppose experience and be the subject of our experience? The self has often been viewed as a specific "thing." Stones are things; the table on which your laptop stands is a thing. And in the same way the table makes it possible for the laptop to stand on it, the self may be a thing that makes experience and consciousness possible. In other words, metaphorically speaking, experience and consciousness stand on the shoulders of the self.

However, another question is whether the self is a thing or, as Western philosophers such as Rene Descartes argued, a substance or a property as it is nowadays formulated in Western philosophy. A substance or property is a specific entity or material that serves as a basis for something like a self. For instance, the body can be considered a physical substance, while the self can be associated with a mental substance. Nowadays one would speak no longer of substance but of properties, like a mental property that is enduring, not subject to change, and that can therefore best account for the continuity of the self over time.

Is our self real and thus does it exist? Or is it just an illusion? Let us compare the situation to perception. When we perceive something in our environment, we sometimes perceive it as not a real thing, but an illusion that does not exist. The question of what exists and is real is what philosophers call an ontological question. Earlier philosophers, such as Rene Descartes, argued that the self is real and exists. Descartes also argued that the self is different from the body. Hence, self and body exist, but differ in their nature and essence. Thus, from this perspective, the self cannot be a physical substance and is a mental substance instead. It is a feature not of the body, but of the mind.

However, the Western characterization of the self as a mental entity has been questioned. For example, the Scottish philosopher David Hume argued that there is no self as a mental entity. There is only a complex set or "bundle" of perceptions of interrelated events that reflect the world in its entirety. There is no additional self in the world; instead, there is nothing but the events we perceive. Everything else, such as the assumption of a self as mental entity, is an illusion. The self as mental entity and thus as a mental substance does not exist and is therefore not real.

To reject the idea of self as mental substance and to dismiss it as mere illusion is currently popular. One major proponent of this view today is the German philosopher Thomas Metzinger (2003). In a nutshell, he argues that through our experience, we develop models of the self, so-called self-models. These self-models are nothing but information processes in our brain. However, since we do not have direct access to these neuronal processes (e.g., all those processes and activities of the cells and neurons in the brain), we tend to assume the presence of an entity that must underlie our own self-model. This entity is then characterized as the self.

Is the Self Based on Integration and Cognition?

What is the self if not a mental entity? Current authors such as Metzinger (2003) and Churchland (2002) argue that the self as mental substance or entity does not exist. How do we come up with the idea of a self, or the self-model as Metzinger calls it? The model of our own self is based on summarizing, integrating, and coordinating all the information from our own body and brain.

What does such integration look like? Take all that information together, coordinate and integrate it, and then you have a self-model of your own brain and body and their respective processes. In more technical terms, our own brain and body are represented in the neuronal activity of the brain. Such representation of our own brain and body amounts then to a model of your self. The self-model is therefore nothing but an inner model of the integrated and summarized version of your own brain and body's information processing. The self is thus a mere model of one's own body's and brain's processes.

The original mental self, the self as mental substance or entity, is in this line of thinking replaced by a self-model. This implies a shift from a metaphysical discussion of the existence and reality of self to the processes that underlie the representation of body and brain as a self-model. Since this representation is based on the coordination and integration of the various ongoing processes in the brain and body, it is associated with specific higher-order cognitive functions such as working memory, attention, executive function, and memory, among others.

What does this imply for the characterization of the self (presupposing a broader concept of self beyond the self as mental substance)? The self is no longer characterized as a mental substance but as a cognitive function. Methodologically, this implies that the self should be investigated empirically rather than metaphysically.

We therefore need to search for the cognitive processes underlying the special self-representation. The self is consequently no longer an issue of philosophy, but rather one of cognitive psychology and ultimately of cognitive neuroscience. According to this model, the self is no longer a metaphysical matter, but merely empirical and, more specifically, cognitive as related to various cognitive functions (Sui & Humphreys, 2015). However, as it will become clear in the following, the self is more than just integrational and cognitive—it extends beyond the cognitive realm to the social and cultural context in which it is situated.

Is the Self Social?

How does the self interact with other selves? So far, we have described the self in an isolated and purely intraindividual way. However, in daily life, the self is not isolated from others but always related to other selves. This is called interindividualism rather than intraindividualism. This raises questions about what is described as the "problem of other minds" or, more generally, questions concerning intersubjectivity. Here we will give a brief description of the problem of intersubjectivity.

How can we make the assumption of attributing mental states and thus self and mind to other people? Philosophy has long relied on what is called the "inference by analogy." What is the inference by analogy? The inference by analogy goes like this. We observe person A to show the behavior of type X. And we know that in our own case the same behavior X goes along with the mental state type M. Since our own behavior and that of the person A are similar, we assume the other person A to show the same mental state type M we experience when exhibiting behavior X.

What kind of inference do we draw here? There is similar or analogous behavior between ourselves and the other person. In addition, my own behavior is associated with a particular mental state. Since now the other person shows the same behavior, I infer that she also shows the same mental state as it is associated with my own behavior. Hence, by indirect inference and analogy via our own case, we claim to obtain knowledge of the other person's mental state. How can we make such inference? We may make it on the basis of our own mental states and their associated behavior. And what we do may also hold true for the other person who in the same way attributes mental states to us by inferring them from the comparison between our behavior and their own mental states.

However, both empathy and the attribution of mental states to another person are puzzling: despite the fact that we do not experience the other's mental states and consciousness, we nevertheless either share them (as in empathy) or infer them (as in inference by analogy). We have no direct access to other persons' experience of a self and its mental states in first-person perspective and nevertheless share their mental states and assume that they have a self. How is that possible?

Different Perspectives of the Self?

This is where we need to introduce yet another perspective. There is the first-person perspective—tied to the self itself and its experience or consciousness of objects, events, or persons in the environment. Additionally, the first-person perspective could also result from the integration of the different selves and their distinct features as described earlier. Then there is the third-person perspective—this perspective allows us to observe the objects, events, or persons in the environment from the outside, rather than from the inside. The picture is not complete though, as it must be complemented by the second-person perspective.

What is the second-person perspective? The second-person perspective has initially been associated in philosophy with the introspection of one's own mental states. Rather than actually experiencing one's own mental states in first-person perspective, the second-person perspective makes it possible to access others' mental states and understand the other as self. At the same time, the second-person perspective also allows one to reflect about one's own self as just another self in the world besides other selves (see also Pfeiffer et al., 2013).

The second-person perspective thus allows us to put the contents of our consciousness as experienced in first-person perspective into a wider context—the context of oneself as related to the environment—as well as to connect that to other persons' mental contents and selves. In other words, the second-person perspective makes it possible to situate and integrate the purely intraindividual self with its first-person perspective into a social context of other persons' selves. This transforms the intraindividual self into an interindividual self, while other selves are also transformed into interindividual selves. Taken together, the second-person perspective allows us to determine the concept of the self as "social self."

How can we define the concept of the social self? The concept of the social self describes the linkage and integration of the self into the social context of other selves. This shifts the focus from experience or consciousness in the first-person perspective to the various kinds of interactions between different selves as associated with the second-person perspective. As we already indicated, there may be different kinds of social interactions including affective precognitive and more cognitive ones that involve meta-representation as described previously.

Independent Versus Interdependent Self?

The social self is closely linked to the culture within which the self socially interacts. Different cultures entail different forms of social interaction and consequently different forms of self. This is most apparent in the distinction between inter- and independent self (Markus & Kitayama, 1991, 2003). Briefly, the independent self is a self that focuses more on itself and its inner states and is also structured more or less independently of the others and the social context—such an independent self is considered to dominate in the Western world. The interdependent self is more focused on social relationships with close others, and especially the family—the self thus structures, stabilizes, and constitutes itself through others and social relationship rather than by and through itself as the independent self. Such an interdependent self is a knot or hub in the social-cultural web—this view of self is more dominant in the Eastern world (Han & Ma, 2016).

However, it must be noted that the distinction between inter- and independent self is not absolute, but relative, where both types are found in Eastern and Western culture to different degrees (Han & Ma, 2016; Han & Northoff, 2009). How is it possible that the self is socially and culturally embedded and thus encultured, while at the same time being embrained? To understand the enculturation and embrainment of the self, we now turn toward neuroscience and what it tells us about the self.

Brain and Self

Cortical Midline Structures and the Self

Anterior midline regions like the ventromedial prefrontal cortex (VMPFC) and perigenual anterior cingulate cortex (PACC) as well as posterior regions such as the posterior cingulate cortex (PCC; as well as other regions inside and outside the cortical midline structure [CMS]) have been most consistently activated during self-related processing (see Araujo et al., 2013; Hu et al., 2016; Murray et al., 2012; Northoff & Bermpohl, 2004; Northoff et al., 2006; van der Meer et al., 2010). Though the VMPFC/PACC and PCC (and other midline regions like the dorsomedial prefrontal cortex, supragenual anterior cingulate cortex, and medial parietal cortex) are related to differential aspects of self-related processing, they are most often conjointly recruited and activated (in different degrees) during different degrees and aspects of self-related processing (Araujo et al., 2013, 2015; Hu et al., 2016; Lou et al., 2016; Murray et al., 2012, 2015; Northoff et al., 2006; van der Meer et al., 2010).

Moreover, data show significant neural overlap between the high resting state and self-related activity levels in the VMPFC/PACC and PCC. Several studies observed that

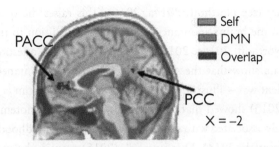

Figure 4.1. Rest-self overlap in default mode network (DMN).

self-specific stimuli did not induce activity change in VMPFC/PACC and PCC during task-evoked activity when compared to their resting state activity levels (D'Argembeau et al., 2005; Davey et al., 2016; Schneider et al., 2008; Whitfield-Gabrieli et al., 2011); such "rest-self overlap" (Bai et al., 2015) was further confirmed by a meta-analysis showing the VMPFC/PACC and PCC as overlapping regions during both resting state and self-related processing (Qin & Northoff, 2011; Figure 4.1).

Recent studies went even one step further, showing that resting state activity and pre-stimulus activity levels predict the degree of self-consciousness, that is, being aware of being a self with certain psychological features (Huang et al., 2016), or self-specificity assigned to subsequent stimuli (see Bai et al., 2015; Qin et al., 2016). If these findings of rest–self-prediction are further confirmed, one may suppose that the resting state itself encodes or contains some information about self-specificity in yet unclear ways. The assumptions of "rest–self overlap" may then be accompanied by the one of "rest–self-containment" (Northoff, 2016), which, reformulated in a cognitive way, amounts to "self-representation" (Sui & Humphreys, 2016, p. 4) or, in a more literary and less tendentious way, "reflection."

The central role of the resting state for mediating self-specificity is further supported by the assumption of a so-called self-network. Based on functional connectivity analysis of a large resting state data set, Murray and colleagues (2012, 2015) demonstrated that anterior midline regions like the PACC and VMPFC together with the anterior insula form a "self-network" in the resting state (see also Huang et al., 2016; Lou et al., 2010, 2016). The co-involvement of the PACC/VMPFC and insula in self-specificity is further supported by these regions' coactivation in task-related studies (see Enzi et al., 2009). The self-network must be distinguished from what they describe as "other network," which includes posterior midline regions like the PCC and the temporoparietal junction (TPJ) (Murray et al., 2015).

Experience Dependence of Cortical Midline Structures

How is it possible that the self is encompassed by the spontaneous activity of the brain (more specifically, the CMS)? The self must have been encoded into the brain's spontaneous activity (see Northoff, 2014a, 2016). This raises the question of how the self is encoded into the brain's spontaneous activity—in addition to the question about the neural code (Northoff, 2014a, 2016), we must address the question of how the self is encoded. The data show that the self is encoded into the spontaneous activity in an experience-dependent way—illustrated by a recent study by Duncan et al. (2015).

Duncan et al. (2015) showed that the CMS resting state's spatiotemporal structure in adulthood is strongly associated with subjects having incurred childhood trauma (Duncan et al., 2015; Nakao et al., 2013). Duncan et al. (2015) employed a measure of entropy, quantifying the degree to which one neuronal state at one specific time point, (e.g., t1) can predict neuronal states at subsequent time points (e.g., t2, t3, etc.), thus describing the degree of order or disorder in neural activity across time. In addition to entropy, they also measured the concentration of glutamate in the same specific core region, the PACC, during the CMS resting state. Adult subjects were investigated whose degree of early childhood trauma was measured with a standard questionnaire, that is, the Child Trauma Questionnaire (CTQ).

The first result was that Duncan et al. (2015) could observe a direct relationship between the degree of early childhood trauma and the entropy in the PACC: the higher the degree of early childhood trauma, the greater the entropy in the PACC resting state's spatiotemporal structure in adulthood (Duncan et al., 2015). This means that higher degrees of early childhood trauma disrupt the order—the degree of prediction of neural activity in the PACC across time—while lower degrees of early childhood trauma lead to a more ordered and stable (i.e., predictable) neural activity pattern in the PACC resting state in adulthood.

Most surprisingly, there was also a relationship between the biochemical and the psychological data. Specifically, the level of glutamate in the PACC was directly related to the degree of early traumatic childhood events: the higher the glutamate in the PACC, the lower the degree of early childhood traumatic life events. This suggests that the early traumatic life events are also encoded at the biochemical level of the brain's neural activity.

Spatiotemporal Memory of the World in the Brain's Spontaneous Activity

What do these data tell us about the brain and the temporal nature of its relation to the world, the world–brain relation (Northoff, 2016, 2018)? First and foremost, the data show the diachronic nature of the brain's spontaneous activity. It contains the traces of the events during early childhood even in adulthood, as Freud and many other early psychologists postulated. The brain's spontaneous or resting state activity can thus be characterized as truly temporal and, more specifically, diachronic with respect to the relation between world and brain (i.e., the world–brain relation).

Second, early life events are encoded in a spatiotemporal way into the brain's spontaneous activity—this is reflected in the measure applied, entropy, which is spatial and temporal at the same time as it describes the degree to which the spatial pattern of neural activity can be predicted across time. One can thus speak of the "spatiotemporal encoding" of experience into the brain's spontaneous activity, which in turn shapes and constitutes the self.

Third, such spatiotemporal encoding must be distinguished from "cognitive encoding." Briefly, cognitive encoding refers to the encoding of specific contents, such as the traumatic events themselves—this amounts to what is generally described as "memory." Specific memories were not investigated in the Duncan et al. study (2015), however. They did not measure task-evoked activity related to specific contents in memory. Instead, they measured only the resting state itself and its spatiotemporal structure. One may now want to distinguish between different memories.

Traditionally, episodic memory is considered as cognitive, in that it is based on specific contents such as the traumatic events themselves. Our data, and those of other researchers, suggest that there is yet another form of episodic memory, namely a noncognitive memory (Sadaghiani & Kleinschmidt, 2013) or, more precisely, "spatiotemporal memory" (Northoff, 2017), where events in the world (like the early childhood traumatic events) are encoded in terms of spatiotemporal features (rather than as cognitive contents). This remains distinct from procedural memory, which is not event related.

Fourth, such spatiotemporal memory does not encode and store contents—it is not declarative, content-based memory. Instead, spatiotemporal memory is probabilistic—it encodes and stores spatiotemporal patterns, based on the statistical frequency distributions that occur in the respective environmental context. Hence, rather than being content based and cognitive, spatiotemporal memory is stochastic, which can be measured statistically. The spontaneous activity's spatiotemporal structure is stochastic, and thereby can be closely related to the statistical frequency distributions in the environment (Northoff, 2014b). Such stochastically based encoding by the brain must necessarily encode the stochastic spatial and temporal differences of the various environmental events as they occur across time and space. Hence, the spatiotemporal nature of the brain's memory and its diachronic features go hand in hand with its essentially stochastic nature.

Why is such spatiotemporal memory relevant for the self? The data on rest–self-containment suggest that the brain's encoding of spatiotemporal memories constitutes the self—the self is the brain's spatiotemporal memory during its interaction with the world. The way in which the brain encodes spatiotemporally the life events in the world constitutes the self. The self is thus based on what conceptually I describe as the world–brain relation (Northoff, 2016, 2018), which can be described by its spatiotemporal structure and memory. The self can consequently also be characterized by spatiotemporal structure and memory, as based on the world–brain relation.

Spatiotemporal Nestedness and Embrainment/Enculturation
Temporal Nestedness of Brain and Self Within the World

Let us consider the empirical data as a whole. The temporal, and more specifically diachronic, nature of the world–brain relation may be manifested in multiple layers of different spatiotemporal scales—the world–brain relation is thus diachronic and spatiotemporal. The most basic and longest spatiotemporal scale is the one of evolution and history—present in the brain's overall organization, including the CMS as the cortical extension of the evolutionarily old limbic system (Northoff, 2011). A shorter time scale, the person's lifespan, is present and manifested in the encoding of early childhood life events into the spontaneous activity's spatiotemporal structure.

One can well assume that the brain's spontaneous activity encodes a wide range of different time scales, from extremely long to very short, for which the brain's own fluctuations in different frequency ranges may be instrumental (Northoff, 2014b). The presence and encoding of multiple time scales in and by the brain's spontaneous activity is empirically well reflected in its high degree of scale-free activity that measures the power relationship between different frequencies (He, 2011, 2014; Huang et al., 2015, 2016; Figure 4.2).

We can now extend these empirical observations within the brain's spontaneous activity itself to the more conceptual level of the world–brain relation. The world–brain relation encodes and is constituted by multiple time scales at one and the same time. Therefore, the world–brain relation can be characterized by what is empirically described as scale-free activity that is characterized by temporal nestedness (Northoff, 2016b, 2018). Temporal nestedness describes the integration and relation between different time scales and, more specifically, that one time scale mirrors and/or is self-similar to the others. That can be compared to the various Russian dolls that, despite their difference in spatial size, show all the same shape—temporal nestedness describes the same principle of self-similarity on the temporal level. Most interestingly, those very same scale-free properties of the spontaneous activity are directly related to—that is, predict—the degree of self-consciousness (Huang et al., 2016; Wolff et al., 2019). The self may thus reflect the temporal nestedness of the brain within the world (i.e., the world–brain relation) and thus the self-similarity between world and brain (Figures 4.3a and 4.3b).

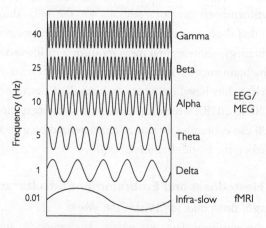

Figure 4.2. Temporal nestedness between different frequencies in the brain's neural activity.

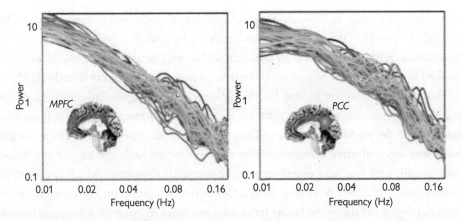

Figure 4.3a. Power spectra in two midline regions in different subjects.

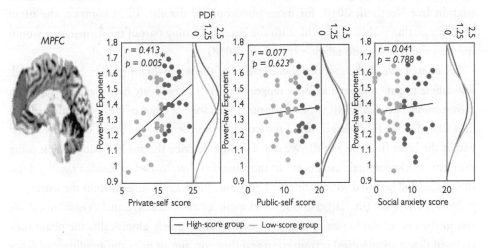

Figure 4.3b. Correlation between power law exponent (y-axis) and self-consciousness scale (x-axis).

In sum, the brain's spontaneous activity can be characterized as temporal, stochastic, and scale-free and as linking the brain in terms of temporal nestedness to its respective environmental context in terms of the world–brain relation. That very same world–brain relation provides the basis for the encoding of life events in terms of experience dependence, which constitutes the self. Therefore, the self may be characterized by temporal nestedness of the brain's spontaneous activity within its respective environmental context. Metaphorically speaking, the self is just a brain-based (temporally) nested and thus self-similar Russian doll within the spatiotemporally more extended world.

World–Brain Relation and Spatiotemporal Nestedness

What exactly do I mean by world–brain relation and nestedness? The world–brain relation is primarily spatiotemporal. More specifically, the world constructs its own time and space, the passage of time and the configuration of space, in a continuous way. One can therefore speak of the world's time and space. As we have seen earlier, the brain and its spontaneous activity construct their own time and space, "inner time and space," as distinguished from the world's "outer time and space," as one may want to say (Northoff, 2018).

This raises the question of how the brain's inner time and space are coordinated with the world's outer time and space. The brain can align and integrate its own inner time and space to the world's outer time and space. For instance, when we listen to music and move our legs and arms automatically in synchronization with the beat of the music, such entrainment has been described as temporospatial alignment, which is central for consciousness (Northoff & Huang, 2017). Conceived on a more conceptual level, temporospatial alignment allows the brain's inner time and space to integrate within and become part of the world's ongoing outer time and space. Since temporospatial alignment allows for spatiotemporal integration of the brain within the world, I speak of the world–brain relation (see Northoff, 2018, for more philosophical details). If, in contrast, the brain were integrating within the world, with the latter becoming part of the former, one would speak of the brain–world relation (Northoff, 2018).

Let us conceive of the spatiotemporal nature of the world–brain relation in more detail. The different spatiotemporal scales or ranges of world and brain are linked and integrated in their relation. Specifically, the smaller spatiotemporal scale or range of the brain is aligned and thus related to the much larger one of the world: the former (i.e., the brain) is thereby nested within the latter (i.e., the world). We can therefore describe the world–brain relation using the term "spatiotemporal nestedness." In the same way that, in a set of Russian nesting dolls, the smaller doll is nested within the next larger one, the brain is nested within the world.

How are different (i.e., larger and smaller) spatiotemporal scales related to each other? We saw in the case of the brain's spontaneous activity that, purely empirically, the phase (i.e., cycles of slower frequencies) is coupled to and thus contains or nests the amplitude of faster frequencies—this is described as cross-frequency coupling (Northoff & Huang, 2017). Taking the different frequencies together results in an elaborate temporal structure where slower frequencies contain or form a nest for the next faster one and so on—one can thus speak of a "slow–fast nestedness" or, better, "spatiotemporal nestedness" (see later), which indicates a certain directedness, that is, from slow to fast, in the brain's spontaneous activity.

I now assume an analogous slow–fast nestedness for spatiotemporal nestedness in the relation between world and brain (see later for details). The world's slower frequencies nest and contain the brain's faster frequencies—taken in purely spatiotemporal terms, the brain is thus nested and contained within the world. This is yet another reason I speak of the world–brain relation rather than the brain–world relation (see later).

World–Brain Relation and Mental Health

The concept of spatiotemporal nestedness can be understood in a purely neuronal sense remaining within the limits of the brain. It then describes how the smaller spatiotemporal scale or range of single stimuli or tasks is integrated, that is, nested, within the relatively larger spatiotemporal scale or range of the brain's spontaneous activity. Taken in this sense, spatiotemporal nestedness must be understood in a purely neuronal sense as confined to the boundaries of the brain.

I here extend the use of the same concept beyond the boundaries of the brain to the brain's relationship with the world. Spatiotemporal nestedness is now no longer purely neuronal, but neuroecological, referring to the neuroecological continuum between world and brain. That very same neuroecological continuum consists in the degree to which different spatiotemporal scales or ranges are linked and integrated and thus nested within each other: the better the brain's smaller spatiotemporal scale is integrated and thus nested within the much larger one of the world, the more continuous the neuroecological continuum is (Figure 4.4).

While being sketched as primarily conceptual (and ontological; Northoff, 2018), the world–brain relation carries major clinical implications. Schizophrenic patients, for instance, suffer from disruption in their world–brain relation—this can be measured by lack of synchronization (as mediated by what can be measured as phase locking or entrainment) of their brain's neural activity with the temporal structure of their respective environment context. The brain's ability to synchronize with its environmental context and thus constitute a world–brain relation may be central when subjects change cultural context. If, for instance, subjects move from east to west while at the same time being prone to labile or unstable synchronization of their brain's neural activity with its novel environmental context, the risk for psychosis among these immigrants may increase. That remains speculative at this point, though, requiring specific empirical testing.

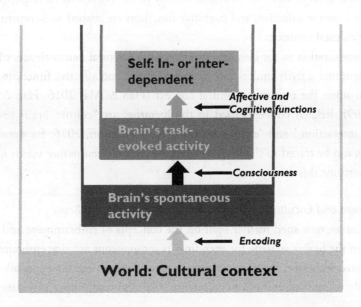

Figure 4.4. Spatiotemporal nestedness of self and brain within the world and its cultural context.

What this example makes clear is that the world–brain relation, despite being a novel and abstract concept, carries major implications for our understanding of the brain's relation to the world and mental health. Especially, the world–brain relation opens the door for a more comprehensive and extended understanding of the spatiotemporal and neuroecological nature of psychopathological symptoms. Psychopathological symptoms, as in schizophrenia and depression, can be conceived as spatiotemporal alterations of the brain's spontaneous activity and its spatiotemporal structure—one can therefore also speak of "spatiotemporal psychopathology" (Northoff, 2016, 2017). Importantly, as the spontaneous activity's spatiotemporal structure extends beyond the brain's boundaries to the respective environmental context, psychopathological symptoms are not only spatiotemporal but also neuroecological (rather than merely neuronal). As culture provides and is part of specific ecological contexts, the neuroecological characterization of psychopathological symptoms is well in line with the cultural effects on mental health (see Scott, "The Cross-National Epidemiology of Mental Health Disorders," this volume).

Embrainment and Enculturation: Brain and Self

How does the spatiotemporal nestedness of the brain within the world stand in relation to the concepts of embrainment and enculturation? Let us briefly define the concepts of embrainment and enculturation.

Briefly, taken in a standard way, the concept of embrainment denotes the encoding of social and cultural contexts by the brain's neuronal activity. Embrainment in this sense, for instance, is manifested in the neuronal differences related to the independent versus the interdependent self (Han & Ma, 2016; Han & Northoff, 2009; Han et al., 2013), while enculturation denotes how the neuronal activity of the brain and its respectively associated sensory, motor, affective, and cognitive functions are shaped and constituted by the respective cultural contexts.

Such enculturation is, for instance, investigated in cultural neuroscience, which shows that the neuronal activity underlying various cognitive and affective functions is strongly dependent upon the respective cultural context (Han & Ma, 2016; Han & Northoff, 2008, 2009). Related concepts used in the literature are "culture–brain nexus," "neuroculture interaction," and "encultured brain" (see Northoff, 2016, for details), which, ultimately, can be traced to the long-standing debate between nature versus nurture and tries to overcome this distinction.

Embrainment and Enculturation: Self-Similarity of Culture and Brain

How can we now shed further light on the concepts of embrainment and enculturation? Given the brain's strategy for encoding its spontaneous activity, embrainment must be considered scale-free; that is, it operates across different time (and spatial) scales. This is especially relevant in cultural neuroscience. Cultural traditions and values have been shaped over thousands of years, thus requiring a rather long-time scale. They are nevertheless entirely present at each moment of time, as, for instance, in our present life span. Importantly, we assume that cultural values are present across time in a more or less self-similar and thus temporally nested way, given that scale-free properties and their spatiotemporal nestedness are ubiquitous in nature and culture and thus in the world in general (He et al., 2010).

This is the moment where cultural context and brain with its spontaneous activity converge. The empirical data, as described earlier, show that the brain, being part of the world, is also characterized by scale-free properties and spatiotemporal nestedness (and consequently our self is too).

Culture and brain may thus be connected intrinsically with each other in terms of self-similarity as manifested in spatiotemporal nestedness, which then accounts for what is described as embrainment. Embrainment of cultural values may thus first and foremost be manifested in the brain's spontaneous activity, which, in a second step, serves as the basis for affective and cognitive functions. Since the spontaneous activity encodes cultural values in a spatiotemporal and self-similar way, the subsequent affective and cognitive function, being based on the spontaneous activity, are affected and shaped by the cultural values in an almost automatic way, that is, by default.

Embrainment and Enculturation: Convergence and Intertwining

What does this imply for the determination of the relationship between embrainment and enculturation? I propose that embrainment and enculturation are necessarily connected with each other. The empirical data suggest that embrainment, the impact of the brain on culture, is closely coupled with enculturation, which describes the impact of culture on the brain's neuronal activity. Why is there such an intrinsic or necessary connection between embrainment and enculturation? The data show that our brain and its spontaneous activity are spatiotemporally nested within the respective cultural context and thus the world. Due to such spatiotemporal nestedness, world/culture and brain are necessarily connected with each other, which I described as the world–brain relation in previous works (Northoff, 2016, 2018).

Such necessary connection between world/culture and brain, that is, the world–brain relation, in turn, makes possible a bidirectional relationship between world/culture and brain—that is, from world/culture to brain (i.e., enculturation), and from brain to world (i.e., embrainment). Therefore, embrainment does not happen without enculturation and related affective and cognitive functions. Conversely, enculturation cannot occur without embrainment and associated affective and cognitive functions. Embrainment and enculturation are thus distinct aspects of one and the same underlying process, the world–brain relation, which, ultimately, can be traced to the self as relational self and its underlying self-related processing.

Embrainment/Enculturation and Our Mental Life

Embrainment and Enculturation of Self and Music

Such view of embrainment carries major empirical and conceptual implications. Let us start with the empirical implications.

Empirically, we may want to investigate the impact of different cultural contexts on the brain's spontaneous activity with the various kinds of temporal (and spatial) measures. One would, for instance, expect that the scale-free properties of spontaneous activity would differ between Eastern and Western cultural contexts, which, psychologically, may be closely related to the self and, more specifically, its degrees of independence versus interdependence. Given that our previous findings show Western subjects' self-consciousness to be predicted by their spontaneous activity's scale-free properties (Huang et al., 2016; Wolff et al., 2019), one would expect the same to occur in Eastern subjects. Moreover, given the presently assumed spatiotemporal nestedness between culture/world and brain (i.e., world–brain relation), one would expect that the degree of scale-free properties (i.e., the exact shape of the power law curve in the power spectrum in the CMS) would differ between Eastern and Western subjects' sense of self (i.e., self-consciousness). Such investigation remains to be done, however.

Yet another empirical example is music, as thematized in the cultural distance hypothesis (CDH) by Demorest and Morrison (2016). The CDH claims that "the degree to which the music of any two cultures differ in the statistical patterns of pitch and rhythm will predict how well a person from one of the cultures can process the music of the other" (Demorest & Morrison, 2016, p. 189). As pointed out previously, scale-free activity and thus self-similarity and spatiotemporal nestedness are stochastically based, which puts them on the same basis as the CDH, which presupposes music to be stochastically based, as it is further supported by its scale-free properties (He et al., 2010). One may consequently assume that the cultural differences in affective and cognitive recruitment and associated neural activity during music may be based on differences in the spontaneous activity's scale-free properties.

Specifically, we expect that the scale-free properties of spontaneous activity are more closely matched with the scale-free properties of the music in the respective cultural context: the more similar the scale-free properties are between the brain's spontaneous activity and music, the better the music will be processed, the more the music will be perceived as self-related, and the more affective and cognitive functions will be recruited. If, in contrast, there is a difference or distance in the scale-free properties between music and the brain, the person may not perceive the music as self-related but strange and non-self-related, and consequently not recruit affective and cognitive functions to the same degree. Accordingly, what Demorest and Morrison (2016) describe as "cultural distance" with respect to music may ultimately be traced down to the degree of statistically and scale-free matching between music and the brain's spontaneous activity, that is, their statistically based scale-free distance or difference.

Concept of Self: Relational and Spatiotemporal

We started the chapter with the concept of self. What does embrainment and enculturation imply for our concept of self? First and foremost, the presence of embrainment and enculturation means that we cannot consider the self to be independent of its respective social and cultural context. The self is thus based on and shaped by the interaction between culture and brain, which we determined to be spatiotemporal, stochastic, and scale-free. If so, the concept of self itself may be described in these terms, that is, as spatiotemporal, stochastic, and scale-free.

The spatiotemporal, stochastic, and scale-free nature of the self situates it neatly between culture (i.e., world) and brain. Importantly, the spatiotemporal, stochastic, and scale-free features constitute or construct a spatiotemporal structure or organization that virtually spans the divides between world, body, and brain. Conceptually, the self may thus be considered a virtual spatiotemporal structure—the self concerns the virtual, that is, spatiotemporal, scale-free, and stochastic, relation between world and brain. Being intrinsically relational, the self signifies the presence of that relation across time and thus its temporal continuity. That is well compatible with the self being closely related to personal identity that describes the temporal continuity of the self across time—temporal continuity of the spatiotemporal, scale-free, and stochastic and culturally sensitive world–brain relation may thus transform on the mental level into the temporal continuity of our self and its personal identity.

Why and how is the relational characterization of the self in this sense relevant for cultural neuroscience? The two culturally differing concepts of self, that is interdependent versus independent self, may be regarded as two possible constellations of the relational self as virtually spanning between world and brain. Independent and interdependent self may thus be two manifestations of one and the same underlying relation (i.e., world–brain relation) that may vary according to the respective cultural context.

This carries major empirical implications. Taken in such a sense, independent and interdependent selves should be characterized by different forms and degrees of spatiotemporal nestedness, which should be manifested in different scale-free properties of the brain's spontaneous activity. The interdependent self is more dependent upon its respective cultural and social context. One would expect the interdependent self to be strongly coupled to those larger and slower-frequency spectra of the respective cultural and social context.

The independent self, in contrast, is more focused on its self and, put empirically, its own frequencies and less on those of its respective cultural and social context. Now, the very slow frequencies of the brain may be not as much needed anymore so that the power is more shifted toward the faster frequencies within the brain. One would consequently expect a less steep power spectrum with lower degrees of scale-free activity in the brain's spontaneous activity in Western subjects that show a strong independent (rather than interdependent) self.

Finally, there are also ethical considerations to consider. There are novel stimulation techniques like deep brain stimulation (DBS) and transcranial magnetic stimulation (TMS) for modulating remedying an altered sense of self (Northoff, 2017). These techniques supposedly modulate the spontaneous activity's spatiotemporal structure and subsequently its encoded information related to the self. However, purely neuronal intervention may be insufficient if the corresponding environmental or cultural context is not properly adapted. Put in a more abstract way, the therapy of the self should not be purely neuronal but better neuroecologically or, more specifically, neuroculturally.

Accordingly, a neurocultural therapy is ethically more proper and appropriate than a purely neuronal therapy as the latter disregards the neuroecological nature of our brain. That also implies that, depending on the respective cultural contexts, one and the same neuronal intervention like DBS or TMS may be applied in different frequency ranges to match the spatiotemporal features of both brain and cultural context. Neuronal or biological intervention may thus be culturally specified and tailored in the same way that we need to strive for individualization of the degree or strength of TMS and/or DBS. Such neurocultural tailoring of biological or neuronal intervention remains speculative at this point, however.

Conclusion

We have discussed the mechanisms of embrainment and enculturation for which we took the self as a paradigmatic example. The self is the basis of our mental health. Different concepts of self in different cultures strongly determine subjects' mental health in different cultures. Moving one's own culturally embedded self into a different culture that portrays and lives a different concept of self can especially impact the subject's mental health, leading to the often-described experience of anomie. To support such cultural appropriations of self, we need to better understand how the self is embrained and which mechanisms are underlying such embrainment of self.

Based on various empirical data, I here suggest spatiotemporal, scale-free, and stochastic embrainment of culture into the brain and, more specifically, its spontaneous activity as featured by its spatiotemporal structure and organization. Such embrainment, in turn, constitutes our self, which therefore, conceptually, can be described as relational, spatiotemporal, scale-free, and stochastic. As our spontaneous activity provides the basis for subsequent affective and cognitive functions, the latter cannot avoid being culturally shaped (i.e., enculturation).

Hence, embrainment and enculturation are two distinct features of one and the same underlying process, the self as relational or social self as mediated by self-related processing. Most importantly, the empirical data show that such intrinsic coupling between embrainment and enculturation (in the gestalt of the self as relational self) occurs by default, as our brain's spontaneous activity is very much tuned to encode its own relationship to its respective cultural and social context. We and our selves are, thus, embrained and encultured by default.

The default character of embrainment and enculturation renders it rather likely that there is a genetic basis for the way the spontaneous activity can develop and construct its spatiotemporal structure (see Greenfield and Vasquez-Salgado, "Sociocultural Developmental Neuroscience," this volume). In that case, one would assume that, for instance, the manifestations of embrainment and enculturation in the spontaneous activity's spatiotemporal structure are inherited between generations. One would then quasi inherit a certain cultural imprinting in one's brain and its spatiotemporal structure from the parents—that could account for intergenerational trauma. Like intrasubject trauma (see Duncan et al., 2015), intergenerational trauma may then be encoded in a spatiotemporal way into the brain's spontaneous activity. The difference between intrasubject and intergenerational trauma would then consist only in the time scale while they would share their spatiotemporal character. This remains rather speculative at this point, though.

The relational and spatiotemporal embrainment of self carries major implications not only for our understanding of the brain in general but also for mental features and their intrinsic cultural dependence. This suggests future empirical investigation as stated in various hypotheses. Moreover, as our self is central for our mental health, its investigation may shed a novel light on global mental health in an age where people including their selves move across the globe—this probes the spontaneous activity's plasticity of its spatiotemporal structure in response to changing cultural contexts (see Goh, "Acculturation by Plasticity and Stability in Neural Processes: Considerations for Global Mental Health," this volume).

We may need to analyze the spatiotemporal features (e.g., spatiotemporal stochastics) of cultural contexts and link them to the subjects' brains with their spontaneous activity's spatiotemporal structure. If cultural adaptation problems occur, resulting in mental health issues (see Scott, "The Cross-National Epidemiology of Mental Health Disorders," this volume), one would expect major misfit or mismatch between the spatiotemporal features of cultural context and the brain's spontaneous activity. These stochastic misfits or mismatches may then be treated by specific training as in music therapy or brain stimulation in an individualized and context-specific way. Accordingly, the here-suggested approach opens the door for the development of completely novel approaches for both prevention and treatment, for example, spatiotemporal intervention or therapy that is intrinsically neurocultural (rather than either exclusively neuronal or cultural). That will also enable us to screen subjects with their brain's spontaneous activity and its scale-free property to detect risk factors of difficulties in cultural adaptation and appropriation of their self to the novel cultural context.

Open Questions and Knowledge Gaps

- Is the self primarily spatiotemporal rather than cognitive?
- Is our brain adapted to and does it integrate culture primarily in a spatiotemporal rather than an affective or cognitive way?

- How can we define and investigate the spontaneous activity's spatiotemporal structure in a more specific and detailed way—what kind of measures do we need to specifically account for the structure and relation?
- How can we better define and operationalize the neuroecological and neurocultural mechanisms as implied by the world–brain relation? This is necessary not only on a conceptual level but also on a more empirical level as mental disorders can be characterized by disruptions in the neuroecological and neurocultural nature of their mental functions, such as sense of self and consciousness.
- What kind of neurocultural therapies with coordination between neuronal and cultural interventions can we develop in the future to better treat mental disorders? This chapter suggests that such neurocultural coordination must be spatiotemporal, but the details of this remain unclear at this point in time.

Acknowledgment

I acknowledge financial support from CIHR (Canada) and NSF (China). Three anonymous reviewers made excellent and very helpful suggestions for improving the text, for which I am grateful.

References

Araujo, H. F., Kaplan, J., & Damasio, A. (2013). Cortical midline structures and autobiographical-self processes: An activation-likelihood estimation meta-analysis. *Frontiers in Humam Neuroscience, 7*, 548. doi:10.3389/fnhum.2013.00548

Araujo, H. F., Kaplan, J., Damasio, H., & Damasio, A. (2015). Neural correlates of different self domains. *Brain and Behavior, 5*(12), e00409. doi:10.1002/brb3.409

Bai, Y., et al. (2015). Pre-stimulus alpha power during self-specific processing is predicted by medial prefrontal cortical glutamate. A combined EEG-MRS study. *Society for Neuroscience, 11*(3), 249–263. doi:10.1080/17470919.2015.1072582

Churchland, P. S. (2002). Self-representation in nervous systems. *Science, 296*(5566), 308–310. doi:10.1126/science.1070564

D'Argembeau, A. Collette, F., Van der Linden, M., Laureys, S., Del Fiore, G., Degueldre, C., Luxen, A., & Salmon, E. (2005). Self-referential reflective activity and its relationship with rest: A PET study. *Neuroimage, 25*(2), 616–624.

Davey, C. G., Pujol, J., & Harrison, B. J. (2016). Mapping the self in the brain's default mode network. *Neuroimage, 132*, 390–397. doi: 10.1016/j.neuroimage.2016.02.022.

Demorest, S. M., & Morrison, S. J. (2016). Quantifying culture: The cultural distance hypothesis of melodic expectancy. In J. Y. Chiao, C. Li, R. Seligman, & R. Turner (Eds.), *The Oxford handbook of cultural neuroscience* (pp. 189–197). Oxford University Press.

Duncan, N. W., Hayes, D., Wiebking, C., & Northoff, G. (2015). Early traumatic life experiences are related to perigenual anterior cingulate entropy and glutamate. *Human Brain Mapping, 204*, 506–510.

Enzi, B., et al. (2009). Is our self nothing but reward? Neuronal overlap and distinction between reward and personal relevance and its relation to human personality. *PLoS One, 4*(12), e8429.

Frings, C., & Wentura, D. (2014). *Self-prioritization processes in action and perception. Journal of Experimental Psychology: Human Perception and Performance, 40*(5), 1737–1740. doi: 10.1037/a0037376

Han, S., & Ma, Y. (2016). Cultural neuroscience studies of self-reflection. In J. Y. Chiao, C. Li, R. Seligman, & R. Turner (Eds.), *The Oxford handbook of cultural neuroscience* (pp. 197–209). Oxford University Press.

Han, S., & Northoff, G. (2008). Culture-sensitive neural substrates of human cognition: A transcultural neu-roimaging approach. *Nature Reviews Neuroscience, 9*(8), 646–654. doi:10.1038/nrn2456

Han, S., & Northoff, G. (2009). Understanding the self: A cultural neuroscience approach. *Progress in Brain Research, 178*, 203–212. doi:10.1016/S0079-6123(09)17814-7

Han, S., Northoff, G., Vogeley, K., Wexler, B. E., Kitayama, S., & Varnum, M. E. (2013). A cultural neuro-science approach to the biosocial nature of the human brain. *Annual Review of Psychology, 64*, 335–359. doi:10.1146/annurev-psych-071112-054629

He, B. J. (2011). Scale-free properties of the functional magnetic resonance imaging signal during rest and task. *Journal of Neuroscience, 31*(39), 13786–13795.

He, B. J. (2014). Scale-free brain activity: Past, present, and future. *Trends in Cognitive Science, 18*(9), 480–487.

He, B. J., Zempel, J. M., Snyder, A. Z., & Raichle, M. E. (2010). The temporal structures and functional sig-nificance of scale-free brain activity. *Neuron, 66*(3), 353–369.

Hiltunen, T., Kantola, J., Abou Elseoud, A., Lepola, P., Suominen, K., Starck, T., Nikkinen, J., Remes, J., Tervonen, O., Palva, S., Kiviniemi, V., & Palva, J. M. (2014). Infra-slow EEG fluctuations are corre-lated with resting-state network dynamics in fMRI. *Journal of Neuroscience, 34*(2), 356–362. doi:10.1523/JNEUROSCI.0276-13.2014

Hu, C., Di, X., Eickhoff, S. B., Zhang, M., Peng, K., Guo, H., & Sui, J. (2016). Distinct and common aspects of physical and psychological self-representation in the brain: A meta-analysis of self-bias in facial and self-referential judgements. *Neuroscience and Biobehavioral Reviews, 61*, 197–207. doi:10.1016/j.neubiorev.2015.12.003

Huang, Z., Obara, N., Davis, H. H., 4th, Pokorny, J., & Northoff, G. (2016). The temporal structure of resting-state brain activity in the medial prefrontal cortex predicts self-consciousness. *Neuropsychologia, 82*, 161–170. doi:10.1016/j.neuropsychologia.2016.01.025

Huang, Z., Zhang, J., Longtin, A., Dumont, G., Duncan, N. W., Pokorny, J., Qin, P., Dai, R., Ferri, F., Weng, X., & Northoff, G. (2015). Is there a nonadditive interaction between spontaneous and evoked activity? Phase-dependence and its relation to the temporal structure of scale-free brain activity. *Cerebral Cortex, 27*(2), 1037–1059. doi:10.1093/cercor/bhv288

Lou, H. C., Changeux, J. P., & Rosenstand, A. (2016). Towards a cognitive neuroscience of self-awareness. *Neuroscience and Biobehavioral Reviews*, 2016 Apr 11. pii: S0149-7634(16)30041-0. doi:10.1016/j.neubiorev.2016.04.004

Lou, H. C., Gross, J., Biermann-Ruben-K, Kjaer, T.W., & Schnitzler, A. (2010). Coherence in consciousness: paralimbic gamma synchrony of self-reference links conscious experiences. *Human Brain Mapping, 31*(2), 185–192.

Markus, H., & Kitayama, S. (1991). Culture and the self: Implications for cognition, emotion, and motiva-tion. *Psychological Review, 98*(2), 224–253.

Markus, H., & Kitayama, S. (2003). Culture, self, and the reality of the social. *Psychological Inquiry, 14*(3/4), 277–283.

Metzinger, T. (2003). *Being no one: The self-model theory of subjectivity*. MIT Press.

Murray, R. J., Debbané, M., Fox, P. T., Bzdok, D., & Eickhoff, S. B. (2015). Functional connectivity map-ping of regions associated with self- and other-processing. *Human Brain Mapping, 36*(4), 1304–1324. doi:10.1002/hbm.22703

Murray, R. J., Schaer, M., & Debbané, M. (2012). Degrees of separation: A quantitative neuroimaging meta-analysis investigating self-specificity and shared neural activation between self- and other-reflection. *Neuroscience and Biobehavioral Review, 36*(3), 1043–1059. doi:10.1016/j.neubiorev.2011.12.013

Nakao, T., et al. (2013). Resting-state EEG power predicts conflict-related brain activity in internally guided but not in externally guided decision-making. *Neuroimage, 66*, 9–21.

Northoff, G. (2011). Self and brain: What is self-related processing? *Trends in Cognitive Science, 15*(5), 186–187; author reply 187–188. doi:10.1016/j.tics.2011.03.001

Northoff, G. (2014a). *Unlocking the brain*. Vol I: *Coding*. Oxford University Press.

Northoff, G. (2014b). *Unlocking the brain*. Vol II: *Consciousness*. Oxford University Press.

Northoff, G. (2016). Cultural neuroscience and neurophilosophy: Does the neural code allow for the brain's enculturation? In J. Y. Chiao, C. Li, R. Seligman, & R. Turner (Eds.), *The Oxford handbook of cultural neu-roscience* (pp. 21–41). Oxford University Press.

Northoff, G. (2017). Personal identity and cortical midline structure (CMS): Do temporal features of CMS neural activity transform into "self-continuity"? *Psychological Inquiry, 28*(2–3), 122–131.

Northoff, G. & Huang, Z. (2017). How do the brain's time and space mediate consciousness and its different dimensions: Temporo-spatial theory of consciousness (TTC). *Neuroscience and Biobehavioral Review, 80,* 630–645.

Northoff, G. (2018). *The spontaneous brain. From the mind-body problem to the world-brain problem.* MIT Press.

Northoff, G., & Bermpohl, F. (2004). Cortical midline structures and the self. *Trends in Cognitive Sciences, 8*(3):102–107. doi: 10.1016/j.tics.2004.01.004

Northoff, G., Heinzel, A., de Greck, M., Bermpohl, F., Dobrowolny, H., & Panksepp, J. (2006). Self-referential processing in our brain—A meta-analysis of imaging studies on the self. *Neuroimage, 31*(1), 440–457.

Pfeiffer, U. J., Timmermans, B., Vogeley, K., Frith, C. D., & Schilbach, L. (2013). Towards a neuroscience of social interaction. *Frontiers in Human Neuroscience, 7,* 22. doi:10.3389/fnhum.2013.00022

Qin, P., Grimm, S., Duncan, N. W., Fan, Y., Huang, Z., Lane, T., Weng, X., Bajbouj, M., & Northoff, G. (2016). Spontaneous activity in default-mode network predicts ascription of self-relatedness to stimuli. *Social Cognitve and Affective Neuroscience, 11*(4), 693–702. doi:10.1093/scan/nsw008

Qin, P., & Northoff, G. (2011). How is our self related to midline regions and the default-mode network? *Neuroimage, 57*(3), 1221–1233.

Sadaghiani, S. & Kleinschmidt, A. (2013). Functional interactions between intrinsic brain activity and behavior. *Neuroimage, 80,* 379–386.

Schneider, F., et al. (2008). The resting brain and our self: Self-relatedness modulates resting state neural activity in cortical midline structures. *Neuroscience, 157*(1), 120–131.

Sui, J., & Humphreys, G. W. (2015). The integrative self: How self-reference integrates perception and memory. *Trends in Cognitive Science, 19*(12), 719–728. doi:10.1016/j.tics.2015.08.015

Sui, J. & Humphreys, G.W. (2016). Introduction to special issue: social attention in mind and brain. *Cognitive Neuroscience, 7*(1–4), 1–4.

van der Meer, L., Costafreda, S., Aleman, A., & David, A. S. (2010). Self-reflection and the brain: A theoretical review and meta-analysis of neuroimaging studies with implications for schizophrenia. *Neuroscience and Biobehavioral Reviews, 34*(6) 935–946. doi:10.1016/j.neubiorev.2009.12.004

Whitfield-Gabrieli, S., et al. (2011). Associations and dissociations between default and self-reference networks in the human brain. *Neuroimage, 55*(1), 225–232.

Wolff, A., Di Giovanni, D. A., Gómez-Pilar, J., Nakao, T., Huang, Z., Longtin, A., & Northoff, G. (2019). The temporal signature of self: Temporal measures of resting-state EEG predict self-consciousness. *Human Brain Mapping, 40*(3), 789–803. doi: 10.1002/hbm.24412.

Cultural Neuroscience

Joan Y. Chiao, Yoko Mano, Zhang Li, Genna M. Bebko, Katherine D. Blizinsky, *and*
Robert Turner

Abstract

Cultural neuroscience is a field of study that examines the bidirectional influences of
cultural and biological factors on the brain and behavior, including mental processes.
Research in cultural neuroscience comprises theoretical and methodological approaches
to understanding how cultural and biological factors affect the etiology of behavior.
Empirical programs in cultural neuroscience seek to determine the root causes and
neurobiological mechanisms underlying the etiology of complex behavior across cultures,
including mental, neurological, and substance abuse (MNS) disorders. This chapter
reviews theoretical, methodological, and empirical advances in cultural neuroscience and
its implications for the discovery of cures and development of effective interventions for
MNS disorders in global mental health.

Key Words: cultural neuroscience, dual inheritance theory, MNS disorders, population
health disparities, global mental health

Global Mental Health

Mental, neurological, and substance abuse (MNS) disorders make up approximately
13% of the global burden of disease (Collins et al., 2011). In 2010, MNS disorders
accounted for approximately 7.4% of global disability-adjusted life-years (DALYs) and
0.5% of global years of life lost to premature mortality (YLLs), and were a leading cause
of global years lived with disability (YLDs; Whiteford et al., 2013). Discovery of cures and
preventions for MNS disorders is necessary to reduce the global burden of disease and to
enhance the understanding of the molecular and cellular mechanisms of the human brain.
The Grand Challenges in Global Mental Health Initiative has identified several research
priorities for the scientific discovery of cures to MNS disorders. The identification of root
causes, risks, and preventative factors of MNS disorders across the life course is a chief
research priority in global mental health.

Research in cultural neuroscience is an evidence-based resource for the scientific discovery of cures, preventions, and interventions in global mental health (Chiao et al., 2017).
Theoretical, methodological, and empirical approaches in cultural neuroscience broaden

the understanding of multilevel mechanisms of the human brain across cultures and time scales. Research in cultural neuroscience aims to the identify biomarkers of MNS disorders throughout the life course across cultures. Cultural neuroscience provides a dimensional approach to the investigation of the etiology of mental health across cultures.

The goal of this chapter is to provide a review of research approaches in cultural neuroscience and discussion of evidence-based research in cultural neuroscience for global mental health. Theoretical approaches in cultural neuroscience provide conceptual frameworks and fundamental principles of cultural and neurobiological explanations of behavior. Methodological approaches in cultural neuroscience consist of standard paradigms that allow for systematic testing of hypotheses through observation and measurement. Empirical approaches in cultural neuroscience include research programs that test specific aspects of conceptual frameworks and fundamental principles. Building research capacity advances international cooperation for the generation of discovery and delivery science in cultural neuroscience and global mental health.

Cultural Neuroscience

Cultural neuroscience addresses universality and cultural differences in human behavior across multiple levels of analysis. Research in cultural neuroscience provides theoretical, methodological, and empirical approaches to the mutually interactive constitution of culture and biology (Chiao & Ambady, 2007). The influence of culture on cognition emerges throughout the life course (D. C. Park & Gutchess, 2002). Cultural approaches to the study of the aging brain illustrate standard paradigms for the study of cognition and aging across cultural settings. Transcultural neuroimaging represents an empirical approach for advancing the study of cultural differences in human cognition with modern neuroimaging techniques (Han & Northoff, 2008). The study of cultural differences in human cognition with neuroimaging reflects the indirect measurement of brain activity for the test of functional relations of brain and behavior across cultural settings.

The neurocultural interaction model serves as a theoretical construct that posits a casual pathway of the influences of cultural and biological adaptations on behavior (Kitayama & Uskul, 2011). The neurocultural interaction model consists of a causal pathway that identifies cultural adaptations as antecedents of neurobiological adaptations that contribute to reproductive success. The framework in cultural neuroscience suggests a causal model for studying how biology and cultural interact to influence behavior (Kim & Sasaki, 2014). The framework in cultural neuroscience provides an interactive model of cultural antecedents that influence genetic and neural processes to produce underlying physiological and psychological responses and behavior.

Theoretical Foundations

Theoretical foundations in cultural neuroscience postulate how cultural and neurobiological systems produce and regulate adaptive behavior. Multilevel theoretical approaches in cultural neuroscience facilitate systematic discovery of frameworks, models, and paradigms that provide parsimonious explanation within cultural and neurobiological systems of behavior. Theoretical frameworks provide schematic descriptions of causal pathways to determine and predict behavioral outcomes. Environmental and developmental approaches serve as antecedents and consequences in theoretical frameworks of cultural and neurobiological systems of behavior. Theoretical approaches in cultural neuroscience investigate multilevel pathways of behavior across distinct time scales, ranging from situational to evolutionary periods. Interactions of cultural and neurobiological systems that occur across short-term and long-term time scales reflect the static and dynamic characteristics of the range of phenomena in the field of cultural neuroscience (Chiao et al., 2013).

Dual Inheritance Theory

Dual inheritance theory proposes that adaptive behavior results from the complementary processes of natural selection and cultural niche construction (Laland et al., 2000). In processes of natural selection, environmental pressures exert influence on specific characteristics of the organism. Cultural niche construction refers to the processes by which organisms change and construct their environment to adapt to ecological conditions. Due to geographic variation in ecological conditions, cultural systems that provide a set of characteristics as adaptation are created and maintained within the social and physical environment.

Coevolutionary theory reflects the interaction of cultural and biological factors in the production of complex behavior (Durham, 1991). Gene–culture coevolutionary models explain cultural adaptations resulting from genetic selection. Culture–gene coevolutionary models assert that genetic adaptations arise through dynamic and cumulative processes of cultural evolution. In culture–gene coevolutionary models, cultural selection alters genetic mechanisms and interactions of culture and genes in the populations. Dual inheritance theory posits that cultural and biological inheritance mutually affect mental and neurobiological architecture to produce and regulate adaptive behavior. Culture and neurobiological systems specialize for adaptive function as a product of genetic and cultural transmission (Boyd & Richerson, 1985; Henrich & McElreath, 2007). Because cultural systems evolve more rapidly relative to genes, the construction of novel environments can create novel selection pressures for genes. Cultural selection also can produce variation in adaptive behavior that is independent of genetic selection, resulting in culturally learned capacities.

Gene–culture coevolutionary theory postulates how cultural adaptations occur from genetic selection. One classic example of coevolutionary theory is gene–culture coevolution of lactose tolerance. In Northern Central Europe, the genetic capacity for milk production in cattle geographically coevolved with genetic and societal tolerance for dairy culture in humans (Beja-Pereira et al., 2003). The geographic prevalence of genes of milk-producing cattle covaries with the geographic prevalence of genes of lactose-tolerant humans. These findings show that human farming practices demonstrate genetic and cultural selection in humans and domesticated animals.

Culture–gene coevolutionary theory posits how genetic adaptations arise from cultural selection. Another example of coevolutionary theory is culture–gene coevolution of individualism–collectivism and the serotonin transporter gene (Chiao & Blizinsky, 2010). Across nations, geographic prevalence of pathogens has led to the geographic prevalence of genetic and cultural selection of collectivistic culture. Cultural collectivism serves an "anti-pathogen" defense, protecting geographic regions from the dispersion of disease-causing pathogens. Across nations, the geographic prevalence of collectivistic cultures has led to reduced prevalence of specific mental health disorders. Cultural collectivism also serves an "anti-psychopathology" defense, protecting geographic regions from prevalence of mental health disorders. Collectivistic social norms, including conformity and hierarchy preference, promote social and health behaviors that prevent disease and mental health disorders.

Coevolutionary theory postulates that genetic and cultural selection lead to adaptive behavior. Through genetic and cultural selection, patterns of neurotransmission tune neural circuitry to encode algorithms and processes in a culture-specific manner. Cultural thinking styles shape neurobiological architecture to respond to and regulate the social and physical environment (Cheon et al., 2018). Cultural and genetic expression adapts to selection pressures, allowing for specialization of mental and neural mechanisms of behavior. Cultural and genetic expression reflects the dynamic aspects of cultural and biological systems that change in response to environmental and ecological demands, such as natural and man-made threats. Throughout evolutionary history, cultural and biological systems have interacted to mutually influence and reinforce adaptive mechanisms of the mind, brain, and behavior.

Cumulative Cultural Evolution

Cumulative cultural evolution reflects the enhancement of cultural processes and capacities due to the accumulation of capacities for cultural adaptation. Cultural evolution may occur more rapidly relative to genetic evolution due to accumulation of cultural traits among nongenetically related individuals through processes of social learning (Boyd & Richerson, 1985; Mesoudi, 2009). The transmission of cultural capacities through social learning allows for the persistence and transfer of cultural information from the model to the nongenetically related learner or a group of learners. The successful transmission of cultural knowledge from model to learner enhances the prestige and knowledge of the model and learners as a group. Cultural adaptations may further spread across the population due to conformity and popularity of cultural thought and processes of population thinking. The frequency of cultural thought within the population may be heightened through social transmission of cultural knowledge due to enhanced cultural contact and positive social relations among ethnic groups. Cultural group selection reflects the adaptation of cultural traits through the cooperation and cohesion of the group. The cohesion of the cultural group for specific cultural knowledge and traits allows for selection of cultural adaptations that strengthen an ingroup advantage for cultural knowledge and representations of the group.

Neurobiological systems of social learning provide mechanisms for processes of cumulative cultural evolution. The mirror neuron system consists of neurons within the left inferior frontal cortex and right superior parietal lobule that are specialized for the acquisition of motor learning. Mirror neurons reflect neural mechanisms for the transmission of simple motor movements from a model to learner, such as nonverbal gestures (Iacoboni et al., 1999). The MNS reflects neural processes that facilitate social learning through imitation or mental processes of observation from action. Observation and imitation of a motor movement elicit neural activity within the MNS due to neural mechanisms that directly match the sensory representation of an observed action within an internal motor representation of that action. The intentional observation of motor movement serves as an antecedent of social learning or the capacity to produce the consequence of motor imitation or identical motor action.

Methodological Foundations

Methodological foundations in cultural neuroscience facilitate the observation and measurement of multilevel systems of natural phenomena across distinct spatial and temporal dimensions. Research methods in cultural neuroscience focus on the empirical study of how culture influences psychological and neurobiological mechanisms of human behavior with qualitative and quantitative methods. Quantitative methods allow for the observation and measurement of culture from a behavioral level of analysis characterized through behavioral surveys or scales. Behavioral paradigms that measure behavior in response to culture that is characterized through simple actions that can be quantified, such as button presses or joystick movement, provide direct and indirect methods for the quantitative study of cultural differences. Qualitative methods allow for the observation and measurement of human behavior from verbal report based on observation and experience. Behavioral paradigms that measure behavior in response to culture that is characterized by unique or distinctive complex action, such as open-ended interviews, may involve the qualitative study of cultural differences to measure behavior.

Culture

Culture is the system of values, beliefs, and practices that maintain and regulate societal behavior at the level of the individual, group, and institution. Cultural systems provide conceptual schemata for the study of culture in relation to behavior across societal levels (Markus & Kitayama, 1991; Oyserman et al., 2002). Cultural systems are characterized through qualitative and quantitative methods for the study of the culture at a particular level of analysis. For the cultural systems of the self, qualitative methods are important for the study of mental processes with open-ended self-responses, such as those measured with cultural priming and daily diary methods.

Cultural priming methods may include essay writing in response to cultural prompts that allow the participant to describe the self in an independent or interdependent manner (Hong et al., 2000; Oyserman & Lee, 2008). Verbal report methods include essay writing in response to cultural prompts that allow the participant to describe the self in general as well as in response to particular contexts or situations. Quantitative methods are utilized to study culture and the self, when the self is characterized in a dimensional manner through self-report behavioral surveys and cultural priming. Behavioral surveys of culture allow the participant to characterize the self along dimensions such as independence and interdependence. Cultural priming methods that are quantitative allow the participant to think about or respond in a culturally congruent manner.

Race refers to the ancestral origin of a cultural group of people that share a geographic origin and characteristic traits based on biological and cultural inheritance. Due to geographic variation in the historical use of race in society, race is a historical concept of biological and social construction (Eberhardt, 2005; Smedley & Smedley, 2005). Race as a biological construction includes the shared physical traits among people in the cultural group; race as a social construction includes the shared social and behavioral traits of people in the cultural group. Race is considered a demographic characteristic, and the societal changes in the use of racial categories reflect the potential for demographic change due to migration and the influence of cultural and political aspects on the history of the characterization.

Racial stereotypes are social categories of character traits and attributes that include the use of generalizations in social inferences about members of the cultural group. The societal use of racial stereotypes can lead to misattribution in social perception of the self and others, affecting the quality of social relations (Fiske et al., 2002) and achievement (Shih et al., 2011; Steele, 1997). Racial attitudes refer to attributes as objects associated with specific racial categories that are observable as unconscious and conscious racial bias (Devine, 1989; Greenwald & Banaji, 1995). Unconscious or implicit racial attitudes reflect the attitudes that are indirectly measured through behavioral measures that assess the strength of an association with reaction time. Conscious or explicit racial attitudes refer to attitudes that are directly measured in behavioral surveys with rating scales. Regulation of racial prejudice through cognitive control enhances the capacity for egalitarianism (Lieberman et al., 2005; Richeson et al., 2003; Shelton et al., 2005).

Ethnicity refers to the societal traditions that make up the heritage of a cultural group of people, including the language, diet, practices, and social norms. Ethnicity includes the characteristics of a cultural group that define social identity, such as the commitment and belonging that a member has to their cultural group demonstrated in cultural practices and community involvement. Ethnic identity is an important component of youth development, as the strengthening ethnic identity through community involvement enhances the feeling of societal commitment and belonging to one's cultural and ethnic heritage in youth (Phinney, 1990; Sellers et al., 1998). The formation of ethnic identity builds from a sense of shared responsibility of the self with others in the cultural group.

Psychology

Research in psychology examines the structure and function of the mind, including antecedent and consequent processes of behavior. Behavioral paradigms, consisting of verbal and nonverbal tasks, include methods for the study of mental processes and behavior. Behavioral responses that are observed and measured allow researchers to infer the types of mental processes associated with a given behavioral paradigm. Spatiotemporal characteristics of behavioral responses, including reaction time and accuracy, allow for the measurement of mental processes during a given task. Mental constructs may be explicit or implicit, such that participants in psychological studies may not necessarily recognize the mental processes that are studied. Behavioral paradigms may be designed to observe mental processes that are not overt, including experimental conditions that measure unconscious processes with behavioral responses as well as mental processes that rely on fictional information. Behavioral paradigms that systematically test theoretical constructs provide effective means for the observation and inference of mental processes.

Neuroscience

Methods in neuroscience allow for the observation of the nervous system across distinct temporal and spatial scales. Neuroscience methods vary in their level of observation as well as in the direct manner of the measurement. Noninvasive methods, such as functional magnetic resonance imaging (fMRI) and event-related potential (ERP), allow for the indirect observation of neural activity. FMRI measures neural response that occurs within regions of brain circuitry, while ERP measures neural response that occurs within brain circuitry close to the scalp. ERP measures changes in neural response within milliseconds of stimulus onset, during recording of cortical activity. Neuroscience methods, such as fMRI and ERP, allow for the study of the direction and magnitude of the association between culture and neural structure and function as well as for the testing of causal models of culture and neural circuitry.

Neuropsychological methods allow researchers to assess the causal relations of a given brain region and mental process. Changes in mental state that occur in neuropsychological populations provide evidence of causal relations between a given brain region and psychological function. Cultural neuropsychology methods provide a means for understanding the causal relation between a given brain region and mental function based on culture, race, or ethnicity (Manly, 2008). The use of race and ethnicity-based norms to assess performance on neuropsychological assessments allows for the evaluation and interpretation of measurement due to cultural factors.

Genetics

Research on culture and genetics ranges from empirical studies of specific genes or single nucleotide proteins (SNPs) to genome-wide association studies (GWASs; Chen et al., 2016; Sasaki et al., 2016). Gene-by-culture interaction studies measure the magnitude of association between a specific gene and mental or behavioral processes due to culture. Cultural neurogenetic studies examine gene-by-culture interaction in neural circuitry across individuals. Cultural genomic studies investigate the association between multiple genes or a set of genes and specific mental processes and behavior. Studies with cross-national genetic indices demonstrate an association between a specific gene or set of genes and cultural processes across nations (Chiao & Blizinsky, 2010). These methodological approaches demonstrate the range of methods for the measurement and observation of interaction in culture and genetics.

Empirical Findings

Empirical findings in cultural neuroscience demonstrate cultural influences on the structure, function, and organization of the nervous system. Cultural systems affect neural mechanisms across a range of psychological domains, from emotion and cognition to social cognition. Culture affects psychological domains located within multilevel mechanisms of brain circuitry observed across distinct spatial and temporal scales.

Emotion

Culture influences the distinct stages of emotion, ranging from antecedent processes to regulatory mechanisms of negative and positive affect. Culture shapes the way that emotional events are perceived, remembered, and responded to (Markus & Kitayama, 1991; Mesquita & Frijda, 1992). Cultural styles of holistic and analytic thinking affect how emotional events are perceived and remembered. Holistic thinking encourages perception of emotional events that includes the focal aspects of the scene as well as the surrounding context, while analytic thinking leads to perception of emotional events that includes primarily the focal aspects of the scene. When events are emotional either in a negative or positive manner, holistic thinking may encourage perception of negative or positive physical events that encodes the focal aspects of the scene within a particular context, while analytic thinking leads to perception of negative or positive physical events that focuses on the focal aspects of the scene. Once emotional events are perceived and remembered, responses may lead to either conscious rethinking about the emotional event or suppression of response to the emotional event depending on cultural display rules (Matsumoto et al., 2008). Due to display rules, individualistic cultures reinforce responses to emotional events that allow for the conscious expression of emotion, while collectivistic cultures encourage responses to emotional events that control or suppress the expression of emotion in a socially appropriate manner.

Emotion Recognition

Culture influences the neural circuitry of emotion. People recognize emotions expressed by members of their own cultural group to a greater extent relative to those expressed by other cultural group members (Elfenbein & Ambady, 2002). The capacity to recognize emotions to a greater extent for ingroup members suggests that the perceptual and recognition memory processes underlying emotional expressions are tuned to the environmental and experiential input of one's culture. In a cross-cultural neuroimaging study of emotion in the United States and Japan, participants viewed and categorized facial expressions of emotion, including fear, anger, happy, and neutral expressions (Chiao et al., 2008; Figure 5.1). Greater bilateral amygdala response to facial expressions of fear was observed for those expressed by members of one's own cultural group. These findings show that neural response with the limbic circuitry is greater for facial expressions of fear.

Culture interacts with genes in the processes of emotion recognition. The serotonin transporter (5-HTTLPR) gene is associated with the regulation of emotion. In a gene-by-culture study of emotion recognition, Japanese and Americans recognized joy and sadness in facial morphs (Ishii et al., 2014). Japanese who carry the short (s) allele of the serotonin transporter gene show greater social sensitivity to facial expressions of emotion relative to Americans and greater efficiency in the detection of changes in emotional expressions.

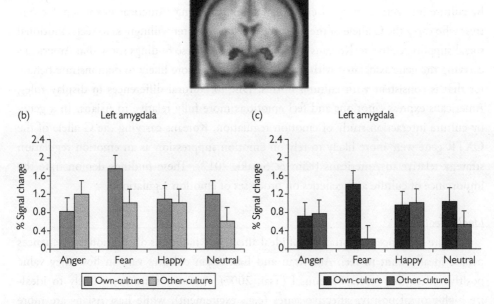

Figure 5.1. Cultural specificity in amygdala response to fear faces. (a) Anatomical definition of left and right amygdala. (b, c) Greater left and right amygdala response to fear expressed by members of one's cultural group.

For interdependent cultures, the capacity to detect subtle emotion expressed by others enhances adaptive behavior that is congruent with the social norms of interdependent cultures. For independent cultures, the capacity to detect subtle emotion of others may be less emphasized in social norms due to the importance of autonomy from others. These findings show the importance of genetic and cultural sensitivity in emotion recognition.

Emotion Regulation

Culture affects how people regulate their emotions. Cultural display rules affect societal norms, regulating the extent to which people express emotions in distinct cultural contexts, and differ for individualistic and collectivistic cultures (Matsumoto et al., 2008). Individualistic cultures encourage expressions of emotion, while collectivistic cultures reinforce suppression of emotional expression. Cultural differences in display rules affect how people regulate their emotions (Ford & Mauss, 2015). When regulating emotional experiences, individualistic cultures are more likely to endorse rethinking feelings, while collectivistic cultures are more likely to strengthen suppression of emotional expression. In a cross-cultural ERP study of emotion regulation, Asian and European Americans were shown unpleasant or neutral pictures and either attended or suppressed emotional response (Murata, Moser, Kitayama, 2013). Asians showed a decrease in late positive potential (LPP) response during emotional suppression relative to attention, while European Americans did not. Cultural differences affect neural response during emotion regulation.

Culture interacts with genetics in the processes of emotion regulation. The oxytocin receptor (OXTR) gene is a gene associated with empathy and social cognition. In a gene-by-culture interaction study of emotional support seeking, Americans experiencing distress who carry the G allele of the OXTR gene show greater willingness to seek emotional social support relative to Koreans (Kim et al., 2010). These findings show that Americans carrying the gene associated with social sensitivity are more likely to demonstrate behavior that is consistent with cultural norms. Due to cultural differences in display rules, Americans express emotions and feel emotions more fully relative to Asians. In a gene-by-culture interaction study of emotion regulation, Koreans carrying the G allele of the OXTR gene were more likely to rely on emotion suppression as an emotion regulation strategy relative to Americans (Kim & Sasaki, 2012). These findings demonstrate the importance of culture and genetics on processes of emotion regulation.

Ideal Affect

Culture influences the processes of ideal affect, or what kinds of emotional experiences people ideally want to feel. American and East Asian cultures vary in how they value positive affect that varies in arousal (Tsai, 2007). Americans are more likely to idealize high-arousal positive affective states (e.g., excitement), while East Asians are more likely to idealize low-arousal positive affective states (e.g., calm). In a neuroimaging study of culture and ideal affect, people viewed positive facial expressions that varied in emotional arousal. Results showed greater neural response in the bilateral ventral striatum when viewing excited relative to calm expressions for European Americans, while greater response in this region was observed for calm relative to excited expressions for East Asians (Park et al., 2016). These findings demonstrate that the cultural idealization of the emotional experience of positive affect is associated with response within neural circuitry of affect and reward. Cultural differences in ideal affect tune neural mechanisms within the reward system.

Culture affects the neurobiological basis of emotion. Cultural variation influences the neural mechanisms associated with the processes of emotional generation, experience, and regulation (Chiao, 2015). Cultural variation also influences the encoding and representation of emotion within limbic and striatal brain circuitry. Cultural influences on the functional organization of neural circuitry of emotion facilitate processes of adaptive behavior.

Cognition

Cultural differences in thinking style are thought to originate from metaphysical and epistemological differences among ancient philosophical traditions of the West and East. Western cultures sustain analytic systems of thought, while Eastern cultures maintain holistic systems of thought (Nisbett et al., 2001). Analytic and holistic styles of thinking constitute cultural influences on cognition. Analytic cognition refers to a system of thought that is field independent, such that the unit of thought is the object independent of the field or context. Holistic cognition refers to a system of thought that is field dependent, such that the object within the field or context is the unit of thought. Cultural influences on neural mechanisms of cognition are affected by the processes of aging (Park & Gutchess, 2002). Cultural variation in thinking style reflects distinct cognitive processes that maintain ancient social organization and practices.

Perception

Culture affects how people perceive and think about the physical environment. East Asians perceive objects within their background, while Westerners are more likely to perceive objects focally in an analytic manner. In a neuroimaging study of culture and perception, European Americans and East Asians in the United States perceived a line within an absolute or relative context (Hedden et al., 2008). European Americans and East Asians show reduced response within the left inferior parietal lobe (l-IPL) and right precentral gyrus (r-PG) when perceiving the line consistent within the cultural context. European Americans show greater neural response within the l-IPL and r-PG during visuospatial judgments in a relative context, while East Asians show greater neural response within these brain regions in an absolute context. These findings suggest efficiency in neural response during perception congruent with the cultural context.

Culture shapes neural mechanisms of global and local perception. In an ERP study of culture and perception, Chinese were primed with independent or interdependent self-construal and completed a global–local perception task (Lin et al., 2008). Chinese primed with independent self-construal showed greater amplitude in the P1 waveform during local perception, while those primed with interdependent self-construal showed greater amplitude in the P1 waveform during global perception. The influence of cultural priming on the electrophysiological mechanisms of attention occurs at an early stage of perception.

Culture and genes affect systems of thought. The serotonin 1A receptor polymorphism (5-HTR1A) is a gene associated with attention, such that the G allele is related to reduced serotonergic neurotransmission. In a gene-by-culture interaction study of cognition, European Americans and East Asians displayed preferences in thinking styles (Kim et al., 2010). European Americans who carry the G allele of the 5-HTR1A showed greater preference for analytic styles of thought in locus of attention, while East Asians who carry the G allele showed preference for holistic styles of thought in locus of attention. People who carry the G allele of the 5-HTR1A showed greater preference for the perception of objects in a manner congruent with the cultural context. These findings demonstrate that cultural variations in attentional style are related to genes and that genetic sensitivity to preferences in thinking style for the locus of attention is congruent with one's culture.

Object Recognition

Culture affects the neural basis of object recognition. In a neuroimaging study of culture and cognition, Americans and East Asians were shown complex visual scenes and encoded objects in a focal or contextual manner (Gutchess et al., 2006). Americans displayed greater neural response in brain regions associated with object processing, including the bilateral middle temporal gyrus, left superior parietal gyrus, and right superior temporal gyrus, relative to East Asians. These findings show cultural variation in object processing within ventral regions of the brain. Due to holistic styles of thinking, East Asians show greater neural sensitivity to cultural context during object processing relative to Westerners (Jenkins et al., 2010). Chinese demonstrate greater neural adaptation in the bilateral occipital complex to incongruent relative to congruent scenes than Americans. Holistic styles of thinking are associated with neural responses during object recognition that are sensitive to context, while analytic styles of thinking are associated with neural responses during object recognition that are independent of context.

Cultural influences on neural processing of objects are also related to the processes of aging. In a neuroimaging study of culture and aging of cognition, East Asian and Westerner young and old adults were shown complex visual scenes and performed scene encoding (Goh et al., 2007). Elderly East Asians show less neural adaptation response in object areas relative to elderly Westerners. Results from this study display the importance of culture on object recognition during aging. Cultural systems of thought tune neural circuitry of object recognition throughout the life course.

Inhibitory Control

Inhibitory control is an important capacity for the regulation of the self that varies across cultures. Interdependent or collectivistic cultures encourage inhibitory control of the self to a greater extent relative to independent or individualistic cultures. Greater reliance on inhibitory control enhances the capacity for flexibility and malleability in response to the cultural context. Independent or individualistic cultures emphasize behavioral consistency of the self including expression of the self relative to interdependent or collectivistic cultures. In a neuroimaging study of culture and inhibitory control, Japanese, Japanese Americans, and Caucasian Americans displayed inhibition in response to verbal information (Pornpattananangkul et al., 2016). Neural response within the left inferior frontal gyrus (l-IFG) was greater for Japanese relative to Japanese Americans and Caucasian Americans. People who showed greater behavioral consistency demonstrated greater anterior cingulate cortex (ACC) response during inhibitory control. These findings display cultural variation in the magnitude of response within the neural circuitry of inhibitory control. The cultural capacity of inhibitory control is associated with neural mechanisms of the prefrontal cortex. Regions of the prefrontal cortex, including the l-IFG and ACC, serve as components of the functional organization of neural mechanisms for cognitive regulation across cultures.

Social Processes
KNOWLEDGE OF SELF AND OTHERS

Culture affects how people think about themselves and their relation to others. Independent or individualistic cultures emphasize autonomy, uniqueness, and distinctness from others, while interdependent or collectivistic cultures define themselves by the social context, including social relations and roles that interconnect them with others (Markus & Kitayama, 1991; Oyserman et al., 2002). Cultural styles of self-construal may be dynamic or malleable to the social context (Hong et al., 2000; Oyserman & Lee, 2008). Temporarily heightening awareness of cultural styles of the self is associated with cultural changes in mental representation of the self.

Culture shapes the concept of the self, which develops early in childhood. Social interaction between parents and children encourages the cultural construction of the self (Wang, 2006). East Asian parents are more likely to reinforce children's thinking of themselves based on their social roles, relationships, and contexts. European parents are more likely to encourage children to think of themselves individually and according to their social attributes, traits, and dispositions. Through interactions with parents, children learn how to remember their social experiences during childhood as unitary features of themselves. During storytelling, East Asian parents reflect on social experiences and describe children's behavior in relation to social norms and expectations. European parents elaborate on stories with their children, emphasizing details of social events related to qualities of their personal actions. Throughout developmental maturation, early cultural experiences coincide with maturational changes in neurobiology. Thus, cultural differences in formation of self-concept are reflected in neural representations of the self.

Neuroimaging studies of the self in adulthood show that culture affects neural representations of the self within the medial prefrontal cortex (MPFC). East Asians and Westerners in China demonstrate greater neural response within the MPFC during self- relative to other judgments (Zhu et al., 2007). Across cultures, people show greater MPFC response when thinking about personal traits, while East Asians have greater MPFC response when thinking about a close other. These findings show that the self is culture specific. That is, neural representations of the self encode information that is independent or interdependent in manner. Findings from a cross-cultural neuroimaging study of the self suggest that Japanese and Caucasian Americans think about themselves in a social context or in a general manner (Chiao et al., 2009). People from individualistic cultures show greater MPFC response when thinking about themselves in a general relative to contextual manner, while people from collectivistic cultures demonstrate greater MPFC response when thinking about themselves in a contextual relative to general manner.

Cultural influences on neural representations of the self are dynamic and malleable. Temporarily heightening awareness of individualism and collectivism modulates neural responses during explicit (Chiao et al., 2010) and implicit (Harada et al., 2010) processing of the self. In a neuroimaging study of culture and self-processes, bicultural individuals primed with individualism showed greater neural response within the MPFC and posterior cingulate cortex (PCC) during general self-processing, while bicultural individuals primed with collectivism showed greater neural response within the MPFC and PCC during contextual self-processing (Chiao et al., 2010). These findings display the cultural malleability of encoding in neural representations of the self. Response within subregions of the MPFC and PCC shows differential sensitivity in neural representations of the self. In a neuroimaging study of cultural priming and self-processes, individuals primed with individualism showed greater neural response within the dorsal, but not ventral, portions of the MPFC (Harada et al., 2010). Cultural encoding is modulated in neural representations associated with processes of evaluation, but not detection, of information related to the self.

Culture tunes social processes of the self across multilevel mechanisms. Culture affects the content and scope of mental representations of the self and others. Independent or individualistic cultural styles of the self emphasize the self as autonomous of others, while interdependent or collectivistic cultural styles of the self conceptualize the self as relational to others. Neural circuitry within the medial portion of the prefrontal cortex encodes and represents social information of the self and others. Cultural variation in subregions of the MPFPC differentiate neural activity related to evaluation of self-relevant information. Cultural styles of self-construal play an important role in the functional organization of the neurobiological basis of knowledge for the self and others.

Empathy

Empathy is the human capacity to share emotional states with others. During empathy, people attend to and perceive the feelings of others, which generates a representation of emotion in the self automatically that is associated with autonomic and physiological processes (Preston & De Waal, 2002). Perceiving the emotional experiences of others is an interdependent process affected by the length and quality of social experience shared by the self and others. Greater interdependence with others is related to the similarity in emotional representation of the self and others.

Neuroimaging studies of empathy show a network of brain regions associated with empathic responding, including the ACC, bilateral anterior insula (AI), and brain regions, including the mirror neuron system, limbic system, and prefrontal cortex (Lamm et al., 2011). The ACC and AI are associated with processes of emotional empathy, including a shared representation of emotion in the self and other. The mirror neuron system includes the pars opercularis of the inferior frontal gyrus and is associated with imitation, action observation, and understanding of intention (Iacoboni, 2009). The limbic system is associated with the perception and recognition of emotion, including emotional responding and emotional memory (Adolphs, 2008). The medial portion of the prefrontal cortex is related to cognitive empathy, including mentalizing and perspective taking. Neuroimaging research on culture and empathy has relied on behavioral paradigms that measure neural response while participants complete empathy tasks of physical (Xu et al., 2009), social (Bruneau et al., 2012; Cikara et al., 2011; Masten et al., 2011), and emotional pain (de Greck et al., 2012; Mathur et al., 2010).

Cultural factors influence the neural mechanisms of imitation. The MNS reflects neural mechanisms within the frontal and parietal lobules specialized for cultural learning. Cultural identity of the model affects the social learning of motor movements through imitation. Observation and motor imitation of African American models show greater neural response within the frontal, parietal, and occipital brain regions than other race ethnic groups, such as European Americans and Chinese Americans, with consistent social learning across models of different ethnic groups (Losin, Iacoboni, Martin, Cross, & Dapretto, 2012). The successful transmission of cultural information from the model to the learner reflects the prestige and knowledge of the cultural group. Successful imitation of cultural information from different ethnic models in the population reflects the popularity of cultural thought and conformity to cultural knowledge within the population.

The gender of learning models affects neural mechanisms of imitation. Successful social learning from models of one's own gender reflects the prestige of cultural acquisition from a model similar to one's own gender identity. Social learning of motor movements from an own-gender relative to an other-gender model is associated with greater neural response within emotional regions such as the striatum, orbitofrontal cortex, and amygdala (Losin, Iacoboni, Martin, & Dapretto, 2012). Neural responses within the ventral striatum are associated with evaluation and reward. Observation of motor action of an own-gender model elicited greater neural processing within reward neural circuitry, suggesting that social learning of motor action from a model of one's own gender is rewarding. Reward learning of motor action from a model of one's gender reflects the selective reinforcement learning of cultural adaptations from one's gender group. The ingroup advantage of gender during social learning reflects the benefits of social cooperation and cohesion among models and learners from the same gender group.

Culture affects the neural basis of empathy. Other-focusedness is a cultural subconstruct of interdependence and is related to the sensitivity to others and primacy of others relative to the self. Thinking about how to understand and help others is necessary to regulate processes related to knowledge of self and others. In a neuroimaging study of culture and empathy, Chinese and Caucasians in China show greater neural response within the ACC and left AI for the physical suffering of group members (Xu et al., 2009). These findings demonstrate an influence of cultural group membership on empathic neural response. People show greater empathic neural response when perceiving the pain and suffering of group members.

Cultural norms of interdependence, such as other-focusedness, which emphasizes sensitivity to and the primacy of others, affect the neural circuitry of empathy. In a cross-cultural neuroimaging study of interdependence and empathy, Koreans and Caucasian Americans viewed scenes of emotional pain or neutral scenes due to a natural disaster (Cheon et al., 2013). Koreans who showed greater other-focusedness had greater neural response within the network for empathy, including the ACC and MPFC, for group members in emotional pain. These findings show that neural response for emotional pain is greater for interdependent Koreans. When members of the cultural group show empathy for pain caused by natural disasters, the empathic neural response for cultural group members is associated with interdependence.

Ethnic identity is an important factor in how people respond to the emotional pain of others. People who identify with their racial or ethnic group feel a sense of belonging or commitment as well as shared values and attitudes with group members (Phinney, 1990; Sellers et al., 1998). People who show strong ethnic identification, such as members of minority groups within the United States, feel a sense of belonging to the social group. In a neuroimaging study of ethnic identity in the United States, African Americans showed greater neural response within cortical midline structures, such as the MPFC, ACC, midcingulate cortex (MCC), and PCC, when perceiving group members in emotional pain, while Caucasian Americans showed greater neural response within bilateral parahippocampal gyri during empathy for group members (Mathur et al., 2012). Racial identification is associated with empathic neural response. The magnitude of cortical midline activity is positively associated, while the magnitude of activity in the bilateral parahippocampus is negatively associated, with magnitude of racial identification during empathic response. These findings show that ethnic identity affects the neurobiological basis of empathy.

Culture and genes interact in processes of empathy. The OXTR gene is a gene associated with social sensitivity and empathic behavior (Kim et al., 2010; Kim et al., 2011). Personal distress is a type of empathic feeling that occurs in response to the pain or suffering of others. In a gene-by-culture interaction study, Americans who experienced personal distress and carry the G allele of the OXTR gene showed greater emotional support seeking relative to Koreans who did not. Americans who are genetically sensitive prefer social contact with others in response to the experience of empathy. These findings show that cultural variation in empathic experience is associated with genetic sensitivity and social behavior. In a neuroimaging study of culture and genes, Chinese were shown group members either in physical pain or neutral conditions (Luo et al., 2015). Interdependent Chinese who carry two copies of the G allele of the OXTR gene displayed greater empathy, such as perspective taking and empathic concern, relative to A-allele carriers. Empathic neural response within brain regions associated with empathy, such as the bilateral insula and adjacent brain regions, shows greater activity for Chinese who carry two copies of the G allele of the OXTR gene. Interdependent Chinese who carry the social sensitivity gene demonstrate greater response in neural mechanisms of empathy for physical pain. These results display the potent role of culture in genetic sensitivity for empathy across levels of analysis.

Arousal and Regulatory Systems

Culture affects psychophysiological arousal to emotional events. Cultural differences affect psychophysiological responses to emotional films. European Americans and Asian Americans were asked to amplify or downregulate emotional responses to emotional films. European Americans show greater skin conductance response during emotion regulation to emotional films relative to Asian Americans, but not neutral films (Soto et al., 2016). These findings show that cultural differences in arousal response to emotional films during emotion regulation are likely due to cultural norms. Given the cultural norm of emotional suppression in East Asia, the regulation of emotion requires less effortful processing for Asian Americans than for European Americans. For European Americans, the motivation to regulate emotions, either amplification or downregulation of emotional experience, may reflect greater effortful processing, requiring enhanced physiological arousal.

The cultural influence on psychophysiological arousal is affected by ethnic group membership. Participants from different ethnic groups—African Americans, Chinese Americans, European Americans, and Mexican Americans—observed emotional film clips with actors from different ethnic groups (Roberts & Levenson, 2006). Participants showed greater psychophysiological responses to ethnically matched film clips relative to ethnically mismatched film clips, or films with actors from other ethnic groups. African Americans and European Americans showed greater psychophysiological arousal for ingroup emotional films. Ethnic differences in arousal response for ingroup emotional films may reflect heightened ethnic identification in emotional responding due to ethnic group membership. Greater ingroup advantage in emotion responding may strengthen the quality of emotional and social understanding of the ethnic group (Elfenbein & Ambady, 2003).

Emotional arousal to negative and positive events enhances the perception of, experience of, and responding to emotional information in the environment. Heightened emotional arousal requires regulation to facilitate emotional responding consistent with cultural norms. Regulatory systems within the brain, such as the neural connectivity of the prefrontal cortex and the amygdala, are related to the capacity for regulation of emotional responding to emotional events (Buhle et al., 2014; Ochsner et al., 2002; Wager et al., 2008). Cultural differences in emotional arousal reflect variation in cultural norms for emotion regulation. Differences in regulation strategies for emotional experience across cultures as well as levels of physiological arousal for the emotional experience of cultural group members reflect the influence of culture on arousal and regulatory systems of emotional experience.

Conclusion

Cultural neuroscience examines the mutual constitution of culture and biology across multiple levels of analysis and time scales. Research in cultural neuroscience provides a life course approach to the study of the etiology of mental health and improves the understanding of environmental influences on culture and biology. Systematic investigation in cultural neuroscience builds resources for use of evidence-based prevention interventions in global mental health. Cultural neuroscience strengthens the understanding of the molecular and cellular mechanisms of the human brain across cultures, enhancing efforts for the scientific discovery of cures, preventions, and interventions in global mental health.

Implications for Global Mental Health

Population Health Disparities

Population health disparities reflect group differences in health outcomes or disease prevalence that are unfair or unjust due to the origin of the difference. Sociocultural factors contribute to population health disparities such as increased exposure to potential risk factors and reduced exposure to protective environmental influences. Members of racial or ethnic minority groups that are historically marginalized may experience greater exposure to negative stereotypes that affect physical health and psychological well-being. Raising awareness of the global burden of MNS disorders provides a means to understanding the factors underlying disparities in global mental health. Research in cultural neuroscience bolsters understanding of the root causes and mechanisms of mental health throughout the life course across cultures. The scientific discovery of identification of biomarkers associated with mental health based on culture, race, or ethnicity provides an evidence-based resource for closing the gap in population health disparities.

Public Policy

The scientific discovery of cures, preventions, and interventions for MNS disorders across cultures is important for addressing chief priorities in global mental health. Building resource capacity in research and education reflects components of policy development for health equity across a range of stakeholders. Infrastructure for research and education in cultural neuroscience and global mental health provides training opportunities and promotes national and international collaboration. Broadening the opportunities for institutions and individuals to build communication and tools through collaboration strengthens international initiatives, programs, and regional networks for cultural neuroscience and global mental health.

Building human resource capacity in international aid and development programs of cultural neuroscience and global mental health enhances opportunities for policy development and implementation to achieve the goal of mental health for all. Investment in mental health policy implementation with international initiatives enhances resources and develops training programs that promote mental health. Regional networks for mental health strengthen support for policy components that respect local ownership and the historical traditions of populations. International cooperation in principles of policy development and implementation promotes the mental health of populations across the globe.

Acknowledgments

Research reported in this publication was supported by the National Institutes of Health under award number R13DA33065. The content is solely the responsibility of the authors and does not necessarily represent the official views of the National Institutes of Health.

References

Adolphs, R. (2008). Fear, faces, and the human amygdala. *Current Opinion in Neurobiology, 18*(2), 166–172.

Beja-Pereira, A., Luikart, G., England, P. R., Bradley, D. G., Jann, O. C., Bertorelle, G., Chamberlain, A. T., Nunes, T. P., Metodiev, S., Ferrand, N., & Erhardt, G. (2003). Gene-culture coevolution between cattle milk protein genes and human lactase genes. *Nature Genetics, 35*(4), 311–313.

Boyd, R., & Richerson, P. J. (1985). *Culture and the evolutionary process.* University of Chicago Press.

Bruneau, E. G., Dufour, N., & Saxe, R. (2012). Social cognition in members of conflict groups: Behavioural and neural responses in Arabs, Israelis and South Americans to each other's misfortunes. *Philosophical Transactions of the Royal Society of London B: Biological Sciences, 367*(1589), 717–730.

Buhle, J. T., Silvers, J. A., Wager, T. D., Lopez, R., Onyemekwu, C., Kober, H., Weber, J., & Ochsner, K. N. (2014). Cognitive reappraisal of emotion: A meta-analysis of human neuroimaging studies. *Cerebral Cortex, 24*(11), 2981–2990.

Chen, C., Moyzis, R. K., Lei, X., Chen, C., & Dong, Q. (2016). The enculturated genome: Molecular evidence for recent divergent evolution in human neurotransmitter genes. In J. Y. Chiao, S.-C. Li, R. Seligman, & R. Turner (Eds.), *The Oxford handbook of cultural neuroscience* (pp. 315–338). Oxford University Press.

Cheon, B. K., Im, D. M., Harada, T., Kim, J. S., Mathur, V. A., Scimeca, J. M., Parrish, T. B., Park, H., & Chiao, J. Y. (2013). Cultural modulation of the neural correlates of emotional pain perception: The role of other-focusedness. *Neuropsychologia, 51*(7), 1177–1186.

Cheon, B. K., Wang, Y., Chiao, J. Y., & Tang, Y. Y. (2018). Cultural neuroscience of dialectical thinking. In Spencer-Rodgers, J. & Peng, K. (Eds.), *The psychological and cultural foundations of East Asian cognition: Contradiction, change and holism* (pp. 181–212). New York: Oxford University Press.

Chiao, J. Y. (2015). Current emotion research in cultural neuroscience. *Emotion Review, 7*(1), 1–14.

Chiao, J. Y., & Ambady, N. (2007). Cultural neuroscience: Parsing universality and diversity across levels of analysis. In S. Kitayama & D. Cohen (Eds.), *Handbook of cultural psychology* (pp. 237–254). Guilford Press.

Chiao, J. Y., & Blizinsky, K. D. (2010). Culture-gene coevolution of individualism-collectivism and the serotonin transporter gene (5-HTTLPR). *Proceedings of the Royal Society (Series B): Biological Sciences, 277*(1681), 529–537.

Chiao, J. Y., Harada, T., Komeda, H., Li, Z., Mano, Y., Saito, D., Parrish, T. B., Sadato N., Iidaka, T. (2010). Dynamic cultural influences on neural representations of the self. *Journal of Cognitive Neuroscience, 22*(1), 1–11.

Chiao, J. Y., Cheon, B. K., Pornpattananangkul, N., Mrazek, A. J., & Blizinsky, K. D. (2013). Cultural neuroscience: Progress and promise. *Psychological Inquiry, 24*(1), 1–19.

Chiao, J. Y., Harada, T., Komeda, H., Li, Z., Mano, Y., Saito, D., Parrish, T. B., Sadato, N., & Iidaka, T. (2009). Neural basis of individualistic and collectivistic views of self. *Human Brain Mapping, 30*(9), 2813–2820.

Chiao, J. Y., Iidaka, T., Gordon, H. L., Nogawa, J., Bar, M., Aminoff, E., Sadato, N., & Ambady, N. (2008). Cultural specificity in amygdala response to fear faces. *Journal of Cognitive Neuroscience, 20*(12), 2167–2174.

Chiao, J. Y., Li, S.-C., Turner, R., Lee-Tauler, S. Y., & Pringle, B. A. (2017). Cultural neuroscience and global mental health. *Culture and Brain, 5*(1), 4–13.

Cikara, M., Botvinick, M. M., & Fiske, S.T. (2011). Bounded empathy: neural responses to outgroup targets' (mis)fortunes. *Journal of Cognitive Neuroscience, 23*(12), 3791–3803.

Collins, P. Y., Patel, V., Joestl, S. S., March, D., Insel, T. R., Daar, A. S., Scientific Advisory Board and the Executive Committee of the Grand Challenges on Global Mental Health, Anderson, W., Dhansay, M. A., Phillips, A., Shurin, S., Walport, M., Ewart, W., Savill, S. J., Bordin, I. A., Costello, E. J., Durkin, M., Fairburn, C., Glass, R. I., . . . Stein, D. J. (2011). Grand challenges in global mental health. *Nature, 475*(7354), 27–30.

De Greck, M., Shu, Z., Wang, G., Zuo, X., Yang, X., Wang, X., Northoff, G., & Han, S. (2012). Culture modulates brain activity during empathy with anger. *Neuroimage, 59*(3), 2871–2872.

Devine, P. G. (1989). Stereotypes and prejudice: Their automatic and controlled components. *Journal of Personality and Social Psychology, 56*(1), 5–18.

Durham, W. H. (1991). *Genes, culture, and human diversity*. Stanford University Press.

Eberhardt, J. L. (2005). Imaging race. *American Psychologist, 60*(2), 181–190.

Elfenbein, H. A., & Ambady, N. (2002). Is there an in-group advantage in emotion recognition? *Psychological Bulletin, 128*(2), 243–249.

Elfenbein, H. A., & Ambady, N. (2003). When familiarity breeds accuracy: Cultural exposure and facial emotion recognition. *Journal of Personality and Social Psychology, 85*, 276–290.

Fiske, S. T., Cuddy, A. J., Glick, P., & Xu, J. (2002). A model of (often mixed) stereotype content: Competence and warmth follow from perceived status and competition. *Journal of Personality and Social Psychology, 82*(6), 878–902.

Ford, B. Q., & Mauss, I. B. (2015). Culture and emotion regulation. *Current Opinion in Psychology, 3*, 1–5.

Goh, J. O., Chee, M. W., Tan, J. C., Venkatraman, V., Hebrank, A., Leshikar, E. D., Jenkins, L., Sutton, B. P., Gutchess, A. H., & Park, D. C. (2007). Age and culture modulate object processing and object-scene binding in the ventral visual area. *Cognitive Affective and Behavioral Neuroscience, 7*(1), 44–52.

Greenwald, A., & Banaji, M. R. (1995). Implicit social cognition: Attitudes, self-esteem, and stereotypes. *Psychological Review, 102*, 4–27.

Gutchess, A.H., Welsh, R.C., Boduroglu, A., Park, D.C. (2006). Cultural differences in neural function associated with object processing. *Cognitive Affective and Behavioral Neuroscience, 6*(2), 102–109.

Han, S., & Northoff, G. (2008). Culture-sensitive neural substrates of human cognition: A transcultural neuroimaging approach. *Nature Reviews Neuroscience, 9*(8), 646–654.

Harada, T., Li, Z., & Chiao, J. Y. (2010). Differential dorsal and ventral medial prefrontal representations of the implicit self modulated by individualism and collectivism: An fMRI study. *Social Neuroscience, 5*(3), 257–271.

Hedden, T., Ketay, S., Aron, A., Markus, H. R., & Gabrieli, J. D. (2008). Cultural influences on neural substrates of attentional control. *Psychological Science, 19*(1), 12–17.

Henrich, J., & McElreath, R. (2007). Dual inheritance theory: The evolution of human cultural capacities and cultural evolution. In R. Dunbar & L. Barrett (Eds.), *Oxford handbook of evolutionary psychology* (pp. 555–570). Oxford University Press.

Hong, Y. Y., Morris, M. W., Chiu, C. Y., & Benet-Martinez, V. (2000). Multicultural minds: A dynamic constructivist approach to culture and cognition. *American Psychologist, 55*(7), 709–720.

Iacoboni, M. (2009). Imitation, empathy, and mirror neurons. *Annual Review of Psychology, 60*, 653–670.

Iacoboni, M., Woods, R. P., Brass, M., Bekkering, H., Mazziotta, J. C., & Rizzolatti, G. (1999). Cortical mechanisms of human imitation. *Science, 286*(5449), 2526–2528.

Ishii, K., Kim, H. S., Sasaki, J. Y., Shinada, M., & Kusumi, I. (2014). Culture modulates sensitivity to the disappearance of facial expressions associated with serotonin transporter polymorphism (5-HTTLPR). *Culture and Brain, 2*, 72–88.

Jenkins, L. J., Yang, Y. J., Goh, J., Hong, Y. Y., & Park, D. C. (2010). Cultural differences in the lateral occipital complex while viewing incongruent scenes. *Social Cognitive and Affective Neuroscience, 5*(2–3), 236–241.

Kim, H. S., Sherman, D. K., Mojaverian, T., Sasaki, J. Y., Park, J., Suh, E. M., & Taylor, S. (2011). Gene-culture interaction: Oxytocin receptor polymorphism (OXTR) and emotion regulation. *Social Psychological and Personality Science, 2*, 665–672.

Kim, H. S., Sherman, D. K., Taylor, S. E., Sasaki, J. Y., Chu, T. Q., Ryu, C., Suh, E. M., & Xu, J. (2010). Culture, serotonin receptor polymorphism and locus of attention. *Social Cognitive and Affective Neuroscience, 5*(2–3), 212–218.

Kim, H. S., & Sasaki, J. Y. (2012). Emotion regulation: The interplay of culture and genes. *Social and Personality Psychology Compass, 6*, 865–877.

Kim, H. S., & Sasaki, J. Y. (2014). Cultural neuroscience: Biology of the mind in cultural context. *Annual Review of Psychology, 65*, 487–514.

Kitayama, S., & Uskul, A. K. (2011). Culture, mind, and the brain: Current evidence and future directions. *Annual Review of Psychology, 62*, 419–449.

Laland, K. N., Olding-Smee, J., & Feldman, M. W. (2000). Niche construction, biological evolution and cultural change. *Behavioural and Brain Sciences, 23*(1), 131–146.

Lamm, C., Decety, J., & Singer, T. (2011). Meta-analytic evidence for common and distinct neural networks associated with directly experienced pain and empathy for pain. *Neuroimage, 54*(3), 2492–502.

Lieberman, M. D., Hariri, A., Jarcho, J. M., Eisenberger, N. I., & Bookheimer, S. Y. (2005). An fMRI investigation of race-related amygdala activity in African-American and Caucasian-American individuals. *Nature Neuroscience, 8*(6), 720–722.

Lin, Z., Lin, Y., & Han, S. (2008). Self-construal priming modulates visual activity underlying global/local perception. *Biological Psychology, 77*(1), 93–97.

Losin, E. A., Iacoboni, M., Martin, A., Cross, K. A., & Dapretto, M. (2012). Race modulates neural activity during imitation. *Neuroimage, 59*(4), 3594–603.

Losin, E. A., Iacoboni, M., Martin, A., & Dapretto, M. (2012). Own-gender imitation activates the brain's reward circuitry. *Social Cognitive and Affective Neuroscience, 7*(7), 804–810.

Luo, S., Ma, Y., Liu, Y., Li, B., Wang, C., Shi, Z., Li, X., Zhang, W., Rao, Y., & Han, S. (2015). Interaction between oxytocin receptor polymorphism and interdependent culture values on human empathy. *Social Cognitive and Affective Neuroscience, 10*(9), 1273–1281.

Manly, J. J. (2008). Critical issues in cultural neuropsychology: Profit from diversity. *Neuropsychological Review, 18*(3), 179–183.

Markus, H. R., & Kitayama, S. (1991). Culture and the self: Implications for cognition, emotion and motivation. *Psychological Review, 8*, 224–253.

Masten, C. L., Telzer, E. H., & Eisenberger, N. I. (2011). An fMRI investigation of attributing negative social treatment to racial discrimination. *Journal of Cognitive Neuroscience, 23*(5), 1042–1051.

Mathur, V. A., Harada, T., Lipke, T., & Chiao, J. Y. (2010). Neural basis of extraordinary empathy and altruistic motivation. *Neuroimage, 51*(4), 1468–1475.

Mathur, V. A. Harada, T., & Chiao, J. Y. (2012). Racial identification modulates default network activity for same and other races. *Human Brain Mapping, 33*(8), 1883–1893.

Matsumoto, D., Yoo, S. H., Fontaine, J., Anguas-Wong, A. M., Arriola, M., Ataca, B., Bond, M. H., Boratav, H. B., Breugelmans, S. M., Cabecinhas, R., Chae, J., Chin, W. H., Comunian, A. L., DeGere, D. N., Djunaidi, A., Fok, H. K., Friedlmeier, W., Ghosh, A., Glamcevski, M., . . . Zebian, S. (2008). Mapping expressive differences around the world: The relationship between emotional display rules and Individualism v. Collectivism. *Journal of Cross-Cultural Psychology*, 39, 55–74.

Mesquita, B., & Frijda, N. H. (1992). Cultural variations in emotions: A review. *Psychological Bulletin, 112*(2), 179–204.

Mesoudi, A. (2009). How cultural evolutionary theory can inform social psychology and vice versa. *Psychological Review, 116*(4), 929–952.

Murata, A., Moser, J. S., & Kitayama, S. (2013). Culture shapes electrocortical responses during emotional suppression. *Social Cognitive and Affective Neuroscience, 8*(5), 595–601.

Nisbett, R. E., Peng, K., Choi, I., & Norenzayan, A. (2001). Culture and systems of thought: Holistic versus analytic cognition. *Psychological Review, 108*(2), 291–310.

Ochsner, K. N., Bunge, S. A., Gross, J. J., & Gabrieli, J. D. (2002). Rethinking feelings: An fMRI study of the cognitive regulation of emotion. *Journal of Cognitive Neuroscience, 14*(8), 1215–1229.

Oyserman, D., Coon, H. M., & Kemmelmeier, M. (2002). Rethinking individualism and collectivism: Evaluation and theoretical assumptions and meta-analyses. *Psychological Bulletin, 128*(1), 3–72.

Oyserman, D., & Lee, S. W. (2008). Does culture influence what and how we think? Effects of priming individualism and collectivism. *Psychological Bulletin, 134*(2), 311–342.

Park, B., Tsai, J. L., Chim, L., Blevins, E., & Knutson, B. (2016). Neural evidence for cultural differences in the valuation of positive facial expressions. *Social Cognitive and Affective Neuroscience, 11*(2), 243–252.

Park, D. C., & Gutchess, A. H. (2002). Aging, cognition, and culture: A neuroscientific perspective. *Neuroscience and Biobehavioral Review, 26*(7), 859–867.

Phinney, J. S. (1990). Ethnic identity in adolescents and adults: Review of research. *Psychological Bulletin, 108*(2), 499–514.

Pornpattananangkul, N., Hariri, A. R., Harada, T., Mano, Y., Komeda, H., Parrish, T. B., Sadato, N., Iidaka, T., & Chiao, J. Y. (2016). Cultural influences on neural basis of inhibitory control. *Neuroimage, 139,* 114–126.

Preston, S. D., & De Waal, F. B. (2002). Empathy: Its ultimate and proximate bases. *Behavioral and Brain Sciences, 25*(1), 1–20.

Richeson, J. A., Baird, A. A., Gordon, H. L., Heatherton, T. F., Wyland, C. L., Trawalter, S., & Shelton, J. N. (2003). An fMRI investigation of the impact of interracial contact on executive function. *Nature Neuroscience, 6*(12), 1323–1328.

Roberts, N. A. & Levenson, R. W. (2006). Subjective, behavioral, and physiological reactivity to ethnically matched and ethnically mismatched film clips. *Emotion, 6*(4), 635–646.

Sasaki, J. Y., LeClair, J., West, A. L., & Kim, H. S. (2016). Application of the gene-culture interaction framework in health contexts. In J. Y. Chiao, S.-C. Li, R. Seligman, & R. Turner (Eds.), *The Oxford handbook of cultural neuroscience* (pp. 279–298). Oxford University Press.

Sellers, R. M., Smith, M. A., Shelton, J. N., Rowley, S. A. J., & Chavous, T. M. (1998). Multidimensional model of racial identity: A reconceptualization of African American racial identity. *Personality and Social Psychological Review, 2,* 18–39.

Shelton, J. N., Richeson, J. A., Salvatore, J., & Trawalter, S. (2005). Ironic effects of racial bias during interracial interactions. *Psychological Science, 16*(5), 397–402.

Shih, M. J., Pittinsky, T. L., & Ho, G. C. (2011). Stereotype boost: Positive outcomes from the activation of positive stereotypes. In Inzlicht, M. & Schmader, T. (Eds.) *Stereotype threat: Theory, process, and application* (pp. 141–158). New York, NY: Oxford University Press.

Smedley, A., & Smedley, B. D. (2005). Race as biology is fiction, racism as a social problem is real: Anthropological and historical perspectives on the social construction of race. *American Psychologist, 60*(10), 16–26.

Soto, J. A., Lee, E. A., & Roberts, N. A. (2016). Convergence in feeling, divergence in physiology: How culture influences the consequences of disgust suppression and amplification among European Americans and Asian Americans. *Psychophysiology, 53,* 41–51.

Steele, C. M. (1997). A threat in the air: How stereotypes shape intellectual identity and performance. *American Psychologist, 52*(6), 613–629.

Tsai, J. L. (2007). Ideal affect: Cultural causes and behavioral consequences. *Perspectives in Psychological Science, 2*(3), 242–259.

Wager, T. D., Davidson, M. L., Hughes, B. L., Lindquist, M. A., & Ochsner, K. N. (2008). Prefrontal-subcortical pathways mediating successful emotion regulation. *Neuron, 59*(6), 1037–1050.

Wang, Q. (2006). Culture and the development of self-knowledge. *Current Directions in Psychological Science, 15*(4), 182–187.

Whiteford, H. A., Degenhardt, L., Rehm, J., Baxter, A. J., Ferrari, A. J., Erskine, H. E., Charlson, F. J., Norman, R. E., Flaxman, A. D., Johns, N., Burstein, R., Murray, C. J., & Vos, T. (2013). Global burden of disease attributable to mental and substance use disorders: Findings from the Global Burden of Disease Study 2010. *Lancet, 382,* 1575–1586.

Xu, X., Zuo, X., Wang, X., & Han, S. (2009). Do you feel my pain? Racial group membership modulates empathic neural responses. *Journal of Neuroscience, 29*(26), 8525–8529.

Zhu, Y., Zhang, L., Fan, J., & Han, S. (2007). Neural basis of cultural influence on self representation. *Neuroimage, 34,* 1310–1317.

Psychophysiological Approaches in Cultural Neuroscience and Global Mental Health

Joan Y. Chiao *and* Norihiro Sadato

Abstract

Advances in cultural neuroscience demonstrate that culture affects how neural systems maintain and regulate social and emotional information. Understanding how neural representations dynamically interact with environmental and cultural factors provides novel insight into how psychophysiological and neural mechanisms encode culture. Research on psychophysiological approaches in cultural neuroscience provide novel ways to observe and measure dynamic cultural influences on the nervous system with temporal precision. Theory and methods on psychophysiological approaches in cultural neuroscience may provide foundational ways of understanding how cultural dynamics shape neural and physiological response and its relation to behavior. Challenges and opportunities for psychophysiological approaches in cultural neuroscience to address issues of population health disparities and global mental health are discussed.

Key Words: cultural neuroscience, psychophysiology, cultural dynamics, population health disparities, global mental health

Introduction

Culture refers to systems of values, practices, and beliefs that are acquired from others and define distinct social groups (Betancourt & Lopez, 1993; Hofstede, 2001; Richerson & Boyd, 2005). Within social groups, culture is transmitted within and across social relationships through social contact, language, diet, and technology. Related to the concept of culture, race as a biological concept typically refers to physical characteristics that are shared among individuals within a given population attributable to shared genetic inheritance, and as a socially constructed concept refers to a cultural inheritance of ideology about groups of people, such as social stereotypes (Helms et al., 2005; Smedley & Smedley, 2005). Ethnicity, a concept associated with both race and culture, refers to the social norms and behaviors that are shared within a group historically defined along demographic terms (e.g., national origin, language, or culture; Helms & Talleyrand, 1997; Phinney, 1996);

ethnic groups may adopt distinct kinds of cultural norms and values, encourage ethnic identity with others within the group, and share experiences and attitudes when defined by minority status (Phinney, 1996). Socioeconomic status (SES) refers to an individual or group's overall status and position in society defined by income, education, and occupation and is consistently associated with health outcomes (Adler et al., 1994; Stephens et al., 2012). People living in low-SES environments, such as the working class and the poor, are at risk for lower health and educational outcomes, due to impoverished conditions including inadequate nutrition, sanitation, education, and medical care (Adler et al., 1994; Hackman et al., 2011).

Cultural dynamics refer to how culture may change across time due to a number of factors (Kashima, 2007, 2014). Macro-level cultural dynamics refer to large-scale, long-term cultural changes that may occur gradually over time or rapidly, such as in the case of punctuated equilibrium (Gould & Eldredge, 1977). Micro-level cultural dynamics refer to cultural change and maintenance including what kinds of factors lead to cultural change and maintenance or stability over time.

There are at least four basic mechanisms of cultural dynamics, including importation, invention, selection, and drift. Cultural importation refers to novel cultural information from a heritage culture that is transmitted into a host culture. Immigrants who migrate to a new nation may import novel cultural information, such as language, diet, technology, and religion, to the host culture, thereby altering cultural dynamics. Cultural invention refers to the introduction of novel cultural information without importation. Cultural selection refers to cultural information that is valued and selectively transmitted or reproduced within a culture. Cultural habits may undergo cultural selection as a means of adaptive health promotion. Cultural drift refers to random processes that produce a change in the prevalence of cultural information across time. Nearly all mechanisms of cultural change require integrating or learning information from other social partners within a given culture.

Early developments in cultural psychology focused on designing methods, such as self-report surveys and archival, longitudinal, and behavioral paradigms, for studying culture. The development of behavioral surveys provides a method for assessment of cultural values, practices, and beliefs with self-report (Gelfand et al., 2011; Markus & Kitayama, 1991; Oyserman et al., 2002). Independent cultural values define the self as autonomous from others, whereas interdependent cultural values define the self in terms of social roles and relationships. Tight culture refers to emphasis on abiding social norms, whereas loose culture refers to tolerance for social norm deviation. Self-report cultural surveys of independence–interdependence and tightness–looseness allow for explicit measurement of cultural values. Self-report indices of SES, including surveys of income, educational attainment, and perceived SES, allow researchers to measure objective and subjective SES to characterize demographic populations defined by ethnicity according to SES (Shavers, 2007). The development of novel behavioral paradigms, such as the frame-line task (Hedden et al., 2008; Kitayama et al., 2003), allowed cultural scientists to test hypotheses about how culture affects the way people think about themselves and the objects around them.

The study of acculturation, or the study of how people migrate and acquire cultural knowledge from the host culture, compares behavioral responses measured at multiple time points before and after people migrate from their heritage culture and learn to adjust to the host culture (Berry, 1997; Telzer, 2011). Cultural priming methods allow cultural scientists to understand how temporal changes in the culture and environment relate to mental states and behavior. Cultural priming or the degree to which a person is exposed consciously or unconsciously to certain kinds of information in the environment can dynamically alter how individuals think and behave by making more accessible given sets of cultural knowledge or beliefs (Hong et al., 2000; Oyserman & Lee, 2008). The use of surveys that assess cultural values, practices, and beliefs allows for quantification of culture and behavior and the integration of cultural information with biological indices. Cross-temporal methods, such as archival and longitudinal research, allow for comparison of cultural norms and trajectories across time. Archival research may, for instance, assess the trajectory of word use related to independence and interdependence or tightness–looseness in public and private records, such as media and diaries. Longitudinal research assesses macro-level cultural dynamics by measuring cultural values, practices, and beliefs repeatedly across a long period of time. The World Value Survey (WVS) is a large-scale longitudinal behavioral survey that assessed cultural values across six time periods, each time period lasting several years, within a nationally representative sample that was administered a survey questionnaire in their native language (Inglehart, 1997; Inglehart et al., 2008). International adoption study design may also allow for longitudinal measurement of macro-level cultural dynamics (McGuinness & Dyer, 2006).

Genetic variation in the human population may also contribute to varying levels of universality and diversity in human brain function. Genes represent the fundamental unit of heredity and substantially influence neurotransmission within the brain. Recent advances in neurogenetics show a genetic contribution to human brain function for specific functional polymorphisms during processing of cognitive, emotional, and social information. The human amygdala shows differential levels of response to emotional faces depending on allelic variation of the serotonin transporter (5-HTTLPR) gene (Hariri, 2009). Short allele carriers of the serotonin transporter gene show increased bilateral amygdala response during emotional processing relative to long allele carriers (Hariri, 2009). Epigenetic variation of the serotonin transporter gene similarly modulates bilateral amygdala response such that increased promoter methylation of the serotonin transporter gene predicts increased amygdala response to threat (Nikolova et al., 2014). Epigenetic variation of the oxytocin receptor (OXTR) gene also influences neural mechanisms in response to perception of anger and fear. High levels of OXTR methylation were associated with increased neural response during face and emotion processing within the amygdala, fusiform, and insula (Puglia et al., 2015). These findings suggest that genetic and epigenetic mechanisms alter neural response during social and emotional processing. The prevalence of allelic variation for the serotonin transporter gene varies across nations such as that East Asian nations (e.g., Japan, Singapore, China) have an increased prevalence of short allele compared to long allele carriers, but a decreased prevalence of mental health disorders, including anxiety and mood disorders; it has been speculated that this is due in part to cultural norms of collectivism (Chiao & Blizinsky, 2010).

Cultural dynamics affect psychophysiological and neurobiological mechanisms of behavior. One of the earliest advances in human neuroscience was the discovery that recordings of brain waves could reveal how the brain gives rise to the mind in a continuous manner (Berger, 1929). Innovations in scientific technology, such as event-related potentials (ERPs), allow scientists to understand how temporal changes in electrical activity relate to mental states and behavior (Galambos & Sheatz, 1962; Walter et al., 1964). The degree of electrical activity near the scalp changes in response to specific events or stimuli in the external environment as well as changes within milliseconds in response to specific events or states within the mind. Despite lack of change in conscious awareness, electrical activity responds to fluctuations within the external and internal environment. How electrical activity modulates across the brain provides clues into what kinds of neural systems or circuitry support distinct kinds of psychological states. While much is known about the role of psychophysiology in understanding mental states and behavior, such methods have less often been employed to understand how culture shapes mind, brain, and behavior. Recent advances in psychophysiological approaches in cultural neuroscience reveal a number of ways that culture modulates brain response in a dynamic manner.

The goal of this chapter is to provide a review of cultural influences on psychophysiological mechanisms and their interaction with neural systems of behavior. Psychophysiological approaches provide novel means to examine how culture shapes brain and behavior within milliseconds of exposure and how the brain embodies culture within milliseconds of response. Psychophysiological approaches facilitate understanding of the neurobiology of cultural dynamics, including the measurement of short- and long-term changes of culture in the brain. Studies integrating psychophysiological approaches in cultural neuroscience may also be able to elucidate for the first time cross-generational and cross-situational effects of culture on the brain. Recent advances in psychophysiology approaches in cultural neuroscience and their implications for understanding population health disparities and global mental health will be discussed.

Cultural Neuroscience and Global Mental Health

Cultural neuroscience and global mental health is a field of study that seeks to identify root mechanisms, causes, and risk factors of mental disorders (Chiao et al., 2017). Research in cultural neuroscience and global mental health provides an evidence-based resource for understanding the cellular and molecular mechanisms of the human brain across cultural settings. Cultural neuroscience examines how culture influences neural mechanisms of behavior across the lifespan to address challenges in global mental health. Theoretical and methodological foundations in cultural neuroscience provide conceptual frameworks and observational tools for the measurement of root causes of mental disorders.

Advances in cultural neuroscience have begun to identify key psychological domains of cultural influences on neural mechanisms of behavior. Cultural neuroscience identifies cultural influences on neurobiological mechanisms of behavior (Chiao, Cheon, Pornpattananankul, Mrazek, Blizinsky, 2013). Cultural influences on neurocognitive mechanisms contribute to the understanding of culture and cognition (Han & Northoff, 2008; Kitayama & Uskul, 2011). Cultural dimensions affect a range of mental processes and neural mechanisms, from emotion and cognition to social and regulatory behavior. Neurodevelopmental trajectories and environmental influences further contribute to the determinants of mental health across cultures. The study of cultural differences in aging contributes to the understanding of culture and cognition across the lifespan (Park & Gutchess, 2002).

Cultural neuroscience as an evidence-based resource contributes to the development and implementation of targeted preventions and interventions in global mental health. Dysregulation of brain regions may differentially affect the etiology of mental disorders across cultural settings. The identification of biomarkers that contribute to health promotion and variation in disease risk across cultural settings contribute to the discovery science and the development of preventions and interventions. Reduction in exposure to societal and environmental risk factors facilitates the delivery science of prevention and intervention of mental disorders. The study of psychophysiological approaches strengthens a dynamical understanding of the human brain in cultural neuroscience and global mental health. Comprehensive integration of cultural neuroscience in global mental health is essential to implementation of the systematic analysis of social and cultural context as risk and protective factors of mental health.

Theoretical Foundations

Theoretical foundations of psychophysiological approaches in cultural neuroscience and global mental health build from the reciprocal interactions of cultural and genetic systems. Dual inheritance theory suggests that cognitive and neural architectures are affected by both cultural and genetic inheritance (Boyd & Richerson, 1985). Not only are cultural habits and practices inherited from parents and caregivers, but also they are inherited within constructed ecological niches (Odling-Smee et al., 2003). One of the most important ways to understand how culture shapes the brain is by studying how culture and genes shape the spatiotemporal dynamics of brain and bodily response (Chiao & Ambady, 2007). Psychophysiology provides theory and methods for understanding how dynamic brain activity affects behavior. Cultural psychology has shown that one of the most important features of culture is its ability to dynamically shape behavior (Hong et al., 2000; Oyserman & Lee, 2008). Priming culture, with visual symbols (e.g., flags) or verbal labels (e.g., pronouns), can alter how people think about themselves and others, cooperate, and make decisions (Hong et al., 2000; Oyserman & Lee, 2008). Priming methods expose people to information in the environment both below and above conscious awareness by changing the amount of exposure to that information. Brief exposure to environmental information, for only approximately 15 or 30 milliseconds, for instance, may not be detectable to a person in their conscious state; however, their behavior or preferences may change as a result. Priming culture with both conscious and unconscious or explicit and implicit methods have been shown to reliably change human behavior. Relatedly, epigenetics research has shown that the level of genetic transmission is alterable, depending on interaction with the environment (Meaney, 2010; Sasaki, LeClair, West, Kim, 2016), within brain regions associated with social (Puglia et al., 2015) and emotional behavior (Nikolova et al., 2014). Conducting research that incorporates culture and epigenetics into psychophysiology research enables us to examine how the environment and cultural and genetic expression alter neural expression within the central and autonomic nervous system in a simultaneous and interactive fashion.

A basic theoretical premise in cultural neuroscience is the notion that culture shapes how the brain and body respond to the environment and produce adaptive behavior (Chiao, Harada et al., 2010). The central nervous system is responsible for the part of the nervous system including the brain and spinal cord that control motor, sensory, and higher-level functioning and interact with other bodily systems such as the autonomic nervous system (Blascovich et al., 2011; Cacioppo et al., 1989); the autonomic nervous system includes the visceral part of the nervous system responsible for bodily changes in response to the environment including temperature, heart rate, digestion, pupillary dilation, arousal, respiratory rate, and perspiration, which are related to social and emotional behavior (Ax, 1953; Levenson, 2014). Depending on cultural values, practices, or beliefs, central and autonomic nervous systems may respond in a distinct manner facilitating adaptive behavior that both constructs and maintains the cultural environment.

Methodological Foundations

Psychophysiological methods in cultural neuroscience integrate key methodological tools from cultural psychology, neuroscience, and psychophysiology. One of the most important discoveries in cultural psychology is the use of cultural priming techniques to show that even brief exposure to cultural information shapes how people think, feel, and behave (Hong et al., 2000; Oyserman & Lee, 2008). Studies by Hong and colleagues (2000), for instance, show that when exposed to visual images that are consistent with individualistic or collectivistic cultural norms, people are more likely to respond in a culturally appropriate manner. Gardner et al. (1999) also showed that when people are exposed to language that promotes either an independent or interdependent cultural norm, people are more likely to respond and think about themselves and others in a culturally appropriate manner. Hence, even brief exposure to cultural information can shape human behavior in an important manner. Additionally, behavioral surveys that measure cultural values, practices, and beliefs are important to assess the explicit preferences, attitudes, or beliefs of others. Responses from cultural surveys have been shown to reliably correlate with neural response within specific brain regions, such as the prefrontal cortex (Chiao, Harada et al., 2009). Combining behavioral responses with temporally sensitive brain recordings, such as those measured with psychophysiological techniques, allows for researchers to make inferences regarding how culture is related to brain responses.

Psychophysiology is one of the most well-studied research areas within human neuroscience. ERP is a well-studied psychophysiological technique that allows researchers to better understand how events in the environment, such as brief exposure to information, shape the magnitude of neural response within a specific time window and brain topography (Luck, 2005). By studying the spatiotemporal dynamics of brain response with ERP, cultural researchers can study when and how neural response changes as a function of processing of social and emotional information and culture. For instance, empathic responses to other emotional states, for example, modulate both early (i.e., N2) and late (i.e., P3) ERP components (Decety et al., 2010; Jiang et al., 2014). Recently, cultural researchers examined which specific time points of empathetic processes are modulated by cultures (Jiang et al., 2014). Similarly, cultural researchers can also focus on specific ERP components that are associated with specific cognitive processes. These ERP components are usually elicited by specific tasks and have a distinct time window and topography (for review, see Luck & Kappenman, 2011). Lewis et al. (2008, see later), for example, were one of the first group of researchers to investigate how cultures differentially influence novelty detection and target categorization by examining two distinct ERP components in the P3 time window: anterior P3a and posterior P3b. By identifying ERP components of interest in one's hypotheses, researchers can make sound predictions or hypotheses regarding how specific neural-cognitive processes are modulated by cultural factors, such as cultural groups, cultural priming, and/or cultural values. Next we provide some empirical advances from recent ERP studies that follow this research approach. Together with behavioral and neuroimaging evidence, ERPs allow cultural researchers to achieve their goals of understanding the mechanisms underlying cultural differences (Heine & Norenzayan, 2006).

Empirical Foundations

One of the earliest ways to understand human emotion was by observing autonomic nervous system or bodily responses during emotional responding, expression, and regulation (Levenson et al., 1992). Early investigations into emotion consisted of examining how facial muscle configurations change in a manner consistent with specific emotion patterns. The rationale for emotion specificity in bodily response still applies to many levels of neural response during emotion, including autonomic and neural physiology

(Levenson et al., 1992). Observations of facial muscle configurations later turned to questions regarding how the underlying bodily physiology, such as finger pulse, blood pressure, heart rate, and skin conductance response, reflects or is modulated by specific emotional responses. Autonomic nervous system activity reflects interaction between neural systems of the brain and internal bodily organs that are interconnected. Autonomic arousal may reflect shifts in bodily states that involve changes in blood flow and sympathetic activity in the heart (Critchley, 2009). While cultures vary in the extent to which people express emotions (Elfenbein & Ambady, 2002), cultural differences in emotional expression are not necessarily observable in autonomic indices during emotion responding (Soto et al., 2005). Similarly, while cultures vary in how and to what extent people regulate emotion (Mauss et al., 2008), little change may be observed in autonomic responses during culturally congruent emotional regulation (Roberts et al., 2008).

Culture and Emotion: Autonomic Response

Nevertheless, recent cultural psychophysiological studies indicate that autonomic responses are heightened when perceiving emotional responses or expressions from people of one's own cultural group, a phenomenon known as the ingroup advantage (Roberts & Levenson, 2006; Soto & Levenson, 2009; Table 6.1). Across four ethnic groups of Americans, Soto and colleagues showed that Chinese Americans exhibit greater autonomic response to Chinese American emotional responding during a naturalistic social interaction, compared to the emotional responding of members of other groups (Soto & Levenson, 2009). This ingroup advantage in emotional responsivity at the autonomic level may reflect early tuning to group members during development, and possibly also positive attitudes for and cultural understanding of or competence with group members that emerge and sustain throughout the lifespan. Relatedly, Roberts and Levenson (2006) observed that across four ethnic groups of Americans, people showed enhanced autonomic response during emotional responses of group members. Butler et al. (2009) found that for Asian Americans, emotional expressivity was positively correlated with heightened blood pressure compared to European Americans possibly due to cultural norms that emphasize emotional suppression or inhibition of emotions that may affect or disrupt social harmony. Mauss and Butler (2010) further showed that emotional control values are related to a challenge pattern of cardiovascular responses in Asian Americans, whereas emotional control values are related to a threat pattern of cardiovascular responses in European Americans. Taken together, these findings demonstrate that cultural group membership plays an important role in shaping psychophysiological responses to emotion.

Electrophysiological measurement of cortical responses provides several distinct ways of understanding how the brain works and its relation to behavior. Given the importance of the human brain in guiding behavior, dynamical changes in electrophysiological responses may provide important clues into complex and subtle mechanisms that shape social and emotional behavior. The relatively enhanced proximity of recording closer to

Table 6.1. Psychophysiological Studies of Culture and Socioemotional Behavior

Study	Participants	Task	Physiological Index	Results[1]
Butler et al. (2009)	Asian Americans, European Americans	Emotional responding	MBP	AA R+ EEB-BP EA R- EEB-BP
Mauss & Butler (2010)	Asian Americans, European Americans	Emotional responding	VC, CO, TPR	AA ECV-Challenge EA ECV-Threat
Roberts & Levenson (2006)	African Americans, Chinese Americans, European Americans, Mexican Americans	Emotional responding	CII, FPT, EPT, FPA, RII	Ingroup > Outgroup
Roberts et al. (2008)	African Americans, Chinese Americans, European Americans, Mexican Americans	Emotional suppression	CII, FPA, FPT, EPT, FT, BP, RII, RSA, SCR, GSA	No differences
Soto et al. (2005)	Chinese Americans, Mexican Americans	Emotional responding	CII, PTT, FPR, EPT, ABP, SCR, FT	No differences
Soto & Levenson (2009)	African Americans, Chinese Americans, European Americans, Mexican Americans	Social interaction	CII, PTT, FPA, EPT, SCR, FT, GSA	$CA^{ingroup} > CA^{outgroup}$

[1] ABP = Arterial blood pressure; BP = blood pressure; CII = cardiac interbeat interval; CO = cardiac output; EPT = ear pulse transmission time; FPA = finger pulse amplitude; FPR = finer pulse response; FT = finger temperature; FPT = finger pulse temperature; GSA = general somatic activity; MBP = mean blood pressure; PTT = pulse transmission time; RII = respiratory intercycle interval; RSA = respiratory sinus arrhythmia; SCR = skin conductance response; TPR = total peripheral resistance; VC = ventricular contractility.

the neural source of psychological and behavioral change is one possible advantage of studying cultural dynamics with electrophysiology. Additionally, the temporal sensitivity of electrophysiological measurement allows for a more detailed understanding of what kinds of processes are antecedents or consequences of a given social and emotional behavior. Determining causality in the relation between brain, body, and behavior in the study of emotion, for instance, has historically been an issue of vast theoretical debate. Cultural psychophysiological theory and methods may provide a novel opportunity to better understand how human emotion unfolds across multiple levels of analysis (Table 6.2).

Culture and Empathy: N2 and Transcranial Magnetic Stimulation/Motor-Evoked Potentials

Numerous neuroimaging studies have recently demonstrated that perceiving others in pain enhances neural responses in the pain matrix, including the anterior cingulate cortex (ACC) and bilateral anterior insula (AI; Decety & Jackson, 2004; Hein & Singer, 2008). Such findings have been taken as evidence for a neural basis of empathy in humans, such

Table 6.2. Psychophysiological Studies of Culture and Socioemotional Behavior

Study	Participants	Task	ERP— Early to Late Components	Results
Jiang et al. (2014)	Chinese, Westerners	Empathy	N2	$INT^{emp} > IND^{emp}$
Murata et al. (2013)	European Americans, Asians	Emotion suppression	LPP	$Asians^{supp} > EA^{supp}$
Kitayama & Park (2014)	European Americans, Asians	Reward Flanker	ERN	$EA^{Self} > AA^{Self}$
Park & Kitayama (2014)	European Americans, Asians	Facial flanker	ERN	$Asians^{face} > EA^{face}$
Goto et al. (2013)	Asian Americans, European Americans	Semantic incongruity of emotion	N400	$AA^{incon} > EA^{incon}$
Goto et al. (2010)	East Asian/ Asian Americans, European Americans	Semantic incongruity	N400	$EA/AA^{incon} > EA^{incon}$
Masuda et al. (2014)	European Americans, Japanese	Analytic attention	N400	$JP^{incon} > EA^{incon}$
Na & Kitayama (2011)	European Americans, Asian Americans	Spontaneous trait inference	N400	$EA^{ant} > AA^{ant}$
Varnum et al. (2012)	Working class, middle class	Spontaneous trait inference	N400	$MC^{ant} > WC^{ant}$

emp = empathy; supp = suppression; incon = incongruity; ant = antonym.

that neural responses during perception of humans are modulated by (a) a cultural group of a victim who is in pain and (b) a cultural value of a perceiver, such as hierarchical preference (Cheon et al., 2013; Chiao, Mathur, et al., 2009; Mathur, Harada, Chiao, 2012). Without ERP evidence, however, researchers would have limited understanding of (a) the temporal sequence of how the brain reacts to the pain of others and (b) the time point at which cultural factors modulate the pain perception processes. Temporal specificity of pain perception has been demonstrated by ERP research, such that pain perception modulates both frontal-central negative-going ERP at around 200 ms and posterior positive-going ERP after 400 ms (Decety et al., 2010; Jiang et al., 2014). These ERPs correspond roughly to the N2 and P3b ERP components. The N2 in particular is thought to involve activity in the ACC, one of the regions in the pain matrix (for a review, see Folstein & Van Petten, 2008). Jiang and colleagues (2014) further demonstrated that cultural factors specifically influence the N2 but not the P3b. Particularly, the influence of pain perception on the N2 was diminished after either (a) Chinese were primed with collectivist values or (b) Westerners were primed with individualistic values, but not vice versa. This suggests that cultural factors modulate early, more automatic processes of pain perception (i.e., N2) rather than the later, more controlled processes (i.e., P3b). Functional magnetic resonance imaging (fMRI) evidence demonstrates *which* pain perception regions in the brain are modulated by cultural factors, whereas ERP evidence provides information regarding *when* these cultural factors modulate the brain.

In addition to pain, a recent cultural psychophysiological study also investigated the influences of cultural priming on another domain of empathy, namely mimicry, that involves cortical excitability of the mirror neuron system (MNS; Obhi et al., 2011). Previous neuroimaging studies of the mirror neuron system show cultural modulation of neural activation during imitation across social groups (Losin, Iacoboni, Martin, Dapretto, 2012; Losin, Cross, Iacoboni, Dapretto, 2014). These findings suggest an important role of cultural and social factors in the neural mechanisms of empathy. In this culture and psychophysiology study, Canadian participants saw either a collectivistic (e.g., a word "together") or individualistic (e.g., a word "alone") prime superimposed on a video of hand movement. During each trial, cortical excitability of the motor cortex was accessed through motor-evoked potentials (MEPs) that resulted from an application of transcranial magnetic stimulation (TMS). Enhanced motor-cortex excitability was found following a collectivistic prime, suggesting that collectivistic cultural values elevate activity in the MNS that underlies behavioral mimicry. Future studies may expand this line of research further using other mimicry indexes, such as electroencephalography (EEG) mu suppression (Pineda, 2005) and heartbeat synchronization (Konvalinka et al., 2011; Pineda, 2005).

Culture and Executive Function: N2

Prior studies in developmental psychology have shown cultural differences in executive function early in childhood. East Asian children typically perform better relative to Western children on executive function tasks, but comparable or worse on social cognition tasks, such as theory of mind (Oh & Lewis, 2008; Sabbagh et al., 2006). One possible explanation for this cultural difference during childhood is that Chinese parents typically expect their children to learn to control their impulses early in development to a greater extent than Western parents (Ho, 1994). ERP studies of impulse control in children have shown that neural activity within the N2 component, recorded from medial-frontal sites between 250 and 500 ms, increases during cognitive inhibition (e.g., no-go trials) relative to noninhibition (e.g., go trials). In a cultural psychophysiological study of executive function in children, Lahat and colleagues (2009) show that Chinese Canadian children show a larger N2 response relative to European Canadian children during inhibition (e.g., no-go trials). Furthermore, Chinese Canadian children showed more activation in the dorsomedial, ventromedial, and bilateral ventrolateral prefrontal cortex during executive function relative to European Canadian children. Results show a cultural difference in N2 response during executive function and identify a neural mechanism underlying executive function performance in children. Parental emphasis on impulse control in Chinese Canadian communities may result in increased recruitment of neurobiological mechanisms for impulse control in children during development compared to European

Canadian communities. These findings demonstrate the viability of studying culture with psychophysiological methods in children and show the importance of utilizing convergent methods with behavioral paradigms to understand how culture affects cognitive development in early childhood.

Culture and Novelty Detection: P3

One of the earliest developments within cultural psychology was the discovery of cultural biases toward contextual information (for review see Nisbett & Miyamoto, 2005). While Westerners usually show a bias toward foreground information, Easterners are often found to have an attentional bias toward background information and toward the relationship between background and foreground. Such behavioral findings are frequently used as evidence for cultural differences in cognition: analytic thinking among Westerners and holistic thinking among Easterners. Moreover, neuroimaging studies that include stimuli with foreground and background information have shown different brain regions associated with such cultural biases, including parietal regions and visual cortices (Goh et al., 2007; Hedden et al., 2008).

Recent ERP evidence complements these behavioral and fMRI findings in many important aspects. Lewis et al. (2008), for example, further examined whether such cultural biases extend beyond attentional biases on objects different in space (i.e., background vs. foreground of a picture) to the biases on objects different in the time of appearance. In a three-stimulus odd-ball task, their participants were asked to respond to designated "target" stimuli (e.g., "six") while ignoring "standard" stimuli (e.g., "eight") and "nontarget" stimuli (e.g., three-character stimuli). That is, the standard stimuli were physically similar to the target, whereas the nontarget stimuli were novel and physically distinct from both the target and nontarget stimuli. Because a posterior, positive-going ERP component, called the P3b, is usually strongest following the target stimuli, the P3b is thought to associate with target categorization processes (Johnson, 1988). Additionally, because an anterior, positive-going ERP component, called the P3a, is mostly enhanced by the nontarget stimuli, the P3a is often associated with novelty detection processes (Polich & Comerchero, 2003). Importantly, compared with classic cultural psychology studies using one image with foreground and background (Nisbett & Miyamoto, 2005), the target stimuli resemble foreground information, while the nontarget stimuli resemble background information. Consistent with behavioral and fMRI findings, Lewis and colleague (2008) demonstrated that the P3a is enhanced for nontarget stimuli among Asian Americans, and the P3b is enhanced for the target stimuli among European Americans. This suggests that culture modulates attentional biases toward context information in both space and time dimensions.

Culture and Congruency: N400

Several recent ERP studies have employed the N400 to investigate cultural biases toward contextual information. The N400 is a negative-deflecting ERP component occurring approximately 400 milliseconds poststimulus at central sites. This component is sensitive to stimuli that are conceptually incongruent to the context (Kutas & Hillyard, 1980). Accordingly, the N400 can be used to index the strength of the relationship between the stimuli of interest and their context. In one of the first studies to examine cultural influences on N400, Goto and colleagues (2010) presented a sequence of context and focal images that are either conceptually congruent (e.g., beach and a crab) or incongruent (e.g., parking lot and a crab) with each other. Their N400 findings show that amplitude for incongruent stimuli was more prominent among Asian Americans than European Americans. Moreover, this enhanced N400 response was associated with less individualistic values. This suggests that Asian Americans and people with low individualistic values are more sensitive to the relationship between the focal stimuli and their context.

Recent studies of culture and the N400 component have further confirmed the sensitivity of this component to culturally congruent information using a spontaneous trait inference task. Na and Kitayama (2011) showed that the N400 is greater in European Americans compared to Asian Americans when people are responding to traits that are the opposite of those paired with faces they have previously seen. European Americans who typically value individualistic cultural norms are more likely to prefer describing others in terms of traits, whereas Asian Americans who typically value collectivistic cultural norms are more likely to describe others in a contextual manner (Chiao, Harada et al., 2010). Hence, when European Americans encounter traits that are incongruent with those paired with previously studied faces, they are more likely to show an increased neural response within approximately 400 milliseconds of exposure to the incongruent social information.

In a novel cultural psychophysiological study of middle-class and working-class Americans, Varnum and colleagues (2012) show that middle-class Americans are more likely to show greater N400 response to incongruent social information compared to working-class Americans. This finding is consistent with prior evidence that middle-class Americans are more likely to show electrophysiological responses consistent with individualistic cultural norms, whereas working-class Americans are more likely to show electrophysiological responses consistent with collectivistic cultural norms. These results represent one of the earliest discoveries of SES affecting a psychophysiological index of social processing and contribute to a growing understanding of how social status is represented in the brain (Harada et al., 2013). These empirical findings of the N400 reveal how an electrophysiological index of incongruity can help to illuminate how culture shapes people's response to social and emotional information in the environment.

Culture and Performance Monitoring: Error-Related Negativity

Cultures vary in the extent to which they emphasize or reward accuracy and attention to detail. The error-related negativity (ERN) refers to a sharp negative deflecting ERP component that responds to errors (Gehring et al., 1990). Occurring approximately 80 to 150 ms after the error occurs at frontal-central sites, the ERN is thought to be associated with processing of errors to monitor one's own performance. The ERN allows recent cultural research to study cultural differences that are difficult to examine with behavioral paradigms. Park and Kitayama (2014), for instance, utilized the ERN to study cultural differences in social-evaluative threats. East Asians, in particular, are thought to be more sensitive to social-evaluative threats than Westerners (Kim & Markman, 2006). Specifically, Park and Kitayama (2014) presented a neutral face before each Flanker stimuli. They found that East Asians enhanced the ERN amplitude to a mistake following a face more so than Westerners. Moreover, the influence of a face on the ERN was associated with more collectivism values. Hence, this pattern of the ERN is consistent with the idea that collectivistic cultures emphasize belongingness in a society (Chiao & Blizinsky, 2010; Kim & Markman, 2006). In fact, the same researchers (Kitayama & Park, 2014) recently showed another situation in which the cultural emphasis on belongingness may have an influence on performance monitoring, as reflected by the ERN. Here, Kitayama and Park (2014) investigated the similarities in performance monitoring between tasks that give reward to the personal self versus to a friend. They found that the self-reward task led to a stronger ERN than the friend-reward task only for European Americans, but not for East Asians. More importantly, the more collectivistic values that the participants had, the fewer the differences in ERN between the self-reward and friend-reward tasks. These findings then are used as evidence for less self-centric motivation among East Asians and people with high collectivistic values. Taken together, these studies show that, depending on the cultural congruence of information attended to, cultural differences in independence and interdependence modulate electrophysiological sensitivity to performance monitoring as indicated by the ERN.

Culture and Emotion Regulation: Late Positive Potential

Culture affects how people respond to and regulate their emotions (Butler et al., 2007). Collectivistic cultures that emphasize social harmony are more likely to endorse emotion regulation strategies that minimize emotional expression that may disrupt the group. Emotional suppression is one kind of strategy that allows people to regulate emotions by minimizing emotional expressions associated with a given emotional state. East Asians may be more successful at suppressing emotions compared to Western Americans, who may find it incongruent with individualistic cultural norms. By contrast, individualistic cultures that emphasize individualism and autonomy are more likely to endorse emotion regulation strategies that promote nonconformity in expression and thought. Cognitive reappraisal is one such emotion regulation strategy that relies on rethinking a person's emotional state to change a negative feeling to a neutral one or a positive feeling to a neutral one. Numerous psychophysiological studies of emotion regulation have identified an ERP component called the late positive potential (LPP) as important in emotion regulation, specifically emotion suppression (Moser et al., 2006; Schonfelder et al., 2014; for review, Hajcak et al., 2010). Occurring around 400 ms after stimuli onset and sustaining for seconds at the central-parietal electrodes, the LPP is thought to reflect sustained cognitive processing or recurring thoughts (Hajcak et al., 2009; Schupp et al., 2000). Murata et al. (2013) recently showed that Asians, but not European Americans, are more likely to show a reduction in LPP during emotional suppression. These findings support the notion that culture shapes how people regulate their emotions and that sustained neural activity within the parietal topography after regulation begins modulates in response to the culturally congruent emotion regulation strategy.

Identification of ERP Components Important to the Study of Culture

One of the main objectives in designing a novel cultural psychophysiological study is to focus a given study on one or two ERP large components and utilize a behavioral paradigm well known for studying culture (Luck, 2005). Prior cultural psychophysiological studies provide an important foundation for future studies that measure culturally mediated constructs with psychophysiological methods. From as early as 200 milliseconds, culturally mediated differences are observed in the degree of amplitude response for a given component. These findings suggest that culturally mediated differences are measurable with psychophysiological methodology and modulate large positive and negative component waves from approximately 200 to 400 ms poststimulus (e.g., N2, P3, N400, LPP, ERN) and reflect largely controlled psychological processes. For instance, the intention to withhold a reflective action (e.g., suppress a laugh) or to not make an error (e.g., concentrate on pressing the right button) may produce variable psychophysiological responses in the LPP and ERN waveforms, respectively, across cultures depending on cultural expectations of appropriate social behavior. Behavioral feedback that results from an intention to conform to one's given cultural norms or practices may in turn lead to changes in psychophysiology, cultural and genetic expression, and the prevalence of man-made environmental pressures. The identification of specific ERP components modulated by culture provide important insights into what specific ERP components may be hypothesized a priori as responding differentially due to cultural factors and behavioral responses that are intended to demonstrate cultural competency and maintenance of cultural niche construction. Understanding the specific relationship between amplitude response within a specific ERP component and explicit or self-reported cultural values, practices, and beliefs, as well as the relation between ERP component modulation, autonomic response, and culture, remains an important open question for future research.

Challenges and Opportunities

There are a number of challenges and opportunities when conducting psychophysiological research in cultural neuroscience. One major advantage of studying how culture shapes the brain with psychophysiology is temporal precision. Psychophysiology enables us to measure autonomic and central neural activity within milliseconds of response, a temporal window that is much closer to actual neural response relative to other kinds of neuroscience methodologies that measure neural activity within only seconds of response. Another major advantage of studying psychophysiological approaches in cultural neuroscience is the practical ability to study neural activity within cultural settings that are not accessible with scientific technology that is not portable. Psychophysiology equipment does not require extensive set-up and can be successfully used in remote, rural, or low-SES cultural regions with minimal technological infrastructure (Chiao & Blizinsky, 2013; Hechtman et al., 2013; Stein et al., 2016). In fact, this practicality aspect of psychophysiological methodologies (e.g., mobility and cost) also allows researchers to conduct large-scale studies that involve a large number of subjects. Iacono (2014) recently conducted a genome-wide study in which psychophysiological methodologies were used to examine endophenotypes among 4,900 twins and parents. Potentially, cultural researchers can employ a similar approach to tackle big questions in cultural science, such as how genes and cultures coevolve or interact across different geographies (Chiao & Blizinsky, 2010).

A third advantage is that there exists a large number of pedagogical resources for learning psychophysiology techniques (Blascovich et al., 2011; Luck, 2005). One of the oldest neuroscience methods for studying the human brain and body, psychophysiology provides scientists with a reliable way of studying well-studied neural phenomena across cultures. A fourth advantage is the potential for empirical findings due to the novelty of the research approach. There have been very few studies designed to study how cultural values, such as individualism–collectivism and tightness–looseness, predict electrophysiological responses to emotion and social behavior; relatedly, there has been little empirical progress made in understanding how cultural values relate to autonomic responses during emotion and social behavior. Prior cultural psychophysiological studies of emotion that did not find ethnic or racial differences in autonomic response during emotion may have not observed a latent relation between cultural and neural response due to instrumentation or the kind of conceptualization of culture. Similar to neuroimaging studies of culture, psychophysiological studies may discover associations between neural biomarkers and culture, even in the absence of behavioral differences, such as lack of cultural differences in reaction time or accuracy. Finally, because numerous initial neuroscientific insights into human behavior have emerged from psychophysiology illustrating the sensitivity of this methodology for measurement of brain–behavior relations, novel neural phenomena may be reliably observed when conducting such studies in novel cultural and environmental settings.

Several challenges may also be encountered when conducting cultural psychophysiological research. One challenge involves the ability to record neural activity within a high level of spatial precision. Scalp EEG, for instance, allows for neural activity recording primarily from the scalp, which does not necessarily allow for measurement of neural activity within brain regions that are located further below the scalp or subcortically. This is perhaps because subcortical neurons are not often arranged in a parallel fashion, and hence are not able to produce a measurable signal at the scalp (Jackson & Bolger, 2014). Intracranial EEG, on the other hand, can give both time and spatial precision, but the technique is too invasive to be used to study group and individual differences, as well as cultural differences. When studying emotional or social representations, for instance, the dynamics of neural response within medial or subcortical regions, such as the human amygdala, may be difficult to measure, thus reducing the kinds of questions or theories of culture that can be tested.

One way to address this challenge is by adopting a multimodal recording strategy when studying how culture affects the brain. By using psychophysiological methods with other kinds of neuroscience methods that have a high degree of spatial precision, such as fMRI, researchers gain the ability to understand how and when the brain responds to the environment and the role of culture in shaping a brain–behavior relation. TMS is a noninvasive method of brain stimulation that measures the function of specific brain circuits and may provide another important convergent method for addressing psychophysiological questions in cultural neuroscience. For instance, temporary stimulation of cortical circuitry within a given brain region that alters behavioral response demonstrates that a given cortical mechanism is necessary for a given psychological function. Identifying with TMS specific cortical regions that may serve as reliable sources of electrophysiological recording is helpful for designing studies that test a priori hypotheses concerning the effects of culture on the spatiotemporal dynamics of cortical response.

Another potential challenge is incorporating the study of culture directly with electrophysiological methods. For instance, behavioral paradigms that have previously demonstrated cultural variation in behavior may need to be adapted or modified when integrated with psychophysiological methods. The ability to continuously measure electrophysiological response from the cortex during completion of a given behavioral paradigm may require additional study trials depending on effect size estimates compared to a behavioral paradigm in order to ensure reliable measurement. Integrating cultural measures before or after psychophysiological measurement may also serve as a potential methodological challenge. While a majority of neuroscience research samples primarily from Western, educated, industrialized, rich democracies (Chiao & Cheon, 2010), little is known about how culture is associated with psychophysiological responses. Rather than assume or infer culture from race or ethnic heritage, measurement of cultural values, beliefs, and norms with validated cultural surveys is needed to integrate cultural data with psychophysiological measurement. Notably, when testing hypotheses regarding how cultural dynamics affect brain response, integrating cultural priming methods prior to measurement of brain response during a given behavioral task may be useful to assess associations between cultural dynamics and brain function (Chiao, Harada et al., 2010; Harada et al., 2010; Varnum et al., 2014).

Future Directions

Very little research has examined autonomic nervous system responses across cultures. While much anthropological and cultural psychological research on emotion details both subtle and large differences in emotional experience across cultures, little evidence yet exists on how culture affects visceral changes in the brain and body to emotional and social information in the environment. One advantage of psychophysiological equipment is the portable nature of the measurement apparatus; the methodological requirements for conducting cultural psychophysiological research may allow for study of remote cultures or cultural-bound syndromes. Hwa-byung or "fire illness" is a culture-bound syndrome that describes the emotional response to chronic social aggression in Korean culture (Min, 1989). While much anthropological description exists of this culture-bound syndrome, it remains unknown whether or not the psychophysiological response associated with this syndrome is similar to or distinct from other ways of describing emotion across cultures (Chiao, 2015). Future research may provide much-needed theoretical and empirical knowledge on how culture shapes the emotional and social brain. While a majority of cultural psychophysiological research has utilized a cross-sectional design to compare psychophysiological responses across racial and ethnic groups, little research has been conducted comparing psychophysiological responses of cultural experts and novices. For instance, earlier neuroimaging findings have shown that the mirror neuron response is enhanced when cultural experts, such as dancers, observe and imitate motor action of other dances, compared to nondancers (Calvo-Merino et al., 2005); however, the temporal onset of this cultural expertise effect within the MNS remains unknown. Another future direction in cultural psychophysiological research may be investigating the neurobiological mechanisms of cultural dynamics.

Additionally, cultural psychophysiological research to date has been conducted within a cross-sectional experimental design. Future studies may allow for cross-temporal experimental design, including archival, longitudinal, and cross-generational studies. Cultural psychophysiological studies conducted with archival research may examine how gradual variation in cultural dynamics within public and private archival records modulates specific electrophysiological responses associated with social and emotional information; relatedly, cultural psychophysiological studies of punctuated equilibrium (Gould & Eldredge, 1977) may utilize the odd-ball paradigm to better understand how rapid cultural change is processed in the brain. Longitudinal cultural psychophysiological studies may involve measurement of psychophysiological response across several time periods such as measurement every year across the first 5 years of an immigrant's acculturation into the host culture. Findings from longitudinal cultural psychophysiological studies of acculturation may address how changes in psychophysiological response across the first 5 years of an immigrant's experience predict acculturation and cultural competence. Cross-generational cultural psychophysiological studies may examine how a grandparent's cultural values, beliefs, and practices predict a parent's psychophysiological mechanisms underlying social and emotional behavior. Relatedly, cross-temporal and cross-sectional studies may examine how culture affects psychophysiological response during specific developmental periods, not only in adulthood, but also during childhood, adolescence, and older age (Lahat et al., 2009).

Finally, there has not yet been cross-cultural empirical investigation into the independent and interactive contribution of both cultural and genetic factors on psychophysiological responses during behavioral tasks. While much is known about the role of the serotonin transporter gene and oxytocin receptor gene in modulating subcortical response during emotion and social cognition, little is known about the extent to which genetic and epigenetic mechanisms alter subcortical response across cultures. Due to the increased prevalence of specific allelic variants within East Asian relative to Western nations or greater genetic homogeneity within the East Asian geographic region, it is possible that the extent to which genetic and epigenetic mechanisms modulate neural response during emotional and social responding varies as a function of culture. Future research integrating cultural and genetic assays with psychophysiological measurement are needed to address how cultural and genetic factors contribute to the dynamics of human brain function (Cheon & Hong, 2016).

Implications

Population Health Disparities

Population health disparities reflect one of the most important and timely issues in health equity. Understanding how and why certain social groups are more vulnerable or resilient to a given disease or disorder provides an opportunity for scientists to better understand and treat such disorders (Chiao & Blizinsky, 2013). Research on affective and social disorders, in particular, may benefit greatly from studies of psychophysiological approaches in cultural neuroscience. For instance, autism as a developmental disorder that is related to difficulties in social cognition or mental state inference varies in prevalence across cultures, possibly due to varying degrees of importance or emphasis of social cognition in the given culture (Baxter et al., 2014). Brief experiences to cultural information strengthen mental capacities for social communication (Adolphs et al., 2005). Understanding how such brief cultural experience affects brain response to social communication may provide important insights into cures for mental disorders.

Research on psychophysiological approaches in cultural neuroscience may contribute to empirical understanding of affective disorders (Gruber et al., 2011; Hechtman et al., 2013). Anxiety and mood disorders have been previously shown to vary in frequency across cultures perhaps due at least in part to the variation in emphasis on vigilance to external threat cues within individualistic and collectivistic cultures (Chiao & Blizinsky, 2010). However, little is known about how central and autonomic nervous system responses fluctuate in response to changes in culture. By studying how the brain dynamically changes due to affective cues in both individualistic and collectivistic cultures, scientists may gain greater insight into how culture buffers individuals from affective disorders and facilitates the maintenance of public health within a given population.

Research on population health disparities in psychopathology may also gain insight from research in cultural neuroscience of moral decision making. Recent research in cultural neuroscience indicates that nations vary in prevalence of psychopathy due in part to cultural variation in tightness–looseness and the serotonin transporter gene (Mrazek et al., 2013). Varying degrees of experience or exposure to tight and loose cultural norms may affect how the brain responds to social and affective information such as moral dilemmas. Studying the temporal dynamics of the brain during moral decision making across cultures may help to better understand global variation in psychopathology.

Global Mental Health

Research in cultural neuroscience has identified specific brain regions that are differentially modulated by specific cultural factors. Understanding the importance of not only genetic but also cultural influences on how the mind and brain work is a fundamental goal of research in cultural neuroscience. A future research development in cultural neuroscience is to identify temporal dynamics of brain systems that are modulated by culture and that contribute to the construction and maintenance of culture. Given that temporal changes in culture and the brain occur with temporal variation, measuring and modeling of temporal dynamics in both cultural and neural systems will allow for greater understanding of how dynamic changes in neurobiology affect mental health across cultural settings.

Cross-national epidemiology shows variation in the prevalence of mental disorders across geographic regions. Geographic variation in the prevalence of mental disorders highlights the importance of cultural settings in the etiology of mental health. Research on culture and global mental health that incorporates psychophysiological and neuroscience foundations may enhance understanding of the molecular and cellular mechanisms of the human brain across cultures. Identifying the root causes and mechanisms underlying mental disorders is a chief goal in the discovery of cures in global mental health. Evidence-based approaches in cultural neuroscience and global mental health provide an important resource for the development and implementation of preventions and interventions in delivery science. Building capacity for psychophysiological research in cultural neuroscience and global mental health is a necessary goal for solving grand challenges in global mental health.

Acknowledgments

We are grateful to Bobby Cheon, Vani Mathur, Alissa Mrazek, Narun Pornpattananangkul, Sarah Heany, and Maria Gendron for their thoughtful insights. D.J.S. is supported by the SAMRC. Research reported in this publication was supported in part by the National Institute of Health Award Numbers R21MH098789 and

R13CA162843. The content is solely the responsibility of the authors and does not necessarily represent the official views of the National Institutes of Health.

References

Adolphs, R., Gosselin, R., Buchanan, T. W., Tranel, D., Schyns, P., & Damasio, A. R. (2005). A mechanism for impaired fear recognition after amygdala damage. *Nature, 433*(7021), 68–72.

Adler, N. E., Boyce, T., Chesney, M. A., Cohen, S., Folkman, S., Kahn, R. L., & Syme, S.L. (1994). Socioeconomic status and health: The challenge of the gradient. *American Psychologist, 49*(1), 15–24.

Ax, A. F. (1953). The physiological differentiation between fear and anger in humans. *Psychosomatic Medicine, 15,* 433–442.

Baxter, A. J., Brugha, T. S., Erskine, H. E., Scheurer, R. W., Vos, T., & Scott, J. G. (2014). The epidemiology and global burden of autism spectrum disorders. *Psychological Medicine, 11,* 1–13.

Berger, H. (1929). Über das elektrenkephalogramm des menschen. *European Archives of Psychiatry and Clinical Neuroscience, 87*(1), 527–570.

Berry, J. W. (1997). Immigration, acculturation, and adaptation. *Applied Psychology, 46*(1), 5–34.

Betancourt, H., & Lopez, S. R. (1993). The study of culture, ethnicity, and race in American psychology. *American Psychologist, 48*(6), 629–637.

Blascovich, J., Mendes, W. B., Vanman, E., & Dickerson, S. (2011). *Social psychophysiology for social and personality psychology.* Affective Science Series. SAGE.

Boyd, R., & Richerson, P. J. (1985). *Culture and the evolutionary process.* University of Chicago Press.

Butler, E. A., Lee, T. L., & Gross, J. J. (2007). Emotion regulation and culture: Are the social consequences of emotion suppression culture-specific? *Emotion, 7*(1), 30–48.

Butler, E. A., Lee, T. L., & Gross, J. J. (2009). Does expressing your emotions raise or lower your blood pressure? The answer depends on cultural context. *Journal of Cross-Cultural Psychology, 40,* 510–517.

Cacioppo, J. T., Petty, R. E., & Tassinary, L. G. (1989). Social psychophysiology: A new look. *Advances in Experimental Psychology, 22,* 39–91.

Calvo-Merino, B., Glaser, D. E., Grezes, J., Passingham, R. E., & Haggard, P. (2005). Action observation and acquired motor skills: An fMRI study with expert dancers. *Cerebral Cortex, 15*(8), 1243–1249.

Cheon, B. K., & Hong, Y. Y. (2016). The cultural neuroscience of intergroup bias. In J. Y. Chiao, S. C. Li, R. Seligman, & R. Turner (Eds.), *The Oxford handbook of cultural neuroscience* (pp. 249–270). New York: Oxford University Press.

Cheon, B. K., Im, D. M., Harada, T., Kim, J. S., Mathur, V. A., Scimeca, J. M., Parrish, T. B., Park, H. W., & Chiao, J. Y. (2013). Cultural modulation of the neural correlates of empathy: The role of other-focusedness. *Neuropsychologia, 51*(7), 1177–1186.

Chiao, J. Y. (2015). Current emotion research in cultural neuroscience. *Emotion Review, 7*(3), 280–293.

Chiao, J. Y., & Ambady, N. (2007). Cultural neuroscience: Parsing universality and diversity across levels of analysis. In S. Kitayama & D. Cohen (Eds.), *Handbook of cultural psychology* (pp. 237–254). New York: Guilford Press.

Chiao, J. Y., & Blizinsky, K. D. (2010). Culture-gene coevolution of individualism-collectivism and the serotonin transporter gene (5-HTTLPR). *Proceedings of the Royal Society B: Biological Sciences, 277*(1681), 529–537.

Chiao, J. Y., & Blizinsky, K. D. (2013). Population disparities in mental health: Insights from cultural neuroscience. *American Journal of Public Health, 103,* S122–S132.

Chiao, J.Y. & Cheon, B.K. (2010). The weirdest brains in the world. *Behavioral and Brain Sciences, 33*(2–3), 88–90.

Chiao, J. Y., Cheon, B. K., Pornpattananangkul, N., Mrazek, A. J., & Blizinsky, K. D. (2013). Cultural neuroscience: Progress and promise. *Psychological Inquiry, 24*(1), 1–19.

Chiao, J. Y., Harada, T., Komeda, H., Li, Z., Mano, Y., Saito, D. N., Parrish, T. B., Sadato, N., & Iidaka, T. (2009). Neural basis of individualistic and collectivistic views of the self. *Human Brain Mapping, 30*(9), 2813–2820.

Chiao, J. Y., Harada, T., Komeda, H., Li, Z., Mano, Y., Saito, D. N., Parrish, T. B., Sadato, N., & Iidaka, T. (2010). Dynamic cultural influences on neural representations of the self. *Journal of Cognitive Neuroscience, 22*(1), 1–11.

Chiao, J.Y., Li, S.C., Turner, R., Lee-Tauler, S.Y., & Pringle, B.A. (2017). Cultural neuroscience and global mental health: Addressing grand challenges. *Culture and Brain, 5*(1), 4–13.

Chiao, J. Y., Mathur, V. A., Harada, T., & Lipke, T. (2009). Neural basis of preference for human social hierarchy versus egalitarianism. *Annals of the New York Academy of Sciences, 1167*, 174–181.

Critchley, H. D. (2009). Psychophysiology of neural, cognitive and affective integration: fMRI and autonomic indicants. *International Journal of Psychophysiology, 73*(2), 88–94.

Decety, J., & Jackson, P. L. (2004). The functional architecture of human empathy. *Behavioral Cognitive Neuroscience Reviews, 3*(2), 71–100.

Decety, J., Yang, C. Y., & Cheng, Y. (2010). Physicians down regulate their pain empathy response: An event-related brain potential study. *NeuroImage, 50*, 1676–1682.

Elfenbein, H. A., & Ambady, N. (2002). On the universality and cultural specificity of emotion recognition: A meta-analysis. *Psychological Bulletin, 129*, 203–235.

Folstein, J. R., & Van Petten, C. (2008). Influence of cognitive control and mismatch on the N2 component of the ERP: A review. *Psychophysiology, 45*(1), 152–170.

Galambos, R., & Sheatz, G. C. (1962). An electroencephalography study of classical conditioning. *American Journal of Physiology, 203*, 173–184.

Gardner, W. L., Gabriel, S., & Lee, A. Y. (1999). "I" value freedom, but "we" value relationships: Self-construal priming mirrors cultural differences in judgment. *Psychological Science, 10*(4), 321–326.

Gehring, W. J., Coles, M., Meyer, D., & Donchin, E. (1990). The error-related negativity: An event-related brain potential accompanying errors. *Psychophysiology, 27*, 34.

Gelfand, M. J., Raver, J. L., Nishii, L., Leslie, L. M., Lun, J., Lim, B. C., Duan, L., Almaliach, A., Ang, S., Arnadottir, J, Aycan, Z., Boehnke, K., Boski, P., Cabecinhas, R., Chan, D., Chhokar, J., D'Amato, A., Ferrer, M., Fischlmayr, I. C., . . . Yamaguchi, S. (2011). Differences between tight and loose cultures: A 33-nation study. *Science, 332*(6033), 1100–1104.

Goh, J. O., Chee, M. W., Tan, J. C., Venkatraman, V., Hebrank, A., Leshikar, E. D., Jenkins, L., Sutton, B.P., Gutchess, A.H. & Park, D. C. (2007). Age and culture modulate object processing and object—scene binding in the ventral visual area. *Cognitive, Affective, & Behavioral Neuroscience, 7*(1), 44–52.

Goto, S. G., Ando, Y., Huang, C., Yee, A., & Lewis, R. S. (2010). Cultural differences in the visual processing of meaning: Detecting incongruities between background and foreground objects using the N400. *Social Cognitive and Affective Neuroscience, 5*(2–3), 242–253.

Goto, S. G., Yee, A., Lowenberg, K., & Lewis, R. S. (2013). Cultural differences in sensitivity to social context: Detecting affective incongruity using the N400. *Social Neuroscience, 8*(1), 63–74.

Gould, S. J., & Eldredge, N. (1977). Punctuated equilibria: The tempo and mode of evolution reconsidered. *Paleobiology, 3*(2), 115–151.

Gruber, J., Dutra, S., Eidelman, P., Johnson, S. L., & Harvey, A. G. (2011). Emotional and physiological responses to normative and idiographic positive stimuli in bipolar disorder. *Journal of Affective Disorders, 133*, 437–442.

Hackman, D. A., Farah, M. J., & Meaney, M. J. (2011). Socioeconomic status and the brain: Mechanistic insights from human and animal research. *Nature Reviews Neuroscience, 11*(9), 651–659.

Hajcak, G., Dunning, J. P., & Foti, D. (2009). Motivated and controlled attention to emotion: Time-course of the late positive potential. *Clinical Neurophysiology, 120*(3), 505–510.

Hajcak, G., Macnamara, A., & Olvet, D. M. (2010). Event-related potentials, emotion and emotion regulation: An integrative review. *Developmental Neuropsychology, 35*(2), 129–155.

Han, S., & Northoff, G. (2008). Culture-sensitive neural substrates of human cognition: A transcultural neuroimaging approach. *Nature Reviews Neuroscience, 9*, 646–654.

Harada, T., Li, Z., Chiao, J.Y. (2010). Differential dorsal and ventral medial prefrontal representations of the self modulated by individualism and collectivism: An fMRI study. *Social Neuroscience, 5*(3), 257–271.

Harada, T., Bridge, D. J., & Chiao, J. Y. (2013). Dynamic social power modulates neural basis of math calculation. *Frontiers in Human Neuroscience (Research Topic on Brains, Genes and the Foundations of Human Society), 6*(350), 1–12.

Hariri, A. R. (2009). The neurobiology of individual differences in complex behavioral traits. *Annual Review of Neuroscience, 32*, 225–247.

Hechtman, L. A., Raila, H., Chiao, J. Y., & Gruber, J. (2013). Positive emotion regulation and psychopathology: A transdiagnostic cultural neuroscience approach. *Journal of Experimental Psychopathology, 4*(5), 502–528.

Hedden, T., Ketay, S., Aron, A., Markus, H. R., & Gabrieli, J. D. (2008). Cultural influences on neural substrates of attentional control. *Psychological Science, 19*(1), 12–17.

Hein, G., & Singer, T. (2008). I feel how you feel but not always: The empathic brain and its modulation. *Current Opinion in Neurobiology, 18*(2), 153–158.

Heine, S. J., & Norenzayan, A. (2006). Toward a psychological science for a cultural species. *Perspectives on Psychological Science, 1*, 251–269.

Helms, J. E., Jernigan, M., & Mascher, J. (2005). The meaning of race in psychology and how to change it: A methodological perspective. *American Psychologist, 60*(1), 27–36.

Helms, J. E., & Talleyrand, R. (1997). Race is not ethnicity. *American Psychologist, 52*, 1246–1247.

Ho, D. Y. F. (1994). Cognitive socialization in Confucian heritage cultures. In P. M. Greenfield & R. R. Cocking (Eds.), *Cross-cultural roots of minority development* (pp. 285–313). Erlbaum.

Hofstede, G. (2001). *Culture's consequences: Comparing values, behaviors, institutions and organizations across nations.* Sage Publications.

Hong, Y. Y., Morris, M. W., Chiu, C. Y., & Benet-Martinez, V. (2000). Multicultural minds: A dynamic constructivist approach to culture. *American Psychologist, 55*(7), 709–720.

Iacono, W. G. (2014). Genome-wide scans of genetic variants for psychophysiological endophenotypes: Introduction to this special issue of Psychophysiology. *Psychophysiology, 51*(12), 1201–1202.

Inglehart, R. (1997). *Modernization and postmodernization: Cultural, economic, and political change in 43 societies.* Princeton University Press.

Inglehart, R., Foa, R., Peterson, C., & Welzel, C. (2008). Development, freedom and rising happiness: A global perspective (1981–2007). *Perspectives in Psychological Science, 3*, 264–285.

Jackson, A. F., & Bolger, D. J. (2014). The neurophysiological bases of EEG and EEG measurement: A review for the rest of us. *Psychophysiology, 51*(11), 1061–1071.

Jiang, C., Varnum, M. E. W., Hou, Y., & Han, S. (2014). Distinct effects of self-construal priming on empathic neural responses in Chinese and Westerners. *Social Neuroscience, 9*(2), 130 138.

Johnson, R. (1988). The amplitude of the P300 component of the event-related potential: Review and synthesis. *Advances in Psychophysiology, 3*, 69–137.

Kashima, Y. (2007). A social psychology of cultural dynamics: Examining how cultures are formed, maintained, and transformed. *Social and Personality Psychology Compass, 2*(1), 107–120.

Kashima, Y. (2014). How can you capture cultural dynamics? *Frontiers in Psychology, 5*(995), 1–16.

Kim, K., & Markman, A. B. (2006). Differences in fear of isolation as an explanation of cultural differences: Evidence from memory and reasoning. *Journal of Experimental Social Psychology, 42*(3), 350–364.

Kitayama, S., Duffy, S., Kawamura, T., & Larsen, J.T. (2003). Perceiving an object and its context in different cultures: a cultural look at new look. *Psychological Science, 14*(3), 201–216.

Kitayama, S., & Park, J. (2014). Error-related brain activity reveals self-centric motivation: Culture matters. *Journal of Experimental Psychology: General, 143*(1), 62–70.

Kitayama, S., & Uskul, A. K. (2011). Culture, mind, and the brain: Current evidence and future directions. *Annual Review of Psychology, 62*, 419–449.

Konvalinka, I., Xygalatas, D., Bulbulia, J., Schjodt, E. M., Jegindo, E. M., Wallot, S., Van Orden, G., & Roepstorff, A. (2011). Synchronized arousal between performers and related spectators. *Proceedings of the National Academy of Sciences, 108*(20), 8514–8519.

Kutas, M., & Hillyard, S. A. (1980). Reading senseless sentences: Brain potentials reflect semantic incongruity. *Science, 207*(4427), 203–205.

Lahat, A., Todd, R. M., Mahy, C. E. V., Lau, K., & Zelazo, P. D. (2009). Neurophysiological correlates of executive function: A comparison of European-Canadian and Chinese-Canadian 5-year-old children. *Frontiers in Human Neuroscience, 3*(72), 1–10.

Levenson, R. W. (2014). The autonomic nervous system and emotion. *Emotion Review, 6*(1), 100–112.

Levenson, R. W., Ekman, P., Heider, K., & Friesen, W. V. (1992). Emotion and autonomic nervous system activity in the Minangkabau of West Sumatra. *Journal of Personality and Social Psychology, 62*, 972–988.

Lewis, R. S., Goto, S. G., & Kong, L. L. (2008). Culture and context: East Asian American and European American differences in P3 event-related potentials and self-construal. *Personality and Social Psychology Bulletin, 34*, 623–634.

Losin, E. A., Cross, K. A., Iacoboni, M., & Dapretto, M. (2014). Neural processing of race during imitation: Self-similarity versus social status. *Human Brain Mapping, 35*(4), 1723–1739.

Losin, E. A., Iacoboni, M., Martin, A., & Dapretto, M. (2012). Own-gender imitation activates the brain's reward circuitry. *Social Cognitive Affective Neuroscience, 7*(7), 804–810.

Luck, S. J. (2005). *An introduction to the event-related potential technique.* MIT Press.

Luck, S. J., & Kappenman, E. S. (Eds.). (2011). *The Oxford handbook of event-related potential components.* Oxford University Press.

Markus, H., & Kitayama, S. (1991). Culture and the self: Implications for cognition, emotion, and motivation. *Psychological Review, 98*, 224–253.

Masuda, T., Russell, M. J., Chen, Y. Y., Hioki, K., & Caplan, J. B. (2014). N400 incongruity effect in an episodic memory task reveals different strategies for handling irrelevant contextual information for Japanese than European Canadians. *Cognitive Neuroscience, 5*(1), 17–25.

Mathur, V. A., Harada, T., & Chiao, J. Y. (2012). Racial identification modulates default network activity for same- and other-races. *Human Brain Mapping, 33*(8), 1883–1893.

Mathur, V. A., Harada, T., Lipke, T., & Chiao, J. Y. (2010). Neural basis of extraordinary empathy and altruistic motivation. *Neuroimage, 51*(4), 1468–1475.

Mauss, I. B., Bunge, S. A., & Gross, J. J. (2008). Culture and autonomic emotion regulation. In S. Ismer, S. Jung, C. Kronast, C. van Scheve, & M. Vanderkerckhove (Eds.), *Regulation emotions: Culture, social necessity and biological inheritance* (pp. 39–60). Blackwell Publishing.

Mauss, I. B., & Butler, E. A. (2010). Cultural background moderates the relationship between emotion control values and cardiovascular challenge versus threat responses to an anger provocation. *Biological Psychology, 84*, 521–530.

McGuinness, T. M., & Dyer, J. G. (2006). International adoption as a natural experiment. *Journal of Pediatric Nursing, 21*(4), 276–288.

Meaney, M. J. (2010). Epigenetics and the biological definition of gene x environment interactions. *Child Development, 81*(1), 41–79.

Min, S. K. (1989). A study on the concept of *Hwa-byung. Journal of Korean Neuropsychiatric Association, 28*, 604–615.

Moser, J. S., Hajcak, G., Bukay, E., & Simons, R. F. (2006). Intentional modulation of emotional responding to unpleasant pictures: An ERP study. *Psychophysiology, 43*(3), 292–296.

Mrazek, A. J., Chiao, J. Y., Blizinsky, K. D., Lun, J., & Gelfand, M. J. (2013). The role of culture-gene coevolution in morality judgment: Examining the interplay between tightness-looseness and allelic variation of the serotonin transporter gene. *Culture and Brain, 1*, 100–117.

Murata, A., Moser, J. S., & Kitayama, S. (2013). Culture shapes electrocortical responses during emotion suppression. *Social Cognitive Affective Neuroscience, 8*(5), 595–601.

Na, J., & Kitayama, S. (2011). Spontaneous trait inferences is culture-specific: behavioral and neural evidence. *Psychological Sciences, 22*(8), 1025–1032.

Nikolova, Y. S., Koenen, K. C., Galea, S., Wang, C. M., Seney, M. L., Sibille, E., Williamson, D. E., & Hariri, A. R. (2014). Beyond genotype: Serotonin transporter epigenetic modification predicts human brain function. *Nature Neuroscience, 17*(9), 1153–1155.

Nisbett, R. E., & Miyamoto, Y. (2005). The influence of culture: Holistic versus analytic perception. *Trends in Cognitive Sciences, 9*(10), 467–473.

Obhi, S. S., Hogeveen, J., & Pascual-Leone, A. (2011). Resonating with others: The effects of self-construal type on motor cortical output. *Journal of Neuroscience, 31*, 14531–14535.

Odling-Smee, F. J., Laland, K. N., & Feldman, M. F. (2003). *Niche construction: The neglected process in evolution.* Monographs in Population Biology 37. Princeton University Press.

Oh, S., & Lewis, C. (2008). Korean preschoolers' advanced inhibitory control and its relation to other executive skills and mental state understanding. *Child Development, 79*, 80–9910.

Oyserman, D., Coon, H., & Kemmelmeier, M. (2002). Rethinking individualism and collectivism: Evaluation of theoretical assumptions and meta-analyses. *Psychological Bulletin, 128*, 3–73.

Oyserman, D., & Lee, S. W. (2008). Does culture influence what and how we think? Effects of priming individualism and collectivism. *Psychological Bulletin, 134*(2), 311–42.

Park, D. C., & Gutchess, A. H. (2002). Aging, cognition and culture: A neuroscientific perspective. *Neuroscience and Biobehavioral Reviews, 26*(7), 859–867.

Park, J., & Kitayama, S. (2014). Interdependent selves show face-induced facilitation of error processing: Cultural neuroscience of self-threat. *Social Cognitive and Affective Neuroscience, 9*(2), 201–208.

Phinney, J. S. (1996). When we talk about American ethnic groups, what do we mean? *American Psychologist*, *51*, 918–927.

Pineda, J. A. (2005). The functional significance of mu rhythms: Translating "seeing" and "hearing" into "doing." *Brain Research Reviews*, *50*, 57–68.

Polich, J., & Comerchero, M. D. (2003). P3a from visual stimuli: Typicality, task, and topography. *Brain Topography*, *15*(3), 141–152.

Pornpattananangkul, N., & Chiao, J. Y. (2014). Affect control theory and cultural priming. *Emotion Review*, *6*(2), 136–137.

Pornpattananangkul, N., Zink, C. F., & Chiao, J. Y. (2014). Neural basis of social status hierarchy. In J. T. Cheng, J. L. Tracy, & C. Anderson (Eds.), *The psychology of social status* (pp. 303–324). Springer Press.

Puglia, M. H., Lillard, T. S., Morris, J. P., & Connelly, J. J. (2015). Epigenetic modification of the oxytocin receptor gene influences the perception of anger and fear in the human brain. *Proceedings of the National Academy of Sciences*, *112*(11), 3308–3313.

Richerson, P. J. & Boyd, R. (2005). *The origin and evolution of cultures*. New York: Oxford University Press.

Roberts, N. A., & Levenson, R. W. (2006). Subjective, behavioral, and physiological reactivity to ethnically matched and ethnically mismatched film clips. *Emotion*, *6*(4), 635–646.

Roberts, N. A., Levenson, R. W., & Gross, J. J. (2008). Cardiovascular costs of emotion suppression cross ethnic lines. *International Journal of Psychophysiology*, *70*(1), 82–87.

Sabbagh, M. A., Xu, F., Carlson, S. M., Moses, L. J., & Lee, K. (2006). The development of executive functioning and theory of mind: A comparison of Chinese and U.S. preschoolers. *Psychological Science*, *17*(1), 74–81.

Sasaki, J. Y., LeClair, J., West, A., & Kim, H. S. (2016). The gene-culture interaction framework and implications for health. In J. Y. Chiao, S. C. Li, R. Seligman, & R. Turner (Eds.), *The Oxford handbook of cultural neuroscience* (pp. 279–298. Oxford University Press.

Schonfelder, S., Kanske, P., Heissler, J., & Wessa, M. (2014). Time course of emotion-related responding during distraction and reappraisal. *Social Cognitive and Affective Neuroscience*, *9*(9), 1310–1319.

Schupp, H. T., Cuthbert, B. N., Bradley, M. M., Cacioppo, J. T., Ito, T., & Lang, P. J. (2000). Affective picture processing: The late positive potential is modulated by motivational relevance. *Psychophysiology*, *37*(2), 257–261.

Shavers, V. L. (2007). Measurement of socioeconomic status in health disparities research. *Journal of the National Medical Association*, *99*(9), 1013–1023.

Smedley, A., & Smedley, B. D. (2005). Race as biology as fiction, racism as a social problem is real: Anthropological and historical perspectives on the social construction of race. *American Psychologist*, *60*(1), 16–26.Soto, J. A., & Levenson, R. W. (2009). Emotion recognition across cultures: The influence of ethnicity on empathic accuracy and physiological linkage. *Emotion*, *9*, 874–884.

Soto, J. A., Levenson, R. W., & Ebling, R. (2005). Cultures of moderation and expression: Emotional experience, behavior and physiology in Chinese Americans and Mexican Americans. *Emotion*, *5*(2), 154–165.

Stein, D. J., Chiao, J. Y., & Van Honk, J. (2016). Cultural neuroscience in South Africa: Promise, pitfalls and framework. In J. Y. Chiao, S. C. Li, R. Seligman, & R. Turner (Eds.), *The Oxford handbook of cultural neuroscience* (pps. 143-154). Oxford University Press.

Stephens, N. M., Markus, H. R., & Fryberg, S.A. (2012). Social class disparities in health and education: Reducing inequality by applying a sociocultural self model of behavior. *Psychological Review*, *119*, 723–744.

Telzer, E. H. (2011). Expanding the acculturation gap-distress model: An integrative review of research. *Human Development*, *53*, 313–340.

Varnum, M. E. W., Na, J., Murata, A., & Kitayama, S. (2012). Social class differences in N400 indicate differences in spontaneous trait inferences. *Journal of Experimental Psychology: General*, *141*, 518–526.

Varnum, M. E. W., Shi, Z., Chen, A., Qiu, J., & Han, S. (2014). When "Your" reward is the same as "My" reward: Self-construal priming shifts neural responses to own vs. friends' rewards. *Neuroimage*, *87*, 164–169.

Walter, W. G., Cooper, R., Aldridge, V. J., McCallum, W. C., & Winter, A. L. (1964). Contingent negative variation: An electric sign of sensori-motor association and expectancy in the human brain. *Nature*, *203*(4943), 380–384.

Culture and Genomics

Joan Y. Chiao, Zhang Li, *and* Norihiro Sadato

Abstract

Cultural and genomic systems maintain and regulate neural systems and behavior underlying mental health. Cultural and genomic systems affect the functional organization of the nervous system. Cultural processes influence the behavioral and genetic expression of functional neural circuitry. Cultural and genetic systems contribute to the neurodevelopmental trajectory of behavioral adaptation. The interaction of genes and environment affects behavioral expression within a cultural context. The goal of this chapter is to provide a review of pathways of interaction in cultural and genomic systems and their influence on the functional organization of the nervous system and behavioral phenotypes of mental health.

Key Words: culture, neuroscience, genetics, epigenetics, genomics, development, environment, population health disparities, global mental health

Introduction

Mental, neurological, and substance abuse (MNS) disorders make up approximately 13% of the burden of disease. The Grand Challenges in Global Mental Health Consortium led by the National Institutes of Health identified research priorities for discovery and delivery science to search for cures to mental disorders as an improvement in human health. The identification of root causes such as biomarkers underlying MNS disorders is a key priority in the discovery of cures, preventions, and interventions for mental health (Collins et al., 2011). Understanding the societal factors and environmental influences that affect resilience and prevention in mental health across the life course is necessary for the translation of discovery science into cures, preventions, and interventions for the amelioration of mental disorders. A comprehensive understanding of the cellular and molecular mechanisms of the human brain is essential to the discovery of cures for mental health. Building the mental capital for the well-being of individuals, societies, and nations enhances the fulfillment of human potential and quality of life as an achievement of the goals of human development.

The mutual influences of cultural and genomic variation contribute to human health. The International Cultural Neuroscience Consortium identified research priorities for addressing issues of global mental health with cultural neuroscience (Chiao et al., 2017). The identification of the root causes of mental health entails the discovery of biomarkers of mental disorders. The mapping of the root causes of mental health and cures for mental disorders builds a fundamental understanding of the sources of human health. Patterns of genetic and cultural variation across geography contribute to the discovery of cures, preventions, and interventions for mental disorders.

The mapping of the human genome provides opportunities for the discovery science of human behavior to identify root causes of mental disorders and underlying cures for the amelioration of mental disorders and the promotion of mental health. The International HapMap Project, designed to understand the patterns of genetic diversity in the human genome, is a fundamental component in the search for root causes of human health (International HapMap Consortium, 2003). The identification of millions of single nucleotide proteins (SNPs) across populations contributes to the understanding of geographic variation of the human genome and the patterns of genetic variation within geographic regions. Genome-wide human genetic maps identify SNPs that affect human health and disease. Genome-wide association studies of human behavior across geographic regions facilitate the discovery of the role of genetic variation in mental health.

The historical differences of ethnocultural groups due to geographic and ancestral origins represent an emergence of cultural and genetic variation in human behavior and their underlying relations. Cultural and genetic variation characterizes the vast range of phenotypic variation across ethnocultural groups of human populations. Cultural and genetic variation construed as the social and biological construction of racial or ethnic differences arises as an emergent property of political context (Bonham et al., 2005). A comprehensive understanding of the human variation of populations arises from the systematic investigation of the role of cultural and genetic variation in human behavior of plural societies.

Human variation of populations consists of variation in groups across levels of analysis. Cultural and genetic systems mutually contribute to the population human variation in phenotypic expression across geography. The geographic variation in environmental or ecological conditions leads to the construction of cultural systems for the production and regulation of behavioral adaptation (Fincher et al., 2008; Gelfand et al., 2011; Markus & Kitayama, 1991; Oyserman et al., 2002). Cultural systems characterize the role of social organization and social practices in the population human variation of genomic and phenotypic expression (Nisbett et al., 2001). Cultural systems influence the genomic expression and developmental pathways of mental constructs and the functional relations of their underlying neural bases (Chiao, 2018). Cultural and genomic variation may guide systems of thought as phenotypic expression in human variation. Genetic variation of populations may guide the social norms of behavioral expression across cultural settings. The behavioral expression of genomic variation as a process of cultural niche construction modifies environmental conditions for psychological and sociocultural adaptation.

Population genetic structure makes up the main genetic clusters of human variation. The genetic structure of populations characterizes the structure of major geographic regions (Rosenberg et al., 2002). The main genetic clusters of human variation are related to geographic regions, with subclusters of genetic variation related to populations within geographic regions. The genetic structure of populations contributes to the human variation in epidemiological prevalence due to the societal exposure to risk and protective factors across cultural settings.

Human population variation in the genome consists of shared genetic ancestry of ethnocultural groups. Genomic variation of populations is related to functional expression of cultural variation. Cultural variation within geographic regions may arise from distinct patterns of geographic, linguistic, or social variation as characteristic sources of genetic variation (Stein, Chiao, van Honk, 2016; Tishkoff et al., 2009). Shared genetic ancestry is related to the shared social practices of indigenous populations. The migration and expansion of the genetic and cultural diversity of the population originate from the genetic and cultural distance of its geographic origin. Geographic and genetic distance are interrelated such that genetic clusters of variation are consistent with the geographic position of populations within geographic regions. Cultural distance as the perceived similarity or difference of ethnocultural groups arises from intercultural contact (Masgoret & Ward, 2006). Geographic distance may contribute to the genetic and cultural distance of ethnocultural groups with shared ancestral origins.

Theoretical Approaches

Dual inheritance theory posits that cultural and genetic selection mutually influence the mental and neural architecture of behavior. Environmental and ecological pressures contribute to the niche construction of cultural systems that produce behavioral adaptations (Boyd & Richerson, 1985). Environmental pressures may exert an influence on behavioral phenotypes, affecting conditions of human survival. In response to environmental pressures, organisms may perform cultural selection, modifying their ecological niche to ensure behavioral adaptation. Both cultural and genetic selection may guide the encoding and regulation of mental and neural mechanisms underlying behavioral adaptation (Chiao et al., 2010).

Gene–culture coevolution postulates that genetic and cultural selection lead to behavioral adaptation. In Northern Europe, the geographic coincidence of cattle milk genes and human lactase encoding genes at European cattle farming sites suggests gene–culture coevolution of tolerance across species (Beja-Pereira et al., 2003). The cultural propensity for cattle farming practices within a geographic location leads to the genetic selection of cattle milk genes and human lactase encoding genes across species as a reinforcement of cultural adaptation.

Culture–gene coevolution posits that cultural adaptations affect the social and physical environments of genetic selection. Cultural systems of individualism and collectivism serve as a protective factor from environmental pressures across nations due in part to genetic selection (Chiao & Blizinsky, 2010). The geographic coincidence of the cultural systems of individualism and collectivism and the allelic frequency of the serotonin transporter gene leads to reduced prevalence of mental disorders across nations. Greater cultural collectivism enhances social vigilance to environmental threats and social harmony for individual and collection action. Cultural systems serve as a protective factor from pathogens and psychopathology in the production of sociocultural adaptation.

The mutual influence of culture and genes may affect the levels of universalism of a given behavioral phenotype. Hierarchical levels of universalism refer to variation in the functional use, ease, and frequency of behavioral expression (Norenzayan & Heine, 2005). Accessibility universalism refers to mental constructs that are present across cultures and perform the same functions to the same degree of ease and frequency. Functional universals are mental constructs that are present across cultures that perform the same functions but show variation in the ease of behavioral expression. Existential universals are mental constructs that are present across cultures but may show variation in functional use and the ease of behavioral expression.

The interplay of genes and culture contributes to psychological adaptation. The genetic sensitivity to environmental factors affects behavioral expression across cultural contexts (Sasaki et al., 2016). The functional ease or frequency of a specific behavioral expression associated with a specific gene may differ across cultural contexts. The genetic sensitivity to risk and preventative factors in the environment modifies the ease of behavioral expression in a manner consistent with the cultural context. The interplay of genes and culture demonstrates the malleability of behavioral expression to the social environment across cultural contexts. The interplay of genes and culture contributes to the capacities for cultural competence.

Culture may affect the epigenetic expression of behavioral adaptation. Epigenetic modification of behavioral expression refers to the variation in the genetic expression of behavioral phenotypes. The malleability of genetic expression may lead to alteration in the ease of behavioral expression due to the social environment (Connelly & Morris, 2016). Theoretical frameworks in cultural epigenetics posit a causal relation between the malleability of genetic and behavioral expression as a function of culture (Chiao & Blizinsky, 2016). The influence of epigenetic variation on the functional processing may affect underlying neural mechanisms of behavioral expression (Canli et al., 2006; Nikolova et al., 2014). When the malleability of genetic expression is regulated by culture, the ease of neural function and behavioral expression may be guided in the social or physical environment by the cultural context. The relation between epigenetic variability and a given behavioral phenotype may be modified by risk and preventative factors in the environment across cultural settings.

Culture characterizes the antecedents and consequences of intercultural contact for relations among ethnocultural groups and the maintenance of cultural heritage. At the level of cultural group, the intercultural contact among the heritage and host culture may lead to cultural change. The cultural change of the heritage and host culture may include patterns of mutual influence in behavior at the group and individual level. Psychological acculturation to cultural change from intercultural contact results in sociocultural and individual adaptation.

Cultural processes characterize the human genome and its relation to behaviors and their underlying mechanisms. Population migration refers to the geographic distance from the ancestral origin. Population migration is related to the allelic variation of the dopamine receptor (DRD4) gene (Chen et al., 1999). Geographic distance from the ancestral origin is associated with variation in the allelic frequency of the DRD4 gene. Population migration shows a positive relation to greater frequency of long alleles of the DRD4 gene.

The enculturated genome characterizes the relations of the genome with sets of behavioral phenotypes of specific ethnocultural groups within a given population. The enculturated genome suggests variation in the relation of the genome with behavioral phenotypes and their underlying endophenotypes (Chen et al., 2016). The functional organization of the nervous system is regulated across specific neurotransmitter systems of the human brain. The variation in the relation of the genome with sets of behavioral phenotypes of specific ethnocultural groups suggests cultural variation in the molecular and cellular mechanisms of the human brain and their relation to mental constructs and behavior.

Methodological Approaches

The relations of cultural and genomic systems are measurable with a range of methodological approaches across levels of the genome. Genes or candidate functional polymorphisms may be characterized as associated with observable behavioral phenotypes across ethnocultural groups. The population allelic frequency of specific genes refers to the frequency of variants of candidate functional polymorphisms within a given population due to selection pressures. The variation of a specific gene may be associated with particular behavioral phenotypes to a varying extent of universalism across ethnocultural groups. Studies of cultural genetics investigate the relation of specific functional polymorphisms to behavioral phenotypes and mental constructs across ethnocultural groups.

Cultural neurogenetics refers to the influence of cultural variation on genetic expression within the structural and functional organization of the nervous system. Cultural systems may modify the ease and frequency of the functional activity related to neural systems regulated by specific genes. The brain activity regulated by specific functional polymorphisms within neural networks may vary across cultures. Cultural influences may modify the efficiency of molecular and cellular mechanisms of the human brain due to allelic variation of specific functional polymorphisms within specific neurotransmitter systems. The mutual influence of cultural and genetic systems maintains and regulates neural systems and their relation to mental constructs and behavior.

Cultural epigenetics characterizes the relation of genetic and behavioral expression of mental constructs across cultures. Studies of cultural epigenetics relate the malleability of genetic expression to behavioral expression of mental constructs across cultures. The frequency and ease of genetic expression and its functional relation to neural and behavioral expression may vary due to environmental factors across ethnocultural groups of populations.

Cultural genomics investigates the relation of the human genome to specific sets of behavioral phenotypes across ethnocultural groups of specific populations. Genome-wide association studies (GWASs) investigate the relation of groups of genes with sets of behavioral phenotypes. Genomic variation across a range of genes may predict variation in the relation of functional genomic patterns to behavioral phenotypes across cultures. Culture may influence the relation of functional genomics to specific behavioral phenotypes. In cultural genomics, GWASs across populations and within a given population may be utilized to investigate the relation of groups of genes with sets of behavioral phenotypes across ethnocultural groups.

Empirical Approaches

Cultural variation influences systems of thought. Analytic thought refers to the perception of objects as independent of the environment, while holistic thought reflects the perception of objects as a part of the environment (Nisbett et al., 2001). Westerners are more likely to perceive objects as independent of the environment, while East Asians are more likely to perceive objects in the environment. Culture affects systems of thought within the level of cognitive processes from perception to cognitive inhibition (Nisbett & Miyamoto, 2005). Westerners are more likely to perceive and remember objects as independent of the environment, while East Asians are more likely to perceive and remember objects within the context of the environment. Cultural differences are also observed in behavioral expression of self-consistency. Westerners are more likely to prefer behavioral consistency across cultural contexts, while East Asians are more likely to prefer inhibitory control and social harmony with the cultural context (Suh, 2002). Cultural variation in systems of thought affect behavioral expression across levels of universalism.

Cultural variation in systems of thought guide the social organization and societal practices that influence cognitive processes. Culture influences the construals of the self that regulate psychological processes (Markus & Kitayama, 1991). Independent self-construal involves the conception of the self as unique, autonomous from others and promoting the goals of the self, while interdependent self-construal includes the conception of the self as belonging, connected and relational to others, promoting the goals of others and the maintenance of social harmony. Cultural variation in the self-system includes characteristic structures and features that function as regulatory mechanisms of social and emotional processes. Cultural processes of the self-system show differential patterns of behavioral expression as a product of emergent mechanisms.

Empirical approaches in cultural genetics investigate cultural influences on the relation of specific genes and behavioral phenotypes. The interplay of genes and culture hypothesizes a differential relation of genes and behavioral phenotypes of social environments across cultural settings. Convergent evidence demonstrates the influence of the environment on gene expression in the behavior (Belsky et al., 2007) and underlying neural mechanisms (Canli et al., 2006; Hariri & Weinberger, 2003). The environmental influences on genetic processes function as the maintenance and production of the behavioral adaptations that reinforce and strengthen the cultural system.

Culture and genes affect the behavioral expression of systems of thought. Cultural variation in systems of thought are related to genes that regulate the behavioral expression of cognitive processes (Kim Sherman Taylor et al., 2010). The serotonin 1A receptor polymorphism (5-HTR1A) regulates gene expression and the efficiency of serotonergic neurotransmission. East Asians who show genetic sensitivity to the social environment display greater behavioral expression of the preference for holistic cognition relative to European Americans. The genetic sensitivity to social norms of the cultural context is shown in cognitive processing as preference in the locus of attention. Holistic styles of thinking arise as behavioral adaptations of culture and systems of thought.

Culture and genes influence the behavioral expression of emotional and social behavior. Cultural norms of East Asians and European Americans differ in patterns of social behavior such as emotional support seeking. European Americans are more likely to seek emotional support when feeling emotional distress relative to East Asians. For East Asians, cultural norms emphasize social harmony and sensitivity to the feelings of others to a greater extent than those of European Americans, while for European Americans, cultural norms encourage uniqueness and self-expression (Markus & Kitayama, 1991; Mesquita & Frijda, 1992; Nisbett et al., 2001). Cultural variation in social norms reflects distinct patterns of social behavior that lead to psychological adaptation.

Cultural variation in emotional social support seeking varies across social environments due in part to genetic variation of the oxytocin receptor (OXTR) gene. The oxytocin receptor genotype (OXTR rs53576) is associated with social sensitivity to cultural norms (Bakermans-Kranenburg & van Ijzendoorn, 2008; Rodrigues et al., 2009). Allelic variation of the OXTR gene is related to differential levels of behavioral expression. The G allele of the OXTR rs53576 is associated with greater levels of social behavioral expression relative to the A allele. In a gene–culture study of emotion, Americans who carried the G allele and showed genetic sensitivity to the social environment and experienced more emotional distress were more likely to seek emotional social support relative to Koreans, who did not (Kim Sherman Sasaki et al., 2010). Cultural influences show a modification of the relation of genotype to social behavioral expression in a manner consistent with the cultural context. Culture acts as a protective factor such that genetic sensitivity to the social environment is expressed to reinforce social norms. Cultural variation in genetic sensitivity to the social environment reflects the mutual influence of cultural and genetic systems in the maintenance and regulation of social behavior.

The interplay of genes and culture shows cultural variation in the ease and frequency of social behavior due to an interaction of genes and the social environment. Culture may serve as a protective factor within the social environment as genetic sensitivity to situational contexts. Cultural influences of religion contribute to the social learning of prosocial behavior and altruism. The cultural acquisition of social thought processes serves as an antecedent to the moral intuitions of charitable behavior. The dopamine receptor (DRD4) gene has previously been associated with variation in novelty-related social behavior and the dopaminergic neurotransmission of cortical neural systems. Allelic variation of the DRD4 gene is associated with varying levels in dopamine signaling within dopaminergic neurotransmitter systems. In a gene–culture study of prosocial behavior, European Americans and Asian Americans who carry the 2- and 7-repeat allele showed genetic sensitivity to the cultural priming of religious social contexts and yielded greater prosocial behavior relative to those who do not (Sasaki et al., 2013). Cultural variation in genetic sensitivity to religious thought strengthens prosocial behavior in a manner consistent with cultural context.

Cultural variation influences genetic sensitivity of social orientation. East Asians who carry the 2-repeat or 7-repeat alleles of the DRD4 gene show genetic sensitivity for the social environment and demonstrate greater interdependent social orientation, while European Americans who carry the 2-repeat or 7-repeat alleles display genetic sensitivity and greater independent social orientation (Kitayama et al., 2014). Cultural variation in genetic sensitivity to social orientation strengthens social norms toward the cultural context. Cultural influences on genetic sensitivity to the social environment arise as distinct patterns of social behavior.

Empirical studies of cultural genetics demonstrate the relation of genetic variation and behavioral expressions across cultures. Cultural variation affects the relation of genetic variation and behavioral expression. Cultural differences in the relation of specific genes and behavior demonstrates the malleability of genes toward the cultural context (Ishii et al., 2014; Kim et al., 2011). Convergent evidence from studies of cultural genetics shows that culture serves as a protective factor strengthening the behavioral expression of genes in a manner consistent with the social norms of the cultural context. The importance of culture in behavior is observed in the ease of behavioral expression from genetic sensitivity to the social environment.

Culture and genes mutually influence the functional organization of the nervous system underlying behavior. Culture influences the functional activity within neural networks of behavior regulated by specific functional polymorphisms. The OXTR gene is associated with functional activity within brain regions of social and emotional neural networks such as the bilateral amygdala, insula, and superior temporal gyri (Michalska et al., 2014). Genetic variation of the OXTR gene shows differential functional neural activity within these cortical and subcortical brain regions of the limbic system during social perception. Cultural variation within neural activity of the social and emotional neural network during empathy is related to genetic sensitivity (Luo et al., 2015). Greater cultural interdependence is associated with genetic sensitivity within the social and emotional neural network during empathy. Cultural variation influences genetic expression within neural circuitry of social and emotional behavior. Cultural and genetic variations maintain and regulate neural mechanisms of social and emotional processes.

Cultural variation in the human genome may guide the functional emergence of mental and neural architecture of behavioral adaptation. The functional organization of the nervous system is regulated across distinct neurotransmitter systems. The genetic expression of specific functional polymorphisms modifies the ease and frequency of neural activity within specialized brain regions dedicated to psychological processes. Evolutionary processes of natural selection alter the population frequency of allelic variation of neurotransmitter systems of the human genome. Natural selection pressures alter the ease of gene flow, affecting the cultural and genetic variation in the population. Cultural and genetic variation may guide behavioral expression as an emergent property of mental and neural architecture related to linguistic or social variation.

Conclusion

In summary, cultural and genetic variations across geographic regions contribute to the behavioral expression of mental health. Patterns of cultural and genetic variations act as sources of cures, preventions, and interventions for mental disorders. Cultural processes act as a guide for social norms to regulate mental and neural mechanisms of behavior. Cultural and genetic variations shape neurobiological mechanisms of human behavior and human potential. Cultural and genetic variations are malleable factors that affect resilience and promotion of mental health.

Implications

Population Health Disparities

Population health disparities refer to differences in prevalence of health risk factors and disease that arise from differences in perceived health status and equitable access to health services across racial and ethnic groups. Racial and ethnic disparities in mental health may lead to more exposure to risk factors but also rely on protective factors such as cultural resources. Patterns of cultural and genetic variation across geographic regions provide insights into the discovery of cures, preventions, and interventions for mental disorders. Cultural and genetic variations in social norms support the notion that reduction in societal exposure to risk factors, such as racial discrimination, may impact population health disparities. The malleability of cultural and genetic variations further suggests the importance of protective factors for the promotion of mental health. Cultural and genetic variations in sensitivity to social support enhance the behavioral expression of cultural competence. Cultural competence strengthens the quality of social relations and ensures effective social communication among racial and ethnic groups.

Global Mental Health

Cross-national epidemiology of mental health disorders demonstrates variation in the prevalence of mental disorders across nations (Kessler & Ustun, 2008). Geographic variation in the prevalence of mental disorders suggests cultural and genetic variations in biomarkers underlying mental disorders. Understanding the mutual influence of cultural and genetic variations on mental processes and the neurobiological mechanisms of behavior contributes to the identification of root causes of mental health and mental disorders. The study of culture and genomics in cultural neuroscience provides a foundation for the systematic investigation into addressing grand challenges in global mental health.

References

Bakermans-Kranenburg, M. J., & van Ijzendoorn, M. H. (2008). Oxytocin (OXTR) and serotonin transporter (5-HTT) genes associated with observed parenting. *Social Cognitive and Affective Neuroscience, 3*(2), 128–134.

Beja-Pereira, A., Luikart, G., England, P.R., Bradley, D.G., Jann, O.C., Bertorelle, G., Chamberlain, A.T., Nunes, T.p., Metodiev, S., Ferrand, N., Erhardt, G. (2003). Gene-culture coevolution between cattle milk protein genes and human lactase genes. *Nature Genetics, 35*(4), 311–313.

Belsky, J., Bakermans-Kranenburg, M. J., & van Ijzendoorn, M. H. (2007). For better or worse: Differential susceptibility to environmental influences. *Current Directions in Psychological Science, 16,* 300–304.

Bonham, V. L., Warshauer-Baker, E., & Collins, F. S. (2005). Race and ethnicity in the genome era: The complexity of the constructs. *American Psychologist, 60*(1), 9–15.

Boyd, R., & Richerson, P. J. (1985). *The origin and evolution of cultures*. Oxford University Press.

Canli, R. Qiu, M., Omura, K., Congdon, E., Haas, B. W., Amin, Z., Herrmann, M. J., Constable, R. T., & Lesch, K. P. (2006). Neural correlates of epigenesis. *Proceedings of the National Academy of Sciences, 103*(43), 16033–16038.

Chen, C., Burton, M., Greenberger, E., & Dmitrieva, J. (1999). Population migration and the variation of dopamine D4 receptor (DRD4) allele frequencies around the globe. *Evolution and Human Behavior 20*(5), 309–324.

Chen, C., Moyzis, R. K., Lei, X., Chen, C., & Dong, Q. (2016). The enculturated genome: Molecular evidence for recent divergent evolution in human neurotransmitter genes. In J. Y. Chiao, S. C. Li, R. Seligman, & R. Turner (Eds.), *The Oxford handbook of cultural neuroscience* (pp. 315–338). Oxford University Press.

Chiao, J. Y. (2018). Developmental aspects in cultural neuroscience. *Developmental Review, 50*(A), 77–89.

Chiao, J. Y., & Blizinsky, K. D. (2010). Culture-gene coevolution of individualism-collectivism and the serotonin transporter gene. *Proceedings of the Biological Sciences B, 277*(1681), 529–537.

Chiao, J. Y., & Blizinsky, K. D. (2016). Cultural neuroscience: Bridging cultural and biological sciences. In E. Harmon-Jones & M. Inzlicht (Eds.), *Social neuroscience: Biological approaches to social psychology* (pp. 247–275). Routledge.

Chiao, J.Y., Hariri, A.R., Harada, T., Mano, Y., Sadato, N., Parrish, T.B., Iidaka, T. (2010). Theory and methods in cultural neuroscience. *Social Cognitive and Affective Neuroscience, 5*(2-3), 356–361.

Chiao, J. Y., Li, S. C., Turner, R., Lee-Tauler, S. Y., & Pringle, B. A. (2017). Cultural neuroscience and global mental health: Addressing grand challenges. *Culture and Brain, 5*(1), 4–13.

Collins, P.Y., Patel, V., Joestl, S.S., March, D., Insel, T.R. Daar, A.S.; Scientific Advisory Board and the Committee of the Grand Challenges on Global Mental health; Anderson, W., Dhansay, M.A., Phillips, A., Shurin, A., Walport, M., Ewart, W., Savill, S.J., Bordin, I.A., Costello, E.J., Durkin, M., Fairburn, C., Glass, R.I., Hall, W., Huang, Y., Hyman, S.E., Jamison, K., Kaaya, S., Kapur, S., Kleinman, A., Ogunniyi, A., Otero-Ojeda, A., Poo, M.M., Ravindranath, V., Sahakian, B.J., Saxena, S., Singer, P.A., Stein, D.J. (2011). Grand challenges in global mental health. *Nature, 475*(7354), 27–30.

Connelly, J. J., & Morris, J. P. (2016). Epigenetics of social behavior. In J. Y. Chiao, S. C. Li, R. Seligman, & R. Turner (Eds.), *The Oxford handbook of cultural neuroscience* (pp. 299–314). Oxford University Press.

Fincher, C. L., Thornhill, R., Murray, D. R., & Schaller, M. (2008). Pathogen prevalence predicts human cross-cultural variability in individualism/collectivism. *Proceedings of the Royal Society B: Biological Sciences, 275*(1640), 1279–1285.

Gelfand, M.J., Raver, J.L., Nishii, L., Leslie, L.M., Lun, J., Lim, B.C., Duan, L., Almaliach, A., Ang, S., Arnadottir, J., Aycan, Z., Boehnke, K., Boski, P., Cabecinhas, R., Chan, D., Chhokar, J., D'Amato, A., Ferrer, M., Fischlmayr, I.C., Fischer, R., Fülöp, M., Georgas, J., Kashima, Y., Kim, K., Lempereur, A., Marquez, P., Othman, R., Overlaet, B., Panagiotopoulou, P., Peltzer, K., Perez-Florizno, L.R., Ponomarenko, L., Realo, A., Schei, V., Schmitt, M., Smith, P.B., Soomro, n., Szabo, E., Taveesin, N., Toyama, M., Van de Vliert, E., Vohra, N., ward, C., Yamaguchi, S. (2011). Differences between tight and loose cultures: a 33-nation study. *Science, 332*(6033), 1100–1104.

Hariri, A. R., & Weinberger, D. R. (2003). Imaging genetics. *British Medical Bulletin, 65,* 259–270.

International HapMap Consortium (2003). The International HapMap Project. *Nature, 426*(6968), 789–796.

Ishii, K., Kim, H. S., Sasaki, J. Y., Shinada, M., & Kusumi, I. (2014). Culture modulates sensitivity to the disappearance of facial expressions associated with serotonin transporter polymorphism (5-HTTLPR). *Culture and Brain, 2*(1), 72–88.

Kessler, R. C., & Ustun, T. B. (2008). *The WHO world mental health surveys: Global perspectives on the epidemiology of mental disorders.* Cambridge University Press.

Kim, H. S., Sherman, D. K., Mojaverian, T., Sasaki, J. Y., Park, J., Suh, E. M., & Taylor, S. E. (2011). Gene-culture interaction: Oxytocin receptor polymorphism (OXTR) and emotion regulation. *Social Psychological and Personality Science, 2,* 665–672.

Kim, H. S., Sherman, D. K., Sasaki, J. Y., Xu, J., Chu, T. Q., Ryu, C., Suh, E. M., Graham, K., & Taylor, S. E. (2010). Culture, distress, and oxytocin receptor polymorphism (OXTR) interact to influence emotional support seeking. *Proceedings of the National Academy of Sciences, 107*(36), 15717–15721.

Kim, H. S., Sherman, D. K., Taylor, S. E., Sasaki, J. Y., Chu, T. Q., Ryu, C., Suh, E. M., & Xu, J. (2010). Culture, serotonin receptor polymorphism and locus of attention. *Social Cognitive and Affective Neuroscience, 5*(2–3), 212–218.

Kitayama, S., King, A., Yoon, C., Tompson, S., Huff, S., & Liberzon, I. (2014). The dopamine D4 receptor gene (DRD4) moderates cultural difference in independent versus interdependent social orientation. *Psychological Science, 25*(6), 1169–1177.

Luo, S., Ma, Y., Liu, Y., Li, B., Wang, C., Shi, Z., Li, X., Zhang, W., Rao, Y., & Han, S. (2015). Interaction between oxytocin receptor polymorphism and interdependent culture values on human empathy. *Social Cognitive and Affective Neuroscience, 10*(9), 1273–1281.

Michalska, K.J., Decety, J., Liu, C.,Chen, Q., Martz, M.E., Jacob, S., Hipwell, A.E., Lee, S.S., Chronis-Tuscano, A., Waldman, I.D., Lahey, B.B. (2014). Genetic imaging of the association of oxytocin receptor gene (OXTR) polymorphisms with positive maternal parenting. *Frontiers in Behavioral Neuroscience, 8,* 21.

Markus, H. R., & Kitayama, S. (1991). Culture and the self: Implications for cognition, emotion, and motivation. *Psychological Review, 98*(2), 224–253.

Masgoret, A. M., & Ward, C. (2006). Cultural learning approach to acculturation. In D. L. Sam & J. W. Berry (Eds.), *The Cambridge handbook of acculturation psychology* (pp. 58–77). Cambridge University Press.

Mesquita, B., & Frijda, N. H. (1992). Cultural variations in emotions: A review. *Psychological Bulletin, 112*(2), 179–204.

Nikolova, Y. S., Koenen, K. C., Galea, S., Wang, C. M., Seney, M. L., Sibille, E., Williamson, D. E., & Hariri, A. R. (2014). Beyond genotype: Serotonin transporter epigenetic modification predicts human brain function. *Nature Neuroscience, 17*(9), 1153–1155.

Nisbett, R. E., & Miyamoto, Y. (2005). The influence of culture: Holistic versus analytic perception. *Trends in Cognitive Science, 9*(10), 467–473.

Nisbett, R. E., Peng, K., Choi, I., & Norenzayan, A. (2001). Culture and systems of thought: Holistic versus analytic cognition. *Psychological Review, 108*(2), 291–310.

Norenzayan, A., & Heine, S. J. (2005). Psychological universals: What are they and how can we know? *Psychological Bulletin, 131*(5), 763–784.

Oyserman, D., Coon, H.M., Kemmelmeier, M. (2002). Rethinking individualism and collectivism: evaluation of theoretical assumptions and meta-analyses. *Psychological Bulletin, 128*(1), 3–72.

Rodrigues, S. M., Saslow, L. R., Garcia, N., John, O. P., & Keltner, D. (2009). Oxytocin receptor genetic variation relates to empathy and stress reactivity in humans. *Proceedings of the National Academy of Sciences, 106,* 21437–21441.

Rosenberg, N. A., Pritchard, J. K., Weber, J. L., Cann, H. M., Kidd, K. K., Zhivotovsky, L. A., & Feldman, M. W. (2002). Genetic structure of human populations. *Science, 298*(5602), 2381–2385.

Sasaki, J. Y., Kim, H. S., Mojaverian, T., Kelley, L. D., Park, I. Y., & Janusonis, S. (2013). Religion priming differentially increases prosocial behavior among variants of the dopamine D4 receptor (DRD4) gene. *Social Cognitive and Affective Neuroscience, 8*(2), 209–215.

Sasaki, J. Y., LeClair, J., West, A., & Kim, H. S. (2016). The gene-culture interaction framework and implications for health. In J. Y. Chiao, S. C. Li, R. Seligman, & R. Turner (Eds.), *The Oxford handbook of cultural neuroscience* (pp. 279–298). Oxford University Press.

Stein, D. J., Chiao, J. Y., & van Honk, J. (2016). Cultural neuroscience in South Africa: Promises and pitfalls. In J. Y. Chiao, S. C. Li, R. Seligman, & R. Turner (Eds.), *The Oxford handbook of cultural neuroscience* (pp. 143–154). Oxford University Press.

Suh, E. M. (2002). Culture, identity consistency, and subjective well-being. *Journal of Personality and Social Psychology, 83*(6), 1378–1391.

Tishkoff, S. A., Reed, F. A., Friedlaender, F. R., Ehret, C., Ranciaro, A., Froment, A., Hirbo, J. B., Awomoyi, A. A., Bodo, J. M., Doumbo, O., Ibrahim, M., Juma, A. T., Kotze, M. J., Lema, G., Moore, J. H., Mortensen, H., Nyambo, T. B., Omar, S. A., Powell, K., . . . Williams, S. M. (2009). The genetic structure and history of Africans and African Americans. *Science, 324*(5930), 1035–1044.

CHAPTER
8

Sociocultural Developmental Neuroscience: Introduction, Implications, and Guiding Principles

Yolanda Vasquez-Salgado *and* Patricia M. Greenfield

Abstract

Neuroscience has been a growing field since the 1940s and, with the advent of new tools for investigating the brain, has skyrocketed in scientific interest. However, most of what is known about human brain development may be applicable only to a restricted set of populations. This situation is problematic because we know cultural features (e.g., values, beliefs, practices) have a profound impact on cognitive, social, and emotional development, yet only recently has research documented the role culture plays in shaping the brain. Though the field of cultural neuroscience has brought promise, it can benefit from the integration of a sociodemographic and developmental lens. This chapter summarizes bodies of multidisciplinary work that integrate sociocultural (sociodemographics, cultural features, or both), developmental research designs (longitudinal, sensitive periods, cross-sectional) and neuroscience research or research that could benefit from this type of multidisciplinary integration. It also discusses the implications of this integration for future research in the new field, sociocultural developmental neuroscience, as well as the implications this integration has for global mental health. The chapter also provides initial, guiding principles for how neuroscientists can go about engaging in this new, emerging field.

Key Words: sociocultural, development, neuroscience, sociodemographic influences, cultural features, sociocultural developmental neuroscience

Neuroscience has been a growing field since the 1940s (electroencephalography [EEG] and event-related potentials [ERPs] being primary tools), and with the advent of new tools for investigating the brain (e.g., magnetic resonance imaging [MRI], functional MRI [fMRI]), scientific interest has skyrocketed (see Figure 8.1). However, the majority of neuroscience studies conducted in humans have taken place in Western, educated, industrialized, rich, and democratic (WEIRD) societies (Chiao & Cheon, 2010; Henrich et al., 2010). For example, if we focus on one type of neuroscience methodology, fMRI, 90% of published peer-reviewed fMRI neuroscience studies have collected their data in Western countries as of 2009 (see Figure 8.2; Chiao, 2009). In addition, much of what we know about human brain development (structure, function) is from convenience samples or samples that lack description (Falk et al., 2013). This is problematic because we know

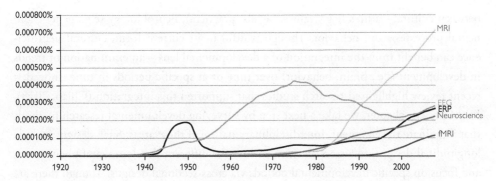

Figure 8.1. Number of books per year from 1920–2008 that mention the terms EEG, ERP, MRI, fMRI and Neuroscience. EEG: electroencephalogram, ERP: event-related-potential, MRI: magnetic resonance imaging, FMRI: functional magnetic resonance imaging. Note: Google N-Gram Viewer was utilized.

from cross-cultural psychology research (research that examines the role of culture and cultural variation in different psychological outcomes) that cultural features (e.g., values, beliefs, practices) have a profound impact on cognitive, social, and emotional development (Greenfield, 2009; Rogoff, 2003), yet only recently has research documented the role culture plays in shaping brain development (Chiao, 2009; Chiao et al., 2013). Thus, most of what we know about human brain development may be applicable only to a restricted set of populations.

The recent birth of *cultural neuroscience* (Chiao, 2009; see the chapter by Chiao et al. on cultural neuroscience, in this volume, for a more recent synthesis) brought promise to this issue. Cultural neuroscience attempts to investigate the interconnected nature

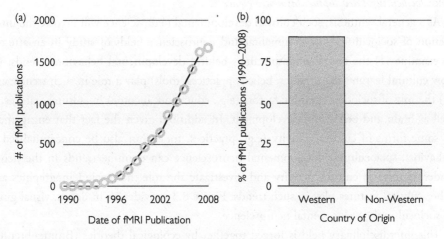

Figure 8.2. "Publication bias in peer-reviewed human neuroimaging (a) Graph illustrating the growth in peer-reviewed human neuroimaging studies from 1990-2008 (b) Graph illustrating the publication bias within the human neuroimaging literature whereby the vast majority (~90%) of publications to date originate from a Western country" (Chiao, 2009).

(Reproduced from Progress in Brain Research, copyright Elsevier 2009).

between cultural features (e.g., values, beliefs, practices), neurobiology (e.g., genetic and neural processes), and behavior. Though fruitful in its current form, cultural neuroscience can benefit from the integration of a developmental lens—an examination of trends in development (i.e., brain, behavior) over time or at specific periods in time. Indeed, a recent review highlighted research studies that supported this integration (Chiao, 2018). In the present chapter, we take a next step by surveying developmental research methods that illuminate the emergent, interdisciplinary nature of these areas. Such designs include longitudinal designs, focus on sensitive periods for different developmental phenomena, and focus on specific developmental periods via cross-sectional designs. Though there are currently developmental neuroscience fields of study (e.g., developmental neuroscience, developmental cognitive neuroscience), fields that focus on neural developmental trajectories, those fields do not necessarily emphasize an integration of cultural features or other forms of diversity that go beyond age. Thus, the integration of developmental research methods into cultural neuroscience is a rather unique element (Miller & Kinsbourne, 2012; Chen & Eisenberg, 2012).

Also of importance, cultural neuroscience has primarily focused its investigation on *cultural features*, which include cultural values, engagement in activities and behaviors that express these values, and engagement in cultural tools such as writing systems and communications technologies (Greenfield, 2009; Markus & Kitayama, 1991; Rogoff, 2003). However, cultural features cannot be taken in isolation; *sociodemographic factors*, such as income, education, and whether one lives in an urban or rural society, must be taken into account (Greenfield, 2009, 2016) as sociodemographics play a role in shaping the cultural features themselves as well as cognitive, social, emotional, and neural development (Greenfield, 2009; Rogoff, 2003). Thus, the outcome of this integration would be a new field: *sociocultural developmental neuroscience*.

As a general synthesis, sociocultural developmental neuroscience will involve the intersection of sociocultural, developmental and neuroscience fields of study in an attempt to examine (1) the neural underpinnings behind developmental behavioral trends; (2) how cultural features (e.g., values, beliefs, practices, tools) play a role in such trends; and (3) the role of sociodemographic factors (e.g., education, income) in cultural features, as well as brain and behavioral development. In addition, given the fact that engagement in some forms of cultural activity (e.g., practices, tools) can also be conceptualized as behaviors, sociocultural developmental neuroscience can examine trends in the neural underpinnings of cultural activity and investigate the role that sociodemographics and other cultural features play in such trends. Figure 8.3 provides an in-depth, visual guide to sociocultural developmental neuroscience.

This interdisciplinary field is forged together by ecological theories (Bronfenbrenner, 1979; Greenfield, 2009) and empirical work in sociocultural, developmental, and neuroscience fields of study (e.g., cultural psychology, cultural neuroscience, developmental neuroscience). Bronfenbrenner's ecological systems theory asserts that development

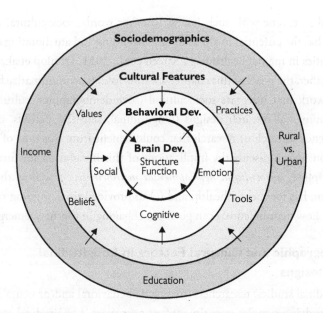

Sociodemographics

Cultural Features

Behavioral Dev.

Values

Practices

Brain Dev.

Income

Structure
Function

Social

Emotion

Rural
vs.
Urban

Beliefs

Tools

Cognitive

Education

Figure 8.3. Sociocultural developmental neuroscience. Sociodemographics may play a direct role in cultural features, behavioral development and brain development. Sociodemographics may play an indirect role in behavioral and brain development through cultural features. Cultural features may play a role in behavioral and brain development. Brain development and behavioral development have an interconnected relationship, as they may both influence each other; variations in this interconnected relationship (e.g., in the form of neural underpinnings of behavior or in relations between neural activity and behavior) may be influenced by sociodemographics and cultural features. Note: Other sociodemographics not in the visual diagram may be incorporated. It is also important to note that sociodemographics and cultural features may be a combination of self and surrounding environmental contexts, contributing to several potential variations in behavioral and brain development. Also, some types of cultural features may also be conceptualized as behaviors and therefore, neural underpinnings of engagement in those features may be examined. Lastly, other patterns within and across the various levels of this diagram may also contribute to variations in behavioral and brain development.

takes place within a nested set of contexts that are both immediate and distal to the individual; variation across those contexts play a role in children's overall development (Bronfenbrenner). Greenfield's theory of social change, culture and human development highlights the role that sociodemographic (e.g., education, income, rural vs. urban settings) shifts in an individual's ecology have in one's cultural values and learning environment as well as the role these three forces play in shaping human development. Thus, this emerging field is theoretically situated and based.

A clear–cut discussion and movement toward a sociocultural developmental neuroscience lens will aid the academic research community in fitting its research practices so that they are aligned with the diverse populations that are growing nationally and that exists internationally. Given the diversity that exists globally, and that global issues, such as mental health, involve examination of behavioral or neural development, a sociocultural developmental neuroscience lens will take into account several sociocultural forces that may be contributing to these issues and, thus, enable us to more effectively understand, pinpoint, and intervene with such issues. In other words, sociocultural developmental neuroscience has the potential to aid us in understanding and ameliorating social class and ethnic disparities in mental health (e.g., Sareen et al., 2011; Dunlop et al., 2003).

Taken together, the goals of this chapter are threefold: (a) to summarize bodies of interdisciplinary work that integrate sociocultural (sociodemographics, cultural features, or both), developmental research designs (longitudinal, sensitive periods, cross-sectional) and neuroscience research or research that could benefit from this type of interdisciplinary integration; (b) to discuss the implications of this integration for future research in the new discipline, *sociocultural developmental neuroscience*, as well as the implications this integration has for mental health; and (c) to provide initial, guiding methodological principles for how neuroscientists can go about engaging in this new, emerging discipline.

Sociodemographic and Cultural Factors In Longitudinal Research Designs

In longitudinal studies, researchers investigate behavioral and/or neural change by following and studying samples over time, often over years. Longitudinal research designs, especially those involving long-term investigations, are a key paradigm in developmental psychology. In the next two sections, we provide examples of how sociodemographic factors have been integrated into long-term and short-term longitudinal research designs.

Long-Term Longitudinal Research: Early Life Deprivation and Emotion Regulation

One area that has been heavily investigated across various stages in development is emotion regulation. *Emotion regulation* involves being able to control one's emotions (e.g., internally decrease an emotional experience; Ochsner et al., 2004). Developmental neuroscience research on the neural underpinnings of emotion regulation has recognized a single normative trajectory. Key areas involved in emotion regulation are the amygdala and prefrontal cortex (PFC; Hare et al., 2008). In neurotypical populations, adults display a negative relationship between amygdala activity and prefrontal cortex when attempting to self-regulate to a fearful stimulus, such that an increase in self-regulation is related to a decrease in amygdala activity and an increase in PFC activity (Hare et al., 2008). In other words, an increase in use of cognitive thinking or strategies (i.e., PFC activity) is typically paired with a decrease in unwanted emotions (i.e., decrease in amygdala activity).

This negative relationship is also present in adolescents (Hare et al., 2008), but to a weaker extent (Gee, Humphreys, et al., 2013). However, children (under age 10) display a different behavioral phenocopy (i.e., a different underlying neural mechanism) when attempting to regulate their emotions—a positive rather than negative relationship— suggesting immaturity (Gee, Humphreys, et al.). This finding makes sense since emotion regulation early in life is supposed to be immature because it is expected that a primary caregiver will be present early in life (Greenough et al., 1987; Moriceau & Sullivan, 2005) to help regulate the environment.

In terms of social context, several studies have focused on *early life deprivation* (Tottenham, 2012). Children who reside in orphanages early in life, and who therefore lack a primary caregiver, reside in an environment with little or no touch, warmth, or intellectual stimulation (Nelson et al., 2014). Among these children, there is consistent evidence that they display larger amygdala cortical volumes (Tottenham et al., 2010) and mature–like amygdala–PFC connectivity in middle childhood (i.e., negative amygdala and PFC connectivity; Gee, Gabard-Durman, et al., 2013). Thus, children who experience this form of early life deprivation begin to utilize adult–like neural strategies to regulate their emotions. In regards to the mental health of these youth, larger amygdala volume has been found to be associated with more internalizing symptoms (e.g., depression) and separation anxiety in middle childhood (Tottenham et al., 2010); a mature amygdala–PFC connectivity earlier than typically displayed has also been found to be associated with more separation anxiety in middle childhood and adolescence (Gee, Gabard-Durman, et al., 2013). The research insights gathered from such longitudinal designs are useful and important because they enable us to understand how early life experiences play a role in neural development and connectivity in later childhood as well as mental health. In referring to Figure 8.3, the work conducted by early deprivation researchers provides evidence for the role of sociodemographic (low resources) and cultural (caregiving practices) contexts on brain (structure, function) and behavioral development.

Integrating sociodemographic factors into developmental neuroscience research on emotion regulation. Though the sociodemographic context in which early life deprivation research was conducted took place within an extreme, low resource context, those resources were not the focus of examination. Additionally, aside from early life deprivation, there is a range of sociodemographic experiences (e.g., living in a rural or urban environment, low income vs. high income, low education vs. high education) within youths' early or current sociodemographic environments that could also be assessed as playing a role in brain and behavioral development (Figure 8.3). Neuroscientists with an early life deprivation emphasis might argue that sociodemographic factors are not specific enough in time to be considered as markers of "early life" experience. However, one study explored the role of income and found interesting results.

Kim et al. (2013) recruited young adults who had taken part in a larger longitudinal study on poverty and child development. Across three different waves of data collection (at about ages 9, 13, and 17), the parents of these young adults had filled out sociodemographic questionnaires that enabled researchers access to the income-to-needs ratio (i.e., family income divided by the poverty threshold) at each point in development. As young adults, they engaged in an fMRI emotion regulation task that required them to look at, maintain, or reappraise images. The findings of this study revealed that childhood family income at age 9 predicted prefrontal (i.e., dorsolateral and ventrolateral PFC) and amygdala activity during the emotion regulation task at age 24. Specifically, lower child-hood income was associated with lower PFC activity and an increase in amygdala activity. In addition, childhood family income at this age predicted the functional connectivity between these areas, with those who experienced lower income in childhood exhibiting a more unsuccessful neural emotion regulation signature and those exposed to higher income exhibiting a more successful neural signature. Adult income was not associated with neural activity. The aforementioned pattern of findings, aligned with use of a socio-cultural developmental lens (Figure 8.3), contribute to the notion that early life experi-ences of poverty may become embedded within individuals and potentially set them on certain developmental, neural paths. However, it is important to mention that when we expand our view to include other sociocultural elements (e.g., parental education, cultural values and practices; Figure 8.3), we will be better able to hone in on variation within these patterns or developmental, neural paths. This notion is supported by theoretical perspectives suggesting that variation in sociodemographic and cultural contexts yields multiple pathways in human development (Bronfenbrenner, 1979; Greenfield, 2009).

Future research. Kim et al.'s study suggests that variations in the sociodemographic environment other than extreme deprivation affect the development of emotion regula-tion. It would therefore be worthwhile to take a sociocultural developmental neuroscience approach by examining the role of income and cultural features in emotion regulation using developmental designs that begin in infancy. It would also be worthwhile to exam-ine how early life experiences with other types of sociodemographic features (e.g., living in a rural vs. urban environment) play a role in shaping neural activity and connectivity between areas critical for emotion regulation. This type of information would broaden the understanding of income and other sociocultural factors in shaping the neural underpin-nings of emotion regulation. It may be, for example, that other sociodemographics (e.g., receiving a certain type of education, living in an urban area or ethnic enclave) and cul-tural features (e.g., cultural values and practices) protect youth against the negative effects of poverty (Jack, 2014). It may also be that, over time, there are shifts in an individual's sociodemographics or cultural features (detailed more in the next section) and those shifts may be linked with neural changes. For more information regarding cultural change, see Varnum and Hampton's chapter on cultural change in this volume.

Integrating cultural values into developmental neuroscience research on emotion regulation. It is promising to integrate cultural values into developmental neuroscience work on emotion regulation because cultural researchers have documented that youth from collectivistic or interdependent cultures (e.g., youth from Asian or Asian American backgrounds) value and behaviorally regulate in a different fashion than youth from indi-vidualistic or independent cultures (e.g., European American youth; Mauss & Butler, 2010; Tsai et al., 2002). In one study, youth watched a neutral film clip and thereafter were exposed to an anger provocation experience that required them to count back in steps of 7 from large numbers (Mauss & Butler, 2010). Throughout the anger provocation experience, participants were interrupted with scripted remarks several times and received feedback of impatience and dissatisfaction from the experimenter.

Participants' values, emotional experience, behavior, and physiological responses were assessed. Their findings indicated that youth from interdependent Asian backgrounds valued, experienced, and behaved with emotional control at significantly higher levels than youth from independent European American backgrounds (Mauss & Butler, 2010). Interestingly, though Asian youth exerted more emotional control, both subjectively and behaviorally, than European American youth, their underlying autonomic physiological responses did not differ. These findings suggest that though self-reports and behaviors vary, underlying autonomic physiological activity does not. Thus, cultural features are important in considering the interconnection between behavioral and physiological responses; this importance is aligned with a sociocultural developmental neuroscience approach (Figure 8.3).

Future research. Even though underlying autonomic physiological activity does not vary, would the cultural differences relating to differences in emotional and behavioral control have a neural signature? And if so, when do these differences emerge and would such neural differences relate to mental health or other behaviors? Neurocultural differences in emotional experience (Immordino-Yang et al., 2016) suggest that it would be worthwhile to explore neurocultural differences in emotion regulation. Central to the interdisciplinary integration of this chapter, a sociocultural developmental neuroscience perspective could explore these relations longitudinally, over time. Specifically, one could investigate whether the neural activity and connectivity associated with emotion regulation exhibits different trajectories or patterns depending on whether one comes from an independent or interdependent family background. One could also examine whether these neural patterns are tied to behaviors that are important for mental health such as depression and anxiety. Such findings could be utilized for intervention.

Implications for mental health. A sociocultural developmental neuroscience approach to emotion regulation would move the field away from the assumption that there is one developmental pathway for emotion regulation. Integrating both sociodemographics and cultural values into neuroscience research on emotion regulation would enable us to understand how different sociocultural groups' emotional regulation registers neurally and the implications of those neural strategies for mental health. It is possible that groups varying in sociodemographics or values also vary in neural strategies and longitudinal trajectories, but that this variation in neural strategies does not necessarily yield differences in mental health. Such findings would provide support for the notion of sociocultural neurodiversity. Understanding the neural strengths that accompany socialization adapted to different ecologies and different sets of cultural values would move the field away from the idea that one pattern of brain development is superior to another.

Shorter-Term Longitudinal Research: Neural Underpinnings of the Cultural Practice of Family Obligation in Emerging Adults

Family obligation values are defined as attitudes towards respecting and assisting family members both now and in the future. The behavioral component of family obligation, known as *family assistance,* consists of spending time with family, running errands for family, helping siblings with homework or helping one's family financially (Fuligni et al., 1999; Telzer & Fuligni, 2009a; Tseng, 2004; Vallejo, 2012). These family obligation values and behaviors, collectivistic in nature, are valued and practiced more highly in the Latinx community than in the European American community (Fuligni et al., 1999). Thus, in discussing the neural underpinnings of the behavioral component of family obligation, we conceptualize it as a cultural practice and a behavior (Figure 8.3).

Telzer et al. (2010) conducted a study in which youth from Latinx and European American backgrounds were exposed to a series of situations that involved giving money to themselves or their family. Though both groups contributed to their families equally, the neural underpinnings of gaining money for themselves (via noncostly reward trials where they would gain money and their family would not lose money) or contributing money to their families (via costly donation trials where they would donate money to their family and lose money in return) operated differently. Latinx participants showed more activity in the ventral striatum, hub of the brain's reward circuitry, when contributing to their family; in contrast, European American participants exhibited more reward activity in the same area when gaining cash for themselves. This finding further demonstrates the need to examine differences at behavioral and neurobiological levels: although engagement of the cultural practice and behavior did not vary, the neural underpinnings provided a different insight.

A separate analysis revealed that heightened bilateral activation in the brain's reward circuitry hub during contributions to family was present among youth with higher family obligation values that centered around assisting one's family (e.g., how often they felt they should eat meals with their family or spend time with their family on weekends). In addition, reward activation exhibited during contributions toward family predicted lower engagement in risk-taking behavior one year later (Telzer et al., 2013). Taken together, results indicate that the cultural practice of contributing material resources to the family was shown to be neurally rewarding for Latinx participants, but not for European American participants. In addition, stronger cultural values for family obligation predicted heightened neural reward when contributing to the family. In terms of mental health, it was the neural reward of giving to family, not behavior in the experiment, that predicted lower risk taking one year later. These findings, aligned with a sociocultural developmental neuroscience lens, demonstrate the importance of examining all four levels of Figure 8.3 (sociodemographics, cultural practices and behavior, brain activity; Figure 8.3).

Together, these studies exemplify a short-term longitudinal design in sociocultural developmental neuroscience. Though Telzer and colleagues assessed neural responses, and one year later gathered survey responses, the same process can be done in reverse, with survey responses being gathered first and neural responses assessed one year later. Specifically, incorporating both orders of assessment would enable sociocultural researchers to explore whether particular behaviors predict particular neural responses or whether particular neural responses predict particular behaviors as the brain and behavioral development are often interconnected in unique ways (Figure 8.3).

Future research. Mechanisms behind Telzer and colleagues' findings (2010, 2013) could be uncovered by delving deeper into the role of both sociodemographics and cultural values in youths' neural response to *prosocial behavior* – engagement in behavior that benefits others (e.g., helping, sharing, donating and comforting others; Dunfield, 2014). In the theory of social change, culture and human development (Greenfield, 2009), greater wealth is linked with more individualistic values and lower levels of family obligation; limited resources are linked with more collectivistic values and higher levels of family obligation. Behaviorally, the theory predicts more generosity to others from people with limited resources and less generosity from individuals with more resources, and this is what Piff et al. (2010) found. In particular, Piff and colleagues (2010) conducted a series of studies that captured the aforementioned notion that individuals of lower socioeconomic status engage in more prosocial behaviors (e.g., donating to charity) and that individuals of higher socioeconomic status engage in less prosocial behavior. Their finding was explained by differences in cultural values. Hence, we would predict that in a socioeconomically diverse sample, there would be greater neural reward for giving to others in the low-socioeconomic-status group and lesser neural reward with the high-socioeconomic-status group, and this would be explained by their cultural values. This examination would be in line with sociocultural developmental neuroscience (Figure 8.3) and would reflect the behavioral findings of Piff et al. at the neural level.

Whereas low socioeconomic status seems to function as a distal mechanism augmenting the neural reward value of making a contribution to family resources, a cultural value—specifically the value of family obligation—might function as the proximal mechanism. These distal (sociodemographics: socioeconomic status) and proximal mechanisms (cultural values: family obligation) could be explored together by assessing participants' socioeconomic status and family obligation values before or after participating in a neural paradigm. The neural paradigm could, perhaps, be extended from the Telzer et al. (2010) and Piff et al. (2010) empirical studies by incorporating prosocial situations (gains, losses) in various contexts (family, close peers, acquaintances, strangers) as different contexts might instigate different prosocial behavioral and neural responses. At the same time, a short-term longitudinal component could be integrated to allow for the relation between these mechanisms and behavioral reports, such as risk taking. Neural responses gathered from this type of sociocultural developmental neuroscience design would enable the field to understand whether neural reward patterns differ depending on context for youth from different sociocultural dispositions and the role of these sociocultural variations in the relation between neural reward circuitry and behavior. Thus, this type of investigation would incorporate all four elements of sociocultural developmental neuroscience (Figure 8.3).

Implications for mental health. Both family obligation (as a cultural value and behavior) in particular and prosocial behavior in general have implications for mental health because both are related to indicators of mental health. Specifically, family obligation values and behaviors are related to positive emotional well-being (Fuligni & Pedersen, 2002; Telzer & Fuligni, 2009) and less risky behaviors (Telzer et al., 2013); engagement in prosocial behaviors is related to more positive affect and less negative affect (Raposa et al., 2006). Thus, there is a need for researchers to continue examining these culturally relevant practices and behaviors neurally as such research can be used for the development of intervention. For example, if the proposed sociocultural developmental neuroscience design outlined in the previous section is successful, it will pinpoint which types of prosocial situations are more rewarding for youth from various sociocultural backgrounds. If one prosocial situation is more rewarding and protective for youth from particular sociocultural backgrounds and another type is more rewarding and protective for youth from other backgrounds, those corresponding prosocial situations can be encouraged as a means to foster positive development.

Sensitive Periods in Development for the Acquisition of Cultural Systems

The notion of a *sensitive period* refers to times in an individual's development when particular experiences or environmental forces play a stronger role in shaping the brain or other aspects of development than at other periods in time. This is also thought of as a time of great "plasticity," the brain's openness to be molded or shaped by one's environment or experiences in a particular domain (Lightfoot et al., 2018). In the next few sections, we provide examples of the role that sociocultural environmental forces (sociodemographics, cultural features) play in shaping cultural systems and brain development. Thus, in terms of Figure 3, our focus will be on the levels pertaining to sociodemographics, cultural features and brain development. For a more thorough review of plasticity, see Goh's chapter, in this volume, that centers around culture and neuroplasticity.

Acquiring a Cultural Meaning System for Interpersonal Relations

Minoura's (1992) research in psychological anthropology suggests that there is a sensitive developmental period for incorporating a cultural meaning system for interpersonal relations. Her research is based on interviews with Japanese families who spent time in the United States and then returned to Japan. She contrasts the more interdependent values of the Japanese meaning system with the more independent values of the meaning system typical in the United States. Her findings suggest that the sensitive period for incorporating one or the other meaning system is between 9 and 15 years of age. Before age 9, she finds that children have not yet solidified their meaning system for social relations and so are open to whatever they encounter between 9 and 15. For example, when a Japanese family moves to the United States with a child under age 9, that child will tend, during the next few years, to acquire the independent social values of the United States. After age 15, teens have solidified their foundational assumptions about normative social relations at a deep level. So, after age 15, they can only acquire a new cultural system on a superficial cognitive level, not on a deep emotional level. This conclusion is based on data showing that if that same child who was in the United States between 9 and 15 moves back with their family to Japan at age 16, they will not feel emotionally comfortable with the Japanese value system, but will retain the U.S. values at a deep emotional level. Minoura's observations imply that the basic cultural value of independence or interdependence is solidified between 9 and 15 years of age. The general outlines of Minoura's conclusion, based on qualitative data, has been reinforced by a subsequent quantitative study of Chinese adolescents in Canada (Kuo & Roysircar, 2004).

Future research. The sensitive period for other areas of development, such as second language acquisition (Hakuta et al., 2003), have been assessed and examined neurally (Thomas & Johnson, 2008). However, the sensitive period for acquiring a cultural meaning system that one carries across interpersonal relations is yet to be examined on the neural level. What brain regions contribute to the acquisition of an independent or interdependent cultural value system between age 9 and 15? Is the functioning of this part of the brain immature before age 9? Does the function of this part of the brain mature around age 9? What brain regions are responsible for the more superficial cognitive acquisition of the value system after age 15? Is this a part of the brain whose functioning matures after age 15? How do these two parts of the brain work together at different ages? Does the neural activity in these areas of the brain relate to social and emotional behaviors, and does this relationship differ depending on whether migration occurs before, during, or after the sensitive period? The answers to these questions are aligned with a sociocultural developmental neuroscience lens and include all levels presented in Figure 8.3. Answering this question will give us insight into the neural foundation of an independent versus interdependent pathway of development (Greenfield, 1994/2014; Greenfield et al., 2003; Stephens, Fryberg et al., 2012; Stephens, Townsend et al., 2012). Given the lack of research in this area, it could potentially be a seminal research program in the emerging field of sociocultural developmental neuroscience.

Implications for mental health. This type of research could lead to better societal understanding of the extent and depth of immigrant adaptation to host society values and the strength of ancestral values at different ages of immigration. Knowledge concerning a sensitive period for acquiring a cultural meaning system for interpersonal relations can contribute to mental health by suggesting ages at which acculturation to host society values would be easier or harder. This knowledge can be utilized by social workers and therapists in mental health counseling as well as language classes for immigrant populations.

Such information can also be used to encourage educational institutions to incorporate interdependent cultural practices into their curriculum so that youth from all cultures and ages of immigration feel comfortable and connected to their learning environment (Trumbull et al., 2001; Stephens, Fryberg et al., 2012; Stephens, Townsend et al., 2012).

Using a Natural Experiment to Explore the Role of a Sensitive Developmental Period and Socioeconomic Status for Acquiring Skill with a Cultural Tool: The Example of Print and the Neural Substrate of Reading

Dehaene and colleagues (2010) compared literate and illiterate adults in Brazil and Portugal. Three of the groups had learned to read as children, two of the groups had learned to read as adults, and one group had never learned to read. Each group was given written sentences to view while in an fMRI scanner. Because the groups learned to read at different ages, the data on brain activation during this task allow us to make inferences about a developmentally sensitive period for learning to read.

The researchers found that the left frontal cortex of the three childhood literacy groups (from both Brazil and Portugal) were the most activated by seeing written sentences; next came the Brazilian and Portuguese groups who had acquired literacy in adulthood; finally, written sentences elicited no frontal cortex activation in the illiterate group, who were from Brazil. The three childhood literacy groups (i.e., the groups who had gone to school as children) also showed the most neural response in the visual word form area, a specialized reading area. The illiterate group showed no response; and the two groups who had learned to read as adults were in the middle.

These findings strongly suggest a sensitive period for acquiring the neural foundation of reading skill. The sensitive period would be a time when neural plasticity for this activity is at its greatest. The evidence suggests that this sensitive period for acquiring the cultural tool of print literacy includes the period between 5 and 7 years of age, the age at which schools typically teach reading. The data do not allow us to make inferences about when it ends.

The results also suggest a connection between reading skill and socioeconomic status (SES), because low-SES Brazilian adults who had learned to read as children showed less activation to written sentences in the visual cortex than did higher-SES literates who had learned to read in childhood. The neural response in the visual cortex for these low-SES adults who had learned to read in childhood was similar to low-SES Brazilian adults who had learned to read as adults. Hence, SES was for this brain area more powerful in determining neural response for acquiring the cultural tool of reading than age of learning. This result suggests the importance of sociodemographic forces in shaping this aspect of neural development. This research aligns with extensive research documenting the role of socioeconomic status in shaping brain development (Hackman et al., 2010). Lastly, in terms of the field of sociocultural developmental neuroscience, Dehaene et al. (2010) utilized three of the levels noted in Figure 8.3 (sociodemographics, cultural features and the development of brain function): They examined the role that socioeconomic status and engagement with the cultural tool of print at different ages had on brain function in adulthood.

Future research and implications for mental health. These two areas of research concerning sensitive periods suggest that each area of cultural knowledge or activity has a distinct sensitive period for its acquisition. Future research in sociocultural developmental neuroscience can explore whether these sensitive developmental periods are linked with important behavioral outcomes (e.g., mental health, academics). This knowledge can be applied to understand what the best age is to initiate instruction or training in various domains of interest to society or to the individual. Central to mental health, we can seek to understand the connection of this neural activity to mental health. A few questions for sociocultural developmental neuroscience would be: What is the sensitive period for acquiring a neural foundation of reading skill (when does it begin, when does it end)? What role does the strength and acquisition of this neural foundation play in mental health? How do sociocultural forces work together to influence this sensitive period? Can sociocultural interventions help strengthen the neural foundation of reading? Can sociocultural interventions help reopen plasticity for acquiring the neural foundation of reading? All of these ideas fit with a sociocultural developmental neuroscience perspective (all levels of Figure 8.3). These are important questions to ask as research has shown that a lack of reading skill is strongly correlated heavily with poor mental health as well as unemployment, lower wages, and fewer advancement opportunities; lack of reading skill is also highly prevalent among the prison population (Boyes et al., 2016; National Endowment for the Arts, 2007).

Specific Developmental Period for Sensitivity to Communication Technologies as a Cultural Tool: Their Neural Attraction for Adolescents and Emerging Adults in a Cross-Sectional Study

Cross-sectional studies involve an examination of different age groups at the same point in time. Differences between the groups are assumed to be the result of age-related developmental changes. In some cases, developmental researchers may choose to examine groups that are vastly different in age, and at other times, they may focus on groups that are only slightly different. The research we now discuss focuses on adolescents and young emerging adults. In a cross-sectional study simulating the photo-sharing app Instagram, in an fMRI scanner, participants viewed a series of Instagram photos that included their own and those of other "peers" (Sherman et al., 2016, 2017). Their photos were manipulated so that some received several "likes" and others received few "likes." High school (adolescent) and college (young, emerging adults) students viewed these stimuli in an fMRI scanner and were instructed to go through each photo and "like" it or click "next" to move on without "liking" the photo. Results revealed that receiving more (vs. fewer) "likes" of one's photos activated the reward centers of the adolescent and emerging adult brain. In addition, the researchers also found a developmental trend that indicated a period of neural sensitivity for usage of this cultural tool. The trend indicated that older adolescents, more so than younger adolescents and emerging adults, displayed greater activation of reward circuitry in viewing their highly "liked" photos. The researchers note that this is connected to a general trend of older adolescents being among the first to gain experience in new media. Together, these findings exemplify the fact that there is often a powerful fit between the use of a cultural tool and the functioning of the human brain. It is thought that the exquisite sensitivity to social reward at this time of life is part and parcel of both the usage and the importance of "likes" to this age group. Hence, in terms of sociocultural developmental neuroscience, the work conducted by Sherman and colleagues (2016, 2017) demonstrates that there is a relation between cultural tool usage and neural function (two levels of Figure 8.3).

Future research and implications for mental health. Though cross-sectional data surrounding adolescents and emerging adults is fruitful, sociocultural developmental neuroscience should incorporate preadolescents into this type of research (with Instagram or other types of apps these youths predominantly use, e.g., YouTube). By including pre-teens, the scientific community would be able to test whether the power of the "like" or other forms of social approval might begin earlier. This type of information would extend our knowledge of this cultural tool and its connection to the human brain; it would also enable us to test whether there is a sensitive period for when this connection takes fold and is at its strongest, across all media types. This question is important as very young children are now using communication media and receiving feedback in various forms (e.g., likes, views, followers). In addition to incorporating younger children, in terms of sociocultural contexts, it would be interesting to examine whether use of mediated cultural tools in different sociodemographic contexts elicit the same neural responses. This is an important question given the ubiquitous presence of remote instruction during the pandemic. Lastly, in connection to mental health, it would also be interesting to know if the brain response to "likes" is related to Internet addiction or to mental health more generally. Future research could also explore the extent to which the neural response to "likes" is related to other behavioral symptoms of addiction. Together, engagement in such inquires would make use of all levels of a sociocultural developmental neuroscience perspective (sociodemographic, cultural features, behavior and the development of neural function; Figure 8.3). This knowledge could perhaps be used to develop standards for healthy use of Facebook and mobile apps such as Instagram and Snapchat. Because teenagers are so sensitive to peer influence, these findings also indicate the dangerous power of perceived social rejection in social networking on the Internet (e.g., in the form of few "likes") as well as the dire need for engagement in further research.

Conclusions from Prior Studies

The field is currently lacking a substantial integration of sociocultural, developmental, and neuroscience fields of study. This situation is problematic because it suggests that our scientific knowledge is largely based on one viewpoint or prototype of development. However, the limited research available that integrates these fields of study suggests that sociocultural forces likely have a significant impact on trajectories of brain and behavioral development around the world. To support this scientific movement, evidence from sociocultural theories and research highlights the substantial influence of sociocultural forces on cognitive, social, and emotional development. Sociocultural developmental neuroscientists can therefore provide insight into the neural substrates that underlie divergent pathways through human development. Thus, sociocultural developmental neuroscience is essential.

Insights from this new field have important implications for uncovering mechanisms that underlie global issues, such as mental health, because sociocultural experiences can serve as both a strength of and a detriment to mental health. Understanding how different sociodemographic and cultural influences work together to impact mental health both behaviorally and neurally will enable researchers to understand the phenomena at a deeper and more complete level (Figure 8.3), yielding the potential for well-informed interventions.

Sociocultural Developmental Neuroscience: Definition and Methodological Principles

At a general level, neuroscience fields of study have operated with universalistic assumptions about development. These universalistic assumptions can best be described by reflecting on the tools that are used to conduct analyses and make inferences about brain response (e.g., a prototype brain structure for all age groups and cultures), as well as the theory behind acquiring a blood oxygen level–dependent (BOLD) signal (i.e., a prototypical hemodynamic pattern and response). Although research has documented that our brains vary in size (Mandal et al., 2011) and in hemodynamic response (e.g., higher rates of metabolism yield differential BOLD signals; Logothetis & Wandell, 2004), the majority of developmental neuroscience studies have ignored this information.

Other fields initially began with universalistic viewpoints as well. For example, although developmental science began with a prototypical theory of development, it soon integrated sociodemographic and cultural variation (Greenfield & Bruner, 1966). The general field of psychology also began with a universalistic stance and later incorporated culture (see Matsumoto & Hwang's chapter, in this volume, that centers around culture and psychology). In a similar way, developmental neuroscience has made great strides in uncovering trends in brain development and linkages to behavioral development. However, as research in developmental neuroscience increases, so should the integration of sociodemographic and cultural factors. This integration of sociocultural diversity will enable researchers, practitioners, and policymakers to understand and pinpoint factors and processes that contribute to and protect against disparities in mental health around the nation and world.

The integration of culture, development, and neuroscience has received some attention (Chen & Eisenberg, 2012; Miller & Kinsbourne, 2012). In fact, the University of California, Los Angeles, created an interdisciplinary center, the Center for Culture, Brain, and Development, which aimed to foster connection between these important topics. Though some researchers have seen the potential for sociocultural developmental neuroscience (Miller & Kinsbourne), the details of what this new field might encompass have not been formally discussed. In the next sections, we define this new field and outline its potential principles.

Definition

As stated in this chapter's introduction, *sociocultural developmental neuroscience* involves the intersection of sociocultural, developmental and neuroscientific fields of study in an attempt to examine (1) the neural underpinnings behind developmental behavioral trends; (2) how cultural features (e.g., values, beliefs, practices, tools) play a role in such trends; and (3) the role of sociodemographic factors (e.g., education, income) in cultural features, as well as brain and behavioral development. In addition, given the fact that engagement in some forms of cultural features (e.g., practices, tools) can also be conceptualized as behaviors (e.g., Telzer et al. 2010; Sherman et al., 2016), sociocultural developmental neuroscience can examine trends in the neural underpinnings of cultural features and investigate the role that sociodemographics and other cultural features play in such trends. Figure 8.3 of this chapter provides an in depth, visual guide and synthesis of sociocultural developmental neuroscience. Though it might not always be possible to integrate all four levels of sociocultural developmental neuroscience into a research design (sociodemographic, cultural features, behavioral and brain development), we encourage this practice where possible. It is important to note that this definition, along with the in-depth, visual guide and synthesis of sociocultural developmental neuroscience (Figure 8.3) is our first attempt at conceptualization. This definition and visual synthesis is expected to evolve over time as do other theories and conceptualizations (Bronfenbrenner, 1979; Greenfield, 2009).

Methodological Principles

Cultural variation within and across national borders: Sociodemographics. The field of sociocultural developmental neuroscience will involve cross-cultural investigation of developmental neuroscience trends to examine how they vary both across and within countries, with a focus on sociodemographic variation. For example, this research strategy could involve a comparison of brain response to a prosocial behavioral task at different ages, between the United States and Mexico, as well as among the various sociodemographic groups (e.g., low vs. high socioeconomic status) within each country. Greenfield's (2009) theory of social change, culture and human development predicts that cultural values vary internationally and within each country due to sociodemographic diversity. For example, although the United States has more economic and educational resources than

Mexico, within each country, there is sociodemographic variability that exists (Greenfield & Quiroz, 2013). The prediction is that this situation may result in differential developmental outcomes within a country (e.g., such as more prosocial behavior among the lower socioeconomic groups) and, therefore, possible differential brain response. Similar comparisons can be made for other aspects of development, such as cognitive or emotional development.

Complete sample characteristics, means, and standard deviations. Sociocultural developmental neuroscience will increase the number of sample characteristics that are included in empirical reports. This outcome will occur because the majority of developmental neuroscience studies and general neuroscience studies conducted in humans lack sample descriptions (Falk et al., 2013). This situation is problematic because it prevents researchers from interpreting the role of cultural factors in past studies and integrating sociodemographic and cultural specificity into future research. The inclusion of tables that provide means and standard deviations of brain and behavioral data across the various sample characteristic would be a useful advance. Inclusion of such information would permit the field to conduct sociocultural meta-analyses of behavioral and neural trends. This type of trend would be especially useful in thinking about global mental health as we would be able to assess how behaviors and neural processes underlying mental health vary within and across cultures on a much larger scale.

Potential new tools for investigating the brain. The tools that we use to conduct fMRI analyses are based on combining all participants' data onto a template that was constructed based on a single adult subject or an average of several adult subjects (Mandal et al., 2012). Although a recent review has suggested the need for age-specific brain templates (Evans et al., 2012), very few researchers have taken on this task (Akiyama et al., 2013). Although some researchers have created appropriate brain templates in different countries (i.e., Korean, Chinese, and French brain templates; Mandal et al., 2012), templates of other countries (e.g., Russia, India, Turkey) remain nonexistent.

But national templates also assume that countries are socioculturally homogenous, which is far from the case, so this is a fallacious assumption. While a standard brain allows researchers to make standardized comparisons of functional activity, it may result in incorrect assumptions about the areas of the brain that are active during behavioral tasks for participants from different sociodemographic and cultural backgrounds. Thus, sociocultural developmental neuroscience should aim to examine sources of neural variability with and without being constrained by standardized templates. Given diversity around the world, this practice would help ensure that the scientific community pinpoints the exact areas of the brain that contribute to neural mechanisms of interest, such as the development of mental health illnesses or mental health disparities in different sociodemographic and cultural settings. If this is not feasible, given the nature of standardization needed in order to conduct comparisons, researchers at the very least should begin to have discussions around this topic.

Neuroscientific methodology. Though much of the selected review in this chapter focused on results from fMRI studies, sociocultural developmental neuroscience will and should encompass all neuroscience techniques for studying brain development (e.g., EEG, ERP, MRI, fMRI, diffusion tensor imaging [DTI]; Goldenberg & Galvan, 2015), as the paucity of studies that take sociodemographic factors and cultural features into account is limited in all techniques. The field will also employ traditional developmental designs for studying age-related differences (i.e., cross-sectional), change over time (i.e., longitudinal designs), and cohort effects (i.e., cohort sequential design). The field will use such designs to answer several questions central to developmental science (e.g., plasticity, continuity, individual differences). The major contribution of the new field will be in its integration of sociodemographic and cultural variation as a major source of comparison of developmental brain and behavioral trends. This integration and triangulation of methods within sociocultural, developmental, and neuroscience fields of study will enable researchers to gain additional perspectives on particular phenomena. For example, the use of multiple methods would enable researchers interested in emotion regulation, a topic central to mental health, to understand neural structure (MRI) and function (fMRI) important for this skill, as well as neural response and timing (ERP) to emotion-related stimuli. Researchers could make sociocultural (sociodemographic and cultural features) comparisons of these neural outcomes across different age groups (cross-sectional), over time (longitudinal), or using both approaches (cohort sequential). There are various combinations of techniques that can be utilized across these fields of study; these combinations will galvanize the field sociocultural developmental neuroscience.

Why Should Sociocultural Developmental Neuroscience Matter to Researchers and How Can It Benefit Society as a Whole?

Researchers. Enhancing our understanding of culture is important given that the world's countries have become increasingly diverse. For example, by 2060, the majority of children in the United States are expected to be from an ethnic minority background (U.S. Census, 2015). Some argue that children from ethnic minority backgrounds are already the majority (U.S. Census Bureau, 2018; Saenz, 2020). Additionally, foreign-born immigrants from various cultural backgrounds make up nearly 14% of the U.S. population (Pew Research Center, 2018). Though current developmental neuroscientists have provided us with a starting point for understanding neural development, much as Piaget did in his cognitive stages of development, now is the time to extend our current knowledge, so that it fits with the diverse populations in our society.

But beyond ethnicity, we need to consider other long-existing sociocultural differences, such as education and neighborhood structure; such contexts have the power to shape brain and behavior and must be examined more extensively. In other words, developmental neuroscientists should integrate sociodemographic and cultural frameworks into their research because most of the world's population is living in diverse societies that will become even more diverse in decades to come.

In a similar vein, cultural neuroscientists must integrate a developmental lens in order to understand the implications of their research findings beyond immediate, one-time-point experiences and must consider sociodemographics in shaping the results of their inquiries. This new field should also matter to sociocultural developmental researchers because it will allow them to extend their current knowledge of sociocultural differences in engagement in practices, tools and other behaviors with new methodological techniques. These extensions will allow sociocultural developmental researchers to understand neural substrates of concepts or frameworks that they have extensively examined with qualitative reports, surveys, and behavioral experiments.

Benefit for society. The field of sociocultural developmental neuroscience has the potential to provide in-depth understanding of social class and ethnic disparities in mental health around the world and pinpoint when these disparities begin to emerge. This information can be useful to practitioners, policymakers, and individuals as they navigate trying to understand the various sociocultural factors that work together to contribute to inequities or that can be leveraged as strengths. This information can be especially useful for nonprofit community organizations around the world that aim to ameliorate mental health disparities that affect disadvantaged communities. These organizations have programs and services in play and may benefit from a connection or link between their community organizations and researchers at academic institutions (Stringer, 2007). This community–academic bridge can work in several ways, such as developing collaboration on evidence–based interventions that aim to dismantle disparities, or as an exchange of knowledge, whereby community organizations aid neuroscientists in understanding the sociocultural populations under study and potentially protective cultural factors while neuroscientists provide insight into the neural mechanisms behind disparities at different points in developmental time.

For neuroscientists, the outcome can be the creation of neural paradigms that have more ecological and cross-cultural validity. For community organizations, the outcome can be the creation of educational campaigns that are tailored for sociocultural groups that are most at risk, as well as campaigns that hone in on particular developmental periods important for mental health disparities. Thus, sociocultural developmental neuroscientists should consider building a connection with nonprofit community and international organizations, as these entities can aid one another in working toward investigating and ameliorating disparities around the world. This type of collaboration, along with the publicizing their scientific findings, will truly benefit our world as a whole.

Overall Conclusion

Sociocultural developmental neuroscience will enable the scientific community to understand how developmental neuroscience trends vary across diverse groups in our society and around the world. This understanding will broaden and integrate the sociocultural, developmental, and neuroscientific fields of study. Sociocultural developmental neuroscience will also extend and merge our theories of biological (Steinberg et al., 2009) and ecological constructs (Bronfenbrenner, 1979; Greenfield, 2009). More importantly, a community of researchers across and within countries will provide descriptive data of their socioculturally diverse samples, permitting a deeper understanding of the role of sociodemographic and cultural context in brain development. These scientific developments will provide ecological validity and developmental sensitivity to neuroscience research, especially for sensitive topics, such as global mental health.

Acknowledgments

The authors would like to thank Shu-Sha Angie Guan, Tara Patterson and Lauren Sherman for their feedback on earlier drafts of this chapter. The development of this chapter was supported by the National Institute of General Medical Sciences of the National Institutes of Health under Award Numbers RL5GM118975 and UL1GM118976. The content is solely the responsibility of the authors and does not necessarily represent the official views of the National Institutes of Health.

References

Akiyama, L. F., Richards, T. R., Imada, T., Dager, S. R., Wroblewski, L., & Kuhl, P. K. (2013). Age-specific average head template for typically developing 6-month-old infants. *PloS One, 8*, e73821.

Bronfenbrenner, U. (1979). *The ecology of human development: Experiments in nature and design*. Harvard University Press.

Chen, X., & Eisenberg, N. (2012). Understanding cultural issues in child development: Introduction. *Child Development Perspectives, 6*, 1–4.

Chiao, J. Y. (2009). Cultural neuroscience: A once and future discipline. *Progress in Brain Research, 178*, 287–304.

Chiao, J. Y. (2018). Developmental aspects in cultural neuroscience. *Developmental Review, 50*, 77–89.

Chiao, J. Y., & Cheon, B. K. (2010). The weirdest brains in the world. *Behavioral and Brain Sciences, 33*, 88–90.

Chiao, J. Y., Cheon, B. K., Pornpattananangkul, N., Mrazek, A. J., & Blizinsky, K. D. (2013). Cultural neuroscience: Progress and promise. *Psychological Inquiry, 24*, 1–19.

Dehaene, S., Pegado, F., Braga, L. W., Ventura, P., Filho, G. N., Jobert, A., Dehaene-Lambertz, G., Kolinsky, R. Morais, J., & Cohen, L. (2010). How learning to read changes the cortical networks for vision and language. *Science, 330*, 1359–1364.

Evans, A. C., Janke, A., Collins, D. L., & Baillet, S. (2012). Brain templates and atlases. *NeuroImage, 62*, 911–922.

Falk, E. B., Hyde, L. W., Mitchell, C., Faul, J., Gonzalez, R., Heitzeg, M. M., Keating, D. P., Langa, K. M., Martz, M. E., Maslowsky, J., Morrison, F. J., Noll, D. C., Patrick, M. E., Pfeffer, F. T., Reuter-Lorenz, P. A., Thomason, M. E., Davis-Kean, P., Monk, C. S., & Schulenberg, J. (2013). What is a representative brain? Neuroscience meets population science. *Proceedings of the National Academy of Sciences, 110*, 17615–17622.

Fuligni, A. J., & Pedersen, S. (2002). Family obligation and the transition to young adulthood. *Developmental Psychology, 38*, 856–868.

Fuligni, A. J., Tseng, V., & Lam, M. (1999). Attitudes toward family obligations among American adolescents with Asian, Latin American, and European backgrounds. *Child Development, 70*, 1030–1044.

Gee, D. G., Gabard-Durnam, L. J., Flannery, J., Goff, B., Humphreys, K. L., Telzer, E. H., Hare, T. A., Bookheimer, S. Y., & Tottenham, N. (2013). Early developmental emergence of human amygdala–prefrontal connectivity after maternal deprivation. *Proceedings of the National Academy of Sciences of the United States of America, 110*, 15638–15643.

Gee, D. G., Humphreys, K. L., Flannery, J., Goff, B., Telzer, E. H., Shapiro, M., Hare, T. A., Bookheimer, S. Y., & Tottenham, N. (2013). A developmental shift from positive to negative connectivity in human amygdala–prefrontal circuitry. *Journal of Neuroscience, 33*, 4584–4593.

Goldenberg, D., & Galvan, A. (2015). The use of functional and effective connectivity techniques to understand the developing brain. *Developmental Cognitive Neuroscience, 12*, 155–164.

Greenfield, P. M. (1994/2014). Independence and interdependence as developmental scripts: Implications for theory, research, and practice. In P. M. Greenfield & R. R. Cocking (Eds.), *Cross cultural roots of minority child development* (pp. 1–37). Erlbaum. Reissued as a Classic Edition by Psychology Press.

Greenfield, P. M. (2009). Linking social change and developmental change: Shifting pathways of human development. *Developmental Psychology, 45*, 401.

Greenfield, P. M. (2016). Social change, cultural evolution, and human development. *Current Opinion in Psychology, 8*, 84–92.

Greenfield, P. M., & Bruner, J. S. (1966). Culture and cognitive growth. *International Journal of Psychology, 1*, 89–107.

Greenfield, P. M., Keller, H., Fuligni, A., & Maynard, A. (2003). Cultural pathways through universal development. *Annual Review of Psychology, 54*, 461–490.

Greenfield, P. M., & Quiroz, B. (2013). Context and culture in the socialization and development of personal achievement values: Comparing Latino immigrant families, European American families, and elementary school teachers. *Journal of Applied Developmental Psychology, 34*, 108–118.

Greenough, W. T., Black, J. E., & Wallace, C. S. (1987). Experience and brain development. *Child Development, 58*, 539–559.

Hackman, D. A., Farah, M. J., & Meaney, M. J. (2010). Socioeconomic status and the brain: Mechanistic insights from human and animal research. *Nature Reviews Neuroscience, 11*, 651–659.

Hakuta, M., Bialystok, E., & Wiley, E. (2003). Critical evidence: A test of the critical period hypothesis for second-language acquisition. *Psychological Science, 14*, 31–38.

Hare, T. A., Tottenham, N., Galvan, A., Voss, H. U., Glover, G. H., & Casey, B. J. (2008). Biological substrates of emotional reactivity and regulation in adolescence during an emotional go-nogo task. *Biological Psychiatry, 63*, 927–934.

Henrich, J., Heine, S. J., & Norenzayan, A. (2010). The weirdest people in the world? *Behavioral and Brain Sciences, 33*, 61–83.

Immordino-Yang, M. H., Yang, X. F., & Damasio, H. (2016). Cultural modes of expressing emotions influence how emotions are experienced. *Emotion, 16*, 1033–1039.

Jack, A. A. (2014). Culture shock revisited: The social and cultural contingencies to class marginality. *Sociological Forum, 29*, 453–475.

Kim, P., Evans, G. W., Angstadt, M., Ho, S. S., Sripada, C. S., Swain, J. E., Liberzon, I., & Phan, K. L. (2013). Effects of childhood poverty and chronic stress on emotion regulatory brain function in adulthood. *Proceedings of the National Academy of Sciences, 110*, 18442–18447.

Kuo, B. C. H. & Roysircar, G. (2004). Predictors of acculturation for Chinese adolescents in Canada: Age of arrival, length of stay, social class, and English reading ability. *Journal of Multicultural Counseling and Development, 32*, 143–154.

Lightfoot, C., Cole, M., & Cole, S. R. (2018). *The development of children* (8th ed.). Worth Publishers.

Logothetis, N. K., & Wandell, B. A. (2004). Interpreting the BOLD signal. *Annual Review of Physiology, 66*, 735–769.

Mandal, P. K., Mahajan, R., & Dinov, I. D. (2012). Structural brain atlases: Design, rationale, and applications in normal and pathological cohorts. *Journal of Alzheimer's Disease, 31*, 169–188.

Markus, H. R., & Kitayama, S. (1991). Culture and the self: Implications for cognition, emotion, and motivation. *Psychological Review, 98*, 224.

Mauss, I. B., & Butler, E. A. (2010). Cultural context moderates the relationship between emotion control values and cardiovascular challenge versus threat response. *Biological Psychology, 84*, 521–530.

Miller, J. G., & Kinsbourne, M. (2012). Culture and neuroscience in developmental psychology: Contributions and challenges. *Child Development Perspectives, 6*, 35–41.

Minoura, Y. (1992). A sensitive period for the incorporation or a cultural meaning system: A study of Japanese children growing up in the United States. *Ethos, 20*, 304–339.

Moriceau, S., & Sullivan, R. M. (2005). Neurobiology of infant attachment. *Developmental Psychobiology, 47*, 230–242.

National Endowment for the Arts. (2007). To read or not to read: A question of national consequence. Retrieved from https://www.arts.gov/sites/default/files/ToRead.pdf

Nelson, C. A., Fox, N. A., & Zeanah, C. H. (2014). *Romania's abandoned children: Deprivation, brain development and the struggle for recovery.* Harvard University Press.

Ochsner, K. N., Ray, R. D., Cooper, J. C., Robertson, E. R., Chopra, S., Gabrieli, J. D. E., & Gross, J. J. (2004). For better or for worse: Neural system supporting cognitive down- and up-regulation of negative emotion. *NeuroImage, 23,* 483–499.

Pew Research Center (2020, August 20). Facts on U.S. Immigrants, 2018. Retrieved from https://www.pewresearch.org/hispanic/2020/08/20/facts-on-u-s-immigrants-current-data/

Piff, P. K., Kraus, M. W., Côté, S., Cheng, B. H., & Keltner, D. (2010). Having less, giving more: The influence of social class on prosocial behavior. *Journal of Personality and Social Psychology, 99,* 771.

Raposa, E. B., Laws, H. B., & Ansell, E. B. (2015). Prosocial behavior mitigates the negative effects of stress in everyday life. *Clinical Psychological Science, 4,* 691–698.

Rogoff, B. (2003). *The cultural nature of human development.* Oxford University Press.

Sanez, R. (2020, January 9). Children of color projected to be majority of U.S. youth this year. The Conversation. https://theconversation.com/children-of-color-already-make-up-the-majority-of-kids-in-inmany-us-states-128499

Sherman, L. E., Greenfield, P. M., Hernandez, L. M., & Dapretto, M. (2017). Peer influence via Instagram: Effects on brain and behavior in adolescence and young adulthood. *Child Development, 1,* 37–47.

Sherman, L. E., Payton, A. A., Hernandez, L. M., Greenfield, P. M., & Dapretto, M. (2016). The power of the like in adolescence: Effects of peer influence on neural and behavioral responses to social media. *Psychological Science, 27,* 10027–10035.

Steinberg, L., Graham, S., O'Brien, L., Woolard, J., Cauffman, E., & Banich, M. (2009). Age differences in future orientation and delay discounting. *Child Development, 80,* 28–44.

Stephens, N. M., Fryberg, S. A., Markus, H. R., Johnson, C. S., & Covarrubias, R. (2012). Unseen disadvantage: how American universities' focus on independence undermines the academic performance of first-generation college students. *Journal of Personality and Social Psychology, 102,* 1178–1197.

Stephens, N. M., Townsend, S. S. M., Markus, H. R., & Phillips, L. T. (2012). A cultural mismatch: Independent cultural norms produce greater increases in cortisol and more negative emotions among first-generation college students. *Journal of Experimental Social Psychology, 48,* 1389–1393.

Stringer, E. T. (2007). *Action research* (3rd ed.). Sage Publications.

Telzer, E. H., & Fuligni, A. J. (2009). Daily family assistance and the psychological well-being of adolescents from Latin American, Asian, and European backgrounds. *Developmental Psychology, 45,* 1177–1189.

Telzer, E. H., Fuligni, A. J., Lieberman, M. D., & Galvan, A. (2013). Ventral striatum activation to prosocial rewards predicts longitudinal declines in adolescent risk taking. *Developmental Cognitive Neuroscience, 3,* 45–52.

Telzer, E. H., Masten, C. L., Berkman, E. T., Lieberman, M. D., & Fuligni, A. J. (2010). Gaining while giving: An fMRI study of the rewards of family assistance among White and Latino youth. *Social Neuroscience, 5,* 508–518.

Thomas, M. S. C., & Johnson, M. H. (2008). New advances in understanding sensitive periods in brain development. *Current Directions in Psychological Science, 17,* 1–5.

Tottenham, N. (2012). Human amygdala development in the absence of species-expected caregiving. *Developmental Psychobiology, 54,* 598–611.

Tottenham, N., Hare, T. A., Quinn, B. T., McCarry, T. W., Nurse, M., Gilhooly, T., Milner, A., Galvan, A., Davidson, M. C., Eigsti, I-M., Thomas, K. M., Freed, P., Booma, E. S., Gunnar, M., Altemus, M., Aronson, J., & Casey, B. (2010). Prolonged institutional rearing is associated with atypically larger amygdala volume and difficulties in emotion regulation. *Developmental Science, 13,* 46.

Tsai, J. L., Chentsova-Dutton, Y., Freire-Bebeau, L., & Przymus, D. E. (2002). Emotional expression and physiology in European Americans and Hmong Americans. *Emotion, 2,* 380–397.

Trumbull, E., Rothstein-Fisch, C., Greenfield, P. M., & Quiroz, B. (2001). Bridging Cultures Between Home and School: A Guide for Teachers. New Jersey: Laurence Erlbaum Associates

U.S. Census Bureau (2015, March 3). Projects of the size and composition of the U.S. Population: 2014 to 2060. Retrieved from https://www.census.gov/library/publications/2015/demo/p25-1143.html

U.S. Census Bureau (2018, March 13). Older people projected to outnumber children for first time in U.S. history. Retrieved from https://www.census.gov/newsroom/press-releases/2018/cb18-41-population-projections.html

Developmental Plasticity and Global Aging

Shu-Chen Li

Abstract

Brain aging at the neurochemical, anatomical, and functional levels has direct implications for various cognitive, motivational, and affective functions in old age. With global population demographics heading towards a faster-growing trend in the population aged 60 and above than all other age groups, the task to maintain and enhance cognitive, motivational, and affective vitality in old age beyond merely reducing or treating physical illnesses plays an increasingly important role for global mental health. Albeit the brain is aging, the aging brain still possesses a substantial amount of plasticity at different levels. Selective recent research findings on cognitive and brain plasticity in old age, focusing on the effects of cognitive and physical fitness interventions as well as lifestyle dietary and social participation factors, are reviewed here. Outlooks on technologies as modern drives for cultural changes as well as prospects of new technological developments in internet-based behavioral interventions are highlighted.

Key Words: aging, demographic change, brain plasticity, developmental plasticity, cognitive intervention, lifestyle intervention, human-technology interactions

What seemingly was often overlooked . . . is that the brain is a dependent variable, something that is co-shaped by experience and culture, something that does not operate within an environmental vacuum, but that at any moment is subject to environmental constraints and affordances.

—Baltes et al. (2006, p. 4)

Recent work in neuroscience, robotics, and psychology . . . stresses the unexpected intimacy of brain, body, and world and invite us to attend to the structure and dynamics of extended adaptive systems. . . . The mind itself . . . is best understood as the activity of an essentially *situated* brain: a brain at home in its proper bodily, cultural and environmental niche.

—Clark (1999, p. 5)

The Challenge of Global Population Aging on Public Mental Health

Through modern health care, medical treatment, and disease prevention, over the past 150 years the human life expectancy at birth has increased from the mid-40s to mid-80s in advanced economies. Such a remarkable increase in lifespan expectancy coupled with a decline in birth rate has resulted in an unprecedented shift in the population demography of many countries in the Organization for Economic Co-operation and Development (OECD): the numbers of individuals aged 60 or above in these societies now are higher than the numbers of individuals aged 15 or younger (Harper, 2014). More recent data from the 2017 revision of the United Nations' population prospects also highlight that the reduction in fertility and increase in life expectancy led to rapidly growing aging populations worldwide. Globally the number of persons aged 60 or above is expected to more than double by 2050 and more than triple by 2100. More specifically, the demographic profiles based on data from the more developed world regions (i.e., Europe, North America, Japan, and Australia/New Zealand) and from the less developed regions (i.e., Africa, Asia excluding Japan, Latin America, the Caribbean, and Oceania) with the anticipated increases in aging populations until 2100 are shown in Figure 9.1. As can be seen, the demographic shift towards a larger proportion of older than younger populations is now already visible in the more developed regions. Taking Europe as an example, currently 25% of the population is already aged 65 years or older, and this percentage is projected to increase to 35% by 2050 (United Nations, Department of Economics and Social Affairs, Population Division, 2017).

Mental Health Implications

According to the World Health Organization (WHO, 1946), health is a state of complete physical, mental, and social well-being and not merely the absence of disease

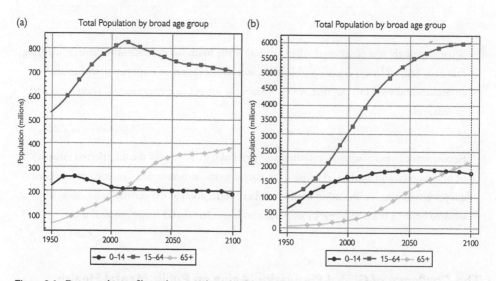

Figure 9.1. Demographic profiles with expected trends of demographic shifts in the 65+/14– ratio in (a) the more developed world regions and in (b) the less developed regions until year 2100 (data from UN *World Population Prospects 2017*, https://esa.un.org/unpd/wpp/; see text for the included regions).

or infirmity. Reflecting this definition, the first motto of the Gerontological Society of America (GSA) in 1946 emphasized "adding life to years, not just more years to life." Thus, maintaining physical and mental functioning and maintaining socioemotional well-being have been considered together as important criteria for successful aging (Baltes & Baltes, 1993; Nyberg & Pudas, 2019; Rowe & Kahn, 1987). The 40-year gain in human physical longevity over the past 150 years is indeed very impressive; however, with the rapid global increase of aging populations, many challenges in terms of maintaining cognitive function, socioemotional well-being, and mental health in general of the elderly populations still lie ahead.

In particular, senile dementia—the decline in mental ability that affects memory, attention, and thinking and problem-solving skills—is a very prominent public mental health concern that has a large socioeconomic impact (the current estimated cost by the WHO is US$818 billion per year). Since dementia is an age-related mental health issue that is associated with neurodegeneration and has a clear increase in prevalence from single- to double-digit percentages in the age range of 80 to 84 years (see data by Prince et al., 2013, replotted in Figure 9.2; Ritchie & Kildea, 1995), the anticipated rapid increase of persons aged 60 and older also predicts a substantial global increase in older populations living with dementia. About 35.6 million people lived with dementia worldwide in 2010, and the numbers are expected to double almost every 20 years, reaching 65.7 million in 2030 and 115.4 million in 2050. Furthermore, the issue is exacerbated in low- and middle-income countries (Prince et al., 2013).

In addition to the need to conduct medical research on treatments and therapies for dementia, the rapid growth of aging populations worldwide calls for more concerted research. Investigations into biocultural co-constructive mechanisms of brain plasticity in old age (e.g., Li, 2003) may provide the global aging populations suitable environmental

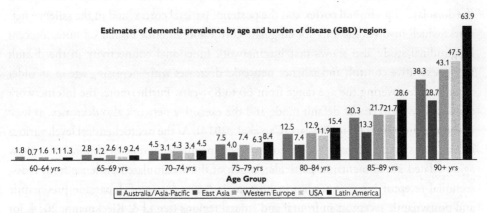

Figure 9.2. Estimates of dementia prevalence by age group and by global burden of disease (GBD) regions (figure plotted based on data from Prince et al. 2013; numbers in million, see text for details).

niches (cf. Clark, 2001; Laland et al., 2000) with the necessary sociocultural affordances to utilize their developmental reserve capacity (Baltes, 1987) to maintain cognitive functions and socioemotional well-being. The following sections review neurocognitive declines during usual aging as well as recent findings on cognitive and brain plasticity in old age, focusing primarily on the effects of cognitive and physical fitness interventions. The effects of lifestyle dietary and social participation factors are briefly highlighted.

The Aging of Brain and Mind

The processes of aging take a toll on the brain at multiple levels (see Jagust & D'Esposito, 2009, for review). At the anatomical level, the structural integrity of various brain regions declines substantially across the adult lifespan (see Fjell & Walhovd, 2010; Raz et al., 2010, for overviews), with the most apparent brain volume shrinkages in several regions (i.e., the frontal and temporal cortex as well as the caudate nucleus and putamen) of the fronto-hippocampal-striatal circuitries (Raz et al., 2010; see Figure 9.3). Aging also affects the structural and functional connectivity between brain regions (see Damoiseaux, 2017, for review). In terms of structural connectivity, other than declines in the integrity of microstructures (Burzynska et al., 2010; Damoiseaux et al., 2009), studies examining structural connectivity networks revealed negative age differences in the efficiency of white matter connections, particularly in the prefrontal and temporal cortices (Zhao et al., 2015). As for functional connectivity, the empirical evidence from cross-sectional functional brain imaging studies consistently shows that during the non-task-related state (commonly known as "resting state"), older adults show lower coherence between temporal fluctuations in the blood oxygen level-dependent (BOLD) signals across brain regions, notably in a network involving the medial prefrontal cortex, lateral parietal cortex, posterior cingulate cortex, and precuneus, which is usually referred to as the default mode network (e.g., Andrews-Hanna et al., 2007; Dennis & Thompson, 2014). Aging also affects the functional connectivity in the executive control network, which encompasses the dorsolateral prefrontal cortex and the posterior parietal cortex, and in the salience network, which involves the anterior cingulate cortex and anterior insula. Of note, a recent longitudinal study also shows that intranetwork functional connectivity in the default mode, executive control, and salience networks decreases with increasing age in an older adult sample covering the age range from 60 to 85 years. Furthermore, the internetwork connectivity between the default mode and the executive network also decreases, at least in the age range from 60 to 70 years (Cao et al., 2014). At the neurochemical level, various transmitter systems (dopamine, serotonin, norepinephrine, and acetylcholine) also show aging-related impairments; in particular, much of the accumulated evidence from cross-sectional receptor imaging studies in humans indicates losses of dopamine presynaptic and postsynaptic receptors in frontal and striatal regions (see Li & Rieckmann, 2014, for review). Moreover, recent research has also started to focus on compromised integrity of the locus coeruleus, which consequently alters noradrenalinergic modulation of cognition and emotion in old age (Hämmerer et al., 2018; Mather & Harley, 2016).

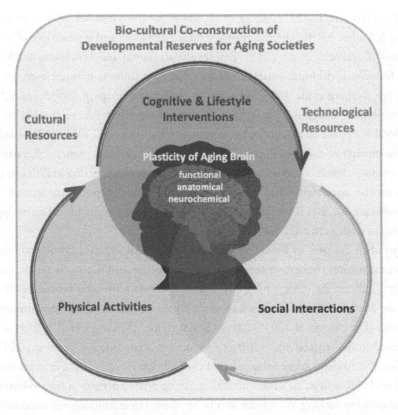

Figure 9.3. Conceptual framework of sociocultural and technological resources channeled through cognitive and physical fitness, lifestyle, as well as social network interventions for co-constructing developmental reserve capacity in old age.

Brain aging at the different levels contributes to gradual declines of multiple basic mental functions in old age: in particular, deficits in attention, executive control, working memory, and episodic memory (see Cabeza et al., 2017, for an overview). Here a few selected links between the aging of the brain and multiple facets of the mind are highlighted. Higher-order cognitive functions that implicate multiple brain regions and the speed of information processing may depend particularly on the structural and functional connectivity between brain regions. Indeed, a recent longitudinal study showed that a substantial amount of change in executive control function (as measured by the Stroop task) over a 3-year period can be accounted for by changes in structural connectivity, particularly changes in micro- and macrostructural connectivity (Fjell et al., 2016). Furthermore, compared to young adults, functional connectivity between the dorsal lateral prefrontal cortex and the right parietal cortex during working memory was compromised in older adults (Rieckmann et al., 2011). Relatedly, aging-related functional changes in the frontal-parietal attentional network are also known to underlie older adults' deficits in top-down attentional control processes, be it in the visual (e.g., Gazzaley et al., 2007; Madden, 2007; Störmer et al., 2013) or auditory domains (e.g., Passow et al., 2014). Episodic memory impairment is another key limitation of older people's mental abilities (e.g., Fandakova et al., 2014; Shing et al., 2008; for overviews see Nyberg et al., 2012; Nyberg & Pudas, 2019), which plays a key role in dementia and is predictive of its clinical diagnosis (Boraxbekk et al., 2015). Besides the structural and functional brain changes in the fronto-hippocampal-striatal circuitries that contribute to episodic memory deficits in old age (Nyberg et al., 2012), findings from receptor imaging (Nyberg et al., 2016), pharmacological imaging (Chowdhury, Guitart-Masip, Bunzeck, et al., 2012), genetic behavioral (Li et al., 2013), and neurocomputational (Li et al., 2001, 2005) studies also point to impacts of deficient dopamine modulation on episodic memory. Related to episodic memory deficit is the impaired spatial learning and navigation abilities in old age, which are also associated with functional alterations in the hippocampal-striatal network (e.g., Schuck et al., 2015; see Lester et al., 2017, for review) and with deficient dopamine modulation of this circuitry (Thurm et al., 2016).

Other than declines in basic cognitive functions, anatomical, network connectional, and neurochemical changes in the aging brain's affective and motivational circuities also have implications for older adults' decision making and affective processing (for overviews see Mather, 2016; Samanez-Larkin & Knutson, 2015). Underrecruitment of the prefrontal (Eppinger et al., 2015) and striatal activities (Eppinger et al., 2013) as well as attenuated frontal-striatal white matter connectivity (Samanez-Larkin et al., 2012) have been found to underlie older adults' altered choice behavior in utilizing information about reward probability to guide decision making. Aging-related deficits in reward-based learning and decision making in part can also be attributed to attenuated neuromodulation of the aging brain, as illustrated in a pharmacological imaging study showing that administering dopamine precursor restored striatal brain activity and improved older adults' reward-based decision making (Chowdhury et al., 2013b). As for socioemotional processing, whereas the cognitive route of the social mind involving mechanisms of theory of mind and metacognition are impaired in old age, the affective route entailing empathy and compassion seems to be relatively preserved (e.g., Reiter et al., 2017; Richter & Kunzmann, 2011). Such findings at the behavioral level parallel well with evidence showing that core brain regions for affective response and valuation (i.e., the amygdala and ventromedial prefrontal cortex) are less affected by aging relative to other brain regions both structurally and functionally (see Mather, 2016, for review). Nevertheless, affective regulation of cognition is affected by aging; in particular, negatively valenced arousal or saliency effects on perception (Lee et al., 2018) and memory (Hämmerer et al., 2018) have been observed and linked to aging-related decline of the locus coeruleus noradrenergic system.

Biocultural Co-Construction of Developmental Plasticity

Developmental processes are inherently "plastic," malleable by experiences and learning. The meta-theoretical framework of biocultural co-construction of developmental plasticity (Li, 2003) highlights interlinked interactions between plasticity across multiple levels (i.e., genetic expressions, neuronal activity, behaviors, and social and cultural processes) during individual lifespan development. Viewed through the lens of this framework, the effects of socioculturally embedded individual experiences that are channeled through cognitive and lifestyle interventions, physical activities, and social interactions on neurocognitive mechanisms of the mind are brought to the foreground (Figure 9.3). In the context of global aging—the multiple levels and facets of neurocognitive aging notwithstanding—the aging human brain, though having more limited developmental reserve than in other life periods (Baltes 1987, 1997), still possesses a certain extent of reserved plasticity at multiple levels (see Li, 2003; Lindenberger et al., 2014; Lövdén et al., 2010, for a variety of concepts along with reviews of empirical findings). The aging brain's reserved plasticity could potentially be mobilized through culturally embedded resources including technology (Murphie & Potts, 2003; Potts, 2015) to support mental functions and well-being in old age. This section selectively highlights evidence that suggests that cultural neuroscience research into biocultural co-constructive processes at the neurochemical, anatomical, and functional levels might open further possibilities besides medical therapeutic approaches for addressing mental health concerns associated with global aging in the 21st century.

Co-Construction of Plasticity Through Cognitive Interventions

Since early research on episodic memory plasticity during adult development (Baltes & Kliegl, 1992), it has been known that although memory plasticity is much more limited in old age relative to young adulthood, older people still could improve their episodic memory performance substantially (Figure 9.4a) after an intensive memory training using a mnemonic (the method of loci) known since ancient Greek times (Bower, 1970; Yates, 1966). The neurocomputational theory of neurocognitive aging (Li et al., 2001) accounts for the negative age differences in memory plasticity at the behavioral level by simulating attenuated neuromodulatory gain control of information processing, mimicking the aging brain's deficient neurotransmitter systems (see Figure 9.4a). Evidence from a functional brain imaging study, which investigated the effect of a cognitive intervention on episodic memory, shows that mnemonic training enhanced functional brain activities in the frontal and parietal regions in young adults. In older adults, however, a training-induced increase in functional brain activity was only observed in the parietal region and only in those older individuals whose memory benefited from the cognitive intervention (Nyberg et al., 2003; see Figure 9.4b).

Beyond episodic memory, older adults' working memory and executive control functions could also benefit from process-based cognitive interventions. Unlike episodic memory, negative adult age differences in the extent of working memory plasticity are less apparent (see Karbach & Verhaeghen, 2014, for a meta-analysis). For instance, a cognitive intervention study that trained the storage and updating aspects of spatial working memory in young (20 to 30 years) and older (70 to 80 years) adults across 45 daily training sessions showed that plasticity (reflected in the effect sizes of training gain) was not less in older adults. After training, older adults could perform at young adults' baseline

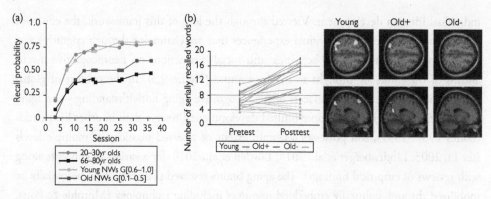

Figure 9.4. Effects of cognitive interventions on (a) empirical and neural network (NW) simulated episodic memory performance (figures adapted from Baltes & Kliegl, Copyright 1992 APA and Li et al., Copyright 2001 Elsevier with permissions) and (b) brain activity (figures adapted from Nyberg et al. with permission, Copyright 2003 the National Academy of Sciences, USA).

levels in terms of both accuracy and speed (see Figure 9.5a; Li et al., 2008). A functional brain imaging study of spatial working memory training in older adults (60 to 70 years) across 5 weeks (Brehmer et al., 2011) showed that concomitant with the performance improvement was increased efficiency of the frontohippocampal attention-memory network as reflected in training-related decreases of task-related activations in various regions of this network. Furthermore, memory improvement was associated with training-related increases in striatal brain activity. Together these findings suggest that cognitive interventions influence the underlying frontal-hippocampal-striatal brain networks in complex manners.

Dopamine modulations of cognitive processes (e.g., cognitive control, working memory, episodic memory, and reward processing) that are subserved by the frontal-hippocampal-striatal circuitries are well established based on accumulated empirical evidence from animal research (see Arnsten et al., 2015; Lisman & Grace, 2015; Schultz, 2013, for reviews). Thus, it is of particular relevance whether the effects of socioculturally embedded cognitive interventions may also impact neuromodulation, beyond behavior performance, brain structural, and functional integrities. Of note, evidence from a receptor imaging study showed that spatial working memory training that lasted for 5 weeks improved spatial working memory of young adults and, at the same time, increased dopamine release in various brain regions in the frontoparietal network. Individuals whose working memory performance benefited more from the training also showed more training-related dopamine release in the right ventral frontal cortex, for instance (see Figure 9.5b; McNab et al., 2009). This finding has been extended in two further receptor imaging studies of working memory training, which showed training-related increases of dopamine release in striatal regions (Bäckman et al., 2011, 2017). Age-related differences in these effects might play a role in an aging-related restriction in transferring working memory intervention effects to other tasks that share similar cognitive processes (Dahlin et al., 2008).

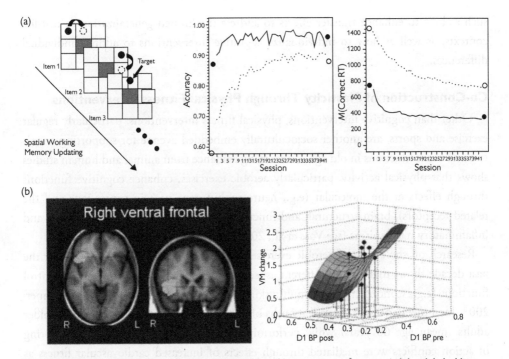

Figure 9.5. Effects of cognitive interventions on (a) spatial working memory performance (solid and dashed lines indicate younger and older adults, respectively; figures adapted from Li et al., Copyright 2008 APA with permission) and (b) brain dopamine release in right ventral frontal region as reflected in dopamine D1 receptor-binding potential (figures adapted from McNab et al. with permission, Copyright 2009 American Association for the Advancement of Science).

Taken together, cognitive interventions seem to be viable socioculturally embedded resources for supporting and maintaining mental functions of the increasing populations of older adults worldwide. However, it needs to be underscored that although current intervention approaches on cognitive and brain functions do induce training-related gains on the trained processes, training benefits usually do not transfer to untrained tasks and mostly do not generalize to real-life contexts (see Simons et al., 2016). Furthermore, individual differences in training effects are substantial (e.g., see Figure 9.3 for positive and no-training effects in two groups of older adults; Nyberg et al., 2003). Regarding brain correlates of individual differences in training gains, the integrity of brain white matter microstructure as measured by mean diffusivity has been shown to be associated with episodic memory plasticity in older adults (aged 68 to 82 years), with individuals who showed higher levels of white matter diffusivity in a widespread region (involving the anterior corpus callosum, the left anterior thalamic radiation, and the right inferior fronto-occipital fasciculus) benefiting less from memory training (de Lange et al., 2016). Furthermore, it has been shown that aging-related reduction in frontoparietal functional connectivity during working memory is related to individual differences in dopamine binding (Rieckmann et al., 2011). Future research still needs to address open questions, such as how to enhance transfer effects to address the limited generalization to real-life contexts, as well as how to individualize cognitive interventions to address individual differences.

Co-Construction of Plasticity Through Physical Fitness Interventions

Other than cognitive interventions, physical fitness interventions, particularly regular exercise and sports, are another socioculturally embedded avenue for supporting cognitive and brain functions in old age. Converging evidence from animal and human studies shows that physical activity, particularly aerobic exercises, enhance cognitive functions through effects at the molecular (e.g., neurotrophin gene protein expressions and the related receptors), brain structural, and functional levels, as well as body metabolic and inflammatory mechanisms (see Voss et al., 2013, for review).

Research on the effects of aerobic exercises on human neurocognitive aging over the past decade shows that among different aspects of cognitive functions, executive control functions (e.g., working memory, multitasking) benefit most (see Colcombe & Kramer, 2003, for a meta-analysis). After 6 months of aerobic exercise, cognitive benefits in older adults (mean age 66 years) while performing a task requiring top-down monitoring of action conflicts were mediated through effects of increased cardiovascular fitness as indexed by maximum oxygen uptake and increased task-related functional brain activations in the attention-memory network, including the medial frontal gyrus, and reduced activity in the anterior cingulate cortex, which is known to underlie conflict monitoring (Colcombe et al., 2004). In addition to benefits on cognitive control processes, aerobic exercises have also been observed to have benefits on episodic memory. Compared to older adults (mean age 68 years) in a control group doing muscle stretching exercises, older adults in the aerobic exercise group showed increased hippocampal volume after 1 year of fitness training. The aerobic exercise-related increase in hippocampal volume effectively reduces the aging-related structural loss by 1 to 2 years (Figure 9.6a; Erickson et al., 2011). Furthermore, the increased hippocampal volume is associated with higher levels of cardiovascular fitness (Figure 9.6b), serum levels of brain-derived neurotrophic factor (BDNF; Figure 9.6c), and episodic memory (Figure 9.6d). Also of relevance here, other than results from randomized controlled studies of physical fitness interventions, self-reported daily physical activity levels have also been found to be associated with brain structural integrity, particularly gray matter volumes in the frontal (e.g., Flöel et al., 2010) and hippocampal regions (Brown et al., 2012). Moreover, a very recent study showed that the intensity of self-rated habitual physical activities (walking, bicycling, jogging, strength training, and other sports) in older adults (64 to 68 years) is positively associated with higher levels of not only working memory and episodic memory but also dopamine (D2/D3) availability in the caudate (a region in the striatum), suggesting that striatal dopamine modulation may underlie the beneficial effects of physical activities on memory performance (Köhncke et al., 2018). Taken together, existing evidence suggests that physical

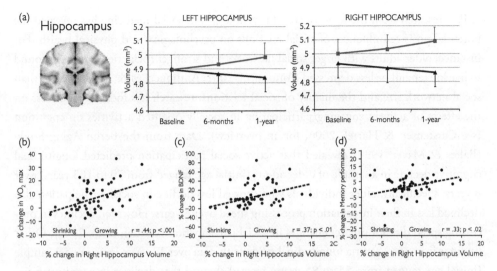

Figure 9.6. Effects of physical fitness interventions on (a) hippocampal volume and the relations between aerobic exercise-related increases in hippocampal volume and (b) cardiovascular fitness as indexed by maximal oxygen uptake, (c) serum level of brain-derived neurotrophic factor, and (d) episodic memory (figures adapted from Erickson et al. with permission, Copyright 2011 the National Academy of Sciences, USA).

exercises have moderate effects on cognition and brain functions at multiple levels. Future research on how to combine physical fitness with other types of interventions to further enhance intervention benefits on mental functioning in old age is important.

Co-Construction of Plasticity Through Lifestyle Interventions and Social Interactions

Although most past intervention research on neurocognitive aging has mainly focused on cognitive and physical fitness interventions, other lines of research have also investigated potential effects of other lifestyle interventions, such as dietary styles and social participation, on cognitive functions in old age. Regarding dietary interventions, the impacts of micronutrients (e.g., zinc, insulin sensitizers), which are important for anti-oxidative effects; flavonoids (found in a variety of fruits and vegetables), which are relevant for synaptic plasticity; omega-3 polyunsaturated fatty acids, which are relevant for anti-inflammatory mechanisms; calorie restriction; and a wide range of other factors have been explored (see Vauzour et al., 2017, for a recent review). To highlight just the effect of dietary L-tyrosine that is converted into the precursor of dopamine (L-Dopa) here, a recent study showed that higher levels of habitual dietary intake of tyrosine was associated with better performance in a variety of cognitive functions, including working memory, episodic memory, and fluid intelligence. Furthermore, the effect was similar for both young and older adults (Kühn et al., 2017). However, in general, current findings about the potential protective effects of the various dietary interventions on neurocognitive aging are still rather inconsistent and fragmented, awaiting further future research.

Past research from the areas of social psychology and social medicine has revealed the potential positive influences of social relations on psychological and physical health. For instance, older adults with larger social networks and stronger social ties have been found to live longer and be less depressed (Antonucci, 2001; Antonucci et al., 1997). Other than social network size and the quality of social relations, research has focused much less on the effects of actively engaging/participating in socially oriented activities on cognition (see Carstensen & Hartel, 2006, for an overview). Data from the Berlin Aging Study (Baltes & Mayer, 1999) revealed that active social participation predicted longitudinal cognitive decline in a sample of older adults (initial age ranged from 70 to 103 years) over 8 years: specifically, older individuals who showed less decline in social participation also declined less in their information processing speed over 8 years. However, declines in processing speed did not predict changes in social participation (Lövdén et al., 2005). Other findings from the Victoria longitudinal study with data over 12 years in a younger sample (initial age ranged from 55 to 85 years) instead showed that declines in cognitive functions predicted declines in social activities (Small et al., 2012). Differences between the ages of the samples as well as measures of social engagement/activity may have contributed to the discrepancies between these two studies. Nevertheless, findings from both studies reveal the intricate dynamic bidirectional relations between staying socially engaged and staying cognitively fit.

Summary and Outlook

The rapidly increasing populations worldwide of people older than 60 years raise big challenges for global mental health. Dementia is an age-related neurodegenerative disorder; its prevalence rate increases drastically after the age of 85. Although usual aging is accompanied by declines in various mental abilities (i.e., attention, executive control, working memory, and episodic memory) even before the onset of dementia, the aging brain still has a certain extent of plasticity at multiple levels that can be mobilized through sociocultural and technological supports.

Existing evidence from neurocognitive research investigating the effects of cognitive, physical fitness, and lifestyle interventions in maintaining cognitive functions, and thus delaying declines of mental abilities, in old age suggests that biocultural co-constructive processes at the neurochemical, anatomical, and functional levels may offer additional possibilities, besides medical therapies, for the global mental health challenges of aging societies. However, the effects of current cognitive interventions are limited, particularly regarding effects that can generalize to real-life benefits. The effects of lifestyle interventions, including dietary supplements and social engagements, are still rather inconsistent. Further research needs, on the one hand, to better understand how intervention effects on multiple levels of brain mechanisms are related to each other and, on the other hand, to systematically develop individualized, composite intervention approaches that combine cognitive, physical fitness, and lifestyle interventions.

Furthermore, biocultural co-constructive processes need to expand and broaden the bases of cultural resources by incorporating new technological developments to support the different types of interventions for aging societies. Culture and technology interact reciprocally; culture shapes societal and technological developments, and technology drives societal and cultural changes (Murphie & Potts, 2003). For instance, although game-based (e.g., Anguera et al., 2013) and/or app-based training bring lab-based cognitive interventions one step closer to real-life contexts, current game-based virtual reality setups are still limited in terms of adaptive, multimodal sensory feedback. To this end, research on age-related differences in the psychophysical principles of multisensory perception (Li et al., 2021), together with breakthroughs in developing new, wearable sensors and softwarized telecommunication networks (e.g., Braun et al., 2017) that allow remote access, manipulation, and control of real and virtual objects and processes (i.e., tactile internet, IEEE P19181: Tactile Internet Standardization Group, http://ti.committees. comsoc.org/), seems promising. In particular, this new line of transdisciplinary research (see Fitzek et al., 2021 for review) might open new possibilities for more flexibly realizing composite intervention approaches in a broader range of virtual reality environments, which hopefully could increase the real-life benefits of interventions.

References

Andrews-Hanna, J. R., Synder, A. Z., Vincent, J. L., Lustig, C., Head, D., Raichle, M. E., & Buckner, R. (2007). Disruption of large-scale brain systems in advanced aging. *Neuron, 56*, 924–935.

Anguera, J. A., Boccanfuso, J., Rintoul, J. L., Al-Hashimi, O., Faraji, F., Janowich, J., Kong, E., Larraburo, Y., Rolle, C., Johnston, E., & Gazaley, A. (2013). Video game training enhances cognitive control in older adults. *Nature, 501*, 97–101.

Antonucci, T. C. (2001). Social relations. In J. E. Birren & K. W. Schaie (Eds.), *Handbook of the psychology of aging* (pp. 427–453). Academic Press.

Antonucci, T. C., Fuhrer, R., & Dartigues, J. F. (1997). Social relations and depressive symptomatology in a sample of community-dwelling French older adults. *Psychology and Aging, 12*, 189–195.

Arnsten, A. F. T., Wang, M., & Paspalas, C. D. (2015). Dopamine's actions in primate prefrontal cortex challenges for treating cognitive disorders. *Pharmacological Reviews, 67*, 681–696.

Baltes, P. B. (1987). Theoretical propositions of life-span developmental psychology—On the dynamics between growth and decline. *Developmental Psychology, 23*, 611–626.

Baltes, P. B. (1997). On the incomplete architecture of human ontogeny: Selection, optimization and compensation as foundation of developmental theory. *American Psychologist, 4*, 366–380.

Baltes, P. B., & Baltes, M. M. (Eds.). (1993). *Successful aging: Perspectives from the behavioral sciences.* Cambridge University Press.

Baltes, P. B., & Kliegl, R. (1992). Further testing of limits of cognitive plasticity: Negative age differences in mnemonic skill are robust. *Developmental Psychology, 28*, 121–125.

Baltes, P. B., & Mayer, K. U. (Eds.). (1999). *The Berlin Aging Study.* Cambridge University Press.

Baltes, P. B., Rösler, F., & Reuter-Lorenz, P. A. (Eds.). (2006). *Lifespan development and the brain: The perspective of biocultural co-construction.* Cambridge University Press.

Bäckman, L., Karlsson, S., Fischer, H., Karlsson, P., Brehmer, Y., Rieckmann, A., MacDonald, S. W. S., Farde, L., & Nyberg, L. (2011). Dopamine D1 receptors and age differences in brain activation during working memory. *Neurobiology of Aging, 32*, 1849–1856.

Bäckman, L., Waris, O., Johansson, J., Anderson, M., Rinne, J. Alakrutti, K., Soveri, A., Laine, M., & Nyberg, L. (2017). Increased dopamine release after working-memory updating training: Neurochemical correlates of transfer. *Scientific Reports, 7*(7160), 1–10.

Boraxbekk, C.-J., Lundquist, A., Nordin, A., Nyberg, L., Nilsson, L.-G., & Adolfsson, R. (2015). Free recall episodic memory performance predicts dementia ten years prior to clinical diagnosis: Findings from the Betula longitudinal study. *Dementia and Geriatric Cognitive Disorders Extra, 5,* 191–202.

Bower, G. H. (1970). Analysis of a mnemonic device: Modern psychology uncovers the powerful components of an ancient system for improving memory. *American Scientist, 58,* 496–510.

Braun, P. J., Pandi, S., Schmoll, R.-S., & Fitzek, Frank, H. P. (2017). On the study of deployment of mobile edge cloud for tactile internet using a 5G gaming application. *In 2017 14th IEEE Annual Consumer Communications & Networking Conference (CCNC)* (pp. 154–159). IEEE.

Brehmer, Y., Rieckmann, A., Bellander, M., Westerberg, H., Fischer, H., & Bäckman, L. (2011). Neural correlates of training-related working-memory gains in old age. *NeuroImage, 58,* 1110–1120.

Brown, B. M., Peiffer, J. J., Sohrabi, H. R., Mondal, A., Gupta, V. B., Rainey-Smith, S. R., et al. (2012). Intense physical activity is associated with cognitive performance in the elderly. *Translational Psychiatry, 2,* e191.

Burzynska, A. Z., Preuschhof, C., Bäckman, L., Nyberg, L., Li, S.-C., Lindenberger, U., & Hekeren, H. R. (2010). Age-related differences in white matter microstructure: Region-specific patterns of diffusivity. *NeuroImage, 40,* 2104–2112.

Cabeza, R., Nyberg, L., & Park, D. C. (Eds.). (2017). *Cognitive neuroscience of aging: linking cognitive and cerebral aging* (2nd Ed.). Oxford University Press.

Cao, M., Wang, J.-H., Dai, Z.-J., Cao, X.-Y., Jiang, L.-L., & Fan, F.-M. (2014). Topological organization of the human functional connectome across the lifespan. *Developmental Cognitive Neuroscience, 7,* 76–93.

Carstensen, L. L., & Hartel, C. R. (Eds.). (2006). *When I'm 64.* National Academies Press.

Chowdhury, R., Guitart-Masip, M., Bunzeck, N., Dolan, R., & Düzel, E. (2013a). Dopamine modulates episodic memory persistence in old age. *Journal of Neuroscience, 32,* 14193–14204.

Chowdhury, R., Guitart-Masip, M., Lambert, C., Dayan, P., Huys, Q., Düzel, E., & Dolan, R. (2013bb). Dopamine restores reward prediction errors in old age. *Nature Neuroscience, 16,* 648–653.

Clark, A. (1999). Where brain, body, and world collide. *Journal of Cognitive Systems Research, 1,* 5–17.

Colcombe, S. J., & Kramer, A. F. (2003). Fitness effects on the cognitive function of older adults: A meta-analytic study. *Psychological Science, 14,* 125–130.

Colcombe, S. J., Kramer, A. F., Erickson, K. I., Scalf, P., McAuley, E., Cohen, N. J., Webb, A., Jerome, G. J., Marquez, D. X., & Elavsky, S. (2004). Cardiovascular fitness, cortical plasticity, and aging. *Proceedings of the National Academy of Sciences USA, 101,* 3316–3321.

Dahlin, E., Neely, A. S., Larsson, A., Bäckman, L., & Nyberg, L. (2008). Transfer of learning after updating training mediated by the striatum. *Science, 320,* 1510–1512.

Damoiseaux, J. S. (2017). Effects of aging on functional and structural connectivity. *NeuroImage, 160,* 32–40.

Damoiseaux, J. S., Smith, S. M., Witter, M. P., Sanz-Arigita, E. J., Barkhof, F., Scheltens, P., Stam, C. J., Zarei, M., & Rombouts, S. A. R. B. (2009). White matter tract integrity in aging and Alzheimer's disease. *Human Brain Mapping, 30,* 1051–1059.

Dennis, E. L., & Thompson, P. M. (2014). Functional brain connectivity using fMRI in aging and Alzheimer's disease. *Neuropsychological Review, 24,* 49–62.

Eppinger, B., Heekeren, H. R., & Li, S.-C. (2015). Age-related prefrontal impairments implicate deficient prediction of future rewards in older adults. *Neurobiology of Aging, 36,* 2380–2390.

Eppinger, B., Schuck, N. W., Nystrom, L. E., & Cohen, J. D. (2013). Reduced striatal responses to reward prediction errors in older compared with younger adults. *Journal of Neuroscience, 33,* 9905–9912.

Fandakova, Y., Lindenberger, U., & Shing, Y. L. (2014). Deficits in process-specific prefrontal and hippocampal activations contribute to adult age differences in episodic memory interference. *Cerebral Cortex, 24,* 1832–1844.

Fitzek, F. H. P., Li, S.-C., Speidel, S., Strufe, T., Simsek, M., & Reisslein, M. (Eds.) (2021). Tactile internet with human-in-the-loop (1st Ed.). New York: Academic Press.

Fjell, A. M., & Walhovd, K. B. (2010). Structural brain changes in aging: Courses, causes and cognitive consequences. *Reviews in Neuroscience, 21,* 187–221.

Fjell, A. M., Sneve, M. H., Grydeland, H., Storsve, A. B., & Walhovd, K. B. (2016). The disconnected brain and executive function decline in aging. *Cerebral Cortex, 27,* 2303–2317.

Flöel, A., Ruscheweyh, R., Kruger, K., Willemer, C., Winter, B., Volker, K., Lohmann, H., Zitzmann, M., Mooren, F., Breitenstein, C., & Knecht, S. (2010). Physical activity and memory functions: Are neurotrophins and cerebral gray matter volume the missing link? *NeuroImage, 49,* 2756–2763.

Erickson, K. J., Voss, M., Prakash, R., Basak, C., Szabo, A., Chaddock, I., Kim, J., Heo, S., Alves, H., White, S.M., Wojcicki, T. R., Mailey, M., Vieira, V. J., Martin, S. A., Pence, B. D., Woods, J. A., McAuley, E., & Kramer, A. F. (2011). Exercise training increases size of hippocampus and improves memory. *Proceedings of the National Academy of Sciences USA, 108*, 3017–3022.

Gazzaley, A., Rissman, J., Conney, J., Rutman, A., Seibert, T., Clapp, W., & D'Esposito, M. (2007). Functional interactions between prefrontal and visual association cortex contribute to top-down modulation of visual processing. *Cerebral Cortex, 17*, i125–i135.

Harper, S. (2014). Economic and social implications of aging societies. *Science, 346*, 587–591.

Hämmerer, D., Callaghan, M. F., Hopkins, A., Kosciessa, J., Betts, M., Cardenas-Blanco, A., Kanowski, M., Weiskopf, N., Dayan, P., Dolan, R. J. & Düzel, E. (2018). Locus coeruleus integrity in old age is selectively related to memories linked to salient negative events. *Proceedings of the National Academy of Sciences USA, 115*, 2228–2233.

Jagust, W., & D'Espositio, M. (Eds.). (2009). *Imaging the aging brain.* Oxford University Press.

Karbach, J., & Verhaeghen, P. (2014). Making working memory work: A meta-analysis of executive control and working memory training in younger and older adults. *Psychological Science, 25*, 2027–2037.

Köhncke, Y., Papenberg, G., Jonasson, L., Karalija, N., Wåhlin, A., Salami, Andersson, M., Axelsson, E., Nyberg, L., Riklund, K., Bäckman, L., Lindenberger, U., & Lövdén, M. (2018). Self-rated intensity of habitual physical activities is positively related with dopamine $D_{2/3}$ receptor availability and cognition. *NeuroImage, 181*, 605–616.

Kühn, S., Düzel, S., Colzato, L., Norman, K., Gallinat, J., Brandmaier, A. M., Lindenberger, U., & Widaman, K. F. (2017). Food for thought: Association between dietary tyrosine and cognitive performance in younger and older adults. *Psychological Research.* Published online December 2017. https://doi.org/10.1007/s00426-017-0957-4

Laland, K. N., Odling-Smee, J., & Feldman, M. W. (2000). Niche construction, biological evolution, and cultural change. *Behavioral and brain sciences, 23*(1), 131–146.

Lee, T.-H., Greening, S. G., Ueno, T., Clewett, D., Ponzio, A., Sakaki, M., & Mather, M. (2018). Arousal increases neural gain via the locus coeruleus-norepinephrine system in younger adults but not in older adults. *Nature Human Behavior, 2*, 356–366.

Lester, A. W., Moffat, S. D., Wiener, J. M., Barnes, C. A., & Wolbers, T. (2017). The aging navigational system. *Neuron, 95*, 1019–1035.

de Lange, A.-M. G., Bråthen, A. C. S., Grydeland, H., Sexton, C., Johansen-Berg, H., Andersson, J. L. R., et al. (2016). White matter integrity as a marker for cognitive plasticity in aging. *Neurobiology of Aging, 47*, 74–82.

Li, S.-C. (2003). Biocultural orchestration of developmental plasticity across levels: The interplay of biology and culture in shaping the mind and behavior across the life span. *Psychological Bulletin, 129*, 171–194.

Li, S.-C., Lindenberger, U., & Sikström, S. (2001). Aging cognition: From neuromodulation to representation. *Trends in Cognitive Sciences, 5*, 479–486.

Li, S.-C., Muschter, E., Limanowski, J., & Hatzipanayioti, A. (2021). Human perception and neurocognitive development across the lifespan. In F. H. P. Fitzek et al. (Eds.), Tactile internet with human-in-the-loop (pp. 203-227). New York: Academic Press.

Li, S.-C., Naveh-Benjamin, M., & Lindenberger, U. (2005). Aging neuromodulation impairs associative memory binding: Neurocomputational account. *Psychological Science, 16*, 445–450.

Li, S.-C., Papenberg, G., Nagel, I. E., Preuschhof, C., Schröder, J., Nietfeld, W., Bertram, L., Heekeren, H. R., Lindenberger, U., & Bäckman, L. (2013). Aging magnifies the effects of dopamine transporter and D2 receptor genes on backward serial memory. *Neurobiology of Aging, 34*, 358.e1–358.e10.

Li, S.-C. & Rieckmann, A. (2014). Neuromodulation and aging: implications of aging neuronal gain control on cognition. *Current Opinion in Neurobiology, 29*, 148–158.

Li, S.-C., Schmiedek, F., Huxhold, O., Röcke, C., Smith, J., & Lindenberger, U. (2008). Working memory plasticity in old age: Practice gain, transfer and maintenance. *Psychology and Aging, 23*, 731–742.

Lindenberger, U., Wenger, E., & Lövdén, M. (2014). Towards a stronger science of human plasticity. *Nature Reviews Neuroscience, 18*, 261–262.

Lisman, J. E., & Grace, A. A. (2015). The hippocampal-VTA loop: Controlling the entry of information into long-term memory. *Neuron, 46*, 703–713.

Lövdén, M., Bäckman, L., Riklund, L., Lindenberger, U., & Schmiedek, F. (2010). A theoretical framework for the study of adult cognitive plasticity. *Psychological Bulletin, 136*, 659–676.

Lövdén, M., Ghisletta, P., & Lindenberger, U. (2005). Social participation attenuates decline in perceptual speed in old and very old age. *Psychology and Aging, 20*, 423–434.

Madden, D. J. (2007). Aging and visual attention. *Current Directions in Psychological Science, 16*, 70–74.

Mather, M. (2016). The affective neuroscience of aging. *Annual Review of Psychology, 67*, 213–238.

Mather, M., & Harley, C. W. (2016). The locus coeruleus: Essential for maintaining cognitive function and the aging brain. *Trends in Cognitive Sciences, 20*, 214–226.

McNab, F., Varrone, A., Farde, L., Jucaite, A., Bystritsky, P. Forssberg, H., & Klingberg, T. (2009). Changes in cortical dopamine D1 receptor binding associated with cognitive training. *Science, 323*, 800–802.

Murphie, A., & Potts, J. (2003). *Culture and technology*. Palgrave Macmillan.

Nyberg, L., Sandblom, J., Jones, S., Neely, A. S., Petersson, K. M. Ingvar, M., & Bäckman, L. (2003). Neural correlates of training-related memory improvement in adulthood and aging. *Proceedings of the National Academy of Sciences USA, 100*, 13728–13733.

Nyberg, L., Lövdén, M., Riklund, K., Lindenberger, U., & Bäckman, L. (2012). Memory aging and brain maintenance. *Trends in Cognitive Sciences, 16*, 292–305.

Nyberg, L., Karalija, N., Salami, A., Andersson, M., Wåhlin, A., Kaboovand, N., Köhncke, Y., Axelsson, J., Rieckmann, A., Papenberg, G., Garrett, D. D., Riklund, K., Lövdén, M., Lindenberger, U., & Bäckman, L. (2016). Dopamine D2 receptor availability is linked to hippocampal-caudate functional connectivity and episodic memory. *Proceedings of National Academy of Sciences USA, 113*, 7918–7923.

Nyberg, L., & Pudas, S. (2019). Successful memory aging. *Annual Review of Psychology, 70*(3), 1–25.

Passow, S., Westerhausen, R., Hugdahl, K., Wartenburger, I., Heekeren, H. R., Lindenberger, U., & Li, S.-C. (2014). Electrophysiological correlates of adult age differences in attentional control of auditory processing. *Cerebral Cortex, 24*, 249–260.

Potts, J. (2015). *The new time and space*. Palgrave Macmillan.

Prince, M., Bryce, R., Albanese, E., Wimo, A., Ribeiro, W., & Ferri, C. P. (2013). The global prevalence of dementia: A systematic review and meta-analysis. *Alzheimer's & Dementia, 9*, 63–75.

Raz, N., Ghisletta, P., Rodrigue, K. M., Kennedy, K. M., & Lindenberger, U. (2010). Trajectories of brain aging in middle-aged and older adults: Regional and individual differences. *NeuroImage, 51*, 501–511.

Reiter, A., Kanske, P., Eppinger, B., & Li, S.-C. (2017). The aging of the social mind—Differential effects on components of social understanding. *Scientific Reports, 7*(11046), 1–8.

Rieckmann, A., Karlsson, S., Fischer, H., & Bäckman, L. (2011). Caudate dopamine D1 receptor density is associated with individual differences in frontoparietal connectivity during working memory. *Journal of Neuroscience, 31*, 14284–14290.

Richter, D., & Kunzmann, U. (2011). Age differences in three facets of empathy: Performance-based evidence. *Psychology and Aging, 26*, 60–70.

Ritchie, K., & Kildea, D. (1995). Is senile dementia "age-related" or "ageing-related—Evidence from metal-analysis of dementia prevalence in the oldest old. *The Lancet, 346*, 931–934.

Rowe, J. W., & Kahn, R. L. (1987). Human aging: Usual and successful. *Science, 237*, 143–149.

Samanez-Larkin, G. R., & Knutson, B. (2015). Decision making in the ageing brain: Changes in affective and motivational circuits. *Nature Reviews Neuroscience, 16*, 278–289.

Samanez-Larkin, G. R., Levens, S. M., Perry, L. M., Dougherty, R. F., & Knutson, B. (2012). Frontostriatal white matter integrity mediates adult age differences in probabilistic reward learning. *Journal of Neuroscience, 32*, 5333–5337.

Schuck, N. W., Doeller, C. F., Polk, T. A., Lindenberger, U., & Li, S.-C. (2015). Human aging alters the neural computation and representation of space. *NeuroImage, 117*, 141–150.

Schultz, W. (2013). Updating dopamine reward signals. *Current Opinion in Neurobiology, 23*, 229–238.

Shing, Y. L., Werkle-Bergner, M., Li, S.-C., & Lindenberger, U. (2008). Associative and strategic components of episodic memory: A life-span dissociation. *Journal of Experimental Psychology: General, 137*, 495–513.

Simons, D. J., Boot, W. R., Charness, N., Gathercole, S. E., Chabris, C. F., Hambrick, D. Z., & Stine-Morrow, E. A. L. (2016). Do "brain-training" programs work? *Psychological Science in the Public Interest, 17*, 103–186.

Small, B., Dixon, R. A., McArdle, J. J., & Grimm, K. J. (2012). Do changes in lifestyle engagement moderate cognitive decline in normal aging? Evidence from Victoria Longitudinal Study. *Neuropsychology, 26*, 144–155.

Störmer, V. S., Li, S.-C., Heekeren, H. R., & Lindenberger, U. (2013). Normal aging delays and compromises early multifocal visual attention during object tracking. *Journal of Cognitive Neuroscience, 25*, 188–202.

Thurm, F., Schuck, N. W., Fauser, M., Doeller, C. F., Stankevich, Y., Evens, R., Riedel, O., Storch, A., Lueken, U., & Li, S.-C. (2016). Dopamine modulation of spatial navigation memory in Parkinson's disease. *Neurobiology of Aging, 38*, 93–103.

United Nations, Department of Economics and Social Affairs, Population Division. (2017). *World population prospects: The 2017 revision.* Retrieved from https://esa.un.org/unpd/wpp/

Vauzour, D., Camprubi-Robles, M., Miquel-Kergoat, S., Andres-Lacueva, C., Bánáti, D., Barberger-Gateau, P., Bowman, G. L., Caberlotto, L., Clarke, R., Hogervorst, E., Kiliaan, A. J., Luca, U., Manach, C., Minihane, A.-M., Mitchell, E. S., Perneczky, R., Perry, H., Roussel, A, M., Schuermans, J., Sijben, J. (2017). Nutrition for the ageing brain: Towards evidence for an optimal diet. *Ageing Research Reviews, 35*, 222–240.

Voss, M. W., Vivar, C., Kramer, A. F., & van Praag, H. (2013). Bridging animal and human models of exercise-induced brain plasticity. *Trends in Cognitive Sciences, 17*, 525–544.

World Health Organization (WHO). (1946). Preamble to the constitution of WHO as adopted by the International Health Conference (New York, June 19–July 22, signed by the representatives of 61 states; WHO Official Records, no. 2, p. 100).

Yates, F. A. (1966). *The art of memory.* University of Chicago Press.

Zhao, T., Cao, M., Niu, H., Zuo, X.-N., Evans, A., He, Y., Dong, Q., & Shu, N. (2015). Age-related changes in the topological organization of the white matter structural connectome across the human lifespan. *Human Brain Mapping, 36*, 3777–3792.

Etiology of Mental Health Disorders

Culture and Emotion

Joan Y. Chiao, Yoko Mano, Dan J. Stein, *and* Norihiro Sadato

Abstract

Culture affects the processes of emotion across multilevel mechanisms. Culture influences distinct stages of emotion, from generation and recognition to experience and regulation of emotion. Theoretical approaches posit causal models of how culture influences mental constructs and neurobiological mechanisms of emotion. Methodological approaches in the study of culture and emotion illustrate the observational tools useful for the measurement of emotion across cultures. Empirical approaches include standard paradigms that allow researchers to test theoretical models of culture and emotion. This chapter examines theoretical, methodological, and empirical approaches in the study of how culture shapes mental constructs and neurobiological mechanisms of emotion. Implications of research on culture neuroscience of emotion for global mental health are discussed.

Key Words: cultural neuroscience, culture, emotion, population health disparities, global mental health

Introduction

The Grand Challenges in Global Mental Health Consortium has identified key priorities for the alleviation of mental, neurological, and substance abuse (MNS) disorders globally (Collins et al., 2011). Among the top challenges are to identify biomarkers of MNS disorders and their social and biological risk factors across the life course. Interactions of social context, genes, and the environment may affect the risk for and persistence of MNS disorders across cultural settings. The identification of cellular and molecular mechanisms in the brain provides important insight into the advancement of cures, preventions, and interventions in global mental health.

The World Health Organization (WHO) Global Burden of Disease (GBD) Study estimates that MNS disorders are considered among the highest-ranked diseases in the world (Kessler & Ustun, 2008). The World Mental Health (WMH) Survey Initiative shows wide variation in cross-national prevalence of MNS disorders. The prevalence of common MNS disorders ranges across nations from 27% in the United States to 6% in Nigeria.

Variation in the cross-national prevalence of MNS disorders may reflect cross-cultural measurement bias or may suggest cultural and social differences in etiology.

Research in cultural neuroscience identifies cellular and molecular mechanisms of emotion in the brain that differentially contribute to mental processes of emotion across cultures. Common MNS disorders, such as mood and substance abuse disorders, are characterized by phenotypes and endophenotypes related to the regulation and dysregulation of processes of emotion and its interaction with cognition in cultural settings. The identification of the modifiable social and biological risk factors for mood and substance abuse disorders requires a comprehensive understanding of the neural mechanisms of regulation and dysregulation of emotion across cultures.

The goal of this chapter is to review theoretical, methodological, and empirical approaches in research on the cultural neuroscience of emotion. First, historical and theoretical perspectives provide insight into the conceptual foundations of the study of culture and emotion that emerged from ancient philosophical thought. Methodological advances in the study of culture and emotion detail considerations regarding the testing of theoretical models using a range of empirical paradigms. Empirical findings in the cultural neuroscience of emotion articulate the advancement of an evidence-based understanding in the study of the neurobiology of culture and emotion (Chiao & Blizinsky, 2013). Implications and future directions in the study of cultural neuroscience of emotion for addressing grand challenges in global mental health are discussed.

Historical Perspective on Culture and Emotion

Historical perspectives of culture and emotion are conceptualized in ancient philosophical theories of the mind. Ancient Western philosophers, such as Plato, posited the self as conscious experience consisting of a discrete form, while ancient Eastern philosophers, such as Confucius, postulated that the self as conscious experience is defined as interconnected with the conscious experience of other minds in the world. While there is overlap in the views of Axial age authors, cultural divergence in notions of the self may also characterize ancient philosophical accounts regarding the properties of the mind that make up the conscious experience of emotion.

Contemporary empiricist accounts of emotion have elaborated the notion of psychological construction as conscious experience of emotion integrative with bodily states of emotion. Psychological theories of emotion consider the causal relation of emotional states with those of cognitive appraisal and bodily states of emotion. Early theories, such as the James–Lange theory of emotion, hypothesized that emotion is caused by bodily changes. Basic emotion theory elaborates on this notion, postulating that specific patterns of emotional states of mind are caused by specific patterns of activity in neural mechanisms of emotion.

While early psychological theories of emotion propose causal models of emotion and the body, cognitive appraisal theories describe causal models that include interaction of properties of conscious experience of emotion and the body with those of cognition. The Cannon–Bard theory of emotion posits that emotion is caused by cognitive appraisal of bodily changes. Cognitive appraisal, as an act of meaning making or way of thinking or interpreting bodily changes, produces emotional states. The psychological construction theory of emotion holds that emotions are emergent properties of coordinated interaction with multiple systems within the mind and brain. Emotions are emergent properties from interactions of mental and neural states of emotion and cognition. The social construction theory of emotion posits that socially learned cultural scripts transmit the properties of mental states of emotion. Social construction theory emphasizes the role of cultural transmission in the acquisition of conscious experiences of emotion through social interaction. Emotions are socially situated, arising from social learning within cultural systems that regulate the generation and expression of emotion. From ancient to contemporary thought, culture plays a fundamental role in the construction of the experience of emotion.

Historical periods represent temporal boundaries of cultural acquisition, when cultural transmission of social norms guides the social construction of emotion (Stein et al., 2016). Universal themes also emerge, for example, historical periods of contemporary intergroup conflict and postconflict recovery have led to unmet needs in mental health and increases in costly expenditures and societal burden due to disease. There is ongoing debate about how best to address the problem of unmet needs, but the development and implementation of programs of research on mental health, such as large-scale cross-national surveys to identify patterns and predictors of mental disorders around the world may be useful in informing such debates. Evidence-based approaches to effectively reduce barriers to recovery and to promote mental health across nations are sorely needed.

Theoretical Approaches in Culture and Emotion

Dual Inheritance Theory

Dual inheritance theory refers to cultural and biological interactions that shape adaptive behavior. The interaction of cultural and biological factors demonstrates a response to environmental pressures (Boyd & Richerson, 1985). Dual inheritance theory maintains and strengthens culture by shaping mental and neural architecture to produce adaptive behavior. An example of dual inheritance theory is lactose tolerance. Gene–culture coevolutionary theory proposes that genetic and cultural inheritance arises from cultural adaptation (Henrich & McElreath, 2007). Geographic prevalence of cattle milk genes in Northern Europe shows geographic concordance with lactose tolerance genes in humans (Beja-Pereira et al., 2003). Human farming practices demonstrate genetic and cultural selection in domesticated animals and humans.

Culture–gene coevolutionary theory posits that genetic and cultural inheritance result from the shaping of mental and neural architecture of adaptive behavior. Another example of dual inheritance theory is cultural collectivism and the serotonin transporter gene

(Chiao & Blizinsky, 2010). There is, however, growing skepticism about the relationship of single candidate gene variants to behavior. The geographic prevalence of pathogens is related to the geographic prevalence of cultural collectivism (Fincher et al., 2008). Cultural collectivism serves as an anti-pathogen defense, such that geographic regions with greater collectivism protect from disease-causing pathogens. Across nations, the speculative hypothesis that geographic prevalence of cultural collectivism leads to greater mental health deserves to be investigated.

Cultural Niche Construction

Cultural niche construction refers to the set of interactive processes such that the organism modifies the environment to produce cultural adaptations that change selection pressures to enhance ecological inheritance (Laland et al., 2000; Mesoudi, 2009). The interaction of the organism with the environment to modify ecological conditions refers to the set of behaviors that construct novel features of the environment to change selection pressures in an adaptive manner that benefits the organism and their ecological inheritance. Cultural niche construction includes the set of interactive processes that range in temporal and spatial scale to produce cultural adaptations, and the mental and neural architecture underlying adaptive behavior. Mental and neural processes of cultural niche construction include the use and invention of language, tools, objects, places, and other features of the social and physical environment to improve the ecological inheritance of the organism.

Psychological Construction

Psychological construction refers to theories that posit that conscious knowledge of emotional experience is acquired through interaction with others (Barrett, 2009). Psychological construction is the set of mental processes that relate the experience of emotion with the physical and social world. The feeling of "what it is like," or qualia, reflects a central component of conscious experience that encompasses sensations and feelings (Nagel, 1997). The mental processes of emotional experience construct a conscious understanding of experience, such as the sensations and feeling shared with others. Emotion recognition, as the psychological capacity to transform the perception of emotions in others into mental representations of emotion that encode valence, intensity, and arousal, reflects the interaction of mental constructs of cognition with emotion. The acquisition of the language of emotion is another means of psychological construction, providing verbal labels as categories to express and regulate basic and self-conscious emotional experience.

Psychological construction of emotion may reflect the set of physical representations of emotion within the human brain. The neural representations of emotion located within brain circuitry, including the limbic system and ventral striatum, encode distinct properties of mental states of emotions, including positive and negative valence, low and high intensity, and low and high arousal. The functional and organizational architecture of emotional brain circuitry consists of distinct mental states of emotion that are consciously experienced as a continuous stream of sensations and feelings. The psychological construction of emotion highlights the role of top-down and bottom-up processes of emotion and its interaction with cognition in the generation, regulation, and maintenance of experience.

Methodological Approaches in Culture and Emotion

Cultural

Cultural neuroscience research of emotion consists of different methodological approaches for observational measurement of neural mechanisms of emotional behavior across cultures. An experimental design that is comparative of two or more cultures enables researchers to test theoretical models and predictions regarding the relation of culture to processes of emotion. Research on the cross-cultural comparison of emotion investigates differences in processes of emotion due to specific factors of culture, rather than to other factors, such as the comparison of data that are from two or more geographic regions, or instruments of two or more languages per se. Methodological instruments that control for method bias or ensure measurement equivalence are necessary to test theoretical models in cross-cultural research of emotion.

Behavioral

Behavioral methodology in culture and emotion consists of behavioral surveys and experimental tasks that measure behavioral responses. The measurement of culture with behavioral surveys allows for the testing of theoretical models regarding cultural systems such as individualism–collectivism or holistic and analytic thought. Cultural factors, such as race and ethnicity, nationality, geographic origin, and native language, may serve as a basis for definition of the cultural group. Culture defined from behavioral surveys may also provide a quantitative index of individual-level endorsement or adherence to cultural systems of behavior.

Behavioral paradigms of culture and emotion include experimental paradigms that measure constructs of emotion, including experience, perception, recognition, and regulation, across cultures. Task paradigms of emotional experience may include behavioral surveys and open-ended interviews that assess how people describe emotional experiences across cultures. Task paradigms of emotional perception and recognition include specific experimental stimuli sets that are standardized across cultures, such as facial expressions of emotion (e.g., Japanese and Caucasian American Facial Expressions of Emotion). Task paradigms of emotion regulation include tasks that assess how people feel during emotion regulation and rest. Across experimental paradigms, stimuli sets and tasks may include back-translation to ensure methodological equivalence across cultures.

Physiological

Physiological methods in culture and emotion measure autonomic responses and their relation to neural activity and behavior. In cultural neuroscience studies of emotions, measurement of the autonomic nervous system records physiological responses that occur during behavioral task paradigms of emotion across cultures. Physiological methods measure responses that reflect characteristics of states of emotion, such as arousal. Physiological methods of culture and emotion include cross-site task paradigms to ensure measurement equivalence. Experimental designs of physiological responses in studies of culture and emotion test theoretical models regarding the identification of physiological indices of culture and emotion as well as the causal role of physiological indices in models of culture and emotion.

Neuroscience

Methods in cultural neuroscience of emotion provide direct and indirect measurement of neural activity and its relation to behavior. Observation of neural activity allows for the testing of theoretical models regarding the identification of causal relation between neural mechanisms and sociocultural mechanisms across cultures. Noninvasive neuroscience methods include functional magnetic resonance imaging (fMRI) and event-related potential (ERP) studies that provide measurement of the structural and functional neural architecture and behavioral performance with structural and functional task paradigms of emotion. Neuroscience studies of culture and emotion include cross-site task paradigms to ensure measurement equivalence of observational instruments across cultures (Chiao et al., 2010). Other neuroscience methods such as neuropsychological studies and transcranial magnetic stimulation (TMS) allow for the testing of causal theories of brain and behavior.

Experimental designs of behavioral task paradigms with neuroscience methods across cultures include measurement of structural and functional components in neural systems of emotion. Neural measurement of the limbic system includes observation of neural signals within the subcortical and orbitofrontal brain circuitry located distal from cortical regions. fMRI studies of the limbic system provide assessment regarding the magnitude of response within the brain regions of interest as well as structural and functional connectivity across brain regions during behavioral paradigms of emotion across cultures.

ERP studies of the limbic system facilitate the direct measurement of neural activity from cortical regions of the brain during behavioral paradigms of emotion across cultures. ERP studies of culture and emotion are designed to compare the electrophysiological response of a waveform recorded from a particular cortical site during a given time window of behavioral response during the task paradigm. Because brain regions of the limbic system are primarily located subcortical to the scalp, fMRI studies of culture and emotion indirectly demonstrate enhanced spatial resolution of the neural response, while ERP studies of culture and emotion show greater temporal resolution of the neural response during task paradigms. Additional neuroscience methods may be utilized to provide enhanced spatial or temporal resolution for a given task paradigm and to test theoretical models regarding the identification and causality of the neural mechanisms and mental constructs of behavioral response.

Methods from neuropsychological and TMS studies test the necessity and causality of brain regions in processes of emotion. Neuropsychological studies of emotion refer to the observation and measurement of mental constructs and behavioral outcomes in patients with focal brain damage within regions associated with social and emotional processes. Neuropsychological studies of emotion in patients with bilateral amygdala damage include testing of emotional capacities, such as emotion recognition (Adolphs et al., 2005). Impairment of emotional processes in patients with specific lesions relative to age-matched controls suggests a necessary and causal role of a focal brain region in processes of emotion. TMS studies refer to the application of brain stimulation to a specific brain region to produce a temporary disruption of neural activity during a given experimental task. Behavioral changes from a given experimental task in accuracy or efficiency that result from brain stimulation suggest a causal relation between brain and behavior. TMS studies of culture and emotion seek to test theories regarding the directional causality of cultural and emotional processes in the brain.

Genetic

Genomic approaches in the study of culture and emotion must increasingly rely on whole genome data Chen et al., 2016; Sasaki et al., 2016). Gene-by-culture studies seek to determine the interaction of cultural and genetic mechanisms on the mind, brain, and behavior. Gene-by-culture interaction studies of behavior identify interactions of specific genetic and cultural factors that influence mental constructs and behavioral outcomes. Gene-by-culture interaction functional neuroimaging studies aim to identify interactions of specific genetic and cultural factors on mental constructs that predict the magnitude of neural activation within a given brain region or the strength of association of neural activation within a network of brain regions. Cross-national cultural genetic studies aim to identify the strength of association between cultural indices, genomic variation, and behavioral outcomes across nations.

Culture and Emotion

Cultural Variation in Emotion

Cultural variation in emotion affects antecedents and consequences of emotion processes. Culture variation is observed in the processes of emotion across distinct cultural dimensions, such as independence and interdependence (Kitayama & Markus, 1994; Mesquita & Frijda, 1992), and individualism and collectivism (Oyserman et al., 2002). Independent or individualistic cultures value self-expression, autonomy from others, and uniqueness, while interdependent or collectivistic cultures emphasize social harmony with others and defining the self by social relations and roles (Markus & Kitayama, 1991). Independent or individualistic cultures encourage expressions of the self, including cultural displays of emotion that are internally generated from experiences of emotion. Interdependent or collectivistic cultures allow for expressions of the self that enhance social norms, such as the regulation of emotion with suppression, and that strengthen social harmony with others, such as social sensitivity to the social and emotional states of others. Cultural variation in emotion demonstrates levels of psychological universalism within the computational components of processes of emotion. Further, cultures are not homogenous so any simplistic generalizations about differences should be regarded as speculative, and this point together with evidence of key overlaps across cultures, requires emphasis.

Culture and Display Rules

Cultures vary in the extent to which they display their emotions. Individualistic and collectivistic cultures vary in their display rules of emotion (Matsumoto et al., 2008). Cultural display rules are social norms guiding the expression of emotion with others across sociocultural contexts. Individualistic cultures prefer self-expression such as facial and vocal expressions of emotion to strengthen the social communication of individuals within the social context. Individualistic cultures enhance the importance of the individual, favoring the pursuit of personal goals relative to ingroup goals. Collectivistic cultures rely on social roles and relationships to guide the relevance and meaning of individual emotions within the social context. Collectivistic cultures encourage maintenance of social harmony, conformity with social norms, and the pursuit of ingroup goals.

Cultures differ in norms of emotional expressivity for ingroup and outgroup members. Across nations, individualistic cultures are associated with social norms of greater emotional expressivity relative to collectivistic cultures. Display rules for individualistic cultures differentially guide norms of emotional expressivity toward group members for negative and positive emotion. For individualistic cultures, expressivity of negative emotions is expected toward members of one's ingroup; however, expressivity of positive emotions is expected toward members of outgroups. Again, however, generalizations about culture may well entail over-simplification, and should be regarded as speculative until there is rigorous replication of findings.

Culture and Emotion Perception

Holistic and analytic perception of facial emotional expressions refers to cultural differences in the emphasis on central and peripheral components of features in emotional expressions (Masuda et al., 2008). Cultural differences in holistic and analytic emotion perception contribute to the intercultural advantage in detection of emotion from facial expressions. Independent cultures show greater emotion recognition accuracy when detecting emotions from faces in the center of a social scene, while interdependent cultures demonstrate enhanced accuracy in emotion recognition when detecting emotion in the social surroundings. Furthermore, East Asians may demonstrate greater attentional deployment to emotions in the surrounding social context relative to Westerners. East Asians may encode emotion from expressions of group members, while Westerners may encode emotions from expressions of individuals. These preliminary findings suggest that Westerners construe emotions as feeling states of the individual, while East Asians conceptualize emotions as interconnected or relational to the feeling states of the group.

Cultural variation in emotion perception is observed not only from holistic and analytic perceptions of the social context but also from patterns of emotional expressions. Westerners may show eye movement patterns that are consistent with the notion of six basic facial expressions of emotion encoded as a regularity in facial muscle patterns, while East Asians may demonstrate eye movement patterns across facial expressions of emotion that suggest encoding of emotional intensity rather than perception of basic emotion categories per se (Jack et al., 2012). Westerners may encode emotions from facial expression patterns as basic emotions, while East Asians may encode emotions from facial expressions as emotional intensity. These preliminary findings suggest that perception of emotion from facial expressions across cultures may reflect components of top-down strategies of culture (e.g., holistic and analytic processing), as well as bottom-up strategies of perception (e.g., patterns of eye movements) such that cultural variation in the perception of emotional expressions may reflects cultural influences on the cognitive construction of emotional dimensions.

Cultures may vary in the perception of emotion across modalities. The Himba are a remote culture of villagers from Namibia who live relatively isolated from Western culture. In studies of culture and emotion with Himba and Westerners, cultural differences are observed in the perception of emotion (Gendron et al., 2014a,b). Preliminary data suggest that Himba may show a perceptual pattern during tasks of emotion perception from vocal and facial cues to encode dimensions of emotion, such as valence and arousal, rather than basic categories of emotion per se, while Westerners may encode basic emotion categories from perceptual cues. Speculatively, the Himba may perceive and encode emotional valence, rather than categories of emotion, from vocal and facial expressions of emotion.

Cultural differences in emotion perception may be observed in visual and auditory systems, suggesting the possibility of the influence of culture on shared mental representations of emotion. While perceptual cues of emotion from the face and voice may communicate feeling states to the perceiver, the mental and neural representations of emotion necessary to decode expressions of emotion and encode the properties of their social significance may rely on cultural context. Cultural learning may play an important role in the transformation of sensory cues of emotional expressions into cognitive representations of emotion categories. Hence, cultural variation in emotion perception from facial and vocal expression possibly suggests cultural influences in top-down and bottom-up strategies for the perceptual encoding of emotional information.

Culture and Emotion Recognition

Cultural group membership influences the accuracy of recognition of emotion for ingroup and outgroup members. The cultural ingroup advantage in emotion recognition refers to the enhanced accuracy in emotion recognition for members of one's cultural group (Elfenbein & Ambady, 2002). Cultural influences on emotion recognition accuracy may reflect cultural learning or the acquisition of mental representations for the recognition of emotion in ingroup members. The cultural ingroup advantage in emotion recognition may result from sensitive periods in development such that mental and neural representations of emotion tune to encode and decode emotion from expressions of members of the cultural ingroup. Top-down strategies in emotion processing may ensure that social categorization of cultural ingroup members facilitates the encoding and decoding of expressions of emotion. Enhanced attentional processing of emotional expressions from cultural ingroup members may serve as an early mechanism for the automatic processing of emotion from expressions of cultural ingroup members. The cultural expectation to understand the mental states of ingroup members may contribute to the cultural ingroup advantage in emotion recognition.

Cultural influences in emotion may also be reflected in recognition of nationality from emotional expressions of cultural ingroup members. People demonstrate enhanced accuracy in recognition of nationality from emotional expressions of the face (Marsh et al., 2003). These preliminary findings suggest that emotional expressions may reflect patterns of facial movement that encode perceptual cues to nationality. The intercultural advantage in the detection of nationality from emotional expressions suggests that the influence of culture arises not only from top-down strategies based on social categorization of cultural ingroup members but also from bottom-up strategies that decode patterns of facial components of emotional expressions that are shared across cultural ingroup members. Across nations, cultures may vary in display rules or norms of emotional expressivity. People of the same nationality may recognize emotions to a greater extent from ingroup members due to shared cultural patterns and expectations of emotional expressivity.

Culture and Ideal Affect

Culture influences ideal affect, or how people want to feel. East Asian cultures may prefer low-arousal positive emotional states, such as feelings of calm, while Western cultures may prefer high-arousal positive emotional states, such as feelings of excitement (Tsai, 2007). The affect valuation theory posits that ideal affect is distinct from actual affect, culture influences ideal affect to a greater extent relative to actual affect, and differences in actual and ideal affect contribute to variation in emotional behavior. Cultural differences in ideal affect extend into mental and neural representations of positive emotion.

Cultural differences in mental and neural representations of positive emotion may reflect information-processing mechanisms toward approach motivations and goal states that reflect ideal affect. East Asian cultures may maintain and enhance practices and norms that strengthen information-processing mechanisms toward goal states of feelings of low arousal, such as calm. By contrast, Western cultures may maintain and encourage practices and norms that enhance information-processing mechanisms toward goal states of feelings of high arousal, such as excitement. Thus, cultural variation in mental and neural representations of ideal affect may produce distinct behavioral consequences related to approach motivation.

Culture and Emotion Regulation

Cultures may differ in the strategies for emotion regulation. Individualistic cultures prefer self-expression and uniqueness of the individual, such as expressions of emotion. Regulation of the experience of emotion in individualistic cultures focuses on cognitive reappraisal or the rethinking of the meaning or significance of the emotional experience (Ford & Mauss, 2015). In individualistic cultures, people are expected to experience and express emotional states and then rely on cognitive strategies, such as thinking about emotional states, to change the intensity or arousal of experiences of emotion. Experiences of negative and positive emotion may vary in intensity and arousal due to cultural expectations and motivations to achieve personal goal states. Through cognitive reappraisal, processes of emotion regulation change the intensity and arousal of emotional experiences to become congruent with the conscious thought of the individual.

By contrast, collectivistic cultures prefer social harmony and conformity with social norms. Depending on the cultural context, regulation of emotion in collectivistic cultures relies on the suppression of emotion in collectivistic cultures. Collectivistic cultures encourage social expectations of sensitivity to the feeling states of others and conforming with the social norms of one's role and social relationships. Expressions of emotion may be considered expressions of the individual, rather than expressions of the cultural group. Thus, in collectivistic cultures, regulation of emotion with expressive suppression serves to maintain the social harmony of the cultural group and to strengthen social roles and relationships by conforming the experience of feeling states of the individual with those of the cultural group. Conformity to social expectations of sensitivity to others changes the intensity and arousal of emotional experiences through minimal expressivity of feeling states of the individual. In collectivistic cultures, cognitive appraisal of the emotional significance of feeling states may occur with social processes of mental state understanding consistent with the social roles and relationships of cultural ingroup members, rather than through the regulation of expression of the emotional experiences unique to the individual. Again, however, generalizations about culture may well entail over-simplification, and should be regarded as speculative until there is rigorous replication of findings.

Culture and Physiology

Culture influences the magnitude of physiological responding to emotional information. Consistent with behavioral studies of the cultural ingroup advantage in emotion recognition accuracy, in a study of culture and emotion, participants viewed emotional film clips with cultural ingroup and outgroup members and subjective experience, behavioral, and physiological responses were measured. African Americans and European Americans show greater subjective, behavioral, and physiological response to the emotional film clips with cultural ingroup members (Roberts & Levenson, 2006). These preliminary findings suggest that subjective, behavioral, and physiological responding is enhanced during the cultural transmission of emotional information across ingroup members. Enhanced physiological response to emotions expressed by cultural ingroup members may reflect an automatic, prepotent response to understand the mental states of others and a behavioral preparedness consistent with those of ingroup members.

Culture also affects physiological responding during emotion regulation. In a study of culture and emotion regulation, European Americans and Asian Americans were shown disgust-eliciting films and regulated their emotions by either dampening or enhancing emotional behavior. European Americans showed greater physiological response during emotion regulation of disgust relative to Asian Americans (Soto et al., 2016). These preliminary results suggest that cultural variation in emotion regulation affects not only cognitive processes but also physiological responding. Despite the absence of cultural differences in emotion regulation strategy, cultural variations in physiological processes of emotion regulation were observed. Baseline differences in emotional arousal from disgust-eliciting films across cultures may contribute to differential physiological responding during emotion regulation.

Culture, Emotion, and Aging

Culture affects processes of emotion during aging. Socioemotional selectivity theory posits that as people become older, the emotional salience of positive events increases relative to those with negative or neutral significance (Carstensen, 1992). Cultural interdependence affects socioemotional selectivity for positive emotions. Older Chinese showed less preference for positive emotion relative to younger Chinese (Fung et al., 2008). The age difference in socioemotional selectivity for positive emotion in Chinese occurs during an early stage of emotion processing, as variation in patterns of eye movements for positive, but not neutral or negative, facial expressions of emotion. Cultural variation in the preference for positive emotion during aging also affects the encoding of positive information. Older Chinese who are more interdependent show less reduction in preference for negative information relative to those who are less interdependent (Fung et al., 2010). Age differences in socioemotional selectivity of positive emotion in interdependent cultures may reflect the maintenance of cognitive processing for negative information in older age.

Cultural emphasis on social harmony and sensitivity to the emotions of others in interdependent cultures may lessen the reliance on positive emotional information in older Chinese. For interdependent cultures, attending to and encoding of negative information may enhance social sensitivity to others and reflect adherence to social norms in older Chinese. Cultural differences in emotion regulation strategies may also contribute to socioemotional selectivity for positive information in older adults of independent and interdependent cultures. Interdependent cultures emphasize the regulation of emotion with expressive suppression, a strategy that lessens the expression and experience of emotion but may not necessarily change the cognitive significance of emotional information. Given the cultural expectations of the elderly in interdependent cultures to serve as a social learning model for the young, maintenance of mental representations of positive and negative emotional information constructs a cultural transmission model of emotion from older to younger Chinese. Similarly, preliminary data on the preference of older Chinese for positive and negative emotional information may enhance cultural expectations for social norms of respect for the elderly in younger Chinese. Cultural variation in positive emotion during aging may have consequences for motivation and approach behaviors. For independent cultures, older adults may perceive the experience of emotion as meaningful to the experience of the individual, and thus socioemotional selectivity for positive emotion enhances the emotional salience for motivation and approach behaviors that strengthen affirmation of the self and positive social experiences. Again, appreciation of cultural heterogeneity and the need for rigorous replication of findings, is important.

Neural Basis of Emotion

The neurobiology of emotion consists of neural systems with cortical and subcortical brain structures dedicated to the generation and regulation of emotional experience. Neural systems of emotion consist of distinct functional properties that guide motivation and behaviors such as approach and withdrawal, as well as anticipation and detection of reward. The magnitude of activity within neural regions of emotion respond to cultural and genetic expression within multiple neurotransmitter systems. Neurobiological mechanisms of emotion represent the physical implementation of emotional processes, including the algorithmic levels of analysis that occur within layers of neuroanatomy.

Limbic System

The limbic system consists of a network of brain regions responsible for the regulation of physiological arousal, including the amygdala, hypothalamus, thalamus, parahippocampal gyrus, cingulate gyrus, and prefrontal cortices. The amygdala is the set of neurons located within the subcortical structure anterior to the hippocampus. The amygdala is composed of molecular and cellular mechanisms regulated by serotonergic neurotransmission. The amygdala is a primary brain region dedicated to the detection of threat and maintenance of vigilance in the social and physical environment. The amygdala functions to respond to threat cues in the environment with automatic, prepotent responses that enhance physiological arousal for withdrawal or avoidance.

The amygdala acts as a neural mechanism that reinforces cultural transmission of social learning. Neuropsychological studies of patients with brain damage in the amygdala and in controls demonstrate deficits in the capacity for emotion recognition, particularly fear faces, suggesting that the brain region is necessary for the understanding of mental states (Adolphs et al., 2005). Notably, when taught to direct attention toward the eye region of fear faces, patients with brain damage and controls show intact capacity to recognize emotions from the face. These findings suggest that the amygdala acts as a neural mechanism guiding attention toward the sensory cues in the social environment that transform emotion percepts into conscious concepts about emotion in others. The amygdala encodes a functional property of emotion that can be independently acquired through cultural transmission of social learning.

The role of the amygdala in the interaction of emotion with cognition is supported by connectivity with other brain regions, such as the medial temporal lobe and prefrontal cortices. The amygdala plays an important role in social learning due to structural and functional connectivity with the medial temporal lobe. Heightened amygdala response enhances the formation of emotional memory. Amygdala response also serves as a precursor to emotional experience that may be dampened or enhanced through processes of emotion regulation. The functional connectivity of the amygdala to regulatory brain regions, such as the prefrontal cortex, is strengthened due to maturation during the development period of adolescence. By adulthood, the functional connectivity of the amygdala and prefrontal cortex contributes to the regulation of emotion, such as processes of cognitive reappraisal. Functional activation within prefrontal-amygdala circuitry illustrates the regulation of neural mechanisms responsible for automatic responses of emotion with those of cognitive control.

Ventral Striatum

The ventral striatum includes a set of brain regions associated with the anticipation and generation of reward (Schultz, 2000). The ventral striatum serves as a brain region that receives neuronal signals of reward detection from previous experience. The magnitude of activity within the ventral striatum is sustained from the detection of the reward-predicting stimulus to the presentation of the reward delivery. Neural representations within the ventral striatum respond to the delivery of reward, distinguishing from the presence of reward from those of nonreward.

Brain dopamine neurons located within the pars compacta of the substantia nigra and the ventral tegmental area demonstrate phasic neural response during detection and perception of rewards. The activity of brain dopamine neurons signal the detection of reward to neurons within the ventral striatum and prefrontal cortex. Neurons within the ventral striatum, amygdala, and orbitofrontal cortex may coordinate for reward-directed learning.

During learning, cortical and subcortical brain structures adapt their reward expectation activity to change in response to reward contingencies.

Delayed reward is associated with greater magnitude of activity within reward expectation neurons within the ventral striatum, while early delivery reduces this activity. Neural activity within the ventral striatum associated with reward expectation occurs independently from the detection of other predictions. The neural activity of the ventral striatum contributes to reward expectation and prediction based on previous experience of reward delivery and the functional use of reward prediction to guide and adapt goal-directed behavior to changes in reward contingencies. Due to motivational value, greater efforts are put forth to direct behavior toward goals with greater reward.

Cultural Influences on Neural Basis of Emotion

Culture and Limbic System

Culture affects neurobiological responses of the amygdala during processes of emotion. The amygdala is a brain region containing a central component of ancient limbic circuitry specialized for the detection of the threat from cues of social communication. The amygdala shows greater neural response to conscious and unconscious perception of threat from negative facial expressions. Functional activity within the amygdala displays genetic variation due to serotonergic neurotransmission. The amygdala is structurally and functionally connected to other brain regions within the limbic system that contribute to arousal, including the parahippocampal gyrus, thalamus, and hypothalamus, as well as regulation, including the prefrontal cortex.

Consistent with behavioral studies of culture and emotion, bilateral amygdala response to fear faces appears greater for members of one's cultural group. In a cross-cultural neuroimaging study, Japanese and Caucasian American participants viewed different types of facial expressions of emotion, including fearful, angry, happy, and neutral faces, during neural measurement (Chiao et al., 2008). Japanese participants showed greater bilateral amygdala response to Japanese fear faces, while Caucasian American participants demonstrated greater bilateral amygdala response to Caucasian American fear faces. This enhanced amygdala response to emotion expressed by members of one's cultural group was specific to fear. These findings are consistent with the notion that the amygdala is specialized for the detection of threat in the environment, such as the expression of fear by members of one's cultural group. Fear expressed in the social environment may signal the detection of perceived or actual physical or social threat for others in the cultural group. Greater bilateral amygdala response for fearful facial expressions of one's cultural group may enhance the ability of others to adaptively respond to the detection of threat in the environment.

Cultural influences on amygdala response to emotional expressions reflect situational readiness to respond to the environment. In a neuroimaging study of culture and emotion, Japanese participants were primed with either individualistic or collectivistic values and then completed threat detection in an emotional dot-probe task during neural measurement (Iidaka & Harada, 2016). Results from the study showed that Japanese participants primed with collectivistic values showed greater amygdala response during threat detection relative to those primed with individualistic values. These findings suggest that cultural priming of collectivistic values enhances amygdala response during threat detection. Temporarily heightened cultural awareness alters the accessibility of neural mechanisms for emotional processing. A dynamic, constructivist account of culture may help explain cultural variation in the functional use of subcortical limbic neural circuitry for emotion.

Culture and Ventral Striatum

Culture modulates neural mechanisms of reward circuitry. Reward circuitry consists of a network of brain regions associated with the processing of reward, including the ventral striatum and adjacent regions, such as the lateral hypothalamus, nucleus accumbens, and medial prefrontal cortex. Neural circuitry of reward is composed of cortical and subcortical regions consisting of midbrain dopamine neurons associated with approach or avoidance behavior. Neural mechanisms of reward processing generate emotional arousal associated with affective anticipation and consequential for motivational outcomes. Affective anticipation, or anticipation of incentive outcomes, alters affective arousal and valence (Knutson & Greer, 2008). The process of affective anticipation leads to the generation of affective arousal and a motivational approach that is consistent in valence.

Cultural resources affect the neural basis of reward. Family obligation is a cultural expectation of Latino culture, in which family members are expected to support each other (Fuligni & Pederson, 2002). During the period of adolescence into adulthood, youth experience heightened value for assistance to family. Youth feel a greater sense of fulfillment and connection to family and demonstrate greater contribution to their family. These preliminary findings suggest that a heightened sense of family obligation in Latino youth encourages social reward for awareness and valuation of family assistance. Cultural differences in family obligation may arise in the reward valuation of altruism for family members.

Cultural resources of familial obligation are associated with neural circuitry of reward valuation. Latino youth show greater mesolimbic response when providing reward to their family relative to White youth participants, who display greater response within mesolimbic regions when receiving reward themselves (Telzer et al., 2010). Latino youth who show greater identification with their family demonstrated greater reward response to family reward. Cultural variation in mesolimbic response may be associated with social reward for Latino youth and personal reward for White youth. Culture may modulate mesolimbic response to personal and social reward in youth.

Cultural variation in ideal affect influences reward neural circuitry. Cultures differ in preferences for ideal emotions (Tsai, 2007). European Americans may prefer to experience high-arousal emotions such as excitement, while Asian Americans may prefer to experience low-arousal emotions, such as calm. Cultural differences in ideal emotions do not necessarily reflect those of actual emotions but refer to affective states that guide motivation, decision making, and social preferences in a cultural context. European Americans and Asian Americans were shown positive emotional expressions during neural measurement (Park et al., 2016). Greater ventral striatal response was observed for positive emotions consistent with cultural ideals. European Americans displayed greater ventral striatal response for excited relative to calm facial expressions, while Asian Americans demonstrated greater ventral striatal response for calm relative to excited facial expressions. Positive emotional expressions consistent with cultural ideals were associated with higher reward valuation. These preliminary findings suggest that enhanced reward processing of positive emotional expressions of one's cultural ideal may reflect a greater propensity to approach emotional signals that are rewarding in one's culture. Cultural differences in ideal affect may shape neural circuitry of reward valuation.

Cultural differentiation in the neurobiological mechanisms of reward processing strengthens distinct cultural values and ideals. For Latino culture, heightened reward processing of familial assistance in youth may reinforce patterns of social and emotional processes among self and close others. Greater neural reward processing in Latino youth due to family obligation may encourage identity formation and self-concept defined by familial culture during the formative period of adolescence. For independent cultures, greater reward processing in youth for personal relative to social reward may reinforce a self-concept that is unique and autonomous from others. Speculatively, ultural variation in enhanced neural response to distinct positive facial expressions may strengthen ideals consistent with one's culture. Cultural norms that encourage emotional experiences of high arousal may enhance motivation for self-expression, while those of low arousal may heighten motivation for social harmony with others.

Culture and Late Positive Potential

Culture affects the neurophysiological processes of emotion regulation. Independent or individualistic cultures prefer to regulate emotions with cognitive reappraisal, while interdependent or collectivistic cultures prefer to regulate emotions with expressive suppression (Ford & Mauss, 2015). Cultural differences in display rules of East Asian and Western cultural contexts may reinforce distinct patterns of social and emotional expression (Matsumoto et al., 2008). The late positive potential (LPP) is an electrophysiological waveform located in the parietal lobe associated with emotional arousal. East Asians show reduced LPP response during expressive suppression relative to attend conditions, relative to European Americans (Murata et al., 2013). Cultural variation in LPP response during emotion regulation supports the notion that the electrophysiological index reflects levels of emotional arousal. These preliminary findings suggest that reduced emotional arousal in East Asians results from emotion regulation, a strategy that is congruent with cultural norms. Cultural variation in emotion regulation strategies occurs in parallel with electro-physiological processes that modulate emotional arousal.

Culture and Serotonin Transporter Gene

Culture affects genetic sensitivity to emotional expressions. The serotonin transporter (5-HTTLPR) gene is an SNP that regulates serotonergic neurotransmission in the mechanisms of cognition and emotion. In a study of cultural and genetic influences on emotion expressions, Japanese and Americans were shown facial morphs of positive and negative emotional expressions and then recognized when emotion was no longer shown (Ishii et al., 2014). Japanese carrying the short (s) allele of the 5-HTTLPR gene demonstrated greater social sensitivity to emotional expressions relative to Americans and detected changes in expressivity of emotion with greater ease. Interdependent cultures emphasize social harmony with and sensitivity to others. These finding demonstrate greater genetic and social sensitivity to changes in emotional expressions in an interdependent culture. There is, however, growing appreciation that candidate gene studies have been underpowered and susceptible to bias; future research may investigate the contribution of multiple genes to cultural sensitivity of emotion expressions using unbiased whole genome approaches. Cultural and genetic selection may speculatively maintain and reinforce social sensitivity to the emotions expressed by others.

Culture and the Oxytocin Receptor Gene

Culture influences genetic mechanisms of emotion regulation. The oxytocin receptor (OXTR) gene is a gene associated with socioemotional processes, including social cognition and empathy. In a gene-by-culture study of emotion regulation, Americans who showed distressed and carried the G allele of the OXTR gene demonstrated enhanced willingness to seek emotional social support, relative to Koreans (Kim et al., 2011). Americans carrying the social sensitivity gene are more likely to express emotional distress and seek social support to regulate their emotions, relative to Koreans. In another gene-by-culture study of emotion regulation, Koreans who carried the G allele of the OXTR gene were more likely to rely on emotion suppression to regulate their emotions, relative to Americans (Kim & Sasaki, 2012). Again such work is underpowered, with findings not yet sufficiently replicated, and future sufficiently powered studies are needed to examine the potential contribution of multiple genes to the sensitivity to cultural strategies of emotion regulation. Arguably, however, these preliminary findings speculatively suggest that culture may affect genetic sensitivity to strategies of emotion regulation.

Conclusion

Research in the cultural neuroscience of emotion has led to preliminary hypotheses about the influence of cultural and genetic variation on neural mechanisms of emotional behavior. Discovery of the relation of mental constructs and neural mechanisms of emotion across cultures has suggested useful phenotypes and endophenotypes of emotional regulation that deserve future study. Cultural differences in emotion may be present in the conceptualization and physical implementation of emotion processes, but further work is needed to move beyond overly simplistic characterization of cultural differences, and to ensure replication of findings. Understanding the neural mechanisms of regulation of emotion across cultures may ultimately contribute to the advancement of discovery and delivery science in global mental health.

Future Directions

Future research in the study of cultural neuroscience of emotion may address several considerations. One future direction is to move beyond under-powered single-gene association studies and towards well-powered unbiased whole genome approaches to study culture and emotion. Future studies in the study of culture and emotion should employ contemporary genomic methods to identify the possible association of genomic variation with specific cultural factors, mental constructs, and behavioral outcomes.

Another direction for future research is to integrate empirical approaches in the study of culture and genes with neuroscience methods to predict behavioral outcomes. Cultural and genetic regulation of neurotransmission occurs within specific neurotransmitter systems. Empirical paradigms that test theoretical models of how cultural and genetic mechanisms regulate the activity within neural networks that predict behavioral outcomes may be of particular interest for the identification of biomarkers underlying complex phenotypes (Chiao, 2015). It is important that such work acknowledge the heterogeneity of different cultures, and require replication before overly simplistic generalizations are made.

A third future direction is the study of cultural influences on the neurobiology of emotion across the lifespan. Culture affects the mental constructs of emotion during aging. Interdependent cultures show less socioemotional selectivity of emotion in older adults relative to independent cultures. However, little is known about how culture influences the neurobiology of emotion in aging. Future studies may examine cultural variation in neural mechanisms of positive and negative emotion in younger and older adults. Future research in the cultural neuroscience of emotion in aging may further test theoretical causal models of culture and the neurobiological mechanisms of emotion on approach motivation and social behavior.

A fourth direction of future research in the study of culture and emotion is the expansion of theoretical, methodological, and empirical approaches at the intersection of cultural neuroscience and global mental health. Theoretical, empirical, and methodological approaches in culture and emotion may contribute to the identification of biomarkers underlying MNS disorders that involve dysregulation of emotion and its regulation. Empirical advances in the study of culture and emotion may ultimately contribute to the advancement of theoretical models, empirical paradigms, and methodological tools for the development of cures, preventions, and interventions in global mental health.

Implications

Global Mental Health

The Grand Challenges in Global Mental Health Initiative provides a set of priorities for discovery and delivery science to undertake toward the goals of reduction of disease burden and improvement in health equity. Research on the cultural neuroscience of emotion potentially contributes to an evidence-based knowledge of the etiology underlying MNS disorders across cultural settings (Chiao, Li, Turner, Lee-Tauler, Pringle, 2017). A comprehensive understanding of the neurobiology of emotion across cultures and the role of culture in the structural and functional organization of the brain may be useful in contributing to efforts in scientific discovery that will ultimately reduce the global burden of MNS disorders. The identification of biomarkers of MNS disorders, and their modifiable social and biological risk factors, addresses one of the top priorities in global mental health, but cultural perspectives emphasize how complex the underlying relevant mechanisms may be, contributing to explaining the current lack of such biomarkers. Advancement in the identification of phenotypes and endophenotypes of emotion across cultural settings may ultimately contribute to efforts toward the amelioration of the global burden of MNS disorders. Sustained investment for research and education in cultural neuroscience may ultimately contribute to efforts in discovery and delivery science for the development of cures, preventions, interventions, and care delivery models in global mental health.

Acknowledgments

We thank Ahmad R. Hariri for helpful suggestions. Research reported in this publication was supported by the National Institutes of Health under award number R21MH098789. The content is solely the responsibility of the authors and does not necessarily represent the official views of the National Institutes of Health.

References

Adolphs, R., Gosselin, F., Buchanan, T. W., Tranel, D., Schyns, P., & Damasio, A. R. (2005). A mechanism for impaired fear recognition after amygdala damage. *Nature, 433*, 68–72.

Barrett, L. F. (2009). Variety is the spice of life: A psychological constructionist approach to understanding variability in emotion. *Cognition and Emotion, 23*, 1284–1306.

Beja-Pereira, A., Luikart, G., England, P. R., Bradley, D. G., Jann, O. C., Bertorelle, G., Chamberlain, A. T., Nunes, T. P., Metodiev, S., Ferrand, N., & Erhardt, G. (2003). Gene-culture coevolution between cattle milk protein genes and human lactase genes. *Nature Genetics, 35*(4), 311–313.

Boyd, R., & Richerson, P. J. (1985). *Culture and the evolutionary process.* University of Chicago Press.

Carstensen, L. L. (1992). Social and emotional patterns in adulthood: Support for socioemotional selectivity theory. *Psychology and Aging, 7*(3), 331–338.

Chen, C., Moyzis, R. K., Lei, X., Chen, C., & Dong, Q. (2016). The enculturated genome: Molecular evidence for recent divergent evolution in human neurotransmitter genes. In J. Y. Chiao, S.-C. Li, R. Seligman, & R. Turner (Eds.), *The Oxford handbook of cultural neuroscience* (pp. 315–338). Oxford University Press.

Chiao, J. Y. (2015). Current emotion research in cultural neuroscience. *Emotion Review, 7*(1), 1–14.

Chiao, J. Y., & Blizinsky, K. D. (2010). Culture-gene coevolution of individualism-collectivism and the serotonin transporter gene (5-HTTLPR). *Proceedings of the Royal Society (Series B): Biological Sciences, 277*(1681), 529–537.

Chiao, J. Y., & Blizinsky, K. D. (2013). Population disparities in mental health: Insights from cultural neuroscience. *American Journal of Public Health, 103*(1), S122–S132.

Chiao, J. Y., Hariri, A. R, Harada, T., Mano, Y., Sadato, N., Parrish, T. B., & Iidaka, T. (2010). Theory and methods in cultural neuroscience. *Social Cognitive and Affective Neuroscience, 5*(2–3), 356–361.

Chiao, J. Y., Iidaka, T., Gordon, H. L., Nogawa, J., Bar, M., Aminoff, E., Sadato, N., & Ambady, N. (2008). Cultural specificity in amygdala response to fear faces. *Journal of Cognitive Neuroscience, 20*(12), 2167–2174.

Chiao, J. Y., Li, S.-C., Turner, R., Lee-Tauler, S. Y., & Pringle, B. A. (2017). Cultural neuroscience and global mental health. *Culture and Brain, 5*(1), 4–13.

Collins, P. Y., Patel, V., Joestl, S. S., March, D., Insel, T. R., Daar, A. S., Scientific Advisory Board and the Executive Committee of the Grand Challenges on Global Mental Health, Anderson, W., Dhansay, M. A., Phillips, A., Shurin, S., Walport, M., Ewart, W., Savill, S. J., Bordin, I. A., Costello, E. J., Durkin, M., Fairburn, C., Glass, R. I., . . . Stein, D. J. (2011). Grand challenges in global mental health. *Nature, 475*(7354), 27–30.

Elfenbein, H. A., & Ambady, N. (2002). Is there an in-group advantage in emotion recognition? *Psychological Bulletin, 128*(2), 243–249.

Fincher, C. L., Thornhill, R., Murray, D. R., & Schaller, M. (2008). Pathogen prevalence predicts human cross-cultural variability in individualism/collectivism. *Proceedings of the Royal Society of London (Series B): Biological Sciences, 275*, 1279–1285.

Ford, B. Q., & Mauss, I. B. (2015). Culture and emotion regulation. *Current Opinion in Psychology, 3*, 1–5.

Fuligni, A. J., & Pederson, S. (2002). Family obligation and the transition to young adulthood. *Developmental Psychology, 38*(5), 856–868.

Fung, H. H., Isaacowitz, D. M., Lu, A. Y., & Li, T. (2010). Interdependent self-construal moderates the age-related negativity reduction effect in memory and visual attention. *Psychology and Aging, 25*, 321–329.

Fung, H. H., Isaacowitz, D. M., Lu, A., Wadliinger, H. A., Goren, D., & Wilson, H. R. (2008). Age-related positivity enhancement is not universal: Older Hong Kong Chinese look away from positive stimuli. *Psychology and Aging, 23*, 440–446.

Gendron, M., Roberson, D., van der Vyver, J. M., & Barrett, L. F. (2014a). Cultural relativity in perceiving emotion from vocalizations. *Psychological Science, 25*(4), 911–920.

Gendron, M., Roberson, D., van der Vyver, J. M., & Barrett, L. F. (2014b). Perceptions of emotion from facial expressions are not culturally universal: Evidence from a remote culture. *Emotion, 14*, 251–262.

Henrich, J., & McElreath, R. (2007). Dual inheritance theory: The evolution of human cultural capacities and cultural evolution. In R. Dunbar & L. Barrett (Eds.), *Oxford handbook of evolutionary psychology* (pp. 555–570). Oxford University Press.

Iidaka, T., & Harada, T. (2016). Cultural values modulate emotional processing in human amygdala. In J. Y. Chiao, S.-C. Li, R. Seligman, & R. Turner (Eds.), *The Oxford handbook of cultural neuroscience* (pp. 107–120). Oxford University Press.

Ishii, K., Kim, H. S., Sasaki, J. Y., Shinada, M., & Kusumi, I. (2014). Culture modulates sensitivity to the disappearance of facial expressions associated with serotonin transporter polymorphism (5-HTTLPR). *Culture and Brain, 2*, 72–88.

Jack, R. E., Garrod, O. G., Yu, H., Caldara, R., & Schyns, P. G. (2012). Facial expressions of emotion are not culturally universal. *Proceedings of the National Academy of Sciences, 109*(19), 7241–7244.

Kessler, R. C., & Ustun, T. B. (Eds.). (2008). *The WHO World Mental Health Surveys: Global perspectives on the epidemiology of mental disorders.* Cambridge University Press.

Kim, H. S., & Sasaki, J. Y. (2012). Emotion regulation: The interplay of culture and genes. *Social and Personality Psychology Compass, 6*, 865–877.

Kim, H. S., Sherman, D. K., Mojaverian, T., Sasaki, J. Y., Park, J., Suh, E. M., & Taylor, S. (2011). Gene-culture interaction: Oxytocin receptor polymorphism (OXTR) and emotion regulation. *Social Psychological and Personality Science, 2*, 665–672.

Kitayama, S., & Markus, H. R. (Eds.). (1994). *Emotion and culture: Empirical investigations of mutual influences.* American Psychological Association.

Knutson, B., & Greer, S. M. (2008). Anticipatory affect: Neural correlates and consequences for choice. *Philosophical Transactions of the Royal Society London B: Biological Sciences, 363*(1511), 3771–3786.

Laland, K. N., Olding-Smee, J., & Feldman, M. W. (2000). Niche construction, biological evolution and cultural change. *Behavioural and Brain Sciences, 23*(1), 131–146.

Markus, H. R., & Kitayama, S. (1991). Culture and the self: Implications for cognition, emotion and motivation. *Psychological Review, 8,* 224–253.

Marsh, A. A., Elfenbein, H. A., & Ambady, N. (2003). Nonverbal "accents": Cultural differences in facial expressions of emotion. *Psychological Science, 14*(4), 373–376.

Masuda, T., Ellsworth, P. C., Mesquita, B., Leu, J., Tanida, S., & Van de Veerdonk, E. (2008). Placing the face in context: Cultural differences in the perception of facial emotion. *Journal of Personality and Social Psychology, 94*(3), 365–381.

Matsumoto, D., Yoo, S. H., Fontaine, J., Anguas-Wong, A. M., Arriola, M., Ataca, B., Bond, M. H., Boratav, H. B., Breugelmans, S. M., Cabecinhas, R., Chae, J., Chin, W. H., Comunian, A. L., DeGere, D. N., Djunaidi, A., Fok, H. K., Friedlmeier, W., Ghosh, A., Glamcevski, M., . . . Zengeya, A. (2008). Mapping expressive differences around the world: The relationship between emotional display rules and Individualism v. Collectivism. *Journal of Cross-Cultural Psychology, 39,* 55–74.

Mesoudi, A. (2009). How cultural evolutionary theory can inform social psychology and vice versa. *Psychological Review, 116*(4), 929–952.

Mesquita, B., & Frijda, N. H. (1992). Cultural variations in emotions: A review. *Psychological Bulletin, 112*(2), 179–204.

Murata, A., Moser, J. S., & Kitayama, S. (2013). Culture shapes electrocortical responses during emotional suppression. *Social Cognitive and Affective Neuroscience, 8*(5), 595–601.

Nagel, T. (1997). What it is like to be a bat? In N. Block, O. Flanagan, & G. Guzeldere (Eds.), *The nature of consciousness: Philosophical debates* (pp. 519–528). MIT Press.

Oyserman, D., Coon, H. M., & Kemmelmeier, M. (2002). Rethinking individualism and collectivism: evaluation of theoretical assumptions and meta-analyses. *Psychological Bulletin, 128*(1), 3–72.

Park, B., Tsai, J. L., Chim, L., Blevins, E., & Knutson, B. (2016). Neural evidence for cultural differences in the valuation of positive facial expressions. *Social Cognitive and Affective Neuroscience, 11*(2), 243–252.

Roberts, N. A., & Levenson, R. W. (2006). Subjective, behavioral and physiological reactivity to ethnically-matched film clips. *Emotion, 6*(4), 635–646.

Sasaki, J. Y., LeClair, J., West, A. L., & Kim, H. S. (2016). Application of the gene-culture interaction framework in health contexts. In J. Y. Chiao, S.-C., Li, R. Seligman, & R. Turner (Eds.), *The Oxford handbook of cultural neuroscience* (pp. 279–298). Oxford University Press.

Schultz, W. (2000). Multiple reward signals in the brain. *Nature Reviews Neuroscience, 1,* 199–207.

Soto, J. A., Lee, E. A., & Roberts, N. A. (2016). Convergence in feeling, divergence in physiology: How culture influences the consequences of disgust suppression and amplification among European Americans and Asian Americans. *Psychophysiology, 53*(1), 41–51.

Stein, D. J., Chiao, J. Y., & van Honk, J. (2016). Cultural neuroscience in South Africa: Promise and pitfalls. In J. Y. Chiao, S.-C., Li, R. Seligman, & R. Turner (Eds.), *The Oxford handbook of cultural neuroscience* (pp. 143–154). Oxford University Press.

Telzer, E. H., Masten, C. L., Berkman, E. T., Lieberman, M. D., & Fuligni, A. J. (2010). Gaining while giving: An fMRI study of the rewards of family assistance among White and Latino youth. *Social Neuroscience, 5,* 508–518.

Tsai, J. L. (2007). Ideal affect: Cultural causes and behavioral consequences. *Perspectives in Psychological Science, 2*(3), 242–259.

CHAPTER

11

How Awe Works in Humanitarian Setting in East Asia: Cultural Differences in Describing the Experience of Awe

Michio Nomura, Ayano Tsuda, *and* Jeremy Rappleye

Abstract

Whether an individual copes with loss in a positive and constructive manner or a negative one depends on cultural values, individual differences, and the quality of support they receive. For example, the experience of awe has been shown to diminish the sense of self, which in turn increases generosity, helping behavior, or healthy mental conditions. To date, however, few studies have examined awe in non-Western contexts. This chapter contributes an empirical study with behavioral methods as well as a theoretical literature review on culture and positive emotion, specifically the awe-related experiences among individuals from East Asia, providing novel insights into how awe experiences work in the face of loss. We found that interpersonal situations and natural disasters (e.g., the earthquake of March 2011) were the most common awe-inspiring events described by the participants, which mostly elicited negative emotions indicating that awe-related experiences may motivate people to connect with others in interdependent contexts and may serve to alleviate negative emotions in the face of natural disasters. The findings from these studies highlight the how culture serves as a protective factor in mental health, particularly for interdependent cultures, and the importance of awe in humanitarian settings, such as natural disasters, were among the most awe-inspiring emotional events.

Key Words: Cultural neuroscience, culture, emotion, loss, global mental health

Theoretical Literature Review on Culture and the Emotion of Awe

Whether an individual copes with loss in a positive and constructive manner or a negative one depends on cultural values, individual differences, and the quality of support they receive. For example, the experience of awe has been shown to diminish the sense of self, which in turn increases generosity, helping behavior, or healthy mental conditions. The psychological definition of awe is an emotion involving both vastness and accommodation (Keltner & Haidt, 2003, Shiota et al., 2007). Vastness can refer to anything that is large in physical size (e.g., a vast landscape) or social status (e.g., one's authority or prestige). Research has proposed that awe may also involve a challenge or contradiction to previous mental structures, which involves a need for accommodation that may or may not be satisfied.

Another characteristic of awe is the "small self" aspect. Piff et al. (2015) describe the small self as a "diminished sense of self (i.e., feeling one's being and goals to be less significant) vis-à-vis something deemed vaster than the individual" (p. 884). In a series of studies, they found evidence that the experience of awe diminishes the sense of self, which in turn increases generosity and helping (i.e., prosocial behavior). They concluded that experiencing awe increases prosocial behavior by widening the concept of the self to include others, while diminishing the importance of the individual or small self.

Despite the growing number of studies on awe experiences, the majority have been conducted in the West (Piff et al., 2015). Few studies have examined awe in non-Western contexts. An exception is Bai et al. (2017), who conducted a series of cross-cultural studies focusing on the small-self aspect of awe. In one such study, they asked Chinese and American participants to write about their awe (or joy) experience at the end of each day, and to rate the size of their sense of self for a 2-week period. They found that on the days in which the individuals experienced awe, their perceived self-size was smaller compared to joy experiences, a finding that was consistent across cultures. Moreover, interpersonal and nature-related awe experiences were the most common elicitors of awe. Nonetheless, Chinese participants reported significantly more interpersonal awe experiences as compared with American participants, whereas the American participants reported awe in relation to the self 20 times more often than their Chinese counterparts.

Bai et al. (2017) also found that nature was recalled by participants when describing their awe experiences. Japanese participants are generally thought to harbor a reverence for nature due to the role of the Shinto religion in Japanese culture (Sugimoto, 2014), and it is thought that this led many Japanese participants to recall many awe experiences related to nature. On the other hand, when participants in the United States were asked to describe in detail an experience in which they felt awe, research found that more than 80% of their recalled awe stories portrayed positive emotions compared to narratives with descriptions involving threats or fear (Gordon et al., 2017). Whereas European Americans typically report experiencing positive emotions more than negative emotions, this positivity bias is atypical for East Asians (Tompson et al., 2018).

Cultural Neuroscience of Positive Emotion

The aforementioned research thus raises the questions: How does culture influence the neurobiological bases of awe? How does culture influence the biomarkers of positive (or negative) emotional experience? There is now a growing literature on the cultural neuroscience of positive emotion, such as empirical investigations identifying cultural influences on neural systems of reward (Telzer et al., 2010). For example, Telzer and colleagues (2010) show that familialism in Latino culture modulates neural responses during reward valuation for self and others. Meanwhile, Park and colleagues (2016) show that ideal affect in East Asian culture affects neural responses during reward valuation of facial expressions of emotion (e.g., joy expressions) and cultural influences on neural mechanisms of reward valuation (ventral striatum; Park et al., 2016).

It should also be noted that analysis of population genetics has revealed that approximately 80% of the Japanese population carries the S-allele polymorphism of the serotonin transporter gene (Kumakiri et al., 1999), while only approximately 40% of Europeans carry it (Gelernter et al., 1997). Interestingly, studies on population genetics imply that the population frequency of S-allele carriers and the population frequency distribution of cultural collectivism are related: higher population frequencies of S-allele carriers are associated with increases in cultural collectivism (Chiao & Blizinsky, 2010). In addition, the relatively effective regulation of behavior in response to punishment that is associated with the S allele (Nomura et al., 2015) may play a major role in the maintenance of social order in Japanese society, which is an example of an interdependent (sometimes called collectivist) and "tight" society (Gelfand et al., 2011; Triandis, 2004) in which those who deviate from social norms are often ostracized. In addition, Mrazek et al. (2013) suggested that the susceptibility of a society to ecological threats can predict its "tightness" or "looseness" via the mediation of S-allele carriers and that, in turn, the frequency of S-allele carriers predicts morally relevant behavior in relation to the society's tightness or looseness.

Not only 5-HTTLPR, dopamine D4 receptor (DRD4) gene polymorphism of which the 7- or 2-repeat allele is more sensitive to environmental influences than those who do not carry this allele. Tompson et al. (2018) found that East Asian carriers of the 7- or 2-repeat allele of the DRD4 gene reported experiencing greater emotional balance (i.e., weaker positivity bias) than noncarriers of these alleles. However, for European Americans, the pattern was reversed such that the positivity bias was stronger among the carriers than among the noncarriers.

Sasaki and colleagues have shown gene-by-environment interaction of religiosity and the dopamine receptor gene (Sasaki et al., 2013): participants with DRD4 susceptibility variants were more prosocial when implicitly primed with religion than not primed with religion, whereas participants without DRD4 susceptibility variants were not impacted by priming. This research has implications for understanding why different people may behave prosocially for different reasons and also integrates gene-by-environment research with experimental psychology (Sasaki et al., 2011). Based on these observations, future research should consider cultural variations in people's perceptions and understandings of awe, as well as the complicated network in which genotype, psychosocial, and cultural factors are in dynamic interaction with one another (Nomura et al., 2006).

Yet discussing cultural variation is complex and challenging. Some explanations rely on physical factors, while others point to ideas and worldviews shaped over long periods of time. In relation to the former, the Japan Institute of Country-ology and Engineering's (JICE's) data derived from the years 2000 to 2009 show that of all the earthquakes occurring worldwide with magnitudes of 6.0 or greater, 20.5% of those took place in Japan, even though Japan's land area makes up only 0.28% of the world's total. In addition, because of the frequency of natural disasters, Japanese individuals are known for their high levels of respect for nature, which is also related to the Shinto religion. Shintoism is based on a creation myth that purports that Japan was created by the sun goddess, and the worship of the supernatural or mystical powers that reside not only in humans but also in the elements of nature is a significant part of the religion (Sugimoto, 2014). Moreover, many people in Japan practice various religions without feeling any sense of inconsistency, such as visiting Shinto shrines during festivals, marrying in Christian churches, and holding funerals in Buddhist temples; this suggests that religious beliefs in Japan are nonexclusive (Sugimoto, 2014), especially compared to other world religions.

In relation to worldviews shaped over long periods of time, it is necessary to consider how different cultures have diverse notions of self that may support or hinder the coupling of awe and "small self." In Western contexts shaped by Platonism, Pauline Christianity, and Stoicism, the ideal of selfhood has been the autonomous individual: that which transcends immediate circumstances and social contexts, developing toward higher levels of understanding and/or freedom from societal demands. With this movement comes greater levels of self-consciousness. Taylor (1989, 2004) has termed this process the "great disembedding," carefully tracing how these early cultural ideals unfolded in subsequent historical phases before eventually culminating in the modern, humanist Western self familiar to us today. The quintessential articulation became the Cartesian self *cogito ergo sum*: skepticism of anything beyond self-reflective thought. The key point is that this "buffered" modern Western self came to see itself as distinct from social and natural contexts enclosing it. Western social practices such as education came to play a major part in reinforcing these ideas, particularly after the Enlightenment, when this ideal of autonomous personhood came to be expressed in terms of *Bildung* (e.g., self-cultivation of each individual toward rational/cultural maturity) or New Education (e.g., Rousseau's notion of freeing the child from societal demands). Under these social institutions the Western self developed in the direction of increasing self-awareness, greater self-consciousness, and increasing emphasis on self-relevant goals. Recent historical-sociological research in the United States has underscored just how much this "big self" has come to dominate the cultural imaginary: "ontological individualism, the idea that the individual is the only firm reality, [has] become widespread" (Bellah et al., 1985, p. 276). Here the valorized themes of selfhood have become acting autonomously, creating a strong separate personal identity, being self-focused and oriented toward the future, being optimistic and expressing positive feelings, and resisting influence from others (Rappleye et al., 2019).

In stark contrast, virtually all of East Asia is without the Platonic or Christian legacy. In China, the cosmos and self were understood predominantly through Daoist and Confucian narratives. Japan was shaped primarily by Buddhism imported around the 8th century but understood on the foundation of an indigenous, nature-oriented animist

Shinto (Kasulis, 2018). Buddhism ideas, forged out of acrimonious but precise debates in India, came to emphasize the doctrine of "no-self" (anatman-vada). More precisely, the Zen schools that would later become dominant in Japan came to emphasize the nonsubstantiality of self: that the self was a momentary phenomenon emerging out of a moment of interaction. Rather than seeking greater self-continuity and self-consciousness, notions of selfhood developed more in the direction of self-negation: the ongoing attempt to reduce or lessen the presence of self, thus opening the door to greater embeddedness in social and natural environments. As one Japanese scholar summarizes:

> Naturally Buddhists do not accept the duality of body and soul, or Plato's idea of the immorality of the soul. In Buddhism it is not the soul that is immutable and self-existing apart from the mutable body. . . . This will be clear when we recall the rejection of Buddhists of the Hindu idea of atman, which is an eternal and unchangeable self. Emphasizing the non-dualistic oneness of body and soul, Buddhists insist that it is an illusion, or at least an unreal conception to believe in the preexistence of the soul. (Abe, 1987)

With the removal of the presumption of an enduring entity called self (i.e., Platonic or Hindu soul), attention would naturally turn to how everything became relationally constituted:

> From the earliest times Buddhists emphasized . . . "dependent origination," relationality, relational origination, and co-arising. This means that everything is dependent upon something else without exception, nothing whatsoever in the universe being independent and self-existing. (Abe, 1987)

This experience of no-self, continual co-arising would shift attention outward: placing the emphasis on attuning to relations, being other-focused, and recognizing similarities. While certainly not all Japanese would understand the depths of the imported Buddhist vision, it already sat well with a pre-existing indigenous animism wherein the natural world was animated and alive. Here too attention was directed outward; animist selves remained "porous" (Taylor, 2004) and responsive to the more-than-human world in which they were embedded. Thus, the ideal Japanese self remained small: self-awareness, self-consciousness, and self-relevant goals had a hard time forming in the porous naturalist cosmos of Shinto and the Buddhist admonishment not to become attached to a consistent self (i.e., limit self-aggrandizement).

When Japan began importing modern institutions in the late 1880s to meet the Western challenge, there was an inevitable clash between these two ideal notions of selfhood. But while Japan would borrow a range of modern Western institutions from the university to the police force to the Western calendar, it did not or could not import the notion of "big self." As early as 1910, there were books, both scholarly and popular, appearing that attempted to historicize and problematize the "big self" presumption embedded in Western modernity (e.g., Tomonaga's *A Self-Aware History of "I" in the Modern Era* and

Soseki's novel *Kokoro*). There was no Japanese equivalent for the philosophical term for self: subjectivity. Yet when an initial translation was made along the lines of then-dominant Neo-Kantianism (shukansei), it felt awkward because of the heavy emphasis on seeing (kan), thus implying a disembedded, disconnected, and thus individualized spectator. It was thus subsequently retranslated (shutaisei), implying an embodied and interconnected notion of subjectivity/self. Put simply, even when facing the modern Western notion of "big self," Japanese thinkers rearticulated their preference for "small self." Still today, the "small self" tends to remain the dominant ideal in Japan, not least because of this deft translation. Meanwhile, numerous social institutions have been constructed without reference to self-conscious, self-directing individuals, including numerous educational practices that focus on self-negation and relational interactions (Komatsu & Rappleye, 2017; Tsuneyoshi, 2001). While the "small self" might be too self-evident for most Japanese to recognize, it is abundantly clear to foreign researchers who visit the country (Kasulis, 1998; Rosenberger, 199). Meanwhile, in a seminal piece, Markus and Kitayama (1991) show the impacts of these fundamentally different forms of self-construal—independent and interdependent—for cognition, emotion, and motivation.

These differences, in physical, historical, and now contemporary, suggest that awe as a complex emotion may manifest differently among individuals (i.e., selves) from interdependent cultures such as Japan in comparison with individuals from individualistic cultures. Indeed, Chinese participants who were reported more interpersonal stories (Bai et al., 2017) have frequently been categorized as more interdependent cultures (Markus & Kitayama, 1991).

Empirical Investigation of Awe Culture in East Asia

To understand how awe is viewed in East Asia, particularly Japan, which has been underresearched to date, we conducted an open-response survey regarding the definition, and experience of awe was included in the questionnaire which was Japanese version of DPES we created (seven-factor model, $\chi2$ likelihood ratios = 3.91, CFI = 0.83, TLI = 0.81, RMSEA = 0.064, AIC = 2786.49; N = 672). (Tsuda & Nomura, in preparation). Participants were asked to identify situations in which they felt awe and the reasons they attributed to experiencing it.

The participants consisted of a sample of university students and other participants recruited through an Internet research firm. A total of 157 participants were students from a university located in Kyoto, enrolled in an educational psychology course (M_{age} = 19.39 years, SD = 2.32; female, 35.67%, did not specify, 1.91%). Additionally, 515 other Japanese participants were recruited through the Internet research firm to answer the online version of the questionnaire in exchange for monetary compensation. The sample consisted of individuals above the age of 20 years (M_{age} = 45.49 years, SD = 12.93; female, 53.60%). This sample will be called the generalized sample from now on and will be referred to as Sample G. The university sample will be referred to as Sample U. Before the experiment, all participants gave informed consent in accordance with the procedures of the internal human ethics review board of Kyoto University.

Define and Describe Awe Experiences in Japan

The participants were asked to write in detail about a situation in which they experienced awe. More specifically, they were asked to describe the situation in terms of (a) the people who were involved, (b) the location, (c) what was going on before awe was felt, (d) what happened that made them feel awe, (e) a description of how they felt using the five senses, and (f) the reason they thought they felt awe. The total number of participants who provided their own definitions of awe was 136 for Sample U and 515 for Sample G. Regarding descriptions of awe-inspiring situations, 84 answered from Sample U, whereas 203 individuals answered from Sample G.

The contents of the participants' descriptions were analyzed using a previously developed coding scheme (Bai et al., 2017) that was adapted to fit the data obtained in the present study. The coding categories included (a) something in nature, (b) another person, (c) the March 2011 earthquake, (d) temples or shrines, (e) art or music, (f) spiritual experiences, (g) some kind of knowledge, (h) monuments, (i) the self, (j) had not experienced it/did not know, (k) accidents, (l) other earthquakes, (m) North Korea, and (n) other. Only those individuals who answered the question were included in the analysis: this amounted to 86 participants from Sample U and 202 from Sample G. During the coding process, (l) other earthquakes and (m) North Korea were mentioned only by participants in Sample G.

The participants' descriptions were also coded for emotions; the emotional categories included (a) negative emotions, (b) positive emotions, (c) mixed emotions, and (d) unknown. Only emotions that were explicitly stated were categorized as negative, positive, or mixed. Distinction between negative and positive emotions was made based on the Geneva Emotion Wheel (Sacharin et al., 2012; Scherer et al., 2013) and the circumplex model of affect (Russell, 1980). For example, emotions such as happiness, amusement, interest, surprise, astonishment, and nostalgia were categorized as positive, whereas emotions such as anger, frustration, envy, fear, sadness, disgust, and worry were categorized as negative. Participants who included both negative and positive emotions in their descriptions were coded as mixed. If no emotions were explicitly described in the description of their experience, it was coded as unknown. Two raters unfamiliar with the objective of the research were trained and then coded 10% of the experience to create interrater reliability, which was established at 91%. Disagreements were resolved through discussion.

As results, regarding the situations described, 38% of all participants stated that at least one other person was involved in their awe experience (Figure 11.1), which supported our hypothesis that situations involving other people would be a common factor among Japanese individuals. Additionally, we also hypothesized that nature-related awe would be

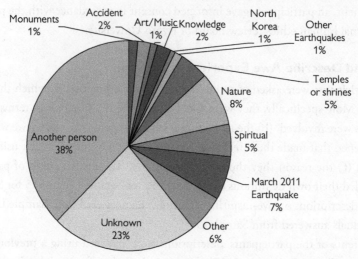

Figure 11.1. The percentages of awe experiences. *Note:* "Other earthquakes" and "North Korea" were only mentioned by participants in Sample G.

a common experience among Japanese individuals. The earthquake of March 11, 2011, was described as an elicitor of awe by 7% of the total sample.

Regarding the emotional aspects of awe experiences, we also examined the frequency of positive and negative emotions used in their descriptions (Figure 11.2), and considered the difference using a chi-square goodness-of-fit test, in which negative, positive, and mixed emotions were compared (the unknown frequencies were not taken into consideration to focus solely on the explicit emotions stated in the narratives). The chi-square analyses

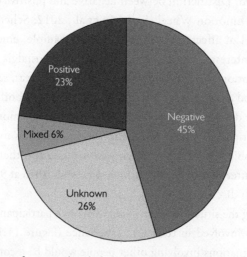

Figure 11.2. The percentages of emotions described in relation to awe experiences.

revealed a significant difference between emotions (χ^2 = 27.46, p < .001). Specifically, negative emotions were mentioned more often than positive or mixed emotions.

Implications for Culture Neuroscience and Global Mental Health

It should be noted that more positive forms of awe existed in the United States than in other countries because of its overall decline in religiosity and the reduction of personal threats in daily life. In Japan, on the other hand, it could be said that there is a constant sense of threat in daily life because of the frequency of natural disasters.

Regarding the cultural aspect, interpersonal situations were found to elicit awe, which is consistent with the findings of Bai et al. (2017). It is important to note that we also included the "self" category in our analysis but no such experiences were identified, which is consistent with the findings of previous research in which U.S. participants described the self as being an elicitor of awe more often than their Chinese counterparts (Bai et al., 2017).

Another finding was that many individuals recalled the earthquake of March 2011 as an awe-inspiring event. The Ministry of Agriculture, Forestry, and Fisheries of Japan (2012) reported that an earthquake with a magnitude of 9.0 hit the Tohoku area on March 11, 2011, which caused a tsunami to hit the east coast of Japan, killing over 20,000 people. Moreover, the tsunami caused nuclear accidents that affected residents living in the area. Some of the participants of the present study mentioned that they experienced the March 2011 earthquake firsthand, while many others described how they experienced the incident by witnessing reports on TV. They also mentioned that the reason they felt awe was because they were astonished by the power of nature and how small and power-less people are in comparison. Although the number of earthquakes occurring in Japan is much higher than any other country in the world (Jishin no Ooi Kuni Nihon, 2017), the impact the March 2011 earthquake had on people was huge, making them realize how small and powerless they were, which is a defining characteristic of awe (Piff et al., 2015).

It was also found that the Japanese participants recalled awe-inspiring moments in which at least one other individual was involved most frequently. Furthermore, the emotions they described were mostly negative, which might imply that awe experiences involving other people in Japan tend to elicit negative emotions. A study comparing the descriptions of daily emotions among Japanese people and Americans found that Japanese people who reported feeling positive emotions during interpersonal experiences, such as respect (see Muto, 2014), reported more positive feelings in general. In contrast, Americans who reported feeling a great deal of positive interpersonally disengaged emotions, such as pride, reported more positive feelings in general, suggesting that Japanese individuals feel positive emotions most often in response to interactions with other people (Kitayama et al., 2000). For instance, many individuals in Sample G mentioned their boss or their superior in their recalled events and that their presence made them feel nervous. Awe is known to make individuals feel subordinate in the presence of others (Stellar et al.,

2017), and by diminishing focus on the self, awe increases the degree to which an individual feels a sense of belonging in their community, as a "small self" mediates the effects of awe on collective cognition and behavior (Bai et al., 2017).

As research has suggested that threat-based awe experiences do not provide momentary well-being like positive awe experiences do because of the heightened sense of powerlessness that people feel (Gordon et al., 2017), the present study's results indicate that people who go out of their way to help others during a time of crisis are ethical and in control of their behavior. As Telzer and colleagues (2010) show that Latino participants who derived greater fulfillment from helping their family 2 years prior to the scan showed increased reward system activation when contributing to their family, these people might identify more with community members and/or others who also suffered from natural disasters.

As pathogen prevalence predicts the endorsement of group-focused moral concerns (van Leeuwen et al., 2012), nations like Japan with a greater historical prevalence of disease-causing infections are more likely to endorse moral concerns about the "community," particularly since the Japanese are an interdependent people. This type of culture and behavior not only may serve an anti-pathogen defense function but also may help people to connect to other people to alleviate their feelings of loss in the face of traumatic events.

Direct comparisons of emotions and experiences were not conducted, so future research should attempt to divide the awe-inspiring situations into several categories and consider what kinds of situations elicit negative or positive emotions to improve our understanding of awe. More cross-cultural research may be required to understand the extent to which awe has a positive or negative impact on individuals.

Since awe is known to help build prosociality, the developmental aspect of awe is also of interest. Previous studies on emotions have shown that in contrast to basic emotions, complex emotions such as pride, envy, and shame develop later in life. Thus, the question arises concerning whether and how awe develops in children as other complex emotions do. For example, the use of children's books would be of interest, since children's books are known to develop vocabulary that may eventually enhance the child's understanding of others' points of view. Creative interventions using awe-inspiring children's books might enhance prosocial behavior in children. Thus, further research is required concerning the developmental aspect of the emotion of awe.

Conclusion

The awe experiences described by the Japanese participants in the present study demonstrate the importance of considering the small-self aspect of awe and feelings of powerlessness, which may enhance the feeling of awe. However, there is still insufficient evidence related to this issue to establish how to best implement social support to alleviate the pain of loss in a given population.

References

Abe, Masao (1987). Sunyata as Formless Form: Plato and Mahayana Buddhism. In Steven Heine (Ed.), *Zen and Comparative Studies* (pp. 139–148). Honolulu: University of Hawaii Press.

Bai, Y., Maruskin, L. A., Chen, S., Gordon, A. M., Stellar, J. E., McNeil, G. D., Peng, K., & Keltner, D. (2017). Awe, the diminished self, and collective engagement: Universals and cultural variations in the small self. *Journal of Personality and Social Psychology*. doi:10.1037/pspa0000087

Bellah, R. N., Madsen, R., Sullivan, W., Swidler, A., & Tipton, S. M. (1985). *Habits of the heart: Individualism and commitment in American life*. University of California Press.

Chiao, J., & Blizinsky, K. D. (2010). Culture-gene coevolution of individualism-collectivism and the serotonin transporter gene. *Proceedings of Biological Sciences, 277*, 529–537.

Gelernter, J., Kranzler, H., & Cubells, J. F. (1997). Serotonin transporter protein (SLC6A4) allele and haplotype frequencies and linkage disequilibria in African- and European-American and Japanese populations and in alcohol-dependent subjects. *Human Genetics, 101*, 243–246.

Gelfand, M. J., Raver, J. L., Nishii, L., Leslie, L. M., Lun, J., Lim, B. C., & Yamaguchi, S. (2011). Differences between tight and loose cultures: A 33-nation study. *Science*, 332, 1100–1104.

Gordon, A. M., Stellar, J. E., Anderson, C. L., McNeil, G. D., Loew, D., & Keltner, D. (2017). The dark side of the sublime: Distinguishing a threat-based variant of awe. *Journal of Personality and Social Psychology, 113*(2), 310–328. http://dx.doi.org/10.1037/pspp0000120.

Jishin no Ooi Kuni Nihon [Japan, a country with earthquakes]. (n.d.). Retrieved December 14, 2017, from http://www.jice.or.jp/knowledge/japan/commentary12

Kasulis, T. (1998). *Intimacy and Integrity: Philosophy and cultural difference*. University of Hawaii Press.

Kasulis, T. (2018). *Engaging Japanese philosophy: A short history*. University of Hawaii Press.

Keltner, D., & Haidt, J. (2003). Approaching awe, a moral, spiritual, and aesthetic emotion. *Cognition & Emotion, 17*(2), 297–314.

Kitayama, S., Markus, H. R., & Kurokawa, M. (2000). Culture, emotion, and well-being: Good feelings in Japan and the United States. *Cognition and Emotion, 14*(1), 93–124.

Komatsu, H., & Rappleye. J. (2017). A PISA paradox? An alternative theory of learning as a possible solution for variations in PISA scores. *Comparative Education Review, 61*(2), 269–297.

Kumakiri, C., Kodama, K., Shimizu, E., Yamanouchi, N., Okada, S., Noda, S., et al. (1999). Study of the association between the serotonin transporter gene regulatory region polymorphism and personality traits in a Japanese population. *Neuroscience Letters, 263*, 205–207.

Markus, H. R., & Kitayama, S. (1991). Culture and the self: Implications for cognition, emotion, and motivation. *Psychological Review, 98*(2), 224–253. doi:10.1037/0033-295x.98.2.224

Mrazek, A. J., Chiao, J. Y., Blizinsky, K. D., Lun, J., & Gelfand, M. J. (2013). The role of culture-gene coevolution in morality judgment: Examining the interplay between tightness-looseness and allelic variation of the serotonin transporter gene. *Culture and Brain, 1*, 110–117.

Ministry of Agriculture, Forestry and Fisheries Japan (2012). FY2011 Annual Report on Food, Agriculture and Rural Areas in Japan (pp. 2–6).

Muto, S. (2014). The concept structure of respect -related emotions in Japanese university students. *Japanese Journal of Psychology, 85*(2), 157–167.

Nomura, M., Kaneko, M., Okuma, Y., Nomura, J., Kusumi, I., Koyama, T., & Nomura, Y. (2015). Involvement of serotonin transporter gene polymorphisms (5-HTT) in impulsive behavior in the Japanese population. *PLoS One, 10*, e0119743. doi:10.1371/journal.pone.0119743

Park, B., Tsai, J. L., Chim, L., Blevins, E., & Knutson, B. (2016). Neural evidence for cultural differences in the valuation of positive facial expressions. *Social Cognitive and Affective Neuroscience, 11*(2), 243–252.

Piff, P. K., Dietze, P., Feinberg, M., Stancato, D. M., & Keltner, D. (2015). Awe, the small self, and prosocial behavior. *Journal of Personality and Social Psychology, 108*(6), 883.

Rappleye, J., Komatsu, H., Uchida, Y., Krys, K., & Markus, H. (2019). "Better policies for better lives"?: Constructive critique of the OECD's (mis)measure of student wellbeing. *Journal of Education Policy*. https://www.tandfonline.com/doi/full/10.1080/02680939.2019.1576923

Rosenberger, N. (Ed.). (1994). *The Japanese sense of self*. Cambridge University Press.

Russell, J. A. (1980). A circumplex model of affect. *Journal of Personality and Social Psychology, 39*, 1161–1178.

Sacharin, V., Schlegel, K., & Scherer, K. R. (2012). *Geneva Emotion Wheel rating study (Report)*. University of Geneva, Swiss Center for Affective Sciences.

Sasaki, J. Y., Kim, H. S., Moraverian, T., Kelley, L. D., Park, I., & Janusonis, S. (2013). Religion priming differentially increases prosocial behavior among variants of dopamine D4 receptor (DRD4) gene. *Social Cognitive and Affective Neuroscience, 8*, 209–215.

Sasaki, J., Kim, H. S., Xu, J. (2011). Religion and well-being: an analysis of an oxytocin receptor polymorphism (OXTR) and culture. *Journal of Cross-Cultural Psychology, 42*, 1394–405.

Scherer, K. R., Schuman, V., Fontaine, J. J. R., & Soriano, C. (2013). The GRID meets the wheel: Assessing emotional feeling via self-report. In J. J. R. Fontaine, K. R. Scherer, & C. Soriano (Eds.), *Components of emotional meaning. A sourcebook* (pp. 281–298). Oxford University Press.

Shiota, M. N., Keltner, D., & Mossman, A. (2007). The nature of awe: Elicitors, appraisals, and effects on self-concept. *Cognition and Emotion, 21*(5), 944–963.

Stellar, J. E., Gordon, A. M., Piff, P. K., Cordaro, D., Anderson, C. L., Bai, Y., Maruskin, L. A., & Keltner, D. (2017). Self-transcendent emotions and their social functions: Compassion, gratitude, and awe bind us to others through prosociality. *Emotion Review, 9*(3), 200–207.

Sugimoto, Y. (2014). *An introduction to Japanese society* (4th ed.). Cambridge University Press.

Taylor, C. (1989). *Sources of self: The making of modern identity*. Harvard.

Taylor, C. (2004). *Modern social imaginaries*. Duke University Press.

Telzer, E. H., Masten, C. L., Berkman, E. T., Lieberman, M. D., & Fuligni, A. J. (2010). Gaining while giving: An fMRI study of the rewards of family assistance among White and Latino youth. *Social Neuroscience, 5*, 508–518.

Tompson, S. H., Huff, S. T., Yoon, C., King, A., Liberzon, I., & Kitayama, S. (2018). The dopamine D4 receptor gene (DRD4) modulates cultural variation in emotional experience. *Culture and Brain, 6*(2), 118–129.

Triandis, H. C. (2004). The many dimensions of culture. *Academy of Management Perspectives, 18*, 88–93.

Tsuda & Nomura, in preparation. Development of Japanese version of the dispositional positive emotion scale.

Tsuneyoshi, R. (2001). *The Japanese model of schooling: Comparison with the United States*. Routledge.

van Leeuwen, F., Park, J. H., Koenig, B. L., & Graham, J. (2012). Regional variation in pathogen prevalence predicts endorsement of group-focused moral concerns. *Evolution and Human Behavior, 33*, 429–437.

Culture, Attention, and Mental Health: Recent Empirical Findings on Visual Scenes and Its Influence on Culture-Bound Syndromes

Takahiko Masuda, Hajin Lee, *and* Matthew J. Russell

Abstract

Under the rubric of interdependent versus independent social orientation and holistic versus analytic cognition, cultural psychologists have demonstrated that there are substantial cultural variations in social cognition. Empirical evidence converges to demonstrate that, in a society where interdependent social orientation and holistic cognition have historically developed, people are more prone to attend to target information, while being sensitive to the context, relationship, and situation that surround the target (context-oriented attention). However, in a society where independent social orientation and analytic cognition have historically developed, people are more prone to attend to what they think is the most salient and important information, while paying little attention to its context, relationship, and situation (object-oriented attention). Until recently, the applications of these findings in the field of mental health science have not been fully discussed. This chapter begins by reviewing the theoretical framework and the cognitive and neural empirical evidence that demonstrate cultural variations in attention. It then introduces a series of studies that examine cross-cultural variations in stress perception between people in independent versus interdependent social orientation. Finally, it reviews a strand of research that could be considered one of many important candidates to further advance basic research on attention to more applied research in the field of mental health, which includes *taijinkyofusho* (TKS), *hikikomori* (social withdrawal)/*NEET* (Not in Education, Employment, or Training) common in Japan, versus social phobia common in North America. The chapter ends with a discussion of a possible collaboration between cultural neuroscience and mental health science.

Key Words: culture, attention, stress, hikikomori, social withdrawal, taijinkyofusho (TKS), NEET, mental health, cultural neuroscience, cultural psychology

Introduction

How does culture influence the human mind? If at all, is cultural influence on the mind superficial or deep? Since the late 1980s, a research field called cultural psychology—an interdisciplinary field that integrates psychology, anthropology, linguistics, philosophy, and neuroscience—has empirically investigated the influence of cultural meaning systems on human psychology (Bruner, 1990; Geertz, 1973; Miller, 1999; Shweder, 1991). While criticizing universalists (Fodor, 2008; Pinker, 1994, 1997, 2007; Pylyshyn, 1999) who selectively focus on innate patterns of behaviors, cultural theorists in this field define culture as a system of meaning shared by people in a given society, and this system shapes people's minds while people intersubjectively sustain the system. Therefore, it is indispensable for cultural psychologists to investigate the mutual constitution of culture and the mind (Shweder, 1991).

Much empirical research for the past three decades has followed theoretical frameworks. More concretely, researchers assume that people in different cultures have different ways of viewing themselves, others, and the world. These different views of the self and the world are associated with culture-specific patterns of cognition and perception. For example, a group of researchers has discussed that there are two types of social orientations: *independent social orientation* and *interdependent social orientation* (Kitayama et al., 2019; Kitayama & Uskul, 2011; Markus & Kitayama, 1991, 2010; Miyamoto, 2013; Nisbett, 2003; Varnum et al., 2010). Those who live in a culture where *independent social orientation* is dominant tend to view themselves as separate from social others and hold cognitive styles that emphasize self-direction, autonomy, and self-expression. In contrast, those who live in a culture where *interdependent social orientation* is dominant tend to view themselves as socially interrelated and connected to significant relationships, and hold cognitive styles that emphasize harmony, relatedness, and connection.

Each type of social orientation develops culturally specific cognitive and perceptual styles. Nisbett and colleagues (Masuda, 2017; Masuda, Russell, et al., 2019; Nisbett, 2003; Nisbett & Masuda, 2003; Nisbett & Miyamoto, 2005; Nisbett et al., 2001) contrasted two kinds of thinking styles: *analytic* and *holistic/dialectic*. The *analytic thinking style* is characterized by an emphasis on taxonomic and rule-based categorization, dispositional orientation in causal attribution and social inference, and formal logic in reasoning. This thinking style is associated with the independent social orientation. Conversely, the *holistic/dialectic thinking style* is characterized by thematic and family resemblance–based categorization of objects, situational orientation in causal attribution and social inference, and dialectical logic in reasoning. This thinking style is associated with the interdependent social orientation.

Several scholars examined how ecology influences people's social orientation, which in turn influences their cognition and perception (Talhelm et al., 2014; Uskul et al., 2008; Varnum et al., 2010). For example, Talhelm et al. (2014) assumed that an interdependent social orientation and holistic thinking style becomes dominant when ecology fosters social cooperation, for example, when ecology forces labor-intensive farming (e.g., rice farming) because people otherwise cannot enjoy harvest without social cooperation. An independent social orientation and analytic cognitive style becomes dominant when ecology encourages less social or more solitary activities such as herding (e.g., wheat farming) because people feel a sense of primary control over the entire farming work. Similarly, Uskul et al. (2008) tested three communities in the Black Sea region of Turkey where people are ethnically similar and speak the same language but differ in their primary economic activities and subsistence systems. They found that herders, who often work alone, tend to hold a more independent social orientation and analytic thinking style, whereas farmers and fishers, whose cooperative works are both valued and required, tend to hold a more interdependent social orientation and holistic/dialectic thinking style.

However, to better understand the cultural transmission process, one should not constrain the antecedents of each social orientation to ecology. In fact, once a civilization is developed based on ecology, the social orientation and associated cognitive and perceptual styles are maintained and even transmitted from one area to other areas of the globe.

The *analytic cognitive and perceptual styles* emerged in an ancient Greece civilization where people emphasized a more independent social orientation. Such a tradition has been sustained in Western cultures such as those in Western Europe and North America, where people emphasize an object-oriented focus in visual attention (selectively focusing more on objects than on context) when they are presented with visual information. In contrast, the *holistic cognitive and perceptual styles* originated from an ancient Chinese civilization and these styles have become dominant in East Asian cultures such as China, Korea, and Japan where people emphasize a context-oriented focus of attention (e.g., Masuda, Russell, et al., 2019).

Much empirical evidence has demonstrated that such differences in thinking styles even influence basic perceptual processes, notably *attention* (Masuda, Russell, et al., 2019; see Masuda, 2017, for review). These studies to date converged to report that there were substantial cultural variations in attention. In the next section we briefly review these studies.

Culture and Attention: Empirical Studies

While there are universal aspects of human attention (Chun & Wolfe, 2001; Posner, 1980), our pattern of attention is often influenced by top-down attention processes—such as knowledge, expectation, motivation, feelings, values, and goals (Bruner, 1957; Bruner & Goodman, 1947). This assertion by the so-called New Look psychologists emerged in the North American academic context, paying little attention to cultural factors. However, this classic approach to human perception works as a foundation of the current research on culture and attention. That is, if our pattern of attention is susceptible to sociocultural factors, it is reasonable to assume that people under a given social orientation attend to the visual scene in a culturally meaningful manner (Senzaki et al., 2014).

Culture and Attention to Nonsocial Scenes

To date, a plethora of attention studies have indeed demonstrated that East Asians are more likely than their North American counterparts to endorse context-sensitive patterns of attention (Boduroğlu & Shah, 2017; Boduroğlu et al., 2009; Doherty et al., 2008; Imada et al., 2013; Ishii & Kitayama, 2002; Ishii et al., 2003; Ji et al., 2000; Kitayama et al., 2003; Kitayama & Ishii, 2002; Masuda, Akase, et al., 2008; Masuda et al., 2016; Masuda & Nisbett, 2001, 2006; Savani & Markus, 2012). Furthermore, developmental researchers reported that such culturally dominant patterns of attention emerge even around 3 to 6 years old (Chiu, 1972; Duffy et al., 2009; Ishii et al., 2017; Kuwabara & Smith, 2012, 2016; Kuwabara et al., 2011), gradually develop around ages 8 to 9 (Imada et al., 2013; Senzaki et al., 2016), and stabilize after age 10 (Ji, 2008; Masuda, Nand, et al., 2019; Miller, 1984).

For example, Masuda and Nisbett (2001) assumed that culturally shared meaning systems would influence people's mode of attention; therefore, even simple narratives based on visual scenes presented on a screen for a short period of time would be affected by such culturally specific modes of attention. By measuring people's narrative styles as an indirect indicator of their attention, they demonstrated that when asked to describe animated vignettes of underwater scenes, European Americans tended to selectively refer more to the focal objects, whereas Japanese participants tended to describe both focal objects and contextual information. These results suggest that European Americans, in keeping with their analytic mode of attention, use a strategy of detecting what they think is important and ignoring the peripheral information in the background. In contrast, Japanese people holistically capture the context as a frame of an event and then develop narratives for the focal objects.

In a subsequent study, Masuda and Nisbett (2001) further tested European American and Japanese recognition styles by targeting their recognition accuracy as an indirect indicator of attention. They first asked participants to evaluate how much they liked animals that appeared in wilderness scenes, and later (in an incidental memory task), to make a recognition judgment and state whether they had seen the animals previously. In this recognition task, the same animals were presented, either in the same wilderness scenes as before or in novel wilderness scenes. The results indicated that both cultures performed well when recognizing congruent images (previously presented animals with their previously matched wilderness scenes). However, when incongruent images were shown (e.g., previously presented animals with novel wildernesses), accuracy decreased for both groups, and accuracy was much poorer for Japanese than for Americans.

Although they use narratives and recognition accuracy that are indirect measurements of one's attention, the findings are the first to show that culture substantially influences human attention. In fact, since then, researchers have further investigated the depth of cultural effects on so-called basic psychological processes by using eye trackers (Chua et al., 2005; Senzaki et al., 2014; Zhang & Seo, 2015). For example, Senzaki et al. (2014)

demonstrated that there was no cultural difference in modes of attention when European Canadians and Japanese simply observed animated vignettes of underwater scenes by selectively focusing on the foreground information rather than background information. However, when Japanese were asked to narrate the story of the scenes, they were more likely than their European Canadian counterparts to allocate their attention to the background.

Recent neuroscience research has also investigated *to what extent* such top-down processes influence the activation of neural responses during attention tasks. By referring to event-related potential (ERP) and functional magnetic resonance imaging (fMRI) research (Goto et al., 2010; Hedden et al., 2008; Masuda et al., 2014), Masuda et al. (2014) assumed that cultural variations in attention are not only observable in people's behavioral responses and patterns of eye movement but also deeply rooted in their neural processing mechanisms. To initiate this investigation, we targeted their neural activities using an ERP methodology, since identifying the neural components that direct variant attention patterns is important to further elucidate mechanisms of culturally specific modes of attention. They analyzed the activation patterns of European Canadians and Japanese during Masuda and Nisbett's (2001) recognition task, through FN400 ERPs, which are thought to indicate memory processes related to the recognition of the discrepancy between old (previously presented) and new (novel) information (e.g., Tsivilis et al., 2001). The results indicated that both European Canadians and Japanese showed increased FN400 responses, reflecting an increased memory processing needed for images with old information. However, the FN400 for new background-incongruent pairs only affected behaviors for the more holistic Japanese, suggesting that the more Japanese processed the background (seen through stronger FN400s), the more likely they were to mistake old information for being new. This provides evidence that Japanese bind contextual information in their memory judgments of target objects.

Similarly, Goto et al. (2010) measured the extent to which people naturally attend to contextual information when asked to make judgments of focal objects. They compared Asian Americans' and European Americans' N400 ERPs to scenes consisting of foreground objects placed on background scenes that were either congruent (e.g., a crab naturally belongs on the beach) or incongruent (e.g., a crab does not fit as well in a parking lot). Related to the properties of the N400, a stronger N400 response to the incongruent objects than to the congruent objects would suggest that the person was taking into consideration the foreground–background semantic fit. The results indicated that Asian Americans showed a stronger N400 response to the incongruent objects (vs. congruent objects) than their North American counterparts, suggesting that Asian Americans are indeed attentive to the relationship between the foreground object and the background.

These findings support the idea that cultural differences in social orientations and thinking styles affect how people perceive visual information. That is, those from more interdependent social orientations tend to see the world holistically, whereas those from more independent social orientations tend to regard people as free from social context.

Culture and Attention to Social Scenes

The social orientation hypothesis (Varnum et al., 2010) assumes that one's cognition and perception are shaped by their reality through social interactions with the members of a society (Varnum et al., 2010). If that is the case, it is reasonable to expect that culturally dominant patterns of attention would be easily observed, especially when the task and the stimuli are more social. In fact, people's attention to a target's facial expression and emotions is subject to substantial cultural variations (Ko et al., 2011; Masuda et al., 2012; Matsumoto et al., 2010; Miyamoto et al., 2011; Stanley et al., 2013).

For example, Miyamoto et al. (2011) demonstrated that holistic thinkers apply a configural-oriented mode of attention (e.g., viewing the face as a whole, and being sensitive to the relationship among facial parts), and analytic thinkers apply a feature-oriented mode of attention (e.g., attending to each facial feature). Similarly, Masuda and colleagues used face lineups to examine the emotional context sensitivity of European Americans and Japanese (Masuda, Ellsworth, et al., 2008; Masuda et al., 2012) and measured the participants' judgment patterns as a cognition. The center person was surrounded by four figures who showed an emotion that was either the same as or different from that of the center person, and participants were asked to judge the intensity of the center person's emotion. This research found that Japanese were more likely than European Americans to take the background people's emotions into account and adjust their ratings of the center person's emotions accordingly. The participants' eye movement patterns were also consistent with this cultural difference in social attention, with Japanese paying more attention to the background faces. Interestingly, Asian Canadians' and Asian international students' eye movement patterns fell between those of European Canadians (who focused their attention exclusively on the center figure) and Japanese (who significantly allocated their attention to the background figures as well). These results support the idea that cultural differences in social orientations and thinking styles also affect how people perceive social scenes. That is, those from a more interdependent social orientation tend to see a target person's emotions as embedded in the social context, and those from a more independent social orientation tend to regard people as free from social context.

Through ERP methods, cultural neuroscientists elucidate how culture influences people's brain activation when they engage in cognitive and perceptual tasks that require participants to pay attention to social events (Fong et al., 2014; Russell et al., 2015). For example, Russell et al. (2015) investigated ERP patterns when European Canadians and Japanese viewed the previously described face lineups created by Masuda and colleagues (Masuda, Ellsworth, et al., 2008; Masuda et al., 2012). They targeted the ERP components known as N400 and late positive complex (LPC), which are related to early processing of semantic incongruities. That is, stronger N400s and LPCs occur when information is considered incongruent. These stronger N400 and LPC patterns might be expected for lineups with differing emotions between the center and background faces when such differences are considered problematic to people's worldviews (i.e., if people are worried about social harmony), and we expected this pattern for holistic cultures. Consistent with this prediction, the results indicated that only Japanese showed stronger N400s and LPCs to differences than European Canadians, between central and background emotions (vs. similar emotions), suggesting that holistic modes of attention also lead to additional neural processing of emotional incongruence.

Furthermore, extending prior research that highlights basic cultural variations in attention to social context (Russell et al., 2015), Russell et al. (2019) investigated how culture influences people's early neural processing of social context for two relationship contexts (i.e., close relationships vs. acquaintances). They compared ERP patterns between European Canadians and Japanese during a face lineup task where participants were asked to rate a center person's emotions (happy vs. sad vs. neutral) surrounded by two background people with congruent or incongruent emotions. To measure how relationship contexts influence early attention processing, they also framed face lineups to be in close or acquaintance relationships. Specifically, they targeted the ERP component known as the N400. The N400 is associated with early processing of semantic incongruities. They predicted that relationship contexts influence when European Canadians and Japanese process incongruent social context differently, due to differences in relationship priorities in the two cultures.

Consistent with their predictions, they found that as interdependent cultures place greater value on considering acquaintance others' views for maintaining their in-group harmony (Leung & Cohen, 2011), only Japanese showed strong N400 processing for incongruent emotions for acquaintances. Conversely, as independent cultures place greater value on personal choice for forming and maintaining their close relationships (Schug et al., 2010), only European Canadians showed strong N400 processing of incongruent emotions for close relationships. These findings have broadened our understanding of how culture influences neural social attention, providing evidence that it depends on relationship type.

Overall, these neuroscientific findings suggest that those who hold an interdependent social orientation are sensitive to interpersonal relationships, especially the relationship with acquaintances, who could be a potential source of stress experiences due to their strong interdependent social norms. If the social norms become salient, people perceive a strong risk in their relationships when they accidentally violate the norms.

Section Summary

As mentioned previously, findings of cultural psychology created the foundation of cultural neuroscience (e.g., Chiao, 2009; Han et al., 2013; Kitayama & Tompson, 2010; Kitayama & Uskul, 2011). Cultural neuroscientists maintain that the human brain is malleable, while also being influenced by external circumstances. Recent evidence in neuroscience that demonstrated that the human brain is malleably influenced by experiences and by the mastering of skills also supports this assertion (Maguire et al., 2000; Scholz et al., 2009).

The range of studies is not limited only to the issue of culture and attention. This new research field has provided scholars with insightful knowledge that culture indeed affects our neural patterns. This has been shown by using the ERP methods (e.g., Goto et al., 2010; Ishii et al., 2010; Kitayama & Murata, 2013; Kitayama & Park, 2014; Lewis et al., 2008; Masuda et al., 2014; Na & Kitayama, 2011; Russell et al., 2015; Varnum et al., 2012), fMRI methods (e.g., Chiao et al., 2009; Goh et al., 2007; Gutchess et al., 2006; Hedden et al., 2008; Zhu et al., 2007), and functional near-infrared spectroscopy (fNIRS) methods (Murata et al., 2015). As such, cultural neuroscience is a wonderful tool for enabling attention researchers to better understand the mechanisms underlying cultural differences in modes of attention.

For example, in the context of self versus significant other perception using the fMRI methods, Zhu et al. (2007) demonstrated that while the Chinese, as holders of interdependent social orientation, activated the *medial prefrontal cortex* (MPFC, which is associated with self-perception) when they thought of the self and the mother, but such a pattern of activation occurred only when Americans thought of the self. The results demonstrated that the Chinese were indeed interdependent, as shown when perceiving the concept of the self and the mother. Chiao et al. (2009) demonstrated that participants who endorse independent social orientation show greater MPFC activation when they judge whether the target word in general is applicable to them (the general self-description task), whereas people who endorse interdependent social orientation show greater MPFC activation when they think of the situation with their mother (the contextual self-description task). These findings suggest that sensitivity to interpersonal relationships is strongly associated with one's social orientation.

Culture, Attention, and Mental Health

Cultural neuroscience also has the potential to elucidate individual differences that mediate cultural beliefs, and to examine how such differences clarify the relationship between behavioral and neural patterns (e.g., Goto et al., 2010; Hedden et al., 2008; Ishii et al., 2010; Na & Kitayama, 2011; Russell et al., 2015). Furthermore, it has the potential to examine the differences among clinical individuals across cultures, while helping the field of culture and mental health flourish. To synthesize research on basic perceptual process and mental health, some researchers have recently initiated research projects. However, to date, only a limited number of studies have examined this possibility, notably the relationship between social orientation, pattern of attention, and well-being.

For example, Lee et al. (2021) investigated whether Japanese are more likely than North American counterparts to feel stress especially when they engage in an interpersonal relationship. Using a situation sampling method (Kitayama et al., 1997), they investigated cultural differences in how nonclinical European Canadians and Japanese evaluate their perceived stress of interpersonal events (which involve interactions with others) versus non-interpersonal events (which do not involve interactions with others). Consistent with prior research on cultural influences in social attention (Masuda, Ellsworth, et al., 2008; Russell et al., 2019), they found that European Canadians, who perceive themselves independent from relationships with others, showed more intense ratings of stress for non-interpersonal events relative to interpersonal ones, whereas Japanese, who perceive themselves embedded in relationships, tended to report interpersonal and non-interpersonal events as more equally stressful.

In a subsequent study, they further investigated the extent to which people manifest mental and physical symptoms of stress in response to culturally dominant interpersonal and non-interpersonal context. Specifically, they asked participants from each culture to imagine themselves experiencing a random selection of the previously collected situations and rate how likely they would be to experience their distress mentally (e.g., feeling depressed) or physically (e.g., having physical fatigue). Informed by the prior findings that the activation of culturally dominant social orientation intensifies emotional reactions (Chentsova-Dutton & Tsai, 2010), their results showed that European Canadians, who have independent social orientation, reported greater mental and physical symptoms of stress when they imagined themselves encountering non-interpersonal events than interpersonal ones. Conversely, Japanese, who have interdependent social orientation, reported greater mental symptoms of stress to interpersonal events than non-interpersonal ones. Notably, social orientation partially mediated the association between culture and mental symptoms from interpersonal events, showing that weaker independence partially explained why Japanese tend to experience stronger mental symptoms of stress from interpersonal events compared to European Canadians.

By broadening the clinical as well as the nonclinical population, this line of research on culture and stress has implications on the development of culturally appropriate stress coping programs for the prevention of clinically diagnosed mental disorders such as depression or anxiety disorder. However, few studies have examined whether basic processes of attention differ between the clinical and the nonclinical population (Amir et al., 2009), which may influence different coping styles between cultures (Lam & Zane, 2004). Thus, further research needs to examine the role of culturally shaped attention styles in coping with stress comparing the clinical versus the nonclinical population.

Researchers on culture-bound syndromes have further reported severely damaged well-being that is stronger than daily stress. In this section, we will review previous works on culture and mental health such as anxiety disorder, notably social phobia, which is dominant in North America, and taijinkyofusho (TKS) and hikikomori/NEET (Not in Employment, Education, or Training), which is dominant in Japan (e.g., Kirmayer, 1991; Kleinknecht et al., 1997; Uchida & Norasakkunkit, 2015).

Taijinkyofusho and Social Phobia

The culture-bound syndrome TKS is defined as a common Japanese psychiatric disorder characterized by a fear of offending or hurting others through one's awkward social behavior or imagined physical defect (Kirkmayer, 1991). People who suffer from this syndrome are likely to be excessively embarrassed about themselves or experience a fearful feeling of annoying others by their own appearances, faces, actions, looks, and even body odor. Kirkmayer (1991) discussed that TKS fits into the scheme of the *Diagnostic and Statistical Manual of Mental Disorders* (DSM) as a form of excessive social anxiety disorder. By contrasting the manifestation of social phobia common in North America and TKS common in Japan, Kleinknecht et al. (1997) discussed that one of the critical differences between social phobia and TKS is the locus of attention: while TKS is understood as a fear that the patients would offend or embarrass others (other-focused social anxiety), social phobia is understood as a fear that the patients would embarrass themselves (self-focused social anxiety). These investigations suggest that the reason TKS is dominant in Japan is due to people's interdependent social orientation.

Why do Japanese individuals with TKS feel their appearances make trouble for others? Why do Japanese individuals with TKS experience such a delusion? One possible answer is that they excessively internalize an interdependent social orientation where social harmony within their in-group is highly valued. In fact, compared to European Americans, Asian Americans' level of social phobia is greater, and their independent versus interdependent social orientation is directly associated with this pattern (Krieg & Xu, 2018). So, it is reasonable to speculate that East Asians feel stress due to their interdependent nature of social expectations. The findings from Lee et al. (2021) gave credence to this speculation—Japanese young adults indeed experience daily stress because of the tension in their public relationships (e.g., acquaintances in the workplace or friends at school settings), which require advanced social skills for conflict resolutions. Japanese participants in the Lee et al. (2021) study indeed described tensions, conflicts, and misunderstandings with their classmates, teammates, and coworkers. If this is the case, there is a strong potential that such stressful experiences lead people to experience more clinical symptoms.

Sato et al. (2014) paid attention to another type of theoretical framework—relational mobility. Relational mobility is defined as the subjective perception of societal dynamics (see Yuki et al., 2007, for review). In some societies, the relationship among others are long term, stable, and exclusive. In such circumstances, it is reasonable to assume that people become careful not to be rejected by others as it is difficult to find a new relationship with their static members in the community. However, in other types of societies, the relationships among others in their environment are short term, unstable, yet accessible, providing many relationship alternatives. In such circumstances, it is reasonable to assume that people do not have to be excessively sensitive to potential social rejection. A plethora of empirical findings suggested that East Asian societies are in general low in social mobility, whereas North American societies are in general high in social mobility. By recruiting the members of the low-mobility society (Japan) and the high-mobility society (United States), Sato et al. demonstrated that Japanese's fear of social rejection was higher than that of Americans. More interestingly, the level of relational mobility is partially mediated by the association between culture and social rejection.

There is an empirical paper that directly investigates the relationship between TKS and patterns of attention. Norasakkunkit et al. (2012) investigated the qualitative differences of these two types of social phobia tendencies: TKS, as a form of other-focused social anxiety common in Japan, and social phobia, as a form of self-focused social anxiety common in the United States. In this study participants completed measures of their social orientation, social phobia, and TKS, and engaged in the Frame and Line test, a context sensitivity test devised by Kitayama et al. (2003) to measure whether individuals find it easier to pay attention holistically or analytically. They demonstrated that social phobia tendencies were associated with decreased levels of holistic cognition. That is, the self-focused social phobia is negatively associated with the performance that requires context sensitivity. In contrast, TKS tendencies were associated with an increased level of holistic cognition, meaning that the other-focused social phobia is positively associated with the context sensitivity task.

Hikikomori/NEET

Hikikomori is another culture-bound syndrome where adolescents and adults withdraw from social life such as school, the workplace, and so on. It is often seen in the subcategory of NEET, the word of which originates from the British government's description of temporary unemployed youth (Department for Education, 2013). Individuals with hikikomori isolate themselves in their own bedrooms for over 6 months or more, with some continuing to practice this behavior for decades (Uchida & Norasakkunkit, 2015). In their report, the Japanese government estimated that there were about 700,000 individuals with hikikomori (Cabinet Office, Japanese Government, 2010). Many scholars have investigated the psychological tendencies of people with hikikomori by using the NEET/Hikikomori Spectrum (Uchida & Norasakkunkit, 2015), by separating hikikomori from depression or other DSM disorders (T. Saito, 1998; K. Saito, 2010), and by assessing a common ground between hikikomori and autism spectrum disorders. These findings suggest that hikikomori is a type of culture-bound syndrome that occurs mostly in postindustrial societies such as Japan. The range of the population who have the potential risk of developing hikikomori is quite broad. It is, of course, difficult to clinically diagnose or survey individuals with hikikomori because of their self-isolating practices. Therefore, researchers target nonclinical individuals and contrast the high-risk group with the low-risk group to delve into the psychological characteristics of individuals with hikikomori.

For example, Norasakkunkit and Uchida (2014) recruited nonclinical Japanese undergraduate students and asked them to fill out the hikikomori scale in order to divide them into the high-risk versus the low-risk group. They then examined their motivation to conform to others' behaviors. As seen previously, Japanese culture is high in interdependent social orientation. Therefore, conformity is often valued as a skill of maintaining harmony, which is an important cultural norm. The results indicated that, while both high- and low-risk participants share the importance of cultural norms, high-risk participants were less likely than their low-risk counterparts to be motivated to conform to others' behaviors. This difference is fully explained by their preferred levels of harmony seeking. That is, the high-risk group, as opposed to the low-risk group, did not value the maintenance of harmony and had a low level of the interdependent social orientation. Furthermore, the high-risk students were less likely to feel ambivalent about their local as well as global identity, indicating that one attribute of hikikomori is their marginalized identity.

Similarly, Ishii and Uchida (2016) recruited individuals who are categorized as NEETs, an upper category of hikikomori, and examined the relationship between NEET tendencies and the desire to engage in social activities. These experiments revealed that individuals with higher levels of NEET tendencies show a lower desire to engage in social activities. In a subsequent study, they recruited non-NEET students and investigated how they spontaneously attend to vocal tones, an indicator that measures context sensitivity and concerns toward others. The results revealed that there was a negative association between the NEET tendencies and attention to vocal tones, suggesting that when NEET tendencies increase, sensitivity to social and contextual factors decreases. Furthermore, NEET tendencies are negatively associated with an interdependent social orientation, which is dominant in Japan. This leaves individuals with higher NEET levels marginalized from the dominant Japanese social orientation.

In Norasakkunkit and Uchida's deceptive experimental setting (2011), Japanese low in NEET risk showed the dominant interdependent motivation; they put in effort to overcome their weaknesses and were more persistent on working on the task. Japanese high in NEET risk showed a completely deviant pattern from the typical Japanese data; they were more persistent when they received positive feedback than when they received negative feedback.

The patterns of effort in NEET individuals are also deviant from that of nonclinical Japanese individuals. In past cross-cultural data with nonclinical participants, Heine et al. (2001) demonstrated that whereas North Americans showed strong persistence to the target task when they received positive feedback, Japanese showed strong persistence to the target task when they received negative feedback. Heine et al. interpret these findings as the difference in their naïve beliefs about their skills and talents and their sense of self-actualization: North Americans share a naïve belief that one's skills and talents are in general innate and fixed, and therefore, to actualize themselves, they are highly motivated to search for their own unique talent and show a self-enhancing tendency. By referring to the findings, Norasakkunkit and Uchida (2011) tested whether NEET individuals' patterns of effort were deviant from that of non-NEET data. As they expected, the results indicated that Japanese participants with a low risk of becoming NEET were more persistent on working on a related task, showing the same motivational pattern as those in the Heine et al. (2001) study. However, NEET individuals' behavior was deviant from the interdependently oriented patterns and rather resembled the patterns observable in societies dominant in the independent social orientation. That is, they were more likely to persist in doing the task when they received positive feedback than when they received negative feedback of failure.

Section Summary

The maintenance of social harmony is one of the key characteristics of an interdependent social orientation (Talhelm et al., 2014; Vernum et al., 2010). East Asian cultures, or cultures that hold an interdependent social orientation, have historically developed a variety of practices for maintaining group harmony. For example, Asian participants are more likely than their North American counterparts to take other people's point of view when remembering memorable scenes (Cohen & Gunz, 2002). In comparison, Japanese people are more likely than European Americans to take a secondary control strategy—they report their willingness to adjust their behavior to match the behavior of others and accommodate themselves to the preset schedule (Morling et al., 2002). Likewise, Japanese people show persistence to the task, especially after receiving information that they have failed in an attempt to meet a standard or others' societal expectations (Heine et al., 2001).

Along with many scholars who have investigated culture-bound syndromes, we maintain that there are two types of clinical tendencies in the contemporary Japanese society: TKS and hikikomori/NEET. These syndromes are deviant from the mainstream interdependent social orientation in the contemporary Japanese culture, but the pattern of deviancy is opposite to each other. In the case of TKS, individuals hold an excessively interdependent social orientation. Therefore, they fail to control the balance between their own will and others' expectations, which leads them to withdraw from society. In contrast, in the case of hikikomori and NEET, individuals hold an excessively independent social orientation, the level of which, we assume, is way higher than North Americans. Therefore, they suffer from accommodating themselves to strong societal expectations in Japan and, at worst, from being unable to experience their own identity and marginalizing themselves in a society where an interdependent social orientation is dominant.

Conclusion

Recent scholars have debated the necessity of an interdisciplinary approach to cultural variations in basic psychological processes, neuroscience, well-being, and mental health. While many scholars have published review articles to overarch the aforementioned fields of research (e.g., Koelkebeck et al., 2017), only a limited number of works to date discuss concrete stories to depict a big picture for the promising field of research. In this chapter, we attempted to provide a brief but detailed report of recent findings in the field of cultural psychology and cultural neuroscience, and nominated two types of culture-bound syndromes, TKS and hikikomori/NEET, which we believe are worth investigating due to their basic psychological mechanisms and their unique attentional characteristics.

To make the story more concrete, we maintain that both individuals who suffer from two extreme patterns of culture-bound syndromes in Japan—taijinkyofusho and hikikomori/NEET individuals may also develop unique patterns of attention to social relationships. For example, different from the findings of Zhu et al. (2007), who conducted a cross-cultural fMRI study regarding Chinese and Americans' MPFC activation with their mother's representation, Japanese high in the hikikomori/NEET risk may reduce the level of MPFC activation even when they live in such a society where an interdependent social orientation is dominant.

Similarly, by using the ERP paradigm of Russell et al. (2019), who examined the differences of N400 activation in participants engaging in an attentional task within a social context, such as with close others and acquaintances, we identified unique brain wave patterns in Japanese at high risk for TKS and hikikomoro/NEET. In their study, Russell et al. (2019) asked participants to engage in an emotion judgment task by presenting a lineup of schematic faces and by manipulating the context of the lineups: acquaintances and close others. They identified that there was cultural variation in the level of N400 activation when participants were prevised with the context of acquaintances: Japanese were more likely than North Americans to activate N400, suggesting that they are especially attentive to the relationships among the lineups partially because their interdependent social norm becomes salient. The data from Lee et al. (2021) gave credence to this assumption—Japanese young adults reported interpersonal stress experiences especially in class, workplace, and public settings. If that is the case, those at high risk for TKS would produce excessively high levels of N400 activation when they perceive a series of face lineup images under the context of acquaintances as well as intimate friends. In contrast, those at high risk for hikikomori/NEET would show a completely different pattern; for example, they would not produce strong N400 activation with acquaintances, and we assume they would not do so even in a significant other condition such as family members, if we were to add such a condition.

As such, we could think of a variety of clinical syndromes that will be targets of research on culture, neuroscience, and mental health. We maintain that such an investigation is the right way to apply basic findings in the field of cultural psychology and cultural neuroscience to concrete clinical issues, and that it has academic and societal implications.

References

Amir, N., Beard, C., Burns, M., & Bomyea, J. (2009). Attention modification program in individuals with generalized anxiety disorder. *Journal of Abnormal Psychology, 118*, 28–33. https://dx.doi.org/10.1037/a0012589

Boduroglu, A., & Shah, P. (2017). Cultural differences in attentional breadth and resolution. *Culture and Brain, 5*, 169–181. https://dx.doi.org/10.1007/s40167-017-0056-9

Boduroğlu, A., Shah, P., & Nisbett, R. E. (2009). Cultural differences in allocation of attention in visual information processing. *Journal of Cross-Cultural Psychology, 40,* 349–360. https://dx.doi.org/10.1177/0022022108331005

Bruner, J. S. (1957). On perceptual readiness. *Psychological Review, 64,* 123–152.

Bruner, J. S. (1990). *Acts of meaning.* Harvard University Press.

Bruner, J. S., & Goodman, C. C. (1947). Value and need as organizing factors in perception. *Journal of Abnormal Social Psychology, 42,* 22–44.

Cabinet Office, Japanese Government. (2010). *Hikikomori ni kansuru jittai chosa* [An investigation of the nature of hikikomori]. Retrieved from http://www8.cao.go.jp/youth/kenkyu/hikikomori/pdf_index.html

Chentsova-Dutton, Y. E., & Tsai, J. L. (2010). Self-focused attention and emotional reactivity: The role of culture. *Journal of Personality and Social Psychology, 98,* 507–519. http://dx.doi.org/10.1037/a0018534

Chiao, J. Y. (2009). Cultural neuroscience: A once and future discipline. *Progress in Brain Research, 178,* 287–304. https://dx.doi.org/10.1016/S0079-6123(09)17821-4

Chiao, J. Y., Harada, T., Komeda, H., Li, Z., Mano, Y., Saito, D., Parrish, T. B., Sadato, N., & Iidaka, T. (2009). Neural basis of individualistic and collectivistic views of self. *Human Brain Mapping, 30,* 2813–2820. https://dx.doi.org/10.1002/hbm.20707

Chiu, L.-H. (1972). A cross-cultural comparison of cognitive styles in Chinese and American children. *International Journal of Psychology, 8,* 235–242.

Chua, F., Boland, J., & Nisbett, R. E. (2005). Cultural variation in eye movements during scene perception. *Proceedings of the National Academy of Sciences of the United States of America, 102,* 12629–12633. https://dx.doi.org/10.1073/pnas.0506162102

Chun, M. M., & Wolfe, J. M. (2001). Visual attention. In E. B. Goldstein (Ed.), *Blackwell's handbook of perception* (pp. 272–310). Blackwell.

Cohen, D., & Gunz, A. (2002). As seen by the other . . . : Perspectives on the self in the memories and emotional perceptions of Easterners and Westerners. *Psychological Science, 13,* 55–59. https://dx.doi.org/10.1111/1467-9280.00409

Department for Education. (2013, June 11). *16- to 18-year-olds not in education, employment or training (NEET).* https://www.gov.uk/government/publications/neet-data-by-local-authority-2012-16-to-18-year-olds-not-in-education-employment-or-training

Doherty, M. J., Tsuji, H., & Phillips, W. A. (2008). The context sensitivity of visual size perception varies across cultures. *Perception, 37,* 1426–1433. https://dx.doi.org/10.1068/p5946

Duffy, S., Toriyama, R., Itakura, S., & Kitayama, S. (2009). The development of culturally-contingent attention strategies in young children in the U.S. and Japan. *Journal of Experimental Child Psychology, 102,* 351–359. https://dx.doi.org/10.1016/j.jecp.2008.06.006

Fodor, J. A. (2008). *LOT 2: The language of thought revisited.* Clarendon Press.

Fong, M. C., Goto, S. G., Moore, C., Zhao, T., Shudson, Z., & Lewis, R. S. (2014). Switching between Mii and Wii: The effects of cultural priming on the social affective N400. *Culture and Brain, 2,* 52–71. https://dx.doi.org/10.1007/s40167-014-0015-7

Geertz, C. (1973). *The interpretation of cultures.* Basic Books.

Goh, J. O., Chee, M. W., Tan, J. C., Venkatraman, V., Hebrank, A., Leshikar, E. D., Jenkins, L., Sutton, B. P., Gutchess, A. H., & Park, D. C. (2007). Age and culture modulate object processing and object-scene binding in the ventral visual area. *Cognitive, Affective & Behavioral Neueroscience, 7,* 44–52. https://dx.doi.org/10.3758/CABN.7.1.44

Goto, S. G., Ando, Y., Huang, C., Yee, A., & Lewis, R. S. (2010). Cultural differences in the visual processing of meaning: Detecting incongruities between background and foreground objects using the N400. *Social Cognitive and Affective Neuroscience, 5,* 242–253. https://dx.doi.org/10.1093/scan/nsp038

Gutchess, A. H., Welsh, R. C., Boduroglu, A., & Park, D. C. (2006). Cross-cultural differences in the neural correlates of picture encoding. *Cognitive, Affective & Behavioral Neuroscience, 6,* 102–109. https://dx.doi.org/10.3758/CABN.6.2.102

Han, S., Northoff, G., Vogeley, K., Wexler, B. E., Kitayama, S., & Varnum, M. E. W. (2013). A cultural neuroscience approach to the biosocial nature of the human brain. *Annual Review of Psychology, 64,* 335–359. https://dx.doi.org/10.1146/annurev-psych-071112-054629

Hedden, T., Ketay, S., Aron, A., Markus, H. R., & Gabrieli, J. D. E. (2008). Cultural influences on neural substrates of attentional control. *Psychological Science, 19,* 12–17. https://dx.doi.org/10.1111/j.1467-9280.2008.02038.x

Heine, S. J., Kitayama, S., Lehman, D. R., Takata, T., Ide, E., Leung, C., & Matsumoto, H. (2001). Divergent consesequences of success and failure in Japan and North America. An investigation of self-improving motivations and malleable selves. *Journal of Personality and Social Psychology, 81*, 599–615. https://dx.doi.org/10.1037/0022-3514.81.4.599

Imada, T., Carlson, S. M., & Itakura, S. (2013). East-West differences in context-sensitivity are evident in early childhood. *Developmental Science, 16*, 198–208. https://dx.doi.org/10.1111/desc.12016

Ishii, K., & Kitayama, S. (2002). Processing of emotional utterances: Is vocal tone really more significant than verbal content in Japanese? *Cognitive Studies, 9*, 67–76.

Ishii, K., Kobayashi, Y., & Kitayama, S. (2010). Interdependence modulates the brain response to word-voice incongruity. *Social Cognitive and Affective Neuroscience, 5*, 307–317. https://dx.doi.org/10.1093/scan/nsp044

Ishii, K., Reyes, J. A., & Kitayama, S. (2003). Spontaneous attention to word content versus emotional tone: Differences among three cultures. *Psychological Science, 14*, 39–46. https://dx.doi.org/10.1111/1467-9280.01416

Ishii, K., Rule, N. O., & Toriyama, R. (2017). Context sensitivity in Canadian and Japanese children's judgments of emotion. *Current Psychology, 36*, 577–584. https://dx.doi.org/10.1007/s12144-016-9446-y

Ishii, K., & Uchida, Y. (2016). Japanese youth marginalization decreases interdependent orientation. *Journal of Cross-Cultural Psychology, 47*, 376–384 https://dx.doi.org/10.1177/0022022115621969

Ji, L. (2008). The leopard cannot change his spots, or can he? Culture and the development of lay theories of change. *Personality and Social Psychology Bulletin, 34*, 613–622. https://dx.doi.org/10.1177/0146167207313935

Ji, L. J., Peng, K., & Nisbett, R. E. (2000). Culture, control, and perception of relationships in the environment. *Journal of Personality and Social Psychology, 78*, 943–955. https://dx.doi.org/10,1037//0022-3514.78.5.943

Kirmayer, L. J. (1991). The place of culture in psychiatric nosology: Taijin kyofusho and DSM-III—R. *Journal of Nervous and Mental Disease, 179*, 19–28. http://dx.doi.org/10.1097/00005053-199101000-00005

Kitayama, S., Duffy, S., Kawamura, T., & Larsen, J. T. (2003). Perceiving an object and its context in different cultures: A cultural look at New Look. *Psychological Science, 14*, 201–206. https://dx.doi.org/10.1111/1467-9280.02432

Kitayama, S., & Ishii, K. (2002). Word and voice: Spontaneous attention to emotional utterances in two languages. *Cognition & Emotion, 16*, 29–59. https://dx.doi.org/10.1080/0269993943000121

Kitayama, S., Markus, H. R., Matsumoto, H., & Norasakkunkit, V. (1997). Individual and collective processes in the construction of the self: Self-enhancement in the United States and self-criticism in Japan. *Journal of Personality and Social Psychology, 72*, 1245–1267. http://dx.doi.org/10.1037/0022-3514.72.6.1245

Kitayama, S., & Murata, A. (2013). Culture modulates perceptual attention: An event-related potential study. *Social Cognition, 31*, 758–769. https://dx.doi.org/10.1521/soco.2013.31.6.758

Kitayama, S., & Park, J. (2014). Error-related brain activity reveals self-centric motivation: Culture matters. *Journal of Experimental Psychology: General, 143*, 62–70. https://dx.doi.org/10.1037/a0031696

Kitayama, S., & Tompson, S. (2010). Envisioning the future of cultural neuroscience. *Asian Journal of Social Psychology, 13*, 92–101. https://dx.doi.org/10.1111/j.1467-839X.2010.01304.x

Kitayama, S., & Uskul, A. K. (2011). Culture, mind, and the brain: Current evidence and future directions. *Annual Review of Psychology, 62*, 419–449. https://dx.doi.org/10.1146/annurev-psych-120709-145357

Kitayama, S., Varnum, M. E. W., & Salvador, C. M. (2019). Cultural neuroscience. In S. Kitayama & D. Cohen (Eds.), *Handbook of cultural psychology.* Guilford Press.

Kleinknecht, R. A., Dinnel, D. L., Kleinknecht, E. E., Hiruma, N., & Harada, N. (1997). Cultural factors in social anxiety: A comparison of social phobia symptoms and Taijin Kyofusho. *Journal of Anxiety Disorders, 11*, 157–177. https://dx.doi.org/10.1016/S0887-6185(97)00004-2

Ko, S. G., Lee, T. H., Yoon, H. Y., Kwon, J. H., & Mather, M. (2011). How does context affect assessments of facial emotion? The role of culture and age. *Psychology and Aging, 26*, 48–59. https://dx.doi.org/10.1037/a0020222.

Koelkebeck, K., Uwatoko, T., Tanaka, J., & Kret, M. E. (2017). How culture shapes social cognition deficits in mental disorders: A review. *Social Neuroscience, 12*, 102–112. https://dx.doi.org/10.1080/17470919.2016.1155482

Krieg, A., & Xu, Y. (2018). From self-construal to threat appraisal: Understanding cultural differences in social anxiety between Asian Americans and European Americans. *Cultural Diversity and Ethnic Minority Psychology.* Advance online publication. http://dx.doi.org/10.1037/cdp0000194

Kuwabara, M., & Smith, L. B. (2012). Cross-cultural differences in cognitive development: Attention to relations and objects. *Journal of Experimental Child Psychology*, *113*, 20–35. https://dx.doi.org/10.1016/j.jecp.2012.04.009

Kuwabara, M., & Smith, L. B. (2016). Cultural differences in visual object recognition in 3-year-old children. *Journal of Experimental Child Psychology*, *147*, 22–38. https://dx.doi.org/10.1016/j.jecp.2016.02.006

Kuwabara, M., Son, J., & Smith, L. B. (2011). Attention to context: U.S. and Japanese children's emotion judgment. *Journal of Cognition and Development*, *12*, 502–517. https://dx.doi.org/10.1080/15248372.2011.554927

Lam, A. G., & Zane, N. W. S. (2004). Ethnic differences in coping with interpersonal stressors: A test of self-construals as cultural mediators. *Journal of Cross-Cultural Psychology*, *35*, 446–459. https://dx.doi.org/10.1177/0022022104266108

Lee, H., Masuda, T., Ishii, K., Yasuda, Y.,& Ohtsubo, Y., (2021). Cultural differences in the perception of daily stress between European Canadian and Japanese undergraduate students. *Personality and Social Psychology Bulletin*.

Leung, A. K., & Cohen, D. (2011). Within- and between-culture variation: Individual differences and the cultural logics of honor, face, and dignity cultures. *Journal of Personality and Social Psychology*, *100*, 507–526. http://dx.doi.org/10.1037/a0022151

Lewis, R. S., Goto, S. G., & Kong, L. (2008). Culture and context: East Asian, American and European American differences in p3 event-related potentials. *Personality and Social Psychology Bulletin*, *34*, 623–634. https://dx.doi.org/10.1177/0146167207313731

Maguire, E. A., Gadian, D. G., Johnsrude, I. S., Good, C. D., Ashburner, J., Frackowiak, R. S., & Frith, C. D. (2000). Navigation-related structural change in the hippocampi of taxi drivers. *Proceedings of the National Academy of Science of the United States of America*, *97*, 4398–4403. https://dx.doi.org/10.1073/pnas.070039597

Markus, H., & Kitayama, S. (1991). Culture and the self: Implications for cognition, emotion, and motivation. *Psychological Review*, *98*, 224–253.

Markus, H. R., & Kitayama, S. (2010). Cultures and selves: A cycle of mutual constitution. *Perspectives on Psychological Science*, *5*, 420–430. https://dx.doi.org/10.1177/1745691610375557Masuda, T. (2017). Culture and attention: Recent empirical findings and new directions in cultural psychology. *Social and Personality Psychology Compass*, *11*, e12363. https://dx.doi.org/10.1111/spc3.12363

Masuda, T., Akase, M., Radford, M. H. B., & Wang, H. (2008). Jokyo youin ga gankyu undo pattern ni oyobosu eikyo: Nihonjin to Seiyojin no syuken jyoho heno binkansa no kikaku kenkyu [Cross-cultural research on the pattern of eye-movement: Comparing the level of concentration between Japanese and Western participants]. *Japanese Journal of Psychology*, *79*, 35–43.

Masuda, T., Ellsworth, P. C., Mesquita, B., Leu, J., Tanida, S., & van de Veerdonk, E. (2008). Placing the face in context: Cultural differences in the perception of facial emotion. *Journal of Personality and Social Psychology*, *94*, 365–381. http://dx.doi.org/10.1037/0022-3514.94.3.365

Masuda, T., Ishii, K., & Kimura, J. (2016). When does the culturally dominant mode of attention appear or disappear? Comparing patterns of eye movement during the visual flicker task between European Canadians and Japanese. *Journal of Cross-Cultural Psychology*, *47*, 997–1014. https://dx.doi.org/10.1177/0022022116653830

Masuda, T., Nand, K., Lee, H., Shimizu, Y., Li, L. M. W., Takada, A., Uchida, Y., Sawa Senzaki, S., & Kodama, M. (2019). *The emergence of culturally dominant modes of attention in 7- to 10-year-old Canadian and Japanese children: The role of reasoning style*. Manuscript submitted for publication. University of Alberta.

Masuda, T., & Nisbett, R. E. (2001). Attending holistically vs. analytically: Comparing the context sensitivity of Japanese and Americans. *Journal of Personality and Social Psychology*, *81*, 922–934.

Masuda, T., & Nisbett, R. E. (2006). Culture and change blindness. *Cognitive Science*, *30*, 381–399. https://dx.doi.org/10.1207/s15516709cog0000_63

Masuda, T., Russell, M. J., Chen, Y. Y., Hioki, K., & Caplan, J. B. (2014). N400 incongruity effect in an episodic memory task reveals different strategies for handling irrelevant contextual information for Japanese than European Canadians. *Cognitive Neuroscience*, *5*, 17–25. https://dx.doi.org/10.1080/17588928.2013.831819

Masuda, T., Russell, M. J., Li, L. M. W., & Lee, H. (2019). Perception and cognition. In S. Kitayama & D. Cohen (Eds.), *Handbook of cultural psychology* (pp. 222–245). Guilford Press.

Masuda, T., Wang, H., Ishii, K., & Ito, K. (2012). Do surrounding figures' emotions affect judgment of the target figure's emotion? Comparing the eye-movement patterns of European Canadians, Asian Canadians, Asian international students, and Japanese. *Frontier in Integrative Neuroscience*, *6*, 72. https://dx.doi.org/10.3389/fnint.2012.00072.

Matsumoto, D., Kwang, H. S., & Yamada, H. (2010). Cultural differences in the relative contributions of face and context to judgments of emotions. *Journal of Cross-Cultural Psychology*, *43*, 198–218. https://dx.doi.org/10.1177/0022022110387426

Miller, J. G. (1984). Culture and the development of everyday social explanation. *Journal of Personality and Social Psychology*, *46*, 961–978.

Miller, J. G. (1999). Cultural psychology: Implications for basic psychological theory. *Psychological Science*, *10*, 85–91. https://dx.doi.org/10.1111/1467-9280.00113

Miyamoto, Y. (2013). Culture and analytic versus holistic cognition: Toward multilevel analyses of cultural influences. *Advances in Experimental Social Psychology*, *47*, 131–188. https://dx.doi.org/10.1016/B978-0-12-407236-7.00003-6

Miyamoto, Y., Yoshikawa, S., & Kitayama, S. (2011). Feature and configuration in face processing: Japanese are more configural than Americans. *Cognitive Science*, *35*, 563–574. https://dx.doi.org/10.1111/j.1551-6709.2010.01163.x

Morling, B., Kitayama, S., & Miyamoto, Y. (2002). Cultural practices emphasize influence in the United States and adjustment in Japan. *Personality and Social Psychology Bulletin*, *28*, 311–323. https://dx.doi.org/10.1177/0146167202286003

Murata, A., Park, J., Kovelman, I., Xiaosu, H., & Kitayama, S. (2015). Culturally non-preferred cognitive tasks require compensatory attention: A functional near infrared spectroscopy (fNIRS) investigation. *Culture and Brain*, *3*, 53–67. https://dx.doi.org/10.1007/s40167-015-0027-y

Na, J., & Kitayama, S. (2011). Spontaneous trait inference is culture-specific behavioral and neural evidence. *Psychological Science*, *22*, 1025–1032. https://dx.doi.org/10.1177/0956797611414727

Nisbett, R. E. (2003). *The geography of thought*. Free Press.

Nisbett, R. E., & Masuda, T. (2003). Culture and point of view. *Proceedings of the National Academy of Sciences of the United States of America*, *100*, 11163–11175. https://dx.doi.org/10.1073/pnas.1934527100

Nisbett, R. E., & Miyamoto, Y. (2005). The influence of culture: Holistic versus analytic perception. *Trends in Cognitive Sciences*, *9*, 467–473. https://dx.doi.org/10.1016/j.tics.2005.08.004

Nisbett, R. E., Peng, K., Choi, I., & Norenzayan, A. (2001). Culture and systems of thought: Holistic vs. analytic cognition. *Psychological Review*, *108*, 291–310. http://dx.doi.org/10.1037/0033-295X.108.2.291

Norasakkunkit, V., Kitayama, S., & Uchida, Y. (2012). Social anxiety and holistic cognition: Self-focused social anxiety in the United States and other-focused social anxiety in Japan. *Journal of Cross-Cultural Psychology*, *43*, 742–757. https://dx.doi.org/10.1177/0022022111405658

Norasakkunkit, V., & Uchida, Y. (2011). Psychological consequences of postindustrial anomie on self and motivation among Japanese youth. *Journal of Social Issues*, *67*, 774–786. https://dx.doi.org/10.1111/j.1540-4560.2011.01727.x

Norasakkunkit, V., & Uchida, Y. (2014). To conform or to maintain self-consistency? Hikikomori risk in Japan and the deviation from seeking harmony. *Journal of Social and Clinical Psychology*, *33*, 918–935. https://dx.doi.org/10.1521/jscp.2014.33.10.918

Pinker, S. (1994). *The language instinct*. Morrow.

Pinker, S. (1997). *How the mind works*. W. W. Norton.

Pinker, S. (2007). *The stuff of thought: Language as a window into human nature*. Viking.

Posner, M. I. (1980). Orienting of attention. *Quarterly Journal of Experimental Psychology*, *32*, 3–25.

Pylyshyn, Z. W. (1999). Is vision continuous with cognition? The case for cognitive impenetrability of visual perception. *Behavioral and Brain Sciences*, *22*, 341–423.

Russell, M. J., Masuda, T., Hioki, K., & Singhal, A. (2015). Culture and social judgments: The importance of culture in Japanese and European Canadians' N400 and LPC processing of face lineup emotion judgments. *Culture and Brain*, *3*, 131–147. https://dx.doi.org/10.1007/s40167-015-0032-1

Russell, M. J., Masuda, T., Hioki, K., & Singhal, A. (2019). Culture and neuroscience: How Japanese and European Canadians process social context in close and acquaintance relationships. *Social Neuroscience*, *14*(4), 484–498. https://dx.doi.org/10.1080/17470919.2018.1511471

Saito, K. (2010). *Guideline of assessment and support for hikikomori*. Ministry of Health, Labour, and Welfare. Retrieved from http://www.ncgmkohnodai. go.jp/pdf/jidouseishin/22ncgm_hikikomori.pdf

Saito, T. (1998). *Shakaiteki hikikomori: Owaranai shishunki* [Social withdrawal: A neverending adolescence]. PHPShinsho.

Sato, K., Yuki, M., & Norasakkunkit, V. (2014). A socio-ecological approach to cross-cultural differences in the sensitivity to social rejection: The partially mediating role of relational mobility. *Journal of Cross-Cultural Psychology*, *45*, 1549–1560. https://dx.doi.org/10.1177/0022022114544320

Savani, K., & Markus, H. R. (2012). A processing advantage associated with analytic perceptual tendencies: European Americans outperform Asians on multiple object tracking. *Journal of Experimental Social Psychology*, *48*, 766–769. https://dx.doi.org/10.1016/j.jesp.2012.01.005

Scholz, J., Klein, M. C., Behrens, T. E. J., & Johansen-Berg, H. (2009). Training induces changes in white-matter architecture. *Nature Neuroscience*, *12*, 1370–1371.

Schug, J., Yuki, M., & Maddux, W. (2010). Relational mobility explains between- and within-culture differences in selfdisclosure to close friends. *Psychological Science*, *21*, 1471–1478. https://dx.doi.org/10.1177/0956797610382786

Senzaki, S., Masuda, T., & Ishii, K. (2014). When is perception top-down and when is it not? Culture, narrative, and attention. *Cognitive Science*, *38*, 1493–1506.

Senzaki, S., Masuda, T., Takada, A., & Okada, H. (2016). The communication of culturally dominant modes of attention from parents to children: A comparison of Canadian and Japanese parent-child conversations during a joint scene description task. *PLoS One*, *11*, e0147199. https://dx.doi.org/10.1371/journal.pone.0147199

Shweder, R. A. (1991). Cultural psychology: What is it? In R. Shweder (Ed.), *Thinking through culture* (pp. 73–110). Harvard University Press.

Stanley, J. T., Zhang, X., Fung, H. H., & Isaacowitz, D. M. (2013). Cultural differences in gaze and emotion recognition: Americans contrast more than Chinese. *Emotion*, *13*, 36–46. http://dx.doi.org/10.1037/a0029209

Talhelm, T., Zhang, X., Oishi, S., Shimin, C., Duan, D., Lan, X., & Kitayama, S. (2014). Large-scale psychological differences within China explained by rice versus wheat agriculture. *Science*, *344*, 603–608. https://dx.doi.org/10.1126/science.1246850

Tsivilis, D., Otten, L. J., & Rugg, M. D. (2001). Context effects on the neural correlates of recognition memory: An electrophysiological study. *Neuron*, *31*, 497–505. https://dx.doi.org/10.1016/S0896-6273(01)00376-2

Uchida, Y., & Norasakkunkit, V. (2015). The NEET and Hikikomori spectrum: Assessing the risks and consequences of becoming culturally marginalized. *Frontiers in Psychology*, *6*, 1117. https://dx.doi.org/10.3389/fpsyg.2015.01117

Uskul, A. K., Kitayama, S., & Nisbett, R. E. (2008). Ecocultural basis of cognition: Farmers and fishermen are more holistic than herders. *Proceedings of the National Academy of Sciences*, *105*, 8552–8556. https://dx.doi.org/10.1073/pnas.0803874105

Varnum, M. E., Grossmann, I., Kitayama, S., & Nisbett, R. E. (2010). The origin of cultural differences in cognition: The social orientation hypothesis. *Current Directions in Psychological Science*, *19*, 9–13. https://dx.doi.org/10.1177/0963721409359301

Varnum, M. E. W., Na, J., Murata, A., & Kitayama, S. (2012). Social class differences in N400 indicate differences in spontaneous trait inference. *Journal of Experimental Psychology: General*, *141*, 518–526. https://dx.doi.org/10.1037/a0026104

Yeung, N., Botvinick, M. M., & Cohen, J. D. (2004). The neural basis of error detection: Conflict monitoring and the errorrelated negativity. *Psychological Review*, *111*, 931–959. http://dx.doi.org/10.1037/0033-295X.111.4.931

Yuki, M., Schug, J., Horikawa, H., Takemura, K., Sato, K., Yokota, K., & Kamaya, K. (2007). *Development of a scale to measure perceptions of relational mobility in society* (CERSS Working Paper 75). Hokkaido University, Center for Experimental Research in Social Sciences.

Zhang, B., & Seo, H. S. (2015). Visual attention toward food-item images can vary as a function of background saliency and culture: An eye-tracking study. *Food Quality and Preference*, *41*, 172–179. https://dx.doi.org/10.1016/j.foodqual.2014.12.004

Zhu, Y., Zhang, L., Fan, J., & Han, S. (2007). Neural basis of cultural influence on self-representation. *Neuroimage*, *34*, 1310–1316. https://dx.doi.org/10.1016/j.neuroimage.2006.08.047

Culture and Numerical Cognition

Rongxiang Tang *and* Yi-Yuan Tang

Abstract

The basic ability to encode numerical information and discriminate numerical quantity can be found in humans as well as certain nonhuman primates. However, humans are unique in that they can perform advanced numerical computation using abstract numerical symbols and number words after receiving formal mathematical instruction. Although similarities exist in numerical cognition and its associated mental processes across people, culture plays a dominant role in shaping how numbers are differentially represented and processed across various cultural groups that speak different languages. Additionally, the development of advanced numeracy skills through formal education is heavily influenced by cultural-specific factors such as parental expectation and societal norms. Understanding such cultural differences would not only profoundly advance the scientific knowledge regarding numerical cognition but also have critical implications for mathematics education and the development of intervention programs for ameliorating potential deficits related to arithmetic ability such as dyscalculia. The focus of this chapter is to provide an overview of how numerical cognition is shaped by culture, discuss pragmatic implications of cultural differences in numerical processing for education and mental health, and conclude with suggestive future directions of research pertaining to cultural differences in numerical cognition.

Key Words: cultural differences, numerical cognition, mathematics education, arithmetic processing, dyscalculia, cognitive neuroscience, cultural neuroscience, global mental health

Introduction

Numerical cognition involves fundamental processes such as the perception, representation, and computation of quantities, which have been extensively studied in psychology and cognitive neuroscience (Göbel et al., 2011). Although research has demonstrated that humans and other primates (i.e., birds, mammals) share the innate ability to discriminate and compare numerical magnitudes (Hubbard et al., 2008), humans are unique in that we are able to compute and perform sophisticated mental arithmetic through learning and developing advanced mathematical skills (Ansari, 2008). For humans in contemporary modern society, numerical cognition relies largely on using numeration systems including abstract numerical symbols such as Arabic numerals or number words to represent and communicate numerical information and to perform mental calculation of mathematical problems. Notably, Arabic numerals, the universal and systematic symbolic representation of numbers, are the result of recent cultural inventions that did not exist back in the beginning of civilization (Göbel et al., 2011). For example, before the widespread implementation of the Arabic numeral system and other similar systems within different cultures, humans had a long history of using body parts such as fingers and hands as convenient tools for representing numbers and their quantities (Butterworth, 1999; Domahs et al., 2010). Nonetheless, as quantities grew in magnitude, humans had to develop alternative and more efficient ways to effectively describe and communicate numerical information.

From an evolutionary perspective, the birth of numeration systems is arguably not an immediate result of natural selection, as we are not born with the innate conceptualization of numeration systems. Instead, we developed these remarkable and sophisticated systems and passed them down to the next generation, for whom the understanding and utilization of such systems must be learned. Therefore, it is evident that numerical cognition is highly culturally dependent, as culture gives rise to not only numeral systems but also languages that allow people to communicate numerical concepts and acquire higher-order numerical abilities and skills (Verguts & Chen, 2017). The present chapter will focus on discussing the processes of numerical cognition that are specifically influenced by culture, with an emphasis on the neural correlates of cultural differences in numerical cognition. The discussion will also extend to cover the implications of cultural differences in numerical cognition for education and mental health by describing possible ways through which mathematics education could be improved by considering cultural factors. Additionally, the potential of developing culture-specific prevention and intervention programs for people with arithmetic deficits will be discussed. Finally, we will provide suggestions of new research directions to facilitate further investigation into culture and numerical cognition.

Cultural Influences on Numerical Cognition

Most fundamental numerical capacities such as the ability to perceive and compare quantities exhibit considerable similarities across people, regardless of their cultural background. Despite these shared basic commonalities, substantial culture-specific variations can be observed both in symbolic representations of numerosity through numeration systems and in brain representations of numerical processing, especially when higher-order cognitive processes such as mental arithmetic and complex calculation are involved (Ansari, 2008; Göbel et al., 2011). As humans learn to acquire basic and advanced numerical skills through daily environmental exposure and formal mathematics education, it is not surprising that culture-specific influences such as language, educational system, and cultural expectation would inevitably contribute to variations in numerical cognition across different cultural groups, as these factors are heavily involved in the development and acquisition of numeracy skills (Tang & Liu, 2009).

One of the notable inventions facilitating complex numerical cognition is numeration systems, which marked a major milestone in human evolution and serve the basis for higher-order cognitive processing of numerical information, as well as interpersonal communication of abstract numerical concepts. Numeration systems, whether notational or purely based on languages (i.e., number words), are indispensable cognitive tools critical for basic numerical ability such as counting (Beller & Bender, 2008). In fact, decades of research have deemed numeration systems as cultural-specific tools that exemplify unique cultural variations, predominately influenced and constrained by linguistic origins and cultural contexts (Bender & Beller, 2011). For instance, the Polynesian and Micronesian cultures and languages shared a common origin—the Oceania, which dates back 6,000 years. Yet while they each evolved and settled into distinct cultural and language groups, their numeration systems also diverged into somewhat different paths, such that Polynesian languages invented specific counting systems for certain objects, whereas Micronesian languages developed the numeral classifier systems (Bender & Beller, 2011). Although it is difficult to pinpoint the exact reasons behind such distinct development of numeration systems for two once-similar cultures, some theorists have suggested that the specific counting systems for objects in Polynesian culture were motivated by socioeconomic reasons, since Polynesian islanders often need to coordinate and redistribute valuable resources within the community to sustain their livelihood (Bender & Beller, 2011). Therefore, the importance of performing complex mental arithmetic in large quantities may likely prompt the gradual cultural-specific development of numeration systems, which undoubtedly facilitate pertinent processes of numerical cognition. Looking at a macro-level, there is similar evidence showing that even when language posits constraints on numeration systems or when the inherited numeration systems are becoming less useful, people within different cultures are often able to flexibly adapt their existing counting systems by extending the limits of counting and developing more creative strategies to cope with potential cognitive challenges associated with complex numerical cognition (Beller & Bender, 2008).

Apart from the cultural evolution of numerical cognition through development of numeration systems, higher-order numeracy skills and abilities can also be significantly influenced by cultural values and norms. One early yet interesting behavioral study conducted nearly two decades ago described the general effects of cultural-related influences on simple arithmetic performance among native Chinese students, Chinese Canadians, and native Canadians. Through multistep arithmetic calculation tasks, the authors showed that native Chinese students outperformed both Chinese Canadians and native Canadians in complex arithmetic calculation such as multiple steps of subtraction, multiplication, and division, indicating that there may be unique cultural effects on educational systems or schooling that induce cross-cultural differences in arithmetic ability (Campbell & Xue, 2001). The authors also demonstrated some nonspecific cultural effects on simple arithmetic ability, such that native Chinese students and Chinese Canadians, despite each receiving different formal education in mathematics, were virtually equivalent in all aspects of simple arithmetic performance in basic operations (i.e., 3 + 4, 7 × 4), whereas native Canadians exhibited poorer performance, even though they received the same mathematical education as Chinese Canadians (Campbell & Xue, 2001). Together, these findings offered one of the first lines of evidence highlighting the role of cultural factors in contributing to differential numerical competencies across unique cultural groups. Additionally, these studies suggested that for simple arithmetic ability, cross-cultural differences in formal education in mathematics do not necessarily account for variations in arithmetic performance, indicating that a vast range of other possibilities including but not limited to extracurricular activities, culturally dependent familial influences, and values may likely put Chinese Canadians in an advantageous situation with regard to numerical abilities.

Indeed, some of the early reports consistently showed that motivational factors, such as proactively seeking out additional academic training in mathematics and positive attitudes toward mathematical learning in Asian Americans, are likely to contribute to superior arithmetic ability when compared to Caucasian Americans (Chen & Stevenson, 1995; Geary et al., 1997). However, it is still inconclusive as to how cultural factors such as values and norms exert the strongest influence over differential arithmetic performance between cultural groups or which cultural factors may act independently or together to interact with other psychological factors to induce such differences in numeracy skills. In this regard, it may be particularly useful to consider cultural factors in conjunction with relevant psychological factors such as motivation and emotion to better understand the role of culture in numerical cognition. For a related discussion regarding culture and psychology, readers can refer to the chapter 3 by Matsumoto and Hwang within this volume.

Following this behavioral report of cultural differences in arithmetic ability, advances in neuroimaging techniques have provided another new avenue for investigating the neural bases of cultural differences in numerical cognition such as mental representation of numbers and mental arithmetic. Almost two decades of research have revealed several key and converging brain regions relevant for numerical processing, including the intraparietal sulcus (IPS) and inferior parietal lobule (IPL; Ansari, 2008; Dehaene et al., 2004), as well as the primary area involving higher-order cognition—the prefrontal cortex. Among these insightful research findings, one neuroimaging study specifically examined differences in neural representations of numerical cognition between native Chinese speakers and native English speakers during simple numerical addition and comparison tasks that involve Arabic numerals. As Arabic numerals are universally used abstract numerical symbols in modern society, they served as excellent stimuli from which cultural differences, if any, can be examined. By comparing brain activation and functional connectivity between these two cultural groups, Tang and colleagues found that English speakers recruited more left perisylvian cortex including Broca's and Wernicke's areas associated with speech production and comprehension during simple addition and comparison tasks, suggesting the putative role of language in numerical processing, while Chinese speakers engaged more frontal-parietal premotor association regions, indicating a distinct neural pathway that may rely on visuospatial processes for numerical tasks (Tang et al., 2006). Further, it was found that as the arithmetic loading increased, there was a trend of increase in the premotor activation of Chinese speakers but not of the English speakers. Together, these results imply that cultural-specific functional differences in numerical cognition can be detected within the brain, especially during mental arithmetic tasks. Furthermore, not only may these specific neurobiological correlates give rise to these observed behavioral differences but also such differences may suggest that culture could possibly lead to dissociable neural mechanisms or pathways of numerical cognition (Tang & Liu, 2009).

Several interpretations could be offered as to why Chinese speakers and English speakers exercise different brain regions and networks during the same arithmetic task. As suggested by Tang and colleagues (2006, 2009), as well as by other researchers, language could be one of the critical cultural factors affecting numerical cognition, as each culture typically has a distinct way of pronouncing and representing numbers (Gelman & Butterworth, 2005). For Chinese speakers, the acquisition of language depends heavily on learning logographic characters and memorizing each stroke and subcharacter making up individual characters, which could result in repeated activation of the visuomotor association area during language processing (Tan et al., 2005; Tang & Liu, 2009). Given that language serves a critical role in facilitating numerical processing, the ancillary engagement of language processes during numerical tasks for Chinese speakers may manifest as increased activation in visuomotor regions of the brain. On the other hand, English is relatively phonetic, which may explain why Broca's area is more engaged during numerical tasks, since Broca's area is associated with speech production. Nonetheless, the scientific research regarding cultural influences on the neural mechanisms of numerical cognition is still in progress, as we often have to infer the role of culture in how it shapes neural processes related to numerical cognition given empirical constraints that preclude us from following the longitudinal development of numerical skills at the individual level within different cultural contexts. Interested readers are encouraged to explore other chapters (chapter 5 by Chiao, Mano, Li, Bebko, Blizinsky, & Turner; chapter 20 by Goh) within this volume that focus primarily on neuroimaging research of culture and how cultural influences may physically shape our brain.

In addition to the role of language in cultural differences of numerical cognition, educational systems add another layer of influence over performance in mental arithmetic, as indicated by the aforementioned findings of Campbell and Xue (2001). In general, mathematical education in kindergarten through 12th grade is far more rigorous in Asian culture than in Western culture, which often includes formal instruction of more complex and advanced mathematical knowledge and problem solving that are not typically found in textbooks or in mathematical curriculum in Western culture (Göbel et al., 2011; Leung, 2001; Tang & Liu, 2009). Lastly, cultural perception of the importance of mathematics could also affect the motivation for learning, as Asian culture typically has a well-established tradition of emphasizing mathematical learning and performing well in examinations compared to Western culture (Hess et al., 1987; Leung, 2001). This unique and culture-dictated conceptualization of the importance of arithmetic competence has integrated excelling in mathematics as a part of Asian identities, which in some sense reinforces the already rigorous educational system toward training numeracy skills, ultimately leading to increased likelihood of superior performance in mathematics for people with an Asian cultural background.

Implications of Cultural Differences in Numerical Cognition for Education and Health

Following the previous discussion, the role of culture in affecting and enhancing arithmetic performance should not be overlooked or underestimated when we consider ways through which we could advance and improve our education in mathematics. Research into cross-cultural differences in numerical cognition have advanced our scientific understanding of how culture shapes numerical processing, yet practical implications of such knowledge are also worth emphasizing, especially since culture-specific influences are ingrained in mathematics education (Leung, 2001, 2006). Therefore, exploiting knowledge of cultural differences in numerical cognition and related processes, specifically between Asian and Western cultures, may help bolster academic performance in mathematics and would allow us to adequately evaluate and adapt useful educational practices from different cultures such as teaching styles and learning attitudes for potential application in real-world educational settings (Leung, 2001, 2006). Although not much has been done in this area of research, it is important to at least start considering these cultural differences with the hope of improving numeracy skills in students from Western cultures.

In two systematic and direct comparisons of mathematics education between Asian and Western cultures, Leung described several important sources of cultural differences in values and practices with regard to mathematics education, which may explain why Asians often excel and outperform their Western counterparts in mathematics. One important difference is the fact that Asians place a particularly strong emphasis on education and gaining competence in the subjects that are being taught in school through hard work and dedication (Leung, 2001, 2006). This emphasis helps establish a positive cycle between teachers and students, in which teachers have the goal of proactively leading and monitoring students toward competence in mathematics, and students have the strong motivation to excel in mathematics, perhaps due to cultural expectation or individual goals of attaining high achievement. However, this cycle could also turn vicious if students do not hold the same cultural values and goals that society expected them to have. Additionally, Leung (2001, 2006) pointed out a key difference in learning strategies between Asian and Western cultures, such that Asian teachers believe in repeated practices with increasing variations that eventually lead to understanding and competence in mathematics, rather than focusing on teaching understanding of the concepts as the priority. This stands in stark contrast to the Western style of teaching, where practicing without thoroughly understanding is not favored as a way of learning. Interestingly, there is some evidence suggesting that the Asian tradition of teaching mathematics may be more effective in enhancing performance (Hess & Azuma, 1991), though this claim remains to be determined by more rigorous research that can directly compare these two distinct learning strategies.

From a developmental perspective, the acquisition of numerical concepts and tools for higher-order numeracy capacities is fundamentally a process of enculturation, as Beller and colleagues (2018) eloquently argued in their most recent review regarding the challenges in numerical cognition and mathematical education. The learning and educative process, as most of us remember, started very early during our childhood with the enculturating practices of collective life, in which siblings and parents participate in daily counting activities and games that involve rudimentary mathematical concepts. An early study by Saxe et al. (1987) described a wide range of practices related to mathematical skills that middle-class parents frequently engaged in with their children, such as learning basic number words and utilizing such words to count objects, or even learning to perform simple arithmetic. Throughout this social interacting process that created numerical environments for children, both parents and children play active roles in facilitating the acquisition of numeracy skills. Additionally, parents are constantly adjusting the content of their interaction in response to the progress of children, which undoubtedly serves a critical role in the initial acquisition and development of numerical abilities (Beller et al., 2018). In cultures where numeracy skills are valued highly, as opposed to cultures that place less emphasis on numeracy skills, one would undoubtedly be exposed in the early stages of life to such enculturating practices of mathematical education, which do not need to happen in formal education settings but do tend to work in one's favor with respect to later structured training and education in mathematics when one enters school. Likewise, in primary education settings, cultural influences are embedded throughout the didactic teaching of numeracy skills, likely resembling the way they exert their influence within the aforementioned familial contexts during the early childhood years, particularly for those cultures that emphasize the importance of numerical abilities.

The implications of culture in the development of numeracy competence and mathematical education can have far-reaching impacts on societal levels as evident from the previous sections. For educators and parents who valued children's competence in mathematics, they face the challenges of increasing the general awareness of their surrounding culture with regard to the importance of numerical competence and creating a "microculture" early in development where positive interaction and values are transmitted to children during the acquisition of numeracy skills. Once children enter into primary education settings, the role of teachers now weighs more heavily than that of parents, who should nonetheless continue to create a "culture" that fosters learning and is dedicated to mathematical education.

Switching from education to global mental health, cultural differences in numerical cognition could also have relevance for understanding and potentially ameliorating deficits in numerosity. While having the ability to be able to process numerical information may be taken for granted, a small portion of the population suffers from arithmetic disability, characterized by difficulties in learning arithmetic and processing numerosity, which can be found in people with normal intelligence and cognitive function, as well as those with other developmental disorders such as attention deficit hyperactivity disorder (Butterworth et al., 2011). This deficit is called dyscalculia, which could result in significant economic consequences for a nation's gross domestic product growth and devastate individuals with low numeracy by limiting their job opportunities and decreasing their mental health (Butterworth et al., 2011). Research thus far has not provided evidence regarding the differential prevalence of dyscalculia or other deficits related to numerical processing across cultures. In fact, research seems to suggest that people from Asian cultures are also not immune to such deficits in processing numerosity and performing arithmetic (Chan et al., 2013; Ho et al., 2015). Therefore, finding ways to prevent and intervene in these deficits would be highly important for promoting global mental health.

Although it may seem as if culture is irrelevant for understanding or developing interventions for deficits in mathematics and numerical processing, education remains the primary approach in improving numeracy skills in children who have dyscalculia (Butterworth et al., 2011; Gifford, 2006). Previous research has suggested that preventative small-group tutoring could be a valuable resource to provide tailored training in mathematics beyond that offered in the general classroom setting (Fuchs et al., 2012). When noticing the first signs of mathematical difficulties, such prevention and intervention approaches could readily help students without leaving them far behind their peers. In addition to dedicating resources to students with deficits in numerical abilities, cultural support could further dissuade students from feeling pressure because of their deficits. As cultural influences are deeply entrenched in mathematical education, being sensitive to popular cultural values and attitudes would undoubtedly benefit the process of intervention. For instance, for children in Asian cultures, those who have dyscalculia may be particularly affected by the cultural expectation of attaining high achievement in mathematics, which could negatively influence their learning and self-perception. It is therefore important to take such cultural factors into account during intervention and targeted education. Nonetheless, existing research into dyscalculia and its interventions is still in its infancy, but subsequent efforts in advancing this field of research would be greatly informed by considering specific cultural factors and differences relevant for numerical cognition and processes.

Conclusions and Future Directions

In this chapter, we reviewed how culture may influence and shape our brain and behavior during numerical processes. The potential implications of cultural differences in numerical cognition for education and mental health were also discussed. It is important to note that culture is a multifaceted concept encompassing a variety of factors that interact with one another and has far-reaching impacts on not only numerical cognition but also other critical aspects of our daily lives. Given that research on cultural differences in numerical processes is still fairly limited within the realm of numerical cognition, there is still a lot to be learned regarding which cultural factors play the greatest role in differentially affecting numerical processing across different cultures. Therefore, future research would need to delineate the exact mechanisms and factors underlying the contribution of culture in shaping the processes of numerical cognition. Another important domain concerns the genetic contribution to numerical cognition, as there is evidence showing high heritability of mathematical abilities (Kovas et al., 2007). The gene-by-environment interaction is not a new concept in cognitive psychology and neuroscience, including the field of numerical cognition, yet since the framework was proposed by Tang and colleagues in 2009, not much has been done with regard to how genetic variations between different cultures may exert influence over the behavioral expression of numerical cognition, or how distinct cultural experiences as part of our environment may reciprocally interact with genes to affect numerical abilities. As such, we are in a stage of research that requires both exploratory and large-scale studies to fill in these research gaps. Without them, we would inadvertently constrain ourselves with the basic yet incomplete knowledge of the relationship between culture and numerical cognition.

Acknowledgment

This work was supported by the Office of Naval Research and Presidential Endowment.

References

Ansari, D. (2008). Effects of development and enculturation on number representation in the brain. *Nature Reviews Neuroscience, 9*(4), 278.

Beller, S., & Bender, A. (2008). The limits of counting: Numerical cognition between evolution and culture. *Science, 319*(5860), 213–215.

Beller, S., Bender, A., Chrisomalis, S., Jordan, F. M., Overmann, K. A., Saxe, G. B., & Schlimm, D. (2018). The cultural challenge in mathematical cognition. *Journal of Numerical Cognition, 4*(2), 448–463.

Bender, A., & Beller, S. (2011). Cultural variation in numeration systems and their mapping onto the mental number line. *Journal of Cross-Cultural Psychology, 42*(4), 579–597.

Butterworth, B. (1999). *The mathematical brain.* Macmillan.

Butterworth, B., Varma, S., & Laurillard, D. (2011). Dyscalculia: From brain to education. *Science, 332*(6033), 1049–1053.

Campbell, J. I., & Xue, Q. (2001). Cognitive arithmetic across cultures. *Journal of Experimental Psychology: General, 130*(2), 299.

Chan, W. W. L., Au, T. K., & Tang, J. (2013). Developmental dyscalculia and low numeracy in Chinese children. *Research in Developmental Disabilities, 34*(5), 1613–1622.

Chen, C., & Stevenson, H. W. (1995). Motivation and mathematics achievement: A comparative study of Asian-American, Caucasian-American, and East Asian high school students. *Child Development, 66*(4), 1215–1234.

Dehaene, S., Molko, N., Cohen, L., & Wilson, A. J. (2004). Arithmetic and the brain. *Current Opinion in Neurobiology, 14*(2), 218–224.

Domahs, F., Moeller, K., Huber, S., Willmes, K., & Nuerk, H. C. (2010). Embodied numerosity: Implicit hand-based representations influence symbolic number processing across cultures. *Cognition, 116*(2), 251–266.

Fuchs, L. S., Fuchs, D., & Compton, D. L. (2012). The early prevention of mathematics difficulty: Its power and limitations. *Journal of Learning Disabilities, 45*(3), 257–269.

Geary, D. C., Hamson, C. O., Chen, G. P., Liu, F., Hoard, M. K., & Salthouse, T. A. (1997). Computational and reasoning abilities in arithmetic: Cross-generational change in China and the United States. *Psychonomic Bulletin & Review, 4*(3), 425–430.

Gelman, R., & Butterworth, B. (2005). Number and language: How are they related? *Trends in Cognitive Sciences, 9*(1), 6–10.

Gifford, S. (2006). Dyscalculia: Myths and models. *Research in Mathematics Education, 8*(1), 35–51.

Göbel, S. M., Shaki, S., & Fischer, M. H. (2011). The cultural number line: A review of cultural and linguistic influences on the development of number processing. *Journal of Cross-Cultural Psychology, 42*(4), 543–565.

Hess, R. D., & Azuma, H. (1991). Cultural support for schooling: Contrasts between Japan and the United States. *Educational Researcher, 20*(9), 2–9.

Hess, R. D., Chang, C. M., & McDevitt, T. M. (1987). Cultural variations in family beliefs about children's performance in mathematics: Comparisons among People's Republic of China, Chinese-American, and Caucasian-American families. *Journal of Educational Psychology, 79*(2), 179.

Ho, C. S. H., Wong, T. T. Y., & Chan, W. W. L. (2015). Mathematics learning and its difficulties among Chinese children in Hong Kong. In S. Chinn (Ed.), *The Routledge international handbook of dyscalculia and mathematical learning difficulties* (pp. 193–202). Routledge.

Hubbard, E. M., Diester, I., Cantlon, J. F., Ansari, D., Van Opstal, F., & Troiani, V. (2008). The evolution of numerical cognition: From number neurons to linguistic quantifiers. *Journal of Neuroscience, 28*(46), 11819–11824.

Kovas, Y., Haworth, C. M., Dale, P. S., & Plomin, R. (2007). The genetic and environmental origins of learning abilities and disabilities in the early school years. *Monographs of the Society for research in Child Development, 72*(3), vii–1.

Leung, K. S. F. (2001). In search of an East Asian identity in mathematics education. *Educational Studies in Mathematics, 47*(1), 35–51.

Leung, K. S. F. (2006). Mathematics education in East Asia and the West: Does culture matter? In Leung, F. K.-S., Graf, Klaus-D., Lopez-Real, Francis J. (Eds.), *Mathematics education in different cultural traditions: A comparative study of East Asia and the West* (pp. 21–46). Springer.

Saxe, G. B., Guberman, S. R., Gearhart, M., Gelman, R., Massey, C. M., & Rogoff, B. (1987). Social processes in early number development. *Monographs of the Society for Research in Child Development, 52*(2), 1–162.

Tan, L. H., Spinks, J. A., Eden, G. F., Perfetti, C. A., & Siok, W. T. (2005). Reading depends on writing, in Chinese. *Proceedings of the National Academy of Sciences, 102*(24), 8781–8785.

Tang, Y. Y., & Liu, Y. (2009). Numbers in the cultural brain. *Progress in Brain Research, 178*, 151–157.

Tang, Y., Zhang, W., Chen, K., Feng, S., Ji, Y., Shen, Ji, Y., Shen, J., Reiman, E. M., & Liu, Y. (2006). Arithmetic processing in the brain shaped by cultures. *Proceedings of the National Academy of Sciences, 103*(28), 10775–10780.

Verguts, T., & Chen, Q. (2017). Numerical cognition: Learning binds biology to culture. *Trends in Cognitive Science, 21*, 409–424.

Influence of Aging on Memory Across Cultures

Angela Gutchess, Nishaat Mukadam, Wanbing Zhang, *and* Xin Zhang

Abstract

This chapter reviews the emerging literature on the ways in which culture can influence memory with age. It first discusses the typical effects of healthy and pathological aging (Alzheimer's disease [AD]) on brain metrics. Next, comparisons of healthy older adults across cultures are reviewed, including studies of brain structure, function, and strategies that yield accurate or erroneous memory. Social influences, such as stereotypes and beliefs about aging, are presented in terms of their direct effects on memory outcomes. The next section considers socioemotional influences more broadly, including social networks and future time perspective that can impact focus on positive information, and how they can impact cognition and memory across cultures with age. The chapter next focuses on AD. Although the work on healthy aging underscores the potential for malleability in memory and cognition across cultures, this may not be possible when pathological changes occur. Thus, this section discusses ways in which culture could impact risk factors for AD and diagnosis, including a number of challenges and considerations for neuropsychological assessment.

Key Words: aging, memory, Alzheimer's disease, culture, cognition

Introduction

The aging of the population seems to be an inevitable trend across the globe. According to the United Nations' "World Population Aging Report," around 962 million people were aged 60 or older in 2017. By 2050, this number is expected to double, reaching about 2.1 billion. The remarkable aging of the population will affect individuals, families, and governments in all aspects, including health care, social security, retirement, caregiving, and the burden of disease and disability. This makes it critical for us to understand the process and mechanisms of aging, with the hope of improving the health and life quality of older people all over the world, and delaying the loss of independence (see Chapter 9 "Developmental Plasticity and Global Aging"). Pronounced cognitive decline occurring as a result of dementia is one of the greatest health threats in the older generation, now affecting nearly 50% of adults over the age of 85 in the United States (Hebert et al., 2003). Advanced age itself is the greatest risk factor for dementia (Guerreiro &

Bras, 2015). Consequently, it is critical to understand the mechanisms of aging and how aging influences cognition.

Although, to date, population aging is most advanced in developed countries, the majority of older adults live in developing countries, which have the fastest growth rate for older populations. For example, India's population over age 65 will number 227 million in 2050, and for China, that number will exceed 330 (United Nation's World Population Ageing Report, 2015). As a result, conducting research on aging across cultures will be important for informing subsequent policies and therapies based on local conditions and unique aspects of the populations. (See Chapter 1 on "The Cross-National Epidemology of Mental Health Disorders" and Chapter 2 on "Cultural Evolutionary Neuroscience") for further discussion of global mental health and epidemiology.)

In this chapter, we will consider the ways that both healthy aging and Alzheimer's disease (AD) could impact memory across cultures. Although there is a dearth of research on cognition across cultures even in younger adults, we will review the emerging literature on cognitive aging across cultures with a focus on long-term memory. The chapter will begin with a review of the brain changes that occur with age. We will then consider how culture can impact healthy aging in terms of brain structure and function, as well as cognitive performance, and the social factors that may impact trajectories with age. We will then turn to pathological aging, with a focus on AD, which leads to pronounced impairment of long-term memory with age. That section will review the contribution of culture to risk factors and neuropsychological assessment for the diagnosis of AD.

Changes to the Brain With Age and Alzheimer's Disease

In this section, we will briefly review some of the changes to the brain that occur with aging, considering changes from the gross level (e.g., gray matter) to the cellular level (e.g., synapses). We will then consider changes that occur with Alzheimer's disease.

Thus far, many magnetic resonance imaging (MRI) studies have examined how typical aging processes influence brain volume and structures, with the general consensus that brain volume shrinks while the ventricles grow in normal aging (Courchesne et al., 2000; Fotenos et al., 2008; Good et al., 2001; Sullivan et al., 2004; Walhovd et al., 2011). However, the rates of atrophy, or shrinkage, vary across regions, with the largest changes observed in the prefrontal cortex and significant but moderate effects in the temporal cortex and thalamus, amygdala, and putamen (Allen et al., 2005; Raz et al., 2004). In contrast, primary sensory regions (e.g., visual and auditory cortex) are relatively well preserved (Fjell & Walhovd, 2010). These findings are in accordance with studies indicating that higher-order executive functions, which mainly rely on regions of the prefrontal cortex, are particularly disrupted by normal aging processes (Schretlen et al., 2000; Yuan & Raz, 2014).

Meanwhile, molecular and cellular studies probe the neurobiological basis of the morphometric changes described earlier. Initially, researchers believed that neuronal death was the major cause of volume reductions and cognitive declines in normal aging (Simic et al., 1997). However, more recent studies found that the number of neurons varies little with age and may even be unchanged in certain brain areas (Freeman et al., 2008; Rapp et al., 2002). Rather, shrinking neuron size, reductions of synapses, and loss of synaptic spines likely account for the reduction in gray matter (Esiri, 2007; Freeman et al., 2008). In addition, the length of myelinated neuron fibers is considerably decreased, up to almost 50%, which is consistent with the decrease of white matter integrity observed in MRI studies (Marner et al., 2003; Peters et al., 2000).

In terms of changes related to AD, AD results in patterns of brain shrinkage distinct from healthy aging processes (see Figure 14.1a). These differences are particularly evident in the hippocampus, a key structure for memory. The atrophy rate of the hippocampus in healthy older adults is 0.84% per year, according to some estimates (Fjell et al., 2009), which is modest compared to the rate of atrophy for some other structures. For patients with AD, however, the rate of atrophy is 4.66% annually, which likely accounts for the patients' deficits in forming new memories as a result of the disease. Moreover, the entire temporal cortex, the lobe surrounding the hippocampus, has a higher-than-average atrophy rate in AD (as depicted in Figure 14.1b), which is seen as a signature of AD (McDonald et al., 2009). Although we noted that the death of neurons does not seem to overall characterize typical aging processes, apoptosis, or cell death, can be severe in brains with AD, with approximately 50% neuronal loss in the entorhinal cortex, a portion of cortex interconnected with the hippocampus and implicated in memory, and 30% in the primary visual cortex (Gomez-Isla et al., 1996; Leuba & Kraftsik, 1994). Lastly, the breakdown of white matter, or demyelination, is significantly faster in AD than typical aging processes (Bartzokis et al., 2003).

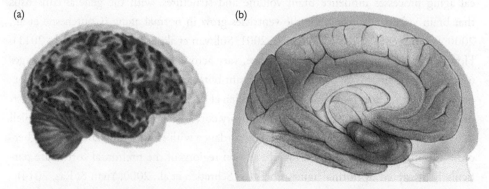

(a)   (b)

Figure 14.1. (a) This panel illustrates how atrophy affects a brain with Alzheimer's disease, compared to a healthy brain. (b) The shading notes the neural regions most affected by Alzheimer's disease, with the most impact on the temporal lobes, including the hippocampus. © 2018 Alzheimer's Association. www.alz.org. All rights reserved. Illustrations by Stacy Jannis.

Cognitive and Cognitive Neuroscience of Aging Across Cultures

This section focuses on comparisons of healthy older adults across cultures. Although our focus is on memory, the small amount of structural and functional neuroimaging research thus far has addressed broader questions about brain health and neural response to viewing pictures. We will review this literature in terms of memory and delve into potential strategies and orientations that can differ across cultures and shape what, how, and under which circumstances information is remembered.

Structural Differences in Brains Across Cultures

Many studies demonstrate that life experiences, from learning to juggle to political affiliation, change brain structures (Draganski et al., 2004; Kanai et al., 2011; Kim et al., 2010). For example, taxi drivers showed increased gray matter in the posterior hippocampus after qualifying to become licensed taxi drivers through 3 to 4 years of training to learn the layout of London. As unqualified trainees experienced no change in hippocampal volume over this time period, it is reasonable to believe that the experience of learning the city is the causal mechanism (Woollett & Maguire, 2011). This kind of structural plasticity as a result of training and life experiences exists in the brains of older adults as well (Boyke et al., 2008). Therefore, we wonder whether the types of neural changes that occur with age are universal across cultures. As culture offers a rich set of life experiences, that begs the question of which aspects of aging are biological imperatives that are unalterable by culture and which aspects can be molded by cultural experiences? (See Chapter 21 for further discussion of plasticity.)

Cross-cultural differences in the aging brain are largely unexplored. The only comparison thus far of MRI structural data was reported by Chee et al. (2011). A large sample of 140 younger and older adults from Singapore and the United States were compared. Results demonstrated that there is noticeable brain volume loss with age, and the extent of decline is similar across the two cultural groups. That is to say, biology plays a dominant role in sculpting aging-related brain changes, rather than culture. Moreover, cortical thickness and density of brain regions also were measured in the study. Young Americans showed greater cortical thickness across many regions when compared with young Singaporeans. However, the cultural differences vanished in older adults, partially due to their high degree of within-group variability (Chee et al., 2011). Another possible explanation is that older adults might diverge more across cultures when they speak different languages. Because the participants from Singapore and the United States are all English native speakers, this could reduce the potential differences that could emerge across cultures with age.

The literature on cross-cultural brain differences in older adults is scant and limited, and there are many unanswered questions. The rich variation in life experiences across cultures, particularly over a lifetime, makes it a rich area worthy of further investigation. As research on the aging brain explodes in Western cultures, it is important to understand to what extent the observed changes with age are universals. Additional cross-cultural study also holds the potential to increase appreciation of factors that impact both the stability and flexibility of aging-brain changes.

Cross-Cultural Comparisons of Memory

There is more study of how culture can affect behavior with age, though the coverage of different memory topics is mixed. There is a rich tradition of considering culture in the study of autobiographical memory (see Chapter 14 for further discussion of auto-biographical memory), a type of memory focused on one's personal past (Ross & Wang, 2010). Although this work has considered child development, much less work considers late-life development and aging. The research incorporating older adults largely focuses on the reminiscence bump (Conway et al., 2005; Rubin et al., 1986), which is the finding that people tend to remember more events from their lives that occurred between the ages of 10 and 30 years, reflecting the timeframe of many formative events for one's self-identity and events corresponding to common cultural life scripts. The reminiscence bump seems to have similar characteristics as observed in Western cultures when tested across older adults drawn from different countries, such as Turkey (Demiray et al., 2009) and Malaysia (Haque & Hasking, 2010). Despite these similarities, some of the functions of autobiographical memory could be influenced by culture. Americans tend to use reminiscing for social bonding more than Trinidadians; despite reductions in this function of memory with age, the cultural differences were consistent across the age groups (Alea et al., 2015). Indigenous Australians tended to use reminiscence for functions such as teaching, maintaining intimacy, and identity more than non-Indigenous Australians, although some functions (e.g., death preparation, teaching) were more common for older adults across cultures compared to younger adults (Nile & Van Bergen, 2015).

Aside from memory for experiences from one's personal past, there have been efforts to compare the effects of aging on memory across cultures when the information to be encoded is presented in a standardized, controlled laboratory setting. Research thus far has concentrated on memory for objects versus contexts, binding, categorization, and self-referencing and has considered social factors, such as stereotypes about aging, that could influence one's memory performance with age.

Cultural differences in memory for objects and contexts have been compared in many studies, with some evidence that compared to Westerners, Easterners preferentially attend to and remember contexts and have difficulty recognizing objects when the context has been removed (Masuda & Nisbett, 2001). Some have discussed this in terms of binding, in that Easterners may bind objects to contexts more than Westerners. Consistent with these notions, some research indicates that Chinese younger and older adults exhibit higher levels of context memory than Canadians, with young adults across cultures performing better than older adults (Yang, Li, et al., 2013). Cultural differences in binding items to sources (e.g., statements to speakers) do not always emerge, though this ability is typically disrupted with age (Chua et al., 2006). Other work has highlighted the difference across cultures in processing objects, rather than contexts or object–context binding. In the only study to compare neural activity across culture and age groups during a cognitive task (Goh et al., 2007), younger and older Americans and Singaporeans passively viewed objects presented on meaningful backgrounds (e.g., a bird in a tree). Repeating elements of the picture allowed adaptation responses to be compared across groups for different aspects of information. For example, repeating the same object four times in a row will lead neural regions responding to objects to adapt, or decrease their response. In contrast, the novel context information presented on each of those four trials would continue to robustly engage regions that respond to contexts. Using this approach, culture was found to impact the engagement of object regions such that Singaporeans exhibited less adaptation to objects than Americans. However, this cultural difference was greater for the older adults, with older Singaporeans showing a reduction in adaptation relative to older Americans, whereas the younger adults did not substantially differ from each other. Although no cultural differences emerged for the backgrounds, the typical reduction with age in regions related to binding items to backgrounds occurred across cultures. Although memory was not assessed in this study, these differences in neural responsivity during this basic stage of processing could have implications for cultural differences in attention and memory.

Another active area of study is in the use of strategies based on categories and relationships. Whereas Americans tend to preferentially sort information on the basis of taxonomic categories (e.g., putting squirrel and cow together because both are animals), Chinese tend to sort based on functional relationships (e.g., putting squirrel and nut together because the squirrel eats the nut; Ji et al., 2004). In terms of memory, presenting words intermixed from a number of categories (e.g., animals, units of time) leads American older adults to recall the information organized by category to a greater extent than the Chinese older adults (Gutchess et al., 2006). Younger adults, in contrast, did not differ across cultures, perhaps reflecting their greater cognitive flexibility to adopt different strategies or recent globalization trends, which could extend to educational practices. Another study was interpreted through the lens of cultural differences in categorization, in that across age groups, Canadians performed better than Chinese at remembering which of two sources was presented with an item (Yang, Chen, et al., 2013). Preferential use of categories is not always an asset in memory, in that the strategy could also lead one astray. After studying word pairs for which half of the trials shared a categorical relationship (e.g., table–chair) and half were unrelated (e.g., table–minute), Americans tended to falsely remember word pairs as sharing categorical relationships to a greater extent than did Turks, a culture shaped by both Eastern and Western influences (Schwartz et al., 2014). When the work was extended to older adults, the tendency persisted for Americans to commit more categorical errors than Turks, despite the tendency across cultures for older adults to exhibit higher levels of false memory for semantically related information

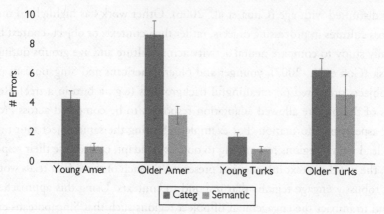

Figure 14.2. Both young and older Americans tend to commit more categorical memory errors (dark bars) than other types of semantic memory errors (light bars). This pattern occurs disproportionately more for Americans than Turks, and despite an overall increase in memory errors for older adults, compared to younger adults. Figure from Gutchess, A., & Boduroglu, A. (2019). Cultural differences in categorical memory errors persist with age. *Aging & Mental Health, 23,* 851-854. doi:10.1080/13607863.2017.1421616, reprinted with permission from Taylor & Francis, Ltd, www.tandfonline.com.

than younger adults (Gutchess & Boduroglu, 2019). This pattern of results is shown in Figure 14.2.

Influence of Values and Beliefs on Memory

Some research examines how well-documented cultural differences in ideas about aging and the self can influence memory. In Western cultures, the self is conceptualized as an independent entity, in which the self is apart from others. In contrast, the Eastern notion of the self is interdependent, tightly connected with and defined through relationships with others (Markus & Kitayama, 1991). Thus, a memory strategy of relating information to oneself, shown to be effective in the West, may be less effective for Easterners. Some research with young adults supports this idea (Sparks et al., 2016; Zhu et al., 2007). In a recent study (W. Zhang et al., 2020) comparing mnemonic benefits of self-referencing across younger and older adults, we found that cultural differences in memory were larger for older adults than younger adults, who performed similarly across cultures.

Focusing on cultural beliefs about age has led to some interesting comparisons of how aging affects memory across cultures. Some early work suggested that negative stereotypes about aging might be responsible for poor cognitive performance with age. Older adults from Chinese and Deaf cultures, which have relatively more positive views of aging, exhibited less memory decline with age than Americans, who have more negative views of aging (Levy & Langer, 1994; see Cavallini et al., 2013, for a related comparison of Sardinian and Milanese older adults). However, a subsequent study comparing American and Chinese cultures did not reach the same conclusion, that negative stereotypes of aging account for memory declines with age. In the follow-up study, memory was poorer with age across both American and Chinese groups (Yoon et al., 2000). Another study found that cultural values influence the performance of Chinese older adults (Barber, 2017). Completing a memory test under conditions of stereotype threat, in which the task was framed as diagnostic of memory declines that occur with age and made negative stereotypes about cognitive aging salient, led older Chinese to perform worse than a control group for which the memory test was described as age-fair. This pattern of performance is in line with a host of stereotype threat research with American older adults. The study went further, however, by adding an intervention condition in which participants first read about cultural values regarding respecting elders, such as filial piety, before completing the memory task. Priming cultural values eliminated the deleterious effects of the stereotype threat instructions, and this group performed as well as the control group. This work suggests that although negative views about cognitive and physical decline with age may be pervasive across cultures (Boduroglu et al., 2006), positive cultural values regarding older adults may offer some protective effects.

Although evidence for cross-cultural differences is converging around some aspects of memory, these topics barely scratch the surface. Thus far, the existing work largely reveals ways in which certain strategies or information-processing biases (e.g., categories, object/context) can improve or impair memory across cultures. In terms of aging, the work thus far largely reveals preservation of cultural differences across the age groups (Gutchess & Boduroglu, 2019; Yang, Chen, et al., 2013; Yang, Li, et al., 2013) or divergence in performance with age across cultures (Goh et al., 2007; Gutchess et al., 2006). The findings of larger cultural differences for older than younger adults may reflect less globalization or shared cultural influences for older cohorts. This pattern could also reflect cognitive resource limitations with age such that older adults are limited to culturally well-practiced strategies rather than flexibly adopting new ones, as young adults might do. Another possible pattern is that cultural differences could emerge in young adults that could be mitigated with aging as cognitive resource limitations eliminate any initial advantages for one group (Park & Gutchess, 2002, 2006; Park et al., 1999). Much more work is needed to understand the interplay of cultural experiences, cognitive resources, and aging across different task demands and neural systems.

Socioemotional Influences on Memory Across Cultures

In addition to the cognitive changes that occur within an individual with age, aging can be associated with alterations in the ways in which people interact with or respond to their environments. As individuals gain awareness of the limited time horizons remaining in their lives, this can lead to transformations in perspectives that impact social and cognitive functions, including memory. This section will discuss the literature on how changes in social and emotional life impact the memory of older adults, as well as how culture influences these changes.

Change in Social Environment and Cognitive Functioning

Older adults are usually found to have narrower social networks and fewer social partners (Charles & Carstensen, 2010), and this trend is similar across cultures (Fung et al., 2001; Fung, Stoeber, et al., 2008). The beginning of this decrease can be traced to midlife, when people start to be more selective in their social interactions (Carstensen, 2006). Past literature on older adults' cognitive health stressed the importance of social activity and maintenance of social structure in old age (Charles & Carstensen, 2010; Wilson et al., 2007). In particular, older males are less likely to suffer from cognitive decline when living with partners compared to when living alone (van Gelder et al., 2006).

Exposure to social activity may serve as a cognitive exercise itself, in terms of engaging in conversation and socializing with others. These cognitive demands could be the core reason social activity benefits older adults' cognitive performance. In a longitudinal study, cognitive activity was found to mediate the relationship between social activity and four domains of cognitive function: cognitive fluency, episodic memory, reasoning, and vocabulary (Brown et al., 2016). Of course, not all social interactions are equally beneficial. Living in a neighborhood with higher socioeconomic status leads to lower likelihood of cognitive decline (Charles & Carstensen, 2010; Lang et al., 2008). Subjective satisfaction with support received from social networks is related to older adults' episodic memory performance over 5 years (Hughes et al., 2008). Another benefit that comes with social networks is emotional support (Blanchard-Fields et al., 2008). High-quality social interactions usually generate positive emotions that are further associated with higher ability in language and abstraction, as well as spatial ability and memory (Seeman et al., 2001). The next section will elaborate more on why emotional support is particularly important to the older population.

Overall, aging is universally perceived to be negatively related to future time perspective across cultures (Fung, Isaacowitz, et al., 2008). However, what is considered socially meaningful may differ across cultures. For Germans, social life revolves less around nuclear family members and more around acquaintances; the pattern is the opposite for Hong Kong Chinese (Fung, Stoeber, et al., 2008). Therefore, from a public health perspective, older adults from different cultures should be encouraged to engage in culturally valued social relationships to maximize the potential cognitive benefits.

Change in Emotional Inclination and Cognitive Functioning

Emotion can have a strong influence on cognition and memory. Greater attention to emotional information can lead to bias in memory, such that emotional information is prioritized over neutral (Mather et al., 1999; Murphy & Isaacowitz, 2008). Some research reveals that older adults attend to emotional information overall (both positive and negative) more than perceptual details because of failure to suppress irrelevant neural activity (Darowski et al., 2008). Though it might be intuitive that positive emotion can enhance mental health, exposure to positive emotion may be particularly important for older adults. A number of studies demonstrate that compared to their younger counterparts, older adults can attend to and remember positive information relatively better than neutral or negative information (Kennedy et al., 2004). According to socioemotional selectivity theory (Carstensen, 1992), changing time perspectives are thought to underlie positivity biases. That is, as people age, their motivations will change to adapt to the foreshortened time remaining in life and declines in their ability to fulfill certain goals. This motivates older adults to invest in emotionally meaningful and positive relationships. Several studies have found evidence for a positivity bias in cognitive domains: older adults outperform younger adults when rating the intensity of positive stimuli (Mikels et al., 2005) and tend to remember relatively more positive than negative images compared to younger adults (Mather & Knight, 2005). However, the positivity bias may be dependent on cognitive control and intentional allocation of attention. When cognitive resources to control attention are limited, older adults exhibit negativity biases similar to younger adults (Mather & Knight, 2005).

In terms of cultural comparisons, evidence of the positivity effect is inconsistent across cultures. Some studies successfully replicated the positivity bias with age in non-Western cultures. A study done in Korea showed that Korean older adults memorize images with positive valence better than negative ones (Kwon et al., 2009). Chinese older adults were found to look at positive images longer than negative images, while their younger counterparts spend equivalent time on both types of images, but this difference in preferential looking failed to lead to any corresponding memory effects (Wang et al., 2015). Other literature failed to find a positivity effect across cultures, and some even found the opposite. In an eye-tracking study, Chinese older adults showed negativity effects rather than positivity effects for attention-related focus on emotional stimuli (Fung, Isaacowitz, et al., 2008). The negativity effects could, in part, reflect the emphasis on interdependence in East Asian cultures, as that self-construal requires awareness of both positive and negative emotions of others, as opposed to the predominant focus on positive emotions in Western cultures (Fung et al., 2010).

More generally, there is also evidence of cultural differences in well-being. Westerners tend to adopt a linear approach to well-being such that American older adults reported less negative emotion in unpleasant situations than American younger adults. In comparison, Japanese older adults reported the same amount of negative emotion as Japanese younger adults, but also more positive emotion under unpleasant situations, which reflects a dialectic approach (Grossmann et al., 2014). Additionally, it is noteworthy that traumatic cultural tragedies or historical conflicts may impact what is considered positive in the present moment as well as cohort differences in the importance placed on thinking positively with age (Gutchess & Huff, 2015). Such lifetime perspectives may influence the degree to which older people in different cultures exhibit positive memory biases.

Potential Influences of Culture on Alzheimer's Disease

Our consideration of healthy aging across cultures underscored the potential malleability and plasticity that could occur in memory for older adults. For example, which brain structures have expanded, or undergone reduced atrophy, as a result of life experiences? How do cultural orientations to information-processing biases or socioemotional priorities shape accurate and inaccurate memory for information and the effectiveness of strategies? In contrast, the flexibility afforded by culture may be eliminated in AD. One might expect that the atrophy of neural regions and reduction in cognitive resources unfold in a set manner due to the biological progression of the disease. Although it may be possible that certain culturally supported strategies or practices help to buffer or alter the course of the disease, this has not been demonstrated at this point in time. Going forward, it will be important to differentiate the neural systems expected to decline in a more fixed and unalterable manner by the disease, such as the medial temporal lobes where the hippocampus is located, compared to regions that undergo less decline and may have more flexibility until late in the disease. Because of the state of the literature, and these likely challenges to finding cultural differences with disease, this section takes a different approach from the previous ones. Although we compare across cultures and ethnic groups in terms of risk factors, we then more broadly consider cultural factors that shape the setting in which diagnosis of dementia or other age-related disorders occurs.

Risk Factors for Alzheimer's Disease

Identifying who is at risk of developing AD is an area of active research. Risk factors range from genetic biomarkers on an individual level (see Chapter 7 for further discussion of cultural genomics) to the types of preferred lifestyle activities or practices on a societal level. Different risk factors could interact in complex ways so that it is possible that some risk factors are more harmful in one culture than another. The following section will introduce a few risk factors of Alzheimer's disease that are relatively well studied across cultures, including both comparisons across nations and across ethnicities within the United States. When reviewing conclusions from this research, we should keep in mind that the diagnostic criteria, measurement tools used, and definition of AD may vary from culture to culture, which is discussed in more detail in the following section. In addition to noting what is different, it is important to attend to what is similar or universal across cultures, as it may have important implications for understanding the effects of and interventions for AD or age-related cognitive decline in general.

In terms of the epidemiology of AD, studies of prevalence across ethnic groups within the United States have found differences between groups. Compared to Caucasians and Asian Americans, who have similar rates, African Americans and Hispanics have a higher prevalence of dementia and AD, whereas Native Americans have a lower risk (Manly & Mayeux, 2004). When comparing the United States to other countries (particularly developing countries), the findings are somewhat mixed. Studies conducted in the 1990s suggested that the frequency of dementia (including AD) in Brazil, Argentina, and other Latin American countries is equivalent to that in countries in Europe and the United States (Mangone & Arizaga, 1999; Nitrini et al., 1995). However, in a survey-based study, African American older adults have been found to have a higher rate of AD than Nigerian elders (Hendrie et al., 2001). There are also countries seeing a change in AD prevalence: Japan used to have a lower AD rate but the frequency began to rise in the late 1990s to a prevalence rate resembling that of America (Yamada et al., 1999). There are many confounds in these comparisons that make it difficult to determine whether there are truly differences in prevalence across cultures or whether they reflect the operation of other factors such as life expectancy (e.g., do people live long enough to exhibit changes warranting a diagnosis of dementia?) and diagnostic method (e.g., do people have to be both structurally *and* functionally impaired to be diagnosed?). But the take-home message from these cross-cultural studies is that systematic difference in AD prevalence exists across countries and ethnic groups within a country. This can then motivate research to examine the causes of these discrepancies. We will now review some of the most commonly known risk factors.

In terms of genetic risk factors, ApoE-ε4 (the ε4 allele of apolipoprotein E) is a genotype known to be related to higher prevalence of AD in all ethnic groups. The negative impact of ApoE-ε4, however, differs across cultures. The relationship between possessing the ε4 allele and developing dementia is the strongest for Japanese individuals, followed by Caucasians, and then followed by Hispanics and African Americans (Farrer et al., 1997). However, genotypes do not tell the whole story. Even taking into account the presence of the ApoE-ε4 allele, people with a higher degree of Cherokee ancestry have a lower likelihood of developing AD than people with less Cherokee lineage (Rosenberg et al., 1996), suggesting there may be factors related to a specific ethnicity that could serve as risk or protective factors for AD. Researchers also demonstrated that a cholesterol-heavy diet may lead to a higher risk of AD, as ApoE is also linked to the clearance of cholesterol, but only for people without the ApoE-ε4 genotype. The risk of AD for people who already have ApoE-ε4 was not affected by cholesterol, which is an example of how genotypes can interact with environmental factors (Hall et al., 2006).

Education is believed to crucially impact not only cognitive development in early life but also cognitive decline in later life. One dominant explanation in the literature is that education facilitates the amassing of cognitive reserve, the amount of resilience one has against cognitive decline (Stern, 2002). Neurologically, it can be viewed as the amount of neural insult one can sustain (e.g., number of synaptic connections one can afford to lose) before being debilitated by cognitive impairments. Most findings with the North American population suggest that years of education are related to higher resilience (Katzman, 1993; Stern et al., 1994; Tucker-Drob et al., 2009). Similar associations were found in China (M. Zhang et al., 1990), Israel (Kahana et al., 2003), and Brazil (Manly & Mayeux, 2004; Nitrini et al., 1995).

A common drawback of these studies is that socioeconomic status (SES) often is unaccounted for in the analyses. One's SES is usually predictive of their literacy because families with higher SES can afford more years of education. This is also true the other way around: people who received extensive education are likely to proceed to have higher SES, through factors such as job attainment and salary. At the same time, higher SES is also related to easier access to health care resources and better nutrition, which are all important factors to consider when making conclusions about the relationship between education and AD. All these factors surrounding material living conditions make up a large portion of risk factors for people living in regions suffering from poverty, famine, and regional conflicts.

Immigration and acculturation experience are additional considerations in terms of risk factors. Interesting research has investigated differences in AD risk between groups of the same ethnicity who immigrated to another country versus remained in the country of origin. AD has a higher prevalence among male Japanese Americans living in Hawaii than among Japanese men living in Japan. The authors suggested that altering the cultural environment by migrating from Japan to Hawaii could influence the development of AD (White et al., 1996), potentially due to adopting a more Westernized diet that is fat and cholesterol heavy (Manly & Mayeux, 2004).

Bilingualism is another common outcome of immigration and acculturation. Research suggests that lifelong bilingualism can serve as a protective mechanism against age-related cognitive decline. Among a group of patients diagnosed with dementia, bilinguals showed a later onset of symptoms than monolinguals (Bialystok et al., 2007; Craik et al., 2010). These findings support the notion that speaking more than one language is a way to increase cognitive reserve and hence helps to maintain cognitive functioning. Taken together, immigration can have a positive or negative impact on the likelihood of developing AD, depending on the lifestyle one is migrating to as well as the linguistic demands of the environment.

Diagnosis of Alzheimer's Disease

The diagnosis of AD is not entirely objective or free from cultural factors. There are no specific tests for a definite diagnosis of AD. Diagnosis is made based on consideration of neuropsychological evaluations and biomarkers (e.g., presence of amyloid, which accumulates into plaques), after ruling out other possible causes of the cognitive decline (e.g., medications, stroke). The diagnosis of AD requires evidence of cognitive decline compared to previous level of functioning. Memory is most affected and must interfere with independence in everyday activities to warrant a diagnosis of AD. The evidence to inform a diagnosis is based on information provided by the individual or a caregiver, alongside evidence of substantial impairment in cognitive performance on neuropsychological tests (American Psychiatric Association, 2013).

Adding cultural considerations to this already complicated diagnostic procedure can lead to additional challenges. As described in the "Neuropsychological Assessment" section, the available diagnostic tools tend to be culturally biased, do not have good construct validity for all cultures, and lack cultural normative data, likely leading to over- or underdiagnosis of cognitive impairment in some cultural groups (Davies et al., 2014; Manly, 2005; Nielsen et al., 2011; Ramirez Gomez et al., 2017). In recent times, race-specific norms have been developed for some tests (Ferman et al., 2005; Pedraza et al., 2005; Rilling et al., 2005), and using such norms would result in more accurate diagnoses (Manly, 2005). However, these norms are not always representative of the minority population (Sayegh, 2016), do not account for all of the differences in group test performance, do not change the inherent bias in testing procedures or familiarity (Manly, 2005), and tend to normalize possible important disparities between cultures (Davies et al., 2014). Besides, the cultural experiences of people from the same racial group vary depending on geographic, socioeconomic, and acculturative factors, making it unfeasible and impractical to create tests and norms for all groups (Brickman et al., 2006; Manly et al., 1998).

As considered in the next section, poorer performance on neuropsychological tests by ethnic minorities due to factors such as health conditions, educational level, socioeconomic status, literacy, language, and acculturation leads to a greater likelihood of misdiagnosis compared to Caucasians (Coffey et al., 2005; Fillenbaum et al., 2001; Ramirez Gomez et al., 2017).

Cultural Differences in Neuropsychological Assessment

Neuropsychological tests are designed to assess cognitive functions including attention, memory, executive functioning, verbal fluency, language, and visuospatial abilities. Tests are often used to identify abnormal levels of cognitive function and help make judgments about differential deficits across abilities, aiding diagnosis. For older adults, this could signify a diagnosable condition (e.g., AD) or other abnormal aging process.

There are a variety of considerations in the use and interpretation of neuropsychological tests. Cultural differences in test performance is one such consideration. Despite the intention for tests to be used across cultures, these tests tend to be culturally biased (Brickman et al., 2006; Rosselli & Ardila, 2003; Weiner, 2008; Whitfield, 2002; Whitfield et al., 2000). In the United States, Caucasians perform better than ethnic minorities (Agranovich & Puente, 2007; Albert et al., 1995; Brickman et al., 2006; Glosser et al., 1993; Loewenstein et al., 1993; Manly et al., 1998; Razani, Burciaga, et al., 2007; Razani, Murcia, et al., 2007; Whitfield et al., 2000). These discrepancies have been seen on both verbal (Carlson et al., 1998; Razani, Burciaga, et al., 2007; Welsh et al., 1995) and nonverbal tasks (Bernard, 1989; Heverly et al., 1986; Razani, Burciaga, et al., 2007) and on a range of cognitive abilities including intelligence (Razani, Murcia, et al., 2007; Touradji et al., 2001), speed of processing (Boone et al., 2007), attention (Boone et al., 2007; Byrd et al., 2004), memory (Manly et al., 2002; Razani, Burciaga, et al., 2007), letter and category fluency (Manly et al., 2002; Touradji et al., 2001), visuospatial abilities (Manly et al., 2002), constructive abilities (Boone et al., 2007; Byrd et al., 2004), and executive functions (Agranovich & Puente, 2007; Boone et al., 2007; Razani, Burciaga, et al., 2007). Education has been considered as a kind of subculture, in which a person learns skills and abilities that influence performance on cognitive tasks, with higher education serving as a protective factor leading to better performance (Albert et al., 1995; Ardila, 2003; Ardila et al., 1989; Rosselli et al., 1990; Unverzagt et al., 1996).

A major reason for this cultural discrepancy is that most neuropsychological tests used have been developed and validated with Caucasian normative groups (Davies et al., 2014). As tests are inherently culturally biased and language dependent, they tend to favor the culture in which they were developed and are likely to measure different constructs across ethnic and cultural groups (Brickman et al., 2006; Jones, 2003; Jones & Gallo, 2002; Manly et al., 2004; Pedraza & Mungas, 2008). There is some support for this from studies showing that there are performance improvements when test material is more culturally relevant to a person (Hayles, 1991). Additional aspects of testing contribute to cross-cultural performance discrepancies, such as prior exposure, test-taking attitudes, cultural values about being assessed one on one in a private setting, participant–examiner interactions, competitiveness of a culture, ability for the examinee to understand and participate in the formal language used during assessment, and familiarity with the test materials used (Ardila, 2005; Manly et al., 1998).

In addition, performance on some neuropsychological tests, including screening instruments (Escobar et al., 1986; Manly et al., 1998) and more specific verbal and nonverbal tasks, may require the use of certain strategies that are not universal (consider examples in the "Cross-Cultural Comparisons of Memory" section), and some that require some formal education (Ramirez Gomez et al., 2017). For example, the complexity of verbal tasks like the digit span or naming months is significantly reduced in languages like Chinese, where each digit is spoken in a single syllable (Hedden et al., 2002), or in Japanese, where the months are in numerical order (Wolfe, 2002). Similarly, nonverbal tasks like drawing a map, copying figures, and timed tests measuring speed of performance are not universal skills and would influence the performance of participants from cultures that do not value or have not honed these skills (Brickman et al., 2006; Rosselli & Ardila, 2003). Cultural differences in preferences for speed versus accuracy could be attributed to cognitive styles (Agranovich et al., 2011) or could be task dependent (Ojeda et al., 2016). For example, Americans were found to be faster but less accurate on timed neuropsychological tests compared to Spanish (Ojeda et al., 2016) and Russian (Agranovich et al., 2011; Agranovich & Puente, 2007) individuals.

A number of factors, both sociological and biological, could contribute to cultural differences in performance on neuropsychological assessment. Cultural differences have been seen in SES, years of education (Braveman et al., 2005; Brickman et al., 2006; Early et al., 2013; Williams, 1999), and quality of education (Byrd et al., 2005; Crowe et al., 2013;

Early et al., 2013; Johnson et al., 2006; Loewenstein et al., 1993; Manly et al., 2002, 2004; Rosselli & Ardila, 2003), which could account for performance discrepancies. Additionally, factors such as the biological differences between cultures in brain organization (Brickman et al., 2006); health conditions like hypertension, diabetes, and cerebrovascular diseases (Nielsen et al., 2011; Ramirez Gomez et al., 2017); literacy (Ardila et al., 2010; Manly et al., 2003); occupation (Le Carret et al., 2003); test-wiseness (Ardila et al., 2010; Manly et al., 2002; Scruggs & Lifson, 1985); and acculturation (Boone et al., 2007; Coffey et al., 2005; Manly et al., 1998, 2004; Ramirez Gomez et al., 2017; Razani, Burciaga, et al., 2007; Schrauf & Iris, 2011) may also account for these differences.

Minimizing Cultural Differences in Assessment

Ideally, assessment would occur with a clinician who is familiar with the client's culture and speaks the language proficiently. Although an interpreter could be used when necessary, this may lose some precision in communicating aspects of the tasks and does not address cultural factors in interpersonal interactions. During cross-cultural assessment, the clinician attempts to accommodate for factors that influence test performance such as SES, education, and acculturation and reduce cultural gaps by explaining concepts such as "best performance" or the importance of speeded tests (Ramirez Gomez et al., 2017).

More long-term solutions to tackle issues of both culture and language would be translation and adaptation of tests, creation of tests for specific cultures, and norming across cultures. Adapting tests to be linguistically and culturally appropriate along with translation is important because simply translating could alter the difficulty of the test or the processes being tested. For instance, translating words to be remembered into another language could alter the number of syllables, making the task more or less difficult (Puente et al., 2013), or the letters provided for a letter fluency task may appear more or less frequently across languages (Loewenstein et al., 1993).

In recent times, tests have been translated and adapted for use in different languages and with different cultures, and new tests for specific cultures have also been developed (e.g., Glosser et al., 1993; Kempler et al., 2010; Prince et al., 2003; Ramirez Gomez et al., 2017). Some tests have even been adapted for use with people with little or no formal education. For instance, the Stick Design Test has been found to be less influenced by formal education than paper-and-pencil tasks such as the Clock Drawing Task. Both tests have similar accuracy for diagnosing AD when used alongside the Mini Mental Status Examination (de Paula et al., 2013), making this test better for older adults with little or no formal education who perform poorer on paper-and-pencil visuospatial tasks (Ardila et al., 2010; Baiyewu et al., 2005).

Societal Factors

The clinician's familiarity with the culture is important in that diagnosing AD depends on the clinician's judgments about what is considered as interfering with functional independence. This is heavily influenced by culture, in terms of the expected role of the individual, and views of aging. Older adults from cultures that emphasize interdependence tend to get more support and assistance from family members for tasks than people from independent cultures (Markus & Kitayama, 1991; Nisbett & Masuda, 2003). This, along with cultural practices like *familism*, solidarity and support among family members (Parveen et al., 2017); *filial piety*, an obligation to care for aging parents (Zimmer, 2005); *respeto*, the importance of hierarchical roles, and *familismo*, the importance of supporting family (Ramirez Gomez et al., 2017), may lead to fewer responsibilities for and expectations from older adults. When assessing functional impairment, families from these cultures may not report an inability to perform a task simply because older adults are not expected or required to perform such tasks. Even when reported, the clinician needs to be aware that not performing the task may be due to these cultural factors rather than an inability to do so. Another gray area would be whether an inability to perform a task but no cultural requirement to do so would be considered as a functional impairment.

In addition, there are cultural differences in the knowledge and awareness about AD, as well as people's perceptions and beliefs. Compared to Caucasians, people from Indian culture (Purandare et al., 2007) and ethnic minorities in the United States (Ayalon & Areán, 2004) and United Kingdom (Parveen et al., 2017) show less accurate knowledge about AD. Indians were also found to have less awareness about memory problems associated with AD than Latin American and Chinese older adults (Mograbi et al., 2012). These cultural differences have been attributed to perceptions and beliefs held by cultures including the stigma associated with AD (Ayalon & Areán, 2004; Mograbi et al., 2012; Mukadam et al., 2011; Parveen et al., 2017), cultural values accepting memory decline as inevitable in old age (Mograbi et al., 2012; Mukadam et al., 2011; Parveen et al., 2017; Purandare et al., 2007; Ramirez Gomez et al., 2017), viewing seeking professional help as a failure to care for a loved one (Lawrence et al., 2008; Mukadam et al., 2011; Ramirez Gomez et al., 2017), and using religious and spiritual practices as treatment (Parveen et al., 2017).

Poor knowledge about AD and cultural beliefs and perceptions serve as barriers to accessing health care services (Connell et al., 2007; Dilworth-Anderson & Gibson, 2002; Lawrence et al., 2008; Nielsen et al., 2011; Purandare et al., 2007). For example, it was found that ethnic minorities in the United States present for dementia evaluations following a longer delay from disease onset compared to Caucasians, scoring significantly lower on cognitive assessments (Sayegh, 2016). Other barriers to treatment could be SES, educational level, poorer access to health care and worse health care coverage (Sayegh, 2016), and negative experiences with general physicians, as well as language, cultural issues, religious beliefs (Parveen et al., 2017), and stigma for the individual and family (Mukadam et al., 2011).

When evaluating clients, clinicians need to be aware of and account for the host of cultural factors that are likely to influence the diagnosis. For all of these reasons, comparisons of memory across different cultures will be exceedingly challenging. For example, is it possible to ensure that samples across cultures are at the same stage of the disorder? As such comparisons are dependent on neuropsychological assessments that are culturally dependent, it may be difficult to match on these measures. Furthermore, the different time courses leading up to diagnosis and stigma across cultures could impact the severity and trajectory of cognitive decline.

Conclusion

Although research investigating the effects of aging on memory across cultures is in its infancy, we hope this chapter has piqued the readers' interest. Studying the ways in which life experiences could shape brain development and memory provides a fertile approach for understanding the malleability of cognition with age. Perhaps certain culturally associated strategies, social structures, or biological risk/protective factors can alter the course of cognitive decline with age, potentially minimizing the loss of some functions with age or delaying the onset of dementia. Such findings could lead to the development of interventions that could be applied more broadly to improve the outcomes for older adults across the globe.

References

Agranovich, A. V., Panter, A. T., Puente, A. E., & Touradji, P. (2011). The culture of time in neuropsychological assessment: Exploring the effects of culture-specific time attitudes on timed test performance in Russian and American samples. *Journal of the International Neuropsychological Society, 17*(4), 692–701. doi:10.1017/S1355617711000592

Agranovich, A. V., & Puente, A. E. (2007). Do Russian and American normal adults perform similarly on neuropsychological tests? Preliminary findings on the relationship between culture and test performance. *Archives of Clinical Neuropsychology, 22*(3), 273–282. doi:10.1016/j.acn.2007.01.003

Albert, M. S., Jones, K., Savage, C. R., Berkman, L., Seeman, T. E., Blazer, D., & Rowe, J. W. (1995). Predictors of cognitive change in older persons: MacArthur studies of successful aging. *Psychology and Aging, 10*(4), 578–589. doi:10.1037/0882-7974.10.4.578

Alea, N., Bluck, S., & Ali, S. (2015). Function in context: Why American and Trinidadian young and older adults remember the personal past. *Memory, 23*(1), 55–68. doi:10.1080/09658211.2014.929704

Allen, J. S., Bruss, J., Brown, C. K., & Damasio, H. (2005). Normal neuroanatomical variation due to age: The major lobes and a parcellation of the temporal region. *Neurobiology of Aging, 26*(9), 1245–1260; discussion 1279–1282. doi:10.1016/j.neurobiolaging.2005.05.023

American Psychiatric Association. (2013). *Diagnostic and statistical manual of mental disorders* (5th ed.). American Psychiatric Publishing.

Ardila, A. (2003). Culture in our brains: Cross-cultural differences in the brain-behavior relationships. In A. Toomela & A. Toomela (Eds.), *Cultural guidance in the development of the human mind.* (pp. 63–78). Ablex Publishing.

Ardila, A. (2005). Cultural values underlying psychometric cognitive testing. *Neuropsychology Review, 15*(4), 185–195. doi:10.1007/s11065-005-9180-y

Ardila, A., Bertolucci, P. H., Braga, L. W., Castro-Caldas, A., Judd, T., Kosmidis, M. H., Matute, E., Nitrini, R., Ostrosky-Solis, F., & Rosselli, M. (2010). Illiteracy: The neuropsychology of cognition without reading. *Archives of Clinical Neuropsychology, 25*(8), 689–712. doi:10.1093/arclin/acq079

Ardila, A., Rosselli, M., & Rosas, P. (1989). Neuropsychological assessment in illiterates: Visuospatial and memory abilities. *Brain and Cognition, 11*(2), 147–166. doi:10.1016/0278-2626(89)90015-8

Ayalon, L., & Areán, P. A. (2004). Knowledge of Alzheimer's disease in four ethnic groups of older adults. *International Journal of Geriatric Psychiatry, 19*(1), 51–57. doi:10.1002/gps.1037

Baiyewu, O., Unverzagt, F. W., Lane, K. A., Gureje, O., Ogunniyi, A., Musick, B., Gao, S., Hall, K., & Hendrie, H. C. (2005). The Stick Design test: A new measure of visuoconstructional ability. *Journal of the International Neuropsychological Society*, *11*(5), 598–605. doi:10.1017/S135561770505071X

Barber, S. J. (2017). An examination of age-based stereotype threat about cognitive decline. *Perspectives on Psychological Science*, *12*(1), 62–90. doi:10.1177/1745691616656345

Bartzokis, G., Cummings, J. L., Sultzer, D., Henderson, V. W., Nuechterlein, K. H., & Mintz, J. (2003). White matter structural integrity in healthy aging adults and patients with Alzheimer disease: A magnetic resonance imaging study. *Archives of Neurology*, *60*(3), 393–398. doi:10.1001/archneur.60.3.393

Bernard, L. C. (1989). Halstead-Reitan Neuropsychological Test performance of Black, Hispanic, and White young adult males from poor academic backgrounds. *Archives of Clinical Neuropsychology*, *4*(3), 267–274. doi:10.1016/0887-6177(89)90017-6

Bialystok, E., Craik, F. I., & Freedman, M. (2007). Bilingualism as a protection against the onset of symptoms of dementia. *Neuropsychologia*, *45*(2), 459–464. doi:10.1016/j.neuropsychologia.2006.10.009

Blanchard-Fields, F., Horhota, M., & Mienaltowski, A. (2008). Social context and cognition. In S. M. Hofer & D. F. Alwin (Eds.), *Handbook of cognitive aging: Interdisciplinary perspectives* (pp. 614–628). Sage Publications.

Boduroglu, A., Yoon, C., Luo, T., & Park, D. C. (2006). Age-related stereotypes: A comparison of American and Chinese cultures. *Gerontology*, *52*(5), 324–333. doi:10.1159/000094614

Boone, K. B., Victor, T. L., Wen, J., Razani, J., & Pontón, M. (2007). The association between neuropsychological scores and ethnicity, language, and acculturation variables in a large patient population. *Archives of Clinical Neuropsychology*, *22*(3), 355–365. doi:10.1016/j.acn.2007.01.010

Boyke, J., Driemeyer, J., Gaser, C., Buchel, C., & May, A. (2008). Training-induced brain structure changes in the elderly. *Journal of Neuroscience*, *28*(28), 7031–7035. doi:10.1523/jneurosci.0742-08.2008

Braveman, P. A., Cubbin, C., Egerter, S., Chideya, S., Marchi, K. S., Metzler, M., & Posner, S. (2005). Socioeconomic status in health research: One size does not fit all. *JAMA: Journal of the American Medical Association*, *294*(22), 2879–2888. doi:10.1001/jama.294.22.2879

Brickman, A. M., Cabo, R., & Manly, J. J. (2006). Ethical issues in cross-cultural neuropsychology. *Applied Neuropsychology*, *13*(2), 91–100. doi:10.1207/s15324826an1302_4

Brown, C. L., Robitaille, A., Zelinski, E. M., Dixon, R. A., Hofer, S. M., & Piccinin, A. M. (2016). Cognitive activity mediates the association between social activity and cognitive performance: A longitudinal study. *Psychology of Aging*, *31*(8), 831–846. doi:10.1037/pag0000134

Byrd, D. A., Sanchez, D., & Manly, J. J. (2005). Neuropsychological test performance among Caribbean-born and U.S.-born African American elderly: The role of age, education and reading level. *Journal of Clinical and Experimental Neuropsychology*, *27*(8), 1056–1069. doi:10.1080/13803390490919353

Byrd, D. A., Touradji, P., Tang, M.-X., & Manly, J. J. (2004). Cancellation test performance in African American, Hispanic, and White elderly. *Journal of the International Neuropsychological Society*, *10*(3), 401–411. doi:10.1017/S1355617704103081

Carlson, M. C., Brandt, J., Carson, K. A., & Kawas, C. H. (1998). Lack of relation between race and cognitive test performance in Alzheimer's disease. *Neurology*, *50*(5), 1499–1501. doi:10.1212/WNL.50.5.1499

Carstensen, L. L. (1992). Motivation for social contact across the life span: A theory of socioemotional selectivity. *Nebraska Symposium on Motivation*, *40*, 209–254.

Carstensen, L. L. (2006). The influence of a sense of time on human development. *Science*, *312*(5782), 1913–1915. doi:10.1126/science.1127488

Cavallini, E., Bottiroli, S., Fastame, M. C., & Hertzog, C. (2013). Age and subcultural differences on personal and general beliefs about memory. *Journal of Aging Studies*, *27*(1), 71–81. doi:10.1016/j.jaging.2012.11.002

Charles, S. T., & Carstensen, L. L. (2010). Social and emotional aging. *Annual Review of Psychology*, *61*, 383–409. doi:10.1146/annurev.psych.093008.100448

Chee, M. W., Zheng, H., Goh, J. O., Park, D., & Sutton, B. P. (2011). Brain structure in young and old East Asians and Westerners: Comparisons of structural volume and cortical thickness. *Journal of Cognitive Neuroscience*, *23*(5), 1065–1079. doi:10.1162/jocn.2010.21513

Chua, H. F., Chen, W., & Park, D. C. (2006). Source memory, aging and culture. *Gerontology*, *52*, 306–313.

Coffey, D. M., Marmol, L., Schock, L., & Adams, W. (2005). The influence of acculturation on the Wisconsin Card Sorting Test by Mexican Americans. *Archives of Clinical Neuropsychology*, *20*(6), 795–803. doi:10.1016/j.acn.2005.04.009

Connell, C. M., Roberts, J. S., & McLaughlin, S. J. (2007). Public opinion about Alzheimer disease among Blacks, Hispanics, and Whites: Results from a national survey. *Alzheimer Disease and Associated Disorders*, *21*(3), 232–240. doi:10.1097/WAD.0b013e3181461740

Conway, M. A., Wang, Q., Hanyu, K., & Haque, S. (2005). A cross-cultural investigation of autobiographical memory: On the universality and cultural variation of the reminiscence bump. *Journal of Cross-Cultural Psychology*, *36*(6), 739–749. doi:10.1177/0022022105280512

Courchesne, E., Chisum, H. J., Townsend, J., Cowles, A., Covington, J., Egaas, B., Harwood, M., Hinds, S., & Press, G. A. (2000). Normal brain development and aging: Quantitative analysis at in vivo MR imaging in healthy volunteers. *Radiology*, *216*(3), 672–682. doi:10.1148/radiology.216.3.r00au37672

Craik, F. I., Bialystok, E., & Freedman, M. (2010). Delaying the onset of Alzheimer disease: Bilingualism as a form of cognitive reserve. *Neurology*, *75*(19), 1726–1729. doi:10.1212/WNL.0b013e3181fc2a1c

Crowe, M., Clay, O. J., Martin, R. C., Howard, V. J., Wadley, V. G., Sawyer, P., & Allman, R. M. (2013). Indicators of childhood quality of education in relation to cognitive function in older adulthood. *Journals of Gerontology: Series A: Biological Sciences and Medical Sciences*, *68*(2), 198–204. doi:10.1093/gerona/gls122

Darowski, E. S., Helder, E., Zacks, R. T., Hasher, L., & Hambrick, D. Z. (2008). Age-related differences in cognition: The role of distraction control. *Neuropsychology*, *22*(5), 638–644. doi:10.1037/0894-4105.22.5.638

Davies, M. S., Strickland, T. L., & Cao, M. (2014). Neuropsychological evaluation of culturally diverse populations. In F. T. L. Leong, L. Comas-Díaz, G. C. Nagayama Hall, V. C. McLoyd, J. E. Trimble, F. T. L. Leong, L. Comas-Díaz, G. C. Nagayama Hall, V. C. McLoyd, & J. E. Trimble (Eds.), *APA handbook of multicultural psychology, Vol. 2: Applications and training* (pp. 231–251). American Psychological Association.

de Paula, J. J., Costa, M. V., Bocardi, M. B., Cortezzi, M., De Moraes, E. N., & Malloy-Diniz, L. F. (2013). The Stick Design Test on the assessment of older adults with low formal education: Evidences of construct, criterion-related and ecological validity. *International Psychogeriatrics*, *25*(12), 2057–2065. doi:10.1017/S1041610213001282

Demiray, B., Gülgöz, S., & Bluck, S. (2009). Examining the life story account of the reminiscence bump: Why we remember more from young adulthood. *Memory*, *17*(7), 708–723. doi:10.1080/09658210902939322

Dilworth-Anderson, P., & Gibson, B. E. (2002). The cultural influence of values, norms, meanings, and perceptions in understanding dementia in ethnic minorities. *Alzheimer Disease and Associated Disorders*, *16*(Suppl 2), S56–S63. doi:10.1097/00002093-200200002-00005

Draganski, B., Gaser, C., Busch, V., Schuierer, G., Bogdahn, U., & May, A. (2004). Neuroplasticity: Changes in grey matter induced by training. *Nature*, *427*(6972), 311–312. doi:10.1038/427311a

Early, D. R., Widaman, K. F., Harvey, D., Beckett, L., Park, L. Q., Farias, S. T., Reed, B., Decarli, C., & Mungas, D. (2013). Demographic predictors of cognitive change in ethnically diverse older persons. *Psychology and Aging*, *28*(3), 633–645. Doi:10.1037/a0031645

Escobar, J. I., Burnam, A., Karno, M., Forsythe, A., Landsverk, J., & Golding, J. M. (1986). Use of the Mini-Mental State Examination (MMSE) in a community population of mixed ethnicity: Cultural and linguistic artifacts. *Journal of Nervous and Mental Disease*, *174*(10), 607–614. doi:10.1097/00005053-198610000-00005

Esiri, M. M. (2007). Ageing and the brain. *Journal of Pathology*, *211*(2), 181–187. doi:10.1002/path.2089

Farrer, L. A., Cupples, L. A., Haines, J. L., Hyman, B., Kukull, W. A., Mayeux, R., Myers, R. H., Pericak-Vance, M. A., Risch, N., & van Duijn, C. M. (1997). Effects of age, sex, and ethnicity on the association between apolipoprotein E genotype and Alzheimer disease. A meta-analysis. APOE and Alzheimer Disease Meta Analysis Consortium. *JAMA*, *278*(16), 1349–1356.

Ferman, T. J., Lucas, J. A., Ivnik, R. J., Smith, G. E., Willis, F. B., Petersen, R. C., & Graff-Radford, N. R. (2005). Mayo's Older African American Normative Studies: Auditory verbal learning test norms for African American elders. *Clinical Neuropsychologist*, *19*(2), 214–227. doi:10.1080/13854040590945300

Fillenbaum, G. G., Heyman, A., Huber, M. S., Ganguli, M., & Unverzagt, F. W. (2001). Performance of elderly African American and White community residents on the CERAD Neuropsychological Battery. *Journal of the International Neuropsychological Society*, *7*(4), 502–509. doi:10.1017/S1355617701744062

Fjell, A. M., & Walhovd, K. B. (2010). Structural brain changes in aging: Courses, causes and cognitive consequences. *Reviews in the Neurosciences*, *21*(3), 187–221.

Fjell, A. M., Walhovd, K. B., Fennema-Notestine, C., McEvoy, L. K., Hagler, D. J., Holland, D., Brewer, J. B., & Dale, A. M. (2009). One year brain atrophy evident in healthy aging. *Journal of Neuroscience*, *29*(48), 15223–15231. doi:10.1523/jneurosci.3252-09.2009

Fotenos, A. F., Mintun, M. A., Snyder, A. Z., Morris, J. C., & Buckner, R. L. (2008). Brain volume decline in aging: Evidence for a relation between socioeconomic status, preclinical Alzheimer disease, and reserve. *Archives of Neurology, 65*(1), 113–120. doi:10.1001/archneurol.2007.27

Freeman, S. H., Kandel, R., Cruz, L., Rozkalne, A., Newell, K., Frosch, M. P., Hedley-Whyte, E. T., Locascio, J. J., Lipsitz, L. A., & Hyman, B. T. (2008). Preservation of neuronal number despite age-related cortical brain atrophy in elderly subjects without Alzheimer disease. *Journal of Neuropathology and Experimental Neurology, 67*(12), 1205–1212. doi:10.1097/NEN.0b013e31818fc72f

Fung, H. H., Carstensen, L. L., & Lang, F. R. (2001). Age-related patterns in social networks among European Americans and African Americans: Implications for socioemotional selectivity across the life span. *International Journal on Aging and Human Development, 52*(3), 185–206. doi:10.2190/1ABL-9BE5-M0X2-LR9V

Fung, H. H., Isaacowitz, D. M., Lu, A. Y., & Li, T. (2010). Interdependent self-construal moderates the age-related negativity reduction effect in memory and visual attention. *Psychology and Aging, 25*(2), 321–329. doi:10.1037/a0019079

Fung, H. H., Isaacowitz, D. M., Lu, A. Y., Wadlinger, H. A., Goren, D., & Wilson, H. R. (2008). Age-related positivity enhancement is not universal: Older Chinese look away from positive stimuli. *Psychology and Aging, 23*(2), 440–446. doi:10.1037/0882-7974.23.2.440

Fung, H. H., Stoeber, F. S., Yeung, D. Y., & Lang, F. R. (2008). Cultural specificity of socioemotional selectivity: Age differences in social network composition among Germans and Hong Kong Chinese. *Journals of Gerontology: Series B: Psychological Sciences and Social Sciences, 63*(3), P156–P164.

Glosser, G., Wolfe, N., Albert, M. L., Lavine, L., Steele, J. C., Calne, D. B., & Schoenberg, B. S. (1993). Cross-cultural cognitive examination: Validation of a dementia screening instrument for neuroepidemiological research. *Journal of the American Geriatrics Society, 41*(9), 931–939. doi:10.1111/j.1532-5415.1993.tb06758.x

Goh, J. O., Chee, M. W., Tan, J. C., Venkatraman, V., Hebrank, A., Leshikar, E. D., Jenkins, L., Sutton, B. P., Gutchess, A. H., & Park, D. C. (2007). Age and culture modulate object processing and object-scene binding in the ventral visual area. *Cognitive, Affective, and Behavioral Neuroscience, 7*, 44–52.

Gomez-Isla, T., Price, J. L., McKeel, D. W., Jr., Morris, J. C., Growdon, J. H., & Hyman, B. T. (1996). Profound loss of layer II entorhinal cortex neurons occurs in very mild Alzheimer's disease. *Journal of Neuroscience, 16*(14), 4491–4500.

Good, C. D., Johnsrude, I. S., Ashburner, J., Henson, R. N., Friston, K. J., & Frackowiak, R. S. (2001). A voxel-based morphometric study of ageing in 465 normal adult human brains. *Neuroimage, 14*(1 Pt 1), 21–36. doi:10.1006/nimg.2001.0786

Grossmann, I., Karasawa, M., Kan, C., & Kitayama, S. (2014). A cultural perspective on emotional experiences across the life span. *Emotion, 14*(4), 679–692. doi:10.1037/a0036041

Guerreiro, R., & Bras, J. (2015). The age factor in Alzheimer's disease. *Genome Medicine, 7*, 106. doi:10.1186/s13073-015-0232-5

Gutchess, A., & Boduroglu, A. (2019). Cultural differences in categorical memory errors persist with age. *Aging and Mental Health, 23*(7), 851–854. doi:10.1080/13607863.2017.1421616

Gutchess, A. H., & Huff, S. (2015). Cross-cultural differences in memory. In J. Chiao, S-C. Li, R. Seligman, & R. Turner (Eds.), *Handbook of cultural neuroscience* (Vol. 1pps. 155–170). Oxford University Press.

Gutchess, A. H., Yoon, C., Luo, T., Feinberg, F., Hedden, T., Jing, Q., Nisbett, R. E., & Park, D. C. (2006). Categorical organization in free recall across culture and age. *Gerontology, 52*(5), 314–323. doi:10.1159/000094613

Hall, K., Murrell, J., Ogunniyi, A., Deeg, M., Baiyewu, O., Gao, S., Gureje, O., Dickens, J., Evans, R., Smith-Gamble, V., Unverzagt, F. W., Shen, J., & Hendrie, H. (2006). Cholesterol, APOE genotype, and Alzheimer disease: An epidemiologic study of Nigerian Yoruba. *Neurology, 66*(2), 223–227. doi:10.1212/01.wnl.0000194507.39504.17

Haque, S., & Hasking, P. A. (2010). Life scripts for emotionally charged autobiographical memories: A cultural explanation of the reminiscence bump. *Memory, 18*(7), 712–729. doi:10.1080/09658211.2010.506442

Hayles, V. R., Jr. (1991). African American strengths: A survey of empirical findings. In R. L. Jones & R. L. Jones (Eds.), *Black psychology* (pp. 379–400). Cobb & Henry Publishers.

Hebert, L. E., Scherr, P. A., Bienias, J. L., Bennett, D. A., & Evans, D. A. (2003). Alzheimer disease in the US population: Prevalence estimates using the 2000 census. *Archives of Neurology, 60*(8), 1119–1122. doi:10.1001/archneur.60.8.1119

Hedden, T., Park, D. C., Nisbett, R., Ji, L.-J., Jing, Q., & Jiao, S. (2002). Cultural variation in verbal versus spatial neuropsychological function across the life span. *Neuropsychology, 16*(1), 65–73. doi:10.1037/0894-4105.16.1.65

Hendrie, H. C., Ogunniyi, A., Hall, K. S., Baiyewu, O., Unverzagt, F. W., Gureje, O., Gao, S., Evans, R. M., Ogunseyinde, A. O., Adeyinka, A. O., Musick, B., & Hui, S. L. (2001). Incidence of dementia and Alzheimer disease in 2 communities: Yoruba residing in Ibadan, Nigeria, and African Americans residing in Indianapolis, Indiana. *JAMA, 285*(6), 739–747.

Heverly, L. L., Isaac, W., & Hynd, G. W. (1986). Neurodevelopmental and racial differences in tactile-visual (cross-modal) discrimination in normal Black and White children. *Archives of Clinical Neuropsychology, 1*(2), 139–145. doi:10.1016/0887-6177(86)90013-2

Hughes, T. F., Andel, R., Small, B. J., Borenstein, A. R., & Mortimer, J. A. (2008). The association between social resources and cognitive change in older adults: Evidence from the Charlotte County Healthy Aging Study. *Journals of Gerontology: Series B: Psychological Sciences and Social Sciences, 63*(4), P241–P244.

Ji, L. J., Zhang, Z. Y., & Nisbett, R. E. (2004). Is it culture or is it language? Examination of language effects in cross-cultural research on categorization. *Journal of Personality and Social Psychology, 87*(1), 57–65. doi:10.1037/0022-3514.87.1.57

Johnson, A. S., Flicker, L. J., & Lichtenberg, P. A. (2006). Reading ability mediates the relationship between education and executive function tasks. *Journal of the International Neuropsychological Society, 12*(1), 64–71. doi:10.1017/S1355617706060073

Jones, R. N. (2003). Racial bias in the assessment of cognitive functioning of older adults. *Aging and Mental Health, 7*(2), 83–102. doi:10.1080/1360786031000045872

Jones, R. N., & Gallo, J. J. (2002). Education and sex differences in the Mini-Mental State Examination: Effects of differential item functioning. *Journals of Gerontology: Series B: Psychological Sciences and Social Sciences, 57*(6), P548–P558. doi:10.1093/geronb/57.6.P548

Kahana, E., Galper, Y., Zilber, N., & Korczyn, A. D. (2003). Epidemiology of dementia in Ashkelon: The influence of education. *Journal of Neurology, 250*(4), 424–428. doi:10.1007/s00415-003-0999-y

Kanai, R., Feilden, T., Firth, C., & Rees, G. (2011). Political orientations are correlated with brain structure in young adults. *Current Biology, 21*(8), 677–680. https://doi.org/10.1016/j.cub.2011.03.017

Katzman, R. (1993). Education and the prevalence of dementia and Alzheimer's disease. *Neurology, 43*(1), 13–20. doi:10.1212/wnl.43.1_part_1.13. PMID: 8423876.

Kempler, D., Teng, E. L., Taussig, M., & Dick, M. B. (2010). The common objects memory test (COMT): A simple test with cross-cultural applicability. *Journal of the International Neuropsychological Society, 16*(3), 537–545. doi:10.1017/S1355617710000160

Kennedy, Q., Mather, M., & Carstensen, L. L. (2004). The role of motivation in the age-related positivity effect in autobiographical memory. *Psychological Science, 15*(3), 208–214. doi:10.1111/j.0956-7976.2004.01503011.x

Kim, P., Leckman, J. F., Mayes, L. C., Feldman, R., Wang, X., & Swain, J. E. (2010). The plasticity of human maternal brain: Longitudinal changes in brain anatomy during the early postpartum period. *Behavioral Neuroscience, 124*(5), 695–700. doi:10.1037/a0020884

Kwon, Y., Scheibe, S., Samanez-Larkin, G. R., Tsai, J. L., & Carstensen, L. L. (2009). Replicating the positivity effect in picture memory in Koreans: Evidence for cross-cultural generalizability. *Psychology and Aging, 24*(3), 748–754. doi:10.1037/a0016054

Lang, I. A., Llewellyn, D. J., Langa, K. M., Wallace, R. B., Huppert, F. A., & Melzer, D. (2008). Neighborhood deprivation, individual socioeconomic status, and cognitive function in older people: Analyses from the English Longitudinal Study of Ageing. *Journal of the American Geriatric Society, 56*(2), 191–198. doi:10.1111/j.1532-5415.2007.01557.x

Lawrence, V., Murray, J., Samsi, K., & Banerjee, S. (2008). Attitudes and support needs of Black Caribbean, South Asian and White British carers of people with dementia in the UK. *British Journal of Psychiatry, 193*(3), 240–246. doi:10.1192/bjp.bp.107.045187

Le Carret, N., Lafont, S., Letenneur, L., Dartigues, J.-F., Mayo, W., & Fabrigoule, C. (2003). The effect of education on cognitive performances and its implication for the constitution of the cognitive reserve. *Developmental Neuropsychology, 23*(3), 317–337. doi:10.1207/S15326942DN2303_1

Leuba, G., & Kraftsik, R. (1994). Visual cortex in Alzheimer's disease: Occurrence of neuronal death and glial proliferation, and correlation with pathological hallmarks. *Neurobiology and Aging, 15*(1), 29–43.

Levy, B., & Langer, E. (1994). Aging free from negative stereotypes: Successful memory in China and among the American deaf. *Journal of Personality and Social Psychology, 66*(6), 989–997.

Loewenstein, D. A., Argüelles, T., Barker, W. W., & Duara, R. (1993). A comparative analysis of neuropsychological test performance of Spanish-speaking and English-speaking patients with Alzheimer's disease. *Journal of Gerontology, 48*(3), P142–P149. doi:10.1093/geronj/48.3.P142

Mangone, C. A., & Arizaga, R. L. (1999). Dementia in Argentina and other Latin-American countries: An overview. *Neuroepidemiology, 18*(5), 231–235. doi:10.1159/000026216

Manly, J. J. (2005). Advantages and disadvantages of separate norms for African Americans. *Clinical Neuropsychologist, 19*(2), 270–275. doi:10.1080/13854040590945346

Manly, J. J., Byrd, D. A., Touradji, P., & Stern, Y. (2004). Acculturation, reading level, and neuropsychological test performance among African American elders. *Applied Neuropsychology, 11*(1), 37–46. doi:10.1207/s15324826an1101_5

Manly, J. J., Jacobs, D. M., Sano, M., Bell, K., Merchant, C. A., Small, S. A., & Stern, Y. (1998). Cognitive test performance among nondemented elderly African Americans and Whites. *Neurology, 50*(5), 1238–1245. doi:10.1212/WNL.50.5.1238

Manly, J. J., Jacobs, D. M., Touradji, P., Small, S. A., & Stern, Y. (2002). Reading level attenuates differences in neuropsychological test performance between African American and White elders. *Journal of the International Neuropsychological Society, 8*(3), 341–348. doi:10.1017/S1355617702813157

Manly, J. J., & Mayeux, R. (2004). Ethnic differences in dementia and Alzheimer's disease. In N. Anderson, R. A. Bulatao, & B. Cohen (Eds.), *Critical perspectives on racial and ethnic differences in health in late life* (pp. 95–145). National Academies Press.

Manly, J. J., Touradji, P., Tang, M.-X., & Stern, Y. (2003). Literacy and memory decline among ethnically diverse elders. *Journal of Clinical and Experimental Neuropsychology, 25*(5), 680–690. doi:10.1076/jcen.25.5.680.14579

Markus, H. R., & Kitayama, S. (1991). Culture and the self: Implications for cognition, emotion, & motivation. *Psychological Review, 98*, 224–253.

Marner, L., Nyengaard, J. R., Tang, Y., & Pakkenberg, B. (2003). Marked loss of myelinated nerve fibers in the human brain with age. *Journal of Comparative Neurology, 462*(2), 144–152. doi:10.1002/cne.10714

Masuda, T., & Nisbett, R. E. (2001). Attending holistically versus analytically: Comparing the context sensitivity of Japanese and Americans. *Journal of Personality and Social Psychology, 81*(5), 922–934. doi:10.1037//0022-3514.81.5.922

Mather, M., Johnson, M. K., & De Leonardis, D. M. (1999). Stereotype reliance in source monitoring: Age differences and neuropsychological test correlates. *Cognitive Neuropsychology, 16*(3–5), 437–458.

Mather, M., & Knight, M. (2005). Goal-directed memory: The role of cognitive control in older adults' emotional memory. *Psychology and Aging, 20*(4), 554–570. doi:10.1037/0882-7974.20.4.554

McDonald, C. R., McEvoy, L. K., Gharapetian, L., Fennema-Notestine, C., Hagler, D. J., Jr., Holland, D., Koyama, A., Brewer, J. B., & Dale, A. M. (2009). Regional rates of neocortical atrophy from normal aging to early Alzheimer disease. *Neurology, 73*(6), 457–465. doi:10.1212/WNL.0b013e3181b16431

Mikels, J. A., Larkin, G. R., Reuter-Lorenz, P. A., & Cartensen, L. L. (2005). Divergent trajectories in the aging mind: Changes in working memory for affective versus visual information with age. *Psychology and Aging, 20*(4), 542–553. doi:10.1037/0882-7974.20.4.542

Mograbi, D. C., Ferri, C. P., Sosa, A. L., Stewart, R., Laks, J., Brown, R., & Morris, R. G. (2012). Unawareness of memory impairment in dementia: A population-based study. *International Psychogeriatrics, 24*(6), 931–939. doi:10.1017/S1041610211002730

Mukadam, N., Cooper, C., & Livingston, G. (2011). A systematic review of ethnicity and pathways to care in dementia. *International Journal of Geriatric Psychiatry, 26*(1), 12–20. doi:10.1002/gps.2484

Murphy, N. A., & Isaacowitz, D. M. (2008). Preferences for emotional information in older and younger adults: A meta-analysis of memory and attention tasks. *Psychology and Aging, 23*(2), 263–286. doi:10.1037/0882-7974.23.2.263

Nielsen, T. R., Vogel, A., Phung, T. K. T., Gade, A., & Waldemar, G. (2011). Over- and under-diagnosis of dementia in ethnic minorities: A nationwide register-based study. *International Journal of Geriatric Psychiatry, 26*(11), 1128–1135.

Nile, E., & Van Bergen, P. (2015). Not all semantics: Similarities and differences in reminiscing function and content between Indigenous and non-Indigenous Australians. *Memory, 23*(1), 83–98. doi:10.1080/09658211.2014.931973

Nisbett, R. E., & Masuda, T. (2003). Culture and point of view. *Proceedings of the National Academy of Sciences of the United States of America*, *100*(19), 11163–11170. doi:10.1073/pnas.1934527100

Nitrini, R., Mathias, S. C., Caramelli, P., Carrilho, P. E., Lefèvre, B. H., Porto, C. S., Magila, M. C., Buchpiguel, C., de Barros, N. G., & Gualandro, S. (1995). Evaluation of 100 patients with dementia in Sao Paulo, Brazil: Correlation with socioeconomic status and education. *Alzheimer Disease and Associated Disorders 9*(3), 146–151.

Ojeda, N., Aretouli, E., Peña, J., & Schretlen, D. J. (2016). Age differences in cognitive performance: A study of cultural differences in Historical Context. *Journal of Neuropsychology*, *10*(1), 104–115. doi:10.1111/jnp.12059

Park, D., & Gutchess, A. (2006). The cognitive neuroscience of aging and culture. *Current Directions in Psychological Science*, *15*(3), 105.

Park, D. C., & Gutchess, A. H. (2002). Aging, cognition, and culture: A neuroscientific perspective. *Neuroscience and Biobehavioral Reviews*, *26*(7), 859–867. doi:S0149763402000726 [pii]

Park, D. C., Nisbett, R. E., & Hedden, T. (1999). Aging, culture, and cognition. *Journals of Gerontology: Series B: Psychological Sciences and Social Sciences*, *54*(2), P75–P84.

Parveen, S., Peltier, C., & Oyebode, J. R. (2017). Perceptions of dementia and use of services in minority ethnic communities: A scoping exercise. *Health & Social Care in the Community*, *25*(2), 734–742. doi:10.1111/hsc.12363

Pedraza, O., Lucas, J. A., Smith, G. E., Willis, F. B., Graff-Radford, N. R., Ferman, T. J., Peterson, R. C., Bowers, D., Ivnik, R. J.,& Ivnik, R. J. (2005). Mayo's Older African American Normative Studies: Confirmatory factor analysis of a core battery. *Journal of the International Neuropsychological Society*, *11*(2), 184–191. doi:10.1017/S1355617705050204

Pedraza, O., & Mungas, D. (2008). Measurement in cross-cultural neuropsychology. *Neuropsychology Review*, *18*(3), 184–193. doi:10.1007/s11065-008-9067-9

Peters, A., Moss, M. B., & Sethares, C. (2000). Effects of aging on myelinated nerve fibers in monkey primary visual cortex. *Journal of Comparative Neurology*, *419*(3), 364–376.

Prince, M., Acosta, D., Chiu, H., Scazufca, M., & Varghese, M. (2003). Dementia diagnosis in developing countries: A cross-cultural validation study. *Lancet*, *361*(9361), 909–917. doi:10.1016/S0140-6736(03)12772-9

Puente, A. E., Perez-Garcia, M., Lopez, R. V., Hidalgo-Ruzzante, N. A., & Fasfous, A. F. (2013). Neuropsychological assessment of culturally and educationally dissimilar individuals. In F. A. Paniagua, A.-M. Yamada, F. A. Paniagua, & A.-M. Yamada (Eds.), *Handbook of multicultural mental health: Assessment and treatment of diverse populations.* (pp. 225–241). Elsevier Academic Press.

Purandare, N., Luthra, V., Swarbrick, C., & Bums, A. (2007). Knowledge of dementia among South Asian (Indian) older people in Manchester, UK. *International Journal of Geriatric Psychiatry*, *22*(8), 777–781. doi:10.1002/gps.1740

Ramirez Gomez, L., Jain, F. A., & D'Orazio, L. M. (2017). Assessment of the Hispanic cognitively impaired elderly patient. *Neurologic Clinics*, *35*(2), 207–229. doi:10.1016/j.ncl.2017.01.003

Rapp, P. R., Deroche, P. S., Mao, Y., & Burwell, R. D. (2002). Neuron number in the parahippocampal region is preserved in aged rats with spatial learning deficits. *Cerebral Cortex*, *12*(11), 1171–1179.

Raz, N., Gunning-Dixon, F., Head, D., Rodrigue, K. M., Williamson, A., & Acker, J. D. (2004). Aging, sexual dimorphism, and hemispheric asymmetry of the cerebral cortex: replicability of regional differences in volume. *Neurobiology and Aging*, *25*(3), 377–396. doi:10.1016/s0197-4580(03)00118-0

Razani, J., Burciaga, J., Madore, M., & Wong, J. (2007). Effects of acculturation on tests of attention and information processing in an ethnically diverse group. *Archives of Clinical Neuropsychology*, *22*(3), 333–341. doi:10.1016/j.acn.2007.01.008

Razani, J., Murcia, G., Tabares, J., & Wong, J. (2007). The effects of culture on WASI test performance in ethnically diverse individuals. *Clinical Neuropsychologist*, *21*(5), 776–788. doi:10.1080/13854040701437481

Rilling, L. M., Lucas, J. A., Ivnik, R. J., Smith, G. E., Willis, F. B., Ferman, T. J., Peterson, R. C., & Graff-Radford, N. R. (2005). Mayo's Older African American Normative Studies: Norms for the Mattis Dementia Rating Scale. *Clinical Neuropsychologist*, *19*(2), 229–242. doi:10.1080/13854040590945328

Rosenberg, R. N., Richter, R. W., Risser, R. C., Taubman, K., Prado-Farmer, I., Ebalo, E., Posey, J., Kingfisher, D., Dean, D., Weiner, M. F., Svetlik, D., Adams, P., Honig, L. S., Cullum, C. M., Schaefer, F. V., & Schellenberg, G. D. (1996). Genetic factors for the development of Alzheimer disease in the Cherokee Indian. *Archives of Neurology*, *53*(10), 997–1000.

Ross, M., & Wang, Q. (2010). Why we remember and what we remember: Culture and autobiographical memory. *Perspectives on Psychological Science, 5*(4), 401–409. doi:10.1177/1745691610375555

Rosselli, M., & Ardila, A. (2003). The impact of culture and education on non-verbal neuropsychological measurements: A critical review. *Brain and Cognition, 52*(3), 326–333. doi:10.1016/S0278-2626(03)00170-2

Rosselli, M., Ardila, A., & Rosas, P. (1990). Neuropsychological assessment in illiterates: II. Language and praxic abilities. *Brain and Cognition, 12*(2), 281–296. doi:10.1016/0278-2626(90)90020-O

Rubin, D. C., Wetzler, S. E., & Nebes, R. D. (1986). Autobiographical memory across the lifespan. In D. C. Rubin & D. C. Rubin (Eds.), *Autobiographical memory* (pp. 202–221). Cambridge University Press.

Sayegh, P. (2016). Cross-cultural issues in the neuropsychological assessment of dementia. In F. R. Ferraro & F. R. Ferraro (Eds.), *Minority and cross-cultural aspects of neuropsychological assessment: Enduring and emerging trends* (pp. 54–71). Taylor & Francis.

Schrauf, R. W., & Iris, M. (2011). A direct comparison of popular models of normal memory loss and Alzheimer's disease in samples of African Americans, Mexican Americans, and refugees and immigrants from the former Soviet Union. *Journal of the American Geriatrics Society, 59*(4), 628–636. doi:10.1111/j.1532-5415.2011.03361.x

Schretlen, D., Pearlson, G. D., Anthony, J. C., Aylward, E. H., Augustine, A. M., Davis, A., & Barta, P. (2000). Elucidating the contributions of processing speed, executive ability, and frontal lobe volume to normal age-related differences in fluid intelligence. *Journal of the International Neuropsychological Society, 6*(1), 52–61.

Schwartz, A. J., Boduroglu, A., & Gutchess, A. H. (2014). Cross-cultural differences in categorical memory errors. *Cognitive Science, 38*(5), 997–1007. doi:10.1111/cogs.12109

Scruggs, T. E., & Lifson, S. A. (1985). Current conceptions of test-wiseness: Myths and realities. *School Psychology Review, 14*(3), 339–350.

Seeman, T. E., Lusignolo, T. M., Albert, M., & Berkman, L. (2001). Social relationships, social support, and patterns of cognitive aging in healthy, high-functioning older adults: MacArthur studies of successful aging. *Health and Psychology, 20*(4), 243–255.

Simic, G., Kostovic, I., Winblad, B., & Bogdanovic, N. (1997). Volume and number of neurons of the human hippocampal formation in normal aging and Alzheimer's disease. *Journal of Comprehensive Neurology, 379*(4), 482–494.

Sparks, S., Cunningham, S. J., & Kritikos, A. (2016). Culture modulates implicit ownership-induced self-bias in memory. *Cognition, 153*, 89–98. doi:10.1016/j.cognition.2016.05.003

Stern, Y. (2002). What is cognitive reserve? Theory and research application of the reserve concept. *Journal of the International Neuropsychological Society, 8*(3), 448–460.

Stern, Y., Gurland, B., Tatemichi, T. K., Tang, M. X., Wilder, D., & Mayeux, R. (1994). Influence of education and occupation on the incidence of Alzheimer's disease. *JAMA, 271*(13), 1004–1010.

Sullivan, E. V., Rosenbloom, M., Serventi, K. L., & Pfefferbaum, A. (2004). Effects of age and sex on volumes of the thalamus, pons, and cortex. *Neurobiology and Aging, 25*(2), 185–192.

Touradji, P., Manly, J. J., Jacobs, D. M., & Stern, Y. (2001). Neuropsychological test performance: A study of non-Hispanic White elderly. *Journal of Clinical and Experimental Neuropsychology, 23*(5), 643–649. doi:10.1076/jcen.23.5.643.1246

Tucker-Drob, E. M., Johnson, K. E., & Jones, R. N. (2009). The cognitive reserve hypothesis: A longitudinal examination of age-associated declines in reasoning and processing speed. *Developmental Psychology, 45*(2), 431–446. doi:10.1037/a0014012

United Nations, Department of Economic and Social Affairs, Population Division (2015). *World Population Ageing 2015 – Highlights.* https://www.un.org/en/development/desa/population/publications/pdf/ageing/WPA2015_Highlights.pdf

Unverzagt, F. W., Hall, K. S., Torke, A. M., Rediger, J. D., Mercado, N., Gureje, O., Osuntokun, B. O., & Hendrie, H. C. (1996). Effects of age, education and gender on CERAD neuropsychological test performance in an African American sample. *Clinical Neuropsychologist, 10*(2), 180–190. doi:10.1080/13854049608406679

van Gelder, B. M., Tijhuis, M., Kalmijn, S., Giampaoli, S., Nissinen, A., & Kromhout, D. (2006). Marital status and living situation during a 5-year period are associated with a subsequent 10-year cognitive decline in older men: The FINE Study. *Journals of Gerontology Series B: Psychological Sciences and Social Sciences, 61*(4), P213–P219.

Walhovd, K. B., Westlye, L. T., Amlien, I., Espeseth, T., Reinvang, I., Raz, N., Agartz, I., Salat, D. H., Greve, D. N., Fischl, B., Dale, A. M., & Fjell, A. M. (2011). Consistent neuroanatomical age-related volume differences across multiple samples. *Neurobiology and Aging, 32*(5), 916–932. doi:10.1016/j.neurobiolaging.2009.05.013

Wang, J., He, L., Jia, L., Tian, J., & Benson, V. (2015). The 'positive effect' is present in older Chinese adults: Evidence from an eye tracking study. *PLoS One, 10*(4), e0121372.

Weiner, M. F. (2008). Perspective on race and ethnicity in Alzheimer's disease research. *Alzheimer's & Dementia: The Journal of the Alzheimer's Association, 4*(4), 233–238. doi:10.1016/j.jalz.2007.10.016

Welsh, K. A., Fillenbaum, G., Wilkinson, W., Heyman, A., Mohs, R. C., Stern, Y., Harrell, L., Edland, S. D., Beekly, D. (1995). Neuropsychological test performance in African-American and White patients with Alzheimer's disease. *Neurology, 45*(12), 2207–2211. doi:10.1212/WNL.45.12.2207

White, L., Petrovitch, H., Ross, G. W., Masaki, K. H., Abbott, R. D., Teng, E. L., Rodriguez, B. L., Blanchette, P. L., Havlik, R. J., Wergowske, G., Chiu, D., Foley, D. J., Murdaugh, C., & Curb, J. D. (1996). Prevalence of dementia in older Japanese-American men in Hawaii: The Honolulu-Asia Aging Study. *JAMA, 276*(12), 955–960.

Whitfield, K. E. (2002). Challenges in cognitive assessment of African Americans in research on Alzheimer disease. *Alzheimer Disease and Associated Disorders, 16*(Suppl 2), S80–S81. doi:10.1097/00002093-200200002-00008

Whitfield, K. E., Fillenbaum, G. G., Pieper, C., Albert, M. S., Berkman, L. F., Blazer, D. G., Rowe, J. W., & Seeman, T. (2000). The effect of race and health-related factors on naming and memory: The MacArthur studies of successful aging. *Journal of Aging and Health, 12*(1), 69–89. doi:10.1177/089826430001200104

Williams, D. R. (1999). Race, socioeconomic status, and health: The added effects of racism and discrimination. In N. E. Adler, M. Marmot, B. S. McEwen, J. Stewart, N. E. Adler, M. Marmot, B. S. McEwen, & J. Stewart (Eds.), *Socioeconomic status and health in industrial nations: Social, psychological, and biological pathways.* (Vol. 896, pp. 173–188). New York Academy of Sciences.

Wilson, R. S., Krueger, K. R., Arnold, S. E., Schneider, J. A., Kelly, J. F., Barnes, L. L., Tang, Y., & Bennett, D. A. (2007). Loneliness and risk of Alzheimer disease. *Archives of General Psychiatry, 64*(2), 234–240. doi:10.1001/archpsyc.64.2.234

Wolfe, N. (2002). Cross-cultural neuropsychology of aging and dementia: An update. In F. R. Ferraro & F. R. Ferraro (Eds.), *Minority and cross-cultural aspects of neuropsychological assessment.* (pp. 285–297). Swets & Zeitlinger Publishers.

Woollett, K., & Maguire, E. A. (2011). Acquiring "the knowledge" of London's layout drives structural brain changes. *Current Biology, 21*(24), 2109–2114. doi:https://doi.org/10.1016/j.cub.2011.11.018

Yamada, M., Sasaki, H., Mimori, Y., Kasagi, F., Sudoh, S., Ikeda, J., Hosoda, Y., Nakamura, S., & Kodama, K. (1999). Prevalence and risks of dementia in the Japanese population: RERF's adult health study Hiroshima subjects. Radiation Effects Research Foundation. *Journal of the American Geriatric Society, 47*(2), 189–195.

Yang, L., Chen, W., Ng, A. H., & Fu, X. (2013). Aging, culture, and memory for categorically processed information. *Journals of Gerontology: Series B: Psychological Sciences and Social Sciences, 68*(6), 872–881. doi:10.1093/geronb/gbt006

Yang, L., Li, J., Spaniol, J., Hasher, L., Wilkinson, A. J., Yu, J., & Niu, Y. (2013). Aging, culture, and memory for socially meaningful item-context associations: An East-West cross-cultural comparison study. *PLoS One, 8*(4), e60703. doi:10.1371/journal.pone.0060703

Yoon, C., Hasher, L., Feinberg, F., Rahhal, T. A., & Winocur, G. (2000). Cross-cultural differences in memory: The role of culture-based stereotypes about aging. *Psychology and Aging, 15*(4), 694–704.

Yuan, P., & Raz, N. (2014). Prefrontal cortex and executive functions in healthy adults: A meta-analysis of structural neuroimaging studies. *Neuroscience and Biobehavioral Reviews, 42*, 180–192. doi:10.1016/j.neubiorev.2014.02.005

Zhang, M., Katzman, R., Salmon, D., Jin, H., Cai, G., Wang, Z., Qu, G., Yu, E., & Levy, P. (1990). The prevalence of dementia and Alzheimer's disease in Shanghai, China: Impact of age, gender, and education. *Annals of Neurology, 27*(4), 428–437.

Zhang, W., Hung, I., Jackson, J., Tai, T.-L., Goh, J. O. S., & Gutchess, A. (2020). Influence of culture and age on the self-reference effect. *Aging, Neuropsychology and Cognition, 27*(3), 370–384. doi: 10.1080/13825585.2019.1620913.

Zhu, Y., Zhang, L., Fan, J., & Han, S. (2007). Neural basis of cultural influence on self-representation. *Neuroimage, 34*(3), 1310–1316.

Zimmer, Z. (2005). Health and living arrangement transitions among China's oldest-old. *Research on Aging, 27*(5), 526–555. doi:10.1177/0164027505277848

Culture and Self-Construal

Sharon G. Goto, Richard S. Lewis, *and* Sarah Grayzel-Ward

Abstract

The construct of self-construal is central to our understanding of cultural differences and similarities in cognition and behavior with implications for the effective prevention, diagnosis, and treatment of major nervous system (MNS) disorders. Self-construal reflects the ways in which a person interacts with others and the environment. Interdependent self-construal refers to individuals whose selves are highly integrated and dependent on their significant social groups. In contrast, independent self-construal refers to those whose selves are less integrated with others and their significant social groups are based on instrumental transactions and goals. The cultural neuroscience literature triangulates the behavioral literature to help understand differences in self-construal across populations, the extent to which self-construal is determined and fluctuates based on situational factors, and the important interactions between genes and culture in understanding behavior. Theory, commonly used research methods, and implications of self-construal for understanding boundary conditions of health conditions, mechanisms of health disparity, and the possibility for intervention and prevention of MNS disorders are discussed.

Key Words: self-construal, individualism, collectivism, interdependence, identity, self

Research on self-construal has spanned more than 40 years, becoming central to our psychological understanding of cultural differences and similarities in cognition and behavior. Today, self-construal continues to expand its scope of influence by inspiring research in the field of cultural neuroscience. Focusing on self-construal to understand cross cultural differences using combinations of behavioral, cognitive, and neural measures has led to perhaps our deepest understanding of the way culture affects individual experiences (see Figure 15.1). Markus and Kitayama (2010) wrote that "the study of culture and self has renewed and extended psychology's understanding of self, identity, or agency and casts it as central to the analysis and interpretation of behavior." (p. 421). Similarly, self-construal has been described as "an interpretive frame for understanding the world," which then affects how individuals shift and prioritize their values and goals (Gardner et al., 1999, p. 322).

What is the self? Self-construal is built upon a fundamental construct, the self, for understanding the way a person interacts with others. S. T. Fiske and Taylor (1991) wrote

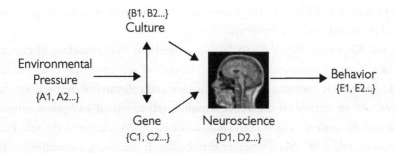

Note: Each factor in the cultural neuroscience model may be composed of a set of variables of each type (e.g., A1, A2 refers to distinct environmental variables; B1, B2 refers to distinct cultural variables).

Figure 15.1. Cultural neuroscience model of human behavior.

of the self as "a collection of at least semi-related and highly domain-specific knowledge structures" (p. 182) that contains information about the "individual person as a physical entity interacting with, and surviving in a particular environment" (Harb & Smith, 2008, p. 178). The self is similar to agency and identity, but agency relates to independence as an actor in the world, and identity refers to how an individual relates to or is influenced by important groups (Markus & Kitayama, 2010). Nonetheless, all of these constructs "attempt to index the dynamic and recursive process of organizing and integrating through which the individual, the biological entity, becomes a meaningful entity—that is a person." (Markus & Kitayama, p. 421).

In the seminal paper "The Self and Social Behavior in Differing Cultural Contexts," Triandis (1989) explored how the construal of the self influences the way an individual interacts with their environment. Triandis identified three different selves (private, public, and collective) that are shaped by cultural variables. From a social cognitive framework, behavior is influenced by sampling of the selves. The more complex the self, the higher probability it will be sampled (Trafimow et al., 1991). Triandis continues by discussing how different aspects of a culture, such as individualism or collectivism, complexity, and tightness or looseness, dictate how the self is developed. The effect of ingroup and outgroup processes are also analyzed, showing that social behavior is more communal with an ingroup member, and that these ingroup and outgroup distinctions are exhibited more strongly in collectivist cultures. Many of these ideas linking an individual's culture, the self, and their social behavior continue to influence the theory and methodologies of researchers in cultural neuroscience. While Triandis focused on public, private, and collective selves, some other types of self-construal include egocentric and sociocentric, autonomous, and independent and interdependent (Gardner et al., 1999). At the same time, Triandis and colleagues (1988) furthered the empirical and theoretical influence of individualism and collectivism that was put forth by Hofstede (1984) as one of four important cultural dimensions useful for differentiating across nations alongside power distance, uncertainty avoidance, and masculinity/femininity.

Markus and Kitayama (1991, 2010) further refined our understanding of culture by more precisely framing independent and interdependent self-construal as constructs at the individual level that correspond to individualism and collectivism, respectively, at the cultural level. As an individual difference variable, self-construal recognizes important culturally based differences in how *individuals* relate to others relative to the self. People, as social animals, relate to others, whether they be family members, communities, racial groups, or nationalities. However, individuals may vary in the *way* they interrelate to these groups, and this is captured by self-construals (see Figure 15.2 for cultural differences in

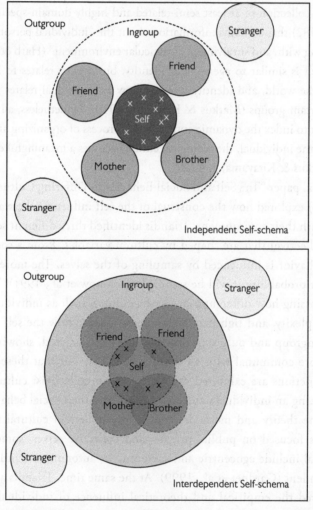

Figure 15.2. Independent and interdependent self-schemas. Figure adapted from Markus and Kitayama (1991) and Heine (2008).

self-construal). Interdependent self-construal refers to individuals whose selves are highly integrated and dependent on their significant social groups. Examples of social groups may include family, as in a related construct, *familisimo*, and workgroups. Labels for such social relations include gemeinschaft, interdependent, sociocentric, communal, and collectivist. Independent self-construal refers to those whose "social relations are formed on the basis of instrumental interests and goals," (p. 423) and the primacy is given to the self over social groups (Markus & Kitayama, 2010).

This seemingly simple distinction has helped to explain differences across a variety of behavioral phenomena (see Markus & Kitayama, 1991, for conceptual links with cognition, emotion, motivation, and social behavior). For example, those with strong independent self-construals tend to value uniqueness and therefore place a high value on choice. Therefore, cognitive dissonance is found to be stronger in those with higher independent self-construals (Kitayama et al., 2004). Additionally, Morris and Peng (1994) found culture to affect fundamental attributions, such that individualists or those high in independence were more likely to make dispositional attributions, whereas collectivists or those high in interdependence were more likely to make situational attributions. As a final example, self-construal affects basic cognitive processing. Interdependent self-construal is associated with more holistic cognitive processing (e.g., taking into account contextual factors) versus independent self-construal, which is associated with a tendency for analytic cognitive processing (e.g., focus on focal objects; see Nisbett et al., 2001). For example, using a change blindness paradigm, East Asians were more sensitive to contextual changes, whereas Americans were more sensitive to changes in focal objects (Masuda & Nisbett, 2006). Many of these studies have relied on self-construal distinctions between East Asian (e.g., Japan, Korea, China) and Western (e.g., United States, Western Europe, Australia) cultures. East Asian individuals tend to show higher levels of interdependent self-construal compared to Western individuals, who tend to have higher levels of independent self-construal. Gender differences have also been found, with women having higher interdependent self-construal compared to men (Cross & Madson, 1997).

Self-construal is primarily measured in two ways: through self-report on Likert scales and through self-generated, open responses. The most commonly used Likert-based scales include Singelis's Self-Construal Scale (1994) based on previous empirical and conceptual work by others (e.g., Hui, 1988; Yamaguchi et al., 1995; Cross & Markus, 1991) and the Cultural Orientation Scale (Triandis & Gelfand, 1998), although others like the Relational-Interdependent Self-Construal Scale (Cross et al., 2000) and Sixfold Self-Construal Scale (Harb & Smith, 2008) are noteworthy alternatives. Beyond Likert scales, Triandis et al. (1990) first adapted Kuhn and MacPartland's (1954) "I am . . ." scale, where participants complete the sentence 20 times. Responses are then coded as reflecting more interdependent (e.g., "I am Japanese American" or "I am a Pomona College student") or independent (e.g., "I am hungry" or "I am curious"). These measures are not without limitations. For example, the "I am" scale is better utilized for understanding cross-cultural, not individual differences (Singelis, 1994), and the Likert-based scales have been questioned for their dimensionality (Oyserman et al., 2002) and the reference group effect (Heine et al., 2002), which recognizes bias in responses due to fluctuating comparison groups (see Cross et al., 2011, for review of measurement issues).

Yet, self-construal is considered to be dynamic. Some studies have found self-construal to change, becoming more interdependent as one acculturates from an East Asian to a North American context (Abe-Kim et al., 2001; P. A. Chen et al., 2015). Here, self-construal is conceptualized and found to be relatively stable across long periods of time, like other individual difference variables. Change occurs slowly, across generations perhaps. However, in a more dynamic framework, all individuals can be conceptualized as possessing construals that are both interdependent and independent (Triandis, 1989; Trafimow et al., 1991). At a given moment, one might have the propensity to sample more independent or interdependent cognitions, depending on context. Thus, individuals with high interdependent self-construal have a higher likelihood of sampling an interdependent cognition but can think and behave independently given independent contextual cues. Y. Hong et al. (2000) called this multiculturalism a "dynamic constructivist approach to culture." (p. 709).

Conceptualizing and operationalizing self-construal as dynamic carries several advantages. "Studying self-construal within a culture is an effective way to investigate the mechanism linking culture, self, and behavior" (Gardner et al., 1999). In effect, one can establish the causal role of self-construal by holding the culture constant and manipulating self-construal. The prototypical method as established by Trafimow et al. (1991) is to prime either interdependent or independent self-construal to understand the effects of self-construal. For example, Kühnen and Oyserman (2002) primed participants interdependently or independently using Gardner's pronoun circling task (circle "I's" or "we's" within a paragraph to prime independent or interdependent self-construal, respectively). They found that independently primed participants were less likely to remember pictorial objects in context compared to those primed interdependently.

Several types of primes have been used to increase the salience or sampling of the different self-construals. The most common primes include relational primes like the pronoun circling task, as already mentioned (Gardner et al., 1999); the Sumerian warrior vignette, where one reads a story of obligation versus personal achievement (Trafimow et al., 1991); and cultural icons, where pictures of Chinese (e.g., Great Wall of China) versus American (e.g., American eagle; Y. Hong et al., 2000) cultural traditions are presented. There is some confusion about the precise nature of the primes, whether they represent and elicit differences in relational self-construal per se or cultural selves (e.g., icons that are likely strongly associated with relational self-construals; for review see Cross et al., 2011; Oyserman & Lee, 2008).

Cultural Neuroscience

The formal beginning of cultural neuroscience can be attributed to Joan Chiao and Nalini Ambady's (2007) influential chapter in the *Handbook of Cultural Psychology*, where they coined and defined the term *cultural neuroscience* and articulated a framework for future research investigating the interrelationship among genetic, neural, psychological, and cultural factors for understanding cognition, affect, and behavior (see in this volume Chiao & Blizinsky).

In the year prior to this chapter a couple of key papers appeared that applied functional magnetic resonance imaging (fMRI) to the study of cultural differences in cognition. Angela Gutchess and colleagues (2006) imaged brain activity while Americans and Chinese observed pictures of target objects and backgrounds. They found different patterns of activity such that Americans showed increased activation of more brain regions than the Chinese when viewing target objects, especially in object-processing regions of the temporal and parietal lobes. This pattern of activity was interpreted as being consistent with the cultural studies of cognition emphasizing the relatively greater attention to focal objects displayed among those from Western cultures (see, e.g., Nisbett et al., 2001). Tang et al. (2006) scanned the brains of Chinese- and English-speaking participants while they performed various arithmetic tasks. They found that English-speaking participants showed greater activation of left hemisphere, perisylvian language-processing areas, suggesting a relatively greater reliance on language areas when processing numbers. In contrast, Chinese-speaking participants showed greater activation of visual premotor areas during numerical tasks, suggesting a relatively greater reliance on visual areas when processing numbers. In both studies, differences in activity between Western and Chinese brains were attributed to *cultural* differences in processing information.

These early studies were intriguing for linking differences in brain activity to differences in culture, but many noncultural genetic and environmental influences were uncontrolled when making comparisons between groups of people raised in different countries. If cultural differences were observed in brain activity, it was unclear which cultural factors would account for the differences.

We attempted to address this limitation by measuring self-construal to see whether it mediated group differences in brain activity. European American and East Asian American undergraduates were recruited to participate in a novelty oddball P3 event-related potential (ERP) study (Lewis et al., 2008). Although both groups showed the expected larger P3 to the target, relative to the distractor, European Americans showed a trend for a relatively greater P3 response to target stimuli. This suggests that the European Americans were allocating greater attention to the targets (see Herrmann & Knight, 2001), consistent with cognitive studies showing that those from individualistic cultures allocate greater attention to focal, target objects (see Nisbett et al., 2001). In the novelty P3 design, additional stimuli are infrequently presented that are not expected, given the task instructions. ERP responses to these stimuli were used to measure attention to stimuli that violate the instructional context of the task. The East Asian Americans showed a greater anterior novelty P3 in response to the contextually novel events, again illustrating greater contextual sensitivity in collectivist (high interdependent self-construal) cultures. Most importantly, we found that collectivism, as measured by the Triandis self-construal scale, mediated the group differences in the novelty P3 ERP.

A similar approach to identifying a cultural construct relating group differences in neural activity was taken by Trey Hedden and colleagues (2008). They scanned the brains of Americans and Chinese while performing an adaptation of Kitayama's framed-line task. In this task, subjects are, in essence, asked to compare the length of lines either relative to the size of the framed line or in absolute terms. They found that East Asians residing in the United States showed greater activation of frontal and parietal areas associated with attention when making the culturally nonpreferred absolute judgments, whereas European Americans showed greater activation of similar brain areas when making culturally nonpreferred relative line judgments. They argued that when participants are making culturally nonpreferred perceptual judgments, they made greater use of attentional networks to solve the task. In contrast, culturally preferred perceptual judgments were more practiced, automatic, and efficient and therefore did not need to rely on effortful attentional networks to the same degree. Importantly, Hedden et al. found that activation of attentional networks during the culturally preferred absolute judgment task was inversely related to independent self-construal in the European Americans. That is, the more independent the European Americans were, the less the activation there was of attentional networks for completing the absolute judgment task. For the East Asians, a similar inverse relationship was found between activation of the attentional network for making absolute judgments and acculturation to the U.S. culture, as measured by length of time in the United States.

Together, these two studies established the importance of self-construal in cultural neuroscience research. First, in both studies the cultural differences found in neural findings were consistent with established cultural differences in cognition. In particular, neural patterns of activity fit within the analytic/holistic dimension of differences proposed by Nisbett and colleagues (2001) and can be interpreted in terms of greater relational or context sensitivity among East Asians relative to European Americans. Moreover, these studies related group differences in brain activity to a specific dimension of culture, refining the connection between the measured differences in brain activity and culture. Conceptions of the self were shown to be a critical factor in cultural differences in brain function. Recently, Han and Humphreys (2016) argued that self-construal was a cultural framework for brain function, stating that "self-construal is a key cultural trait that activates a cognitive framework that constrains neural strategies and modulates the neural processes underlying cognition and emotion" (p. 10).

Indeed, self-construal has served as the dominant framework for understanding cultural neuroscience research utilizing diverse methodologies investigating cognitive, affective, and social domains. Not surprisingly, the bulk of these studies have investigated the neural representation of the self. Most of these studies have participants reflect on attributes of the self in comparison to attributes of others, often a close other, such as "mother," and/or a well-known public figure, such as a political leader. For example, in a study of Chinese and Danes, Ma et al. (2014) measured medial prefrontal cortex (PFC) and temporoparietal junction (TPJ) activity during mental, social, and physical attribute judgments about self and a public figure. Across all subjects increased interdependent self-construal was related to decreased medial PFC activity during social judgments of the self, which was consistent with their hypothesis of a lessened encoding of self-reflection in the medial PFC of interdependents. Ma et al. also found that interdependency was positively related to social judgments of the self, which may reflect a greater tendency to think about others when making judgments of the self due to the proposed role of the TPJ in mentalization about others (Saxe & Kanwisher, 2003). In a study of Japanese and European Americans, Chiao et al. (2009) found that medial PFC activity was positively correlated with interdependent self-construal during contextual judgments of the self (e.g., "When talking to my mother I am casual") versus more general judgments of the self (e.g., "In general I am assertive"). Together, these results reveal different patterns of self-reflection-related neural activity that is related to cultural differences in self-construal. Those high in interdependent self-construal may have a reduced neural representation of the self and view themselves in the context of others. These neural activation patterns are "dynamic" and can be influenced by situational priming (see next section) and acculturation (P. A. Chen et al., 2015).

Interestingly, self-construal has also been a dominant framework for understanding the neural basis of cultural differences in cognition beyond concepts of the self, and has been found for studies of attention, perception, and social cognition. In a series of ERP studies, Goto and colleagues used an N400 design to assess the degree to which European American and East Asian Americans would spontaneously assess semantic relationships between central target objects and background images, reflecting holistic processing of objects within the visual field. In contrast with many cross-cultural studies, these studies compared cultural values between ethnicity of participants living in the same country, thereby somewhat controlling for exposure to the dominant culture. In the first of these, participants made incidental judgments of a central object (e.g., a crab) and the N400 was used to index the degree to which participants spontaneously processed the semantic incongruity between the central target and the surrounding image (e.g., a parking lot; Goto et al., 2010). East Asian Americans displayed a greater N400 in response to incongruent foreground and background semantic relationships than did European Americans. This suggests that the East Asian Americans were spontaneously processing the semantic relationship between the focal target and the background, reflecting greater context sensitivity, and is consistent with a holistic style of perception (Nisbett et al., 2001). Among all participants, smaller N400s, reflecting less semantic incongruity, were associated with greater independent self-construal. A follow-up study investigated the processing of affective incongruities between focal target stimuli and backgrounds (Goto et al., 2013). East

Asian and European Americans judged whether focal faces were happy or sad against positive and negative background scenes. Similar to the previous study, Asian Americans displayed a larger N400 to affective incongruities between the central, target face and the affective background. Again, among all participants, interdependent self-construal was related to the magnitude of the N400 such that greater N400s, reflecting greater semantic incongruity, were associated with greater interdependent self-construal. These studies highlight self-construal as an important cultural construct that can frame neural differences between ethnic groups, as well as individual differences within cultures.

The N400 ERP design has been shown to be an effective paradigm in cultural neuroscience self-construal research. Na and Kitayama (2011) found that European Americans were more likely to spontaneously develop trait inferences in face–trait pairings. European Americans were also more likely to show an N400 in response to a subsequent lexical decision task when an "incongruent trait" was primed by a previously presented face. Among all participants, the magnitude of the N400 was correlated with independent self-construal. These findings are consistent with independents' greater tendency toward trait attributions of others and interdependents' greater tendency to see personal characteristics as being situationally and contextually determined.

Cultural neuroscience research has begun to explore the neural mechanisms associated with long-standing psychological conceptions of culture and self associated with cognition, affect, and social cognition. Neural measures have been shown to be particularly sensitive to cultural differences in processing information, even in the absence of differences in behavior. With additional research, neuroscience methods promise to uniquely contribute to our increased understanding of culture and conceptions of the self.

Priming

In a series of studies of Chinese university students, self-construal priming was shown to alter neural activity across a wide variety of tasks. C. Wang et al. (2013) attempted to determine the effect of self-construal priming on resting state activity relative to a calculation task. They found that both interdependent and independent priming activated the ventromedial PFC and the posterior cingulate, both part of the midline self-referential network (see Northoff et al., 2006). In addition, they found that interdependent, relative to independent, priming activated the dorsomedial PFC and the left middle PFC. However, priming did not seem to alter functional connectivity during the resting state. These results suggest that there may be both situation-variant and situation-invariant aspects of neural patterns of activation related to self-construal priming relative to baseline brain states.

Self-construal priming has also resulted in task-dependent activations. For example, priming interdependent relative to independent self-construal has resulted in relatively greater activity of the middle frontal cortex when viewing a familiar face (Sui & Han, 2007); the P1 ERP in response to global processing (Lin et al., 2008); the ventral striatum in response to a reward to a close other (Varnum et al., 2014); the cingulate, insula, and supplementary motor area in response to videos of ingroup members in pain (W. Wang et al., 2015); and a smaller N130 ERP amplitude in response to painful stimuli (C. Wang et al., 2014). Situational priming of self-orientation clearly influences the way the brain processes information, even within a culture.

Biculturals theoretically have two equally strong independent and interdependent selves and may dynamically alter activation of self-related frames according to situational demands (Y. Hong et al., 2000). Therefore, biculturals are a particularly interesting group in which to explore self-construal priming on neural activity. Chiao et al. (2010) investigated priming of self-identified bicultural Asian Americans on neural activation in relation to general trait attributes and situational contextual attributes of the self. Interdependent priming was associated with relatively greater activation of the medial PFC and posterior cingulate in response to judgments of the self in contextually situated circumstances than when making more general trait judgments. This is consistent with interdependent people being more contextually sensitive (Masuda & Nisbett, 2006).

Zhu et al. (2007) reported that there was greater overlapping activity of the ventromedial PFC when Chinese were thinking about self and mother than when Westerners were thinking about self and mother. This is consistent with cultural differences in the relationship between self and close others proposed by Markus and Kitayama (1991), where the separation between self and close others is more distinct in independents. In Hong Kong biculturals, Ng et al. (2010) found that Chinese primes resulted in greater overlap of activation of the ventromedial PFC when making trait judgments about self and other than when primed with Western primes.

In a study comparing biculturals and monoculturals, self-construal was primed in East Asian Americans and European Americans during an N400 ERP task (Fong et al., 2014). The N400 was used to measure subjects' incidental perception of incongruities between the facial expressions of a central, target figure and the facial expressions of surrounding distractor figures. Following an interdependent prime, the East Asian Americans displayed a greater N400 during incongruent trials compared to the independent prime condition. In contrast, the European Americans did not show a greater N400 during incongruent trials following either prime. This suggests that biculturals may show greater facility in shifting neural activity according to situational primes than monoculturals.

Jiang et al. (2014) measured ERP responses to pictures of painful and nonpainful situations and found that Western subjects showed an increased N2 to painful relative to nonpainful situations following interdependent priming. This suggests that interdependent priming increases an empathic pain response in Western subjects. However, it is not clear to what extent these subjects represented monoculturals. The Western subjects were a diverse group of students residing in China for a short period of time, most of whom were English speaking. Interestingly, interdependent self-construal priming primarily *reduced* the empathic pain response in Chinese. Jiang et al. suggested that interdependent priming in an interdependent culture may enhance the boundary between ingroup and outgroup members, resulting in a decreased empathic pain response to pictures of strangers.

These self-construal priming studies illustrate the influence that attention to different conceptions of the self can have on activation of neural systems. Together they demonstrate that activation of different schemas of self will selectively influence how the brain processes information across a wide range of tasks. The dynamic nature of priming has been well established in monocultural brains, suggesting multiple neural representations of selves within individuals. Furthermore, there is some evidence that biculturals may have a relatively greater fluency in shifting among these multiple representations.

Neural Architecture

Experience has been shown to alter the gross size of brain structures in rather remarkable ways. In some of the most highly publicized of these studies, the size of the right posterior hippocampus was associated with time spent driving a London taxi and proficiency on the demanding "Knowledge of London" driving licensing test (Maguire et al., 2000; Wollett & Maguie 2011), and juggling resulted in an increase in visual temporal and parietal lobe areas (Draganski et al., 2004). Therefore, it follows, as Kitayama and Tompson (2010) have argued, that cultural practices should also influence brain structure development. F. Wang et al. (2017) proposed that the ventromedial PFC, an area shown to be involved in self-referential thought (e.g., Kelley et al., 2002; Mitchell et al., 2005), would be greater in those showing increased independent self-construal. Consistent with their hypothesis, in a study of Chinese undergraduates, greater interdependent self-construal scores were associated with decreased ventromedial PFC volume (as well as greater dorso- and rostro-lateral prefrontal cortical volumes). In a study of Japanese, interdependent self-construal was also inversely correlated with PFC volume (Kitayama et al., 2017). However, their correlation was found with the orbitofrontal PFC, which is associated with valuation and decision making (see, e.g., Packer et al., 2011). Kitayama et al. interpreted these findings as being consistent with the notion that interdependent self-construal is associated with a reduced self-interest, which follows from a greater sense of obligation and duties toward others. Together, these studies indicate that the size of prefrontal cortical areas associated with self-related processing is correlated with self-construal such that a greater sense of independence of self is associated with greater representation of self-processing regions in the prefrontal cortex. However, it remains unclear what cellular elements underlie differences in cortical volume associated with self-related processing. Plausible candidates include the number of neurons or glial cells, greater branching of neuronal processes, or simply greater interstitial volumes.

Kitayama and Tompson (2010) have also argued that connectivity of brain areas, even more so than brain activation, should be influenced by cultural practices. During a resting state connectivity analysis, C. Wang et al. (2013) found a positive relationship between independent self-construal and ventromedial PFC–posterior cingulate cortex synchronization in Chinese university students. These two structures represent the ventral and posterior components of the proposed midline self-referential processing system (Northoff et al., 2006), respectively. The posterior cingulate has been related to self-referential memory processing and together with the ventromedial PFC's association with self-referential external and internal perception represents a critical system connecting stimulus-driven and memorial self-referential thought. They found that interdependent self-construal was positively related to ventromedial PFC–dorsomedial PFC synchronization. Monitoring the self in relation to others is highly valued among interdependents, and it is interesting that increased synchronization among the ventromedial PFC, associated with self-referential processing, and the dorsomedial PFC, associated with thinking about others (Mitchell et al., 2005), is associated with greater interdependence. Importantly, the functional connectivity patterns were not affected by independent and interdependent priming conditions, suggesting that these connectivity patterns represent more chronic aspects of culture.

More recently, Li et al. (2018) partially replicated these findings in a resting state analysis of Chinese university students and similarly found that independent self-construal was positively correlated with synchronization between the posterior cingulate cortex/cuneus and medial PFC. Interestingly, the PCC/cuneus synchronization with the right temporal parietal junction, associated with theory of mind (Saxe & Kanwisher, 2003), was correlated with interdependent self-construal. In addition, they also found that independent self-construal was positively correlated with the inferior frontal gyrus and its connectivity with the middle and superior frontal gyrus and right temporal parietal junction. They attributed these findings to greater connectivity of executive control system among independents. Lastly, they found evidence for a negative relationship between the self-related default mode network and the executive control network, and this may represent a fundamental trade-off between external and internal focus of attention, which may be key to understanding individual differences in self-construal.

The brain volume and connectivity studies represent a productive area of future investigation of the neural basis of self-construal and would greatly benefit from cross-cultural comparisons since all of these studies rely on East Asian samples, and it is not clear whether we can extrapolate from these studies to volume and connectivity patterns of those from individualistic cultures.

Culture × Gene Interactions

Advances in our understanding of how genes regulate brain processes has led to new perspectives on the relationship between culture and cognition. Some of this work has focused on explorations of cultural variations in functional single nucleotide polymorphisms (SNPs) and self-construal. SNPs consist of variations in alleles that code for a single nucleotide. Those that have functional implications for neurotransmission have been of particular interest to the study of cognitive, affective, and social neuroscience.

This work is in its earliest stages, and the complexity of issues relating SNPs, culture, and behavior cannot be overemphasized (see Dick et al., 2011). Several examples of gene × culture interactions have been identified in the literature, with the greatest attention being paid to SNPs associated with serotonin, dopamine, and oxytocin transmission. For instance, in a cross-national study of the serotonin transporter polymorphism, Chiao and Blizinsky (2009) found a positive association between the frequency of the short allele for the serotonin transporter and collectivism, which was inversely related to the prevalence of affective disorders. The short allele has been linked to decreased transcription efficiency and associated with decreased serotonergic receptor binding in humans (David et al., 2005). Given the interest in the involvement of serotonin in mood disorders, this finding was interpreted in light of culture–gene coevolution theory, whereby collectivistic values coevolve to buffer against a genetic susceptibility toward affective disorders.

In contrast, Ma et al. (2013) did not find a difference in self-construal between those with short alleles and long alleles within a sample of Chinese college students. However, they did find that long-allele subjects, but not short-allele subjects, showed a relationship between interdependent self-construal and social brain activity when thinking about self and a close other ("mother"). Among the long-allele subjects, there was a tendency for a positive association with interdependent self-construal in more medial brain areas when thinking about self (middle frontal, medial prefrontal, insula, and hippocampus) and mother (left frontal, medial prefrontal, and insula), and an inverse relationship in more lateral areas when thinking about self (middle frontal, superior parietal, temporoparietal junction, and middle temporal gyrus) and mother (superior parietal). This pattern of results may reflect a greater activation of the midline self-referential network when thinking about self and a close other in those that are more highly interdependent and relatively less activation of a more lateral mentalizing network, at least in long-allele individuals.

In another cross-national study, Luo and Han (2014) investigated the relationship between the frequency of the OXTR rs53576 oxytocin receptor polymorphism, which has been associated with social cognition and self-construal. They found a correlation between the percent of the A allele and collectivism, and similar to Chiao and Blizinsky (2009), they found that collectivism mediated the relationship between OXTR rs535765 and mood disorder. Within a Chinese population, Luo et al. (2015) found evidence for the G-allele carriers showing a positive relationship between interdependent self-construal and empathy, and a positive relationship between interdependent self-construal and activity of the amygdala, insula, and superior temporal gyrus in response to video clips of others in pain. Together, these studies suggest that variations in oxytocin may account for neural differences in social cognition that are fundamental to individual differences and cultural differences in interdependent self-construal.

In a comparative study of European Americans and East Asians, the dopamine D4 receptor gene was found to moderate cultural differences in self-construal (Kitayama et al., 2014). The 7- and 2-repeat allele polymorphisms have been associated with increased dopaminergic signaling and varies across cultures (C. Chen et al., 1999). Among those with the 7- and 2-repeat alleles, there were marked differences in self-construal between the two groups such that the European Americans were significantly more independent than the East Asians. In contrast, there was no significant difference in self-construal among noncarriers. Given that the 7/2-repeat D4 polymorphism has been proposed to be associated with increased reward sensitivity to the environment (Bakermans-Kranenburg et al., 2008), it is interesting, in the context of this study, that carriers are the ones with the greatest adherence to the social orientation of the dominant culture, independent of whether the dominant culture is a collectivist or individualist culture.

In summary, the cultural neuroscience literature builds upon the psychological research on self-construal in three important ways. First, the literature based upon neural measures is consistent with the behavioral literature and provides clues as to the biological underpinnings. Together, they provide confirmation of the central role that self-construal plays in understanding cultural effects on cognition, brain, and behavior. It is important and indeed useful to note differences in self-construal across populations. These stable differences can reasonably predict behavioral predispositions through the sampling of culturally influenced selves (e.g., default network, neural architecture, or connectivity based on differences in experience). Second, because of the sensitive and dynamic nature of neural measures, the cultural neuroscience literature has shed light on the extent to which self-construal is determined and fluctuates based on situational factors. These cultural differences should be understood as not immutable. That is, they can change based on cultural or situational influences, resulting in changes to social cognition. Third, the cultural neuroscience literature sheds light on the important interactions between genes and culture in understanding behavior. Again, self-construal plays a central role in understanding the coevolution of culture based on population-based genetics. Collective social environments may be particularly protective for those with a genetically based predisposition for affective disorders.

Global Health

Within a cultural neuroscience framework, understanding the neural mechanisms and cultural context of self-construal are essential aspects of effective prevention, diagnosis, and treatment. Major nervous system (MNS) disorders, such as schizophrenia, affective disorders, epilepsy, dementia, and substance abuse, are a significant global burden (Collins et al., 2011). An important challenge is to minimize national, racial, cultural, and socioeconomic class disparities in preventative and treatment interventions to effectively meet the mental health needs of all (Chiao et al., 2013; see in this volume Greenfield & Vasquez-Salgado). The cultural factor of self-construal is known to mediate and moderate neural systems of human behavior in a variety of ways and can influence conceptions of the self and interactions with others, which may play a critical role in addressing mental health challenges across the globe (see in this volume, Blais; Chiao et al., 2016).

Self-construal has implications for understanding the boundary conditions for when a disorder is more or less likely to occur in a culture. For example, controlling for stressful environmental influences, affective disorders may not be equally distributed across populations. Highlighting a direct relationship between self-construal and health, the gene × culture interaction involving the serotonin transporter 5-HTTLPR allele has been proposed to explain variations in the prevalence of affective disorders across the globe. As previously discussed, Chiao and Blizinsky (2013) found that the genetic selection of the S allele of the serotonin transporter gene, which is higher in East Asian regions, was associated with a lower prevalence of affective disorders compared with geographic regions that showed no genetic selection. The selection of the S allele, which is thought to be a risk factor for mood disorders, was buffered by collectivistic cultural values of East Asian cultures. This is consistent with research using solely self-reports where interdependent self-construal was positively correlated with social anxiety disorder (SAD) and independent self-construal was negatively correlated with SAD in a sample of native-born Israelis and immigrants from Ethiopia and the former Soviet Union (Hasenson-Atzmon et al., 2016).

Similarly, posttraumatic stress disorder (PTSD) has also been linked to self-construal and cultural identity. Trauma survivors with PTSD from independent cultures reported more mental defeat, more alienation, permanent change, and fewer control strategies than non-PTSD trauma survivors from independent cultures. However, only alienation appraisals differed among independent survivors with and without PTSD (Jobson, 2009). Therefore, all populations should not be assumed as similar, and knowing a population's self-construal levels may shed light on the likelihood of affective disorders or predisposition toward affective disorders.

Self-construals also have implications for understanding the mechanism for the prevalence of MNS disorders within a given culture. For example, J. J. Hong and Woody (2007) found that views of self fully mediate differences in self-reported anxiety between East Asians and Westerners. In addition, two factors (interdependent self-construal and self-criticism) were partial mediators for ethnic differences. Dinnel et al. (2002) explored social phobia and anxiety as defined by the *Diagnostic and Statistical Manual of Mental Disorders*, fourth edition (DSM-IV), and taijinkyofusho (TKS), which is a Japanese form related to social anxiety. TKS was first identified in Japan and is described as an obsession of shame, manifested by a morbid fear of embarrassing or offending others by blushing, improper facial expressions, a blemish, a physical deformity, staring inappropriately, or emitting offensive odors or flatulence. TKS symptoms were more likely to be found in Japanese students as well as those students who scored high on interdependence and low on independence. For both Japanese and American students, those who scored higher for social phobia were also high on interdependence and low on independence. J. J. Hong and Woody (2007) acknowledge that "conceptualizations of pathological social anxiety may need to be revised to be useful for studying individuals in East Asian cultures"

(p. 1786). The increased social demands for those with higher interdependent self-construals may lead to greater social unease.

Electrophysiological methods are useful for pinpointing the stage of processing information, and therefore in the identification of mechanisms, that may mediate the relationship between self-construal and affective disorders. In a study of East Asian Americans, G. Park et al. (2018) found that an early ERP (P1) was an indirect mediator of the relationship between self-construal and social anxiety. Increasing interdependent self-construal was negatively related to the P1 amplitude to angry faces, which in turn was negatively associated with social anxiety. The cultural value of interdependence emphasizing the importance of accurately reading others' emotions in conjunction with cultural factors interfering with the accurate reading of others (not looking directly at the eyes, emotion suppression, and reading outgroup members) may explain the double bind that Asian Americans experience (see Lau et al., 2009).

Self-construal may also play a critical role in emotion regulation. Cheung and Park (2010) investigated whether anger would mediate family structure/temperament with depressive symptoms across race and self-construal. Based on their findings, anger was a significant mediator for the indirect effects of depressive symptoms. Moreover, race and interdependent self-construal moderated the suppression of depression symptoms. Those who identified as Asian Americans and had high interdependent self-construal showed attenuated symptoms of depression. Being able to regulate one's emotions was dependent in part on cultural identity and self-construal. In terms of fear, bilateral amygdala responses can be modulated by culture. Those who were native to Japan and the United States showed greater activation to fear in members of their own groups.

Beyond predicting cultural differences in the experience of MNS disorders, self-construal can help understand disparities in help-seeking behavior. Negative stereotypes can affect assumptions of treatment efficacy or perceptions of health care providers' willingness to treat patients. Indeed, 50% of European immigrants were unwilling to use mental health services (Barry & Grilo, 2002). Along with English-language proficiency, lower adherence to Asian values, and lower levels of stigma, interdependent self-construal was associated with higher help-seeking behaviors in Asian Americans (Shea & Yeh, 2008).

We caution against an interpretation that increased interdependent self-construal leads to greater MNS disorders. Much research exists on the benefits of interdependence such as providing a protective social code of caring for ingroup members. We mean only to suggest that regardless of the specific MNS disorder, knowing levels of interdependent self-construal can provide insight into the reasons for health disparity and ultimately preventative strategies. Furthermore, self-construal is evidenced to be mutable and dynamic. In populations immigrating from more strongly collectivist cultures to more individualistic cultures, one might expect levels of independent self-construal to increase with prolonged cultural exposure and across generations. Likewise, one might expect that increased environmental cues of interdependence may lead to greater empathy and augmentation of emotion, both positive and negative. Conversely, exposure to environmental cues of independence may reduce such effects.

There is a striking paucity of research in global mental health that takes advantage of the advances in our understanding of neural mechanisms associated with cultural differences in self-construal. For example, given the interrelations that have been well documented among poverty, education, stress, brain development, and well-being (see, e.g., Blair & Raver, 2018), we have little understanding of the direct and indirect effects between these factors, self-construal, and global mental health. Furthermore, much of the research is still being conducted within the United States. Studies based on American samples are not accurate representations of the world's population (Henrich et al., 2010). Some researchers, like Arnett (2008), have posited that this narrowness in the research cannot be justified by science. Interventions that take advantage of our understanding of the neural mechanisms involved in self-construal and mental disorders are largely lacking but hold great promise. For example, the overlap in medial forebrain structures involved in self-construal and affective disorders (see, e.g., Price & Drevets, 2012) suggests that there could be intervention strategies based on our knowledge of culturally specific genetic and neural activity relationships. Such strategies may range from intraindividual to community-based approaches. To be sure, it is important for clinicians, therapists, public health practitioners, and policymakers to be aware of cultural differences in the genetic and neural mechanisms associated with mental health outcomes. Self-construal should play a central role in the informed consideration of these factors, leading the way to a greater variety of innovative and effective treatment approaches.

References

Abe-Kim, J., Okazaki, S., & Goto, S. G. (2001). Unidimensional versus multidimensional approaches to the assessment of acculturation for Asian American populations. *Cultural Diversity and Ethnic Minority Psychology, 7*(3), 232.

Arnett, J. J. (2008). The neglected 95%: Why American psychology needs to become less American. *American Psychologist, 63*(7), 602–614. doi:10.1037/0003-066x.63.7.602

Bakermans-Kranenburg, M. J., van IJzendoorn, M. H., Pijlman, F. T. A., Mesman, J., & Juffer, F. (2008). Differential susceptibility to intervention: Dopamine D4 receptor polymorphism (DRD4 VNTR) moderates effects on toddlers' externalizing behavior in a randomized control trial. *Developmental Psychology, 44*, 293–300.

Barry, D. T., & Grilo, C. M. (2003). Cultural, self-esteem, and demographic correlates of perception of personal and group discrimination among East Asian immigrants. *American Journal of Orthopsychiatry, 73*(2), 223–229. doi:10.1037/0002-9432.73.2.223.

Blair, C., & Raver, C. C. (2016). Poverty, stress, and brain development: New directions for prevention and intervention. *Academic Pediatrics, 16*(3), S30–S36. http://doi.org/10.1016/j.acap.2016.01.010

Chen, C., Burton, M., Greenberger, E., & Dmitrieva, J. (1999). Population migration and the variation of dopamine D4 receptor (DRD4) allele frequencies around the globe. *Evolution and Human Behavior, 20*(5), 309–324.

Chen, P. A., Wagner, D. D., Kelley, W. M., & Heatherton, T. F. (2015). Activity in cortical midline structures is modulated by self-construal changes during acculturation. *Culture and Brain, 3*(1), 39–52. doi:10.1007/s40167-015-0026-z

Cheung, R. Y., & Park, I. J. (2010). Anger suppression, interdependent self-construal, and depression among Asian American and European American college students. *Cultural Diversity and Ethnic Minority Psychology, 16*(4), 517–525. doi:10.1037/a0020655

Chiao, J. Y., & Ambady, N. (2007). Cultural neuroscience: Parsing universality and diversity across levels of analysis. In S. Kitayama & D. Cohen (Eds.), Handbook of Cultural Psychology (pp. 237–254). The Guilford Press.

Chiao, J. Y., & Blizinsky, K. D. (2009). Culture-gene coevolution of individualism-collectivism and the serotonin transporter gene. *Proceedings of the Royal Society B: Biological Sciences, 277*(1681), 529–537. http://doi.org/10.1098/rspb.2009.1650

Chiao, J. Y., Cheon, B. K., Pornpattananangkul, N., Mrazek, A. J., & Blizinsky, K. D. (2013). Cultural Neuroscience: Progress and Promise. *Psychological inquiry, 24*(1), 1–19. https://doi.org/10.1080/1047840X.2013.752715

Chiao, J. Y., & Blizinsky, K. D. (2013). Population disparities in mental health: Insights from cultural neuroscience. *American Journal of Public Health, 103*(S1), S122–S132. doi:10.2105/ajph.2013.301440

Chiao, J. Y., Harada, T., Komeda, H., Li, Z., Mano, Y., Saito, D., Parish, T. B., Sadato, N. & Iidaka, T. (2009). Neural basis of individualistic and collectivistic views of self. *Human brain mapping, 30*(9), 2813–2820.

Chiao, J. Y., Iidaka, T., Gordon, H. L., Nogawa, J., Bar, M., Aminoff, E, Sadato, N., & Ambady, N. (2008). Cultural specificity in amygdala response to fear faces. *Journal of Cognitive Neuroscience, 20*(12), 2167–2174. doi:10.1162/jocn.2008.20151

Collins, P. Y., Patel, V., Joestl, S. S., March, D., Insel, T. R., Daar, A. S., Scientific Advisory Board and the Executive Committee of the Grand Challenges on Global Mental Health, Anderson, W., Dhansay, M. A., Phillips, A., Shurin, S., Walport, M., Ewart, W., Savill, S. J., Bordin, I. A., Costello, E. J., Durkin, M., Fairburn, C., Glass, R. I., Hall, W., . . . Stein, D. J. (2011). Grand challenges in global mental health. *Nature, 475*(7354), 27–30. https://doi.org/10.1038/475027a

Cross, S., & Markus, H. (1991). Possible selves across the life span. *Human Development, 34*(4), 230–255. doi:10.1159/000277058

Cross, S. E., Bacon, P. L., & Morris, M. L. (2000). The relational-interdependent self-construal and relationships. *Journal of Personality and Social Psychology, 78*(4), 791.

Cross, S. E., Hardin, E. E., & Gercek-Swing, B. (2011). The what, how, why, and where of self-construal. *Personality and Social Psychology Review, 15*(2), 142–179. doi:10.1177/1088868310373752

Cross, S. E., & Madson, L. (1997). Models of the self: Self-construals and gender. *Psychological Bulletin, 122*(1), 5–37. doi:10.1037//0033-2909.122.1.5

David, S. P., Murthy, N. V., Rabiner, E. A., Munafò, M. R., Johnstone, E. C., Jacob, R., Walton, R.T., Grasby, P. M. (2005). A functional genetic variation of the serotonin (5-HT) transporter affects 5-HT1A receptor binding in humans. *Journal of Neuroscience: The Official Journal of the Society for Neuroscience, 25*(10), 2586–2590. http://doi.org/10.1523/JNEUROSCI.3769-04.2005

Dick, D. M., Latendresse, S. J., & Riley, B. (2011). Incorporating genetics into your studies: a guide for social scientists. *Frontier in Psychiatry, 2,* 17.

Dinnel, D., Kleinknecht, R. M., & Tanaka-Matsumi, J. (2002). A cross-cultural comparison of social phobia symptoms. *Journal of Psychopathology and Behavioral Assessment, 24*(2), 75–84. doi:10.1023/A:1015316223631

Draganski, B., Gaser, C., Busch, V., Schuierer, G., Bogdahn, U., & May, A. (2004). Neuroplasticity: Changes in grey matter induced by training. *Nature, 427*(6972), 311.

Fiske, S. T., & Taylor, S. E. (1991). *McGraw-Hill series in social psychology* (2nd ed., Social cognition). McGraw-Hill Book Company.

Fong, M. C., Goto, S. G., Moore, C., Zhao, T., Schudson, Z., & Lewis, R. S. (2014). Switching between Mii and Wii: The effects of cultural priming on the social affective N400. *Culture and Brain, 2*(1), 52–71. http://doi.org/10.1007/s40167-014-0015-7

Gardner, W. L., Gabriel, S., & Lee, A. Y. (1999). "I" value freedom, but "we" value relationships: Self-construal priming mirrors cultural differences in judgment. *Psychological Science, 10*(4), 321–326. doi:10.1111/1467-9280.00162

Goto, S. G., Ando, Y., Huang, C., Yee, A., & Lewis, R. S. (2010). Cultural differences in the visual processing of meaning: Detecting incongruities between background and foreground objects using the N400. *Social Cognitive and Affective Neuroscience, 5*(2–3), 242–253. http://doi.org/10.1093/scan/nsp038

Goto, S. G., Yee, A., Lowenberg, K., & Lewis, R. S. (2013). Cultural differences in sensitivity to social context: Detecting affective incongruity using the N400. *Social Neuroscience, 8*(1), 63–74. http://doi.org/10.1080/17470919.2012.739202

Gutchess, A. H., Welsh, R. C., Boduroglu, A., & Park, D. C. (2006). Cultural differences in neural function associated with object processing. *Cognitive, Affective & Behavioral Neuroscience, 6*(2), 102–109.

Han, S., & Humphreys, G. (2016). Self-construal: A cultural framework for brain function. *Current Opinion in Psychology, 8*, 10–14. http://doi.org/10.1016/j.copsyc.2015.09.013

Harb, C., & Smith, P. B. (2008). Self-construals across cultures. *Journal of Cross-Cultural Psychology, 39*(2), 178–197. doi:10.1177/0022022107313861

Hasenson-Atzmon, K., Marom, S., Sofer, T., Lev-Ari, L., Youngmann, R., Hermesh, H., & Kushnir, J. (2016). Cultural impact on SAD: Social anxiety disorder among Ethiopian and Former Soviet Union immigrants to Israel, in comparison to native-born Israelis. *Israel Journal of Psychiatry and Related Sciences, 53*, 48–54.

Hedden, T., Ketay, S., Aron, A., Markus, H. R., & Gabrieli, J. D. E. (2008). Cultural influences on neural substrates of attentional control. *Psychological Science: A Journal of the American Psychological Society / APS, 19*(1), 12–17. http://doi.org/10.1111/j.1467-9280.2008.02038.x

Heine, S. J., Lehman, D. R., Peng, K., & Greenholtz, J. (2002). What's wrong with cross-cultural comparisons of subjective Likert scales?: The reference-group effect. *Journal of Personality and Social Psychology, 82*(6), 903–918. doi:10.1037/0022-3514.82.6.903

Henrich, J., Heine, S. J., & Norenzayan, A. (2010). The weirdest people in the world? *Behavioral and Brain Sciences, 33*(2–3), 61–83. http://doi.org/10.1017/S0140525X0999152X

Herrmann, C. S., & Knight, R. T. (2001). Mechanisms of human attention: Event-related potentials and oscillations. *Neuroscience & Biobehavioral Reviews, 25*(6), 465–476.

Hofstede, G. (1984). *Culture's consequences: International differences in work-related values* (Vol. 5). Sage.

Hong, J. J., & Woody, S. R. (2007). Cultural mediators of self-reported social anxiety. *Behaviour Research and Therapy, 45*(8), 1779–1789. doi:10.1016/j.brat.2007.01.011

Hong, Y., Morris, M. W., Chiu, C., & Benet-Martínez, V. (2000). Multicultural minds: A dynamic constructivist approach to culture and cognition. *American Psychologist, 55*(7), 709–720. doi:10.1037/0003-066x.55.7.709

Hui, C. (1988). Measurement of individualism-collectivism. *Journal of Research in Personality, 22*(1), 17–36. doi:10.1016/0092-6566(88)90022-0

Jiang, C., Varnum, M. E. W., Hou, Y., & Han, S. (2014). Social neuroscience. *Social Neuroscience, 9*(2), 130–138. http://doi.org/10.1080/17470919.2013.867899

Jobson, L. (2009). Drawing current posttraumatic stress disorder models into the cultural sphere: The development of the 'threat to the conceptual self' model. *Clinical Psychology Review, 29*(4), 368–381. doi:10.1016/j.cpr.2009.03.002

Kelley, W., Macrae, C., Wyland, C., Caglar, S., Inati, S., & Heatherton, T. (2002). Finding the self? An event-related fMRI study. *Journal of Cognitive Neuroscience, 14*(5), 785–794.

Kitayama, S., King, A., Yoon, C., Tompson, S., Huff, S., & Liberzon, I. (2014). The dopamine D4 receptor gene (DRD4) moderates cultural difference in independent versus interdependent social orientation. *Psychological Science: A Journal of the American Psychological Society / APS, 25*(6), 1169–1177. http://doi.org/10.1177/0956797614528338

Kitayama, S., Snibbe, A. C., Markus, H. R., & Suzuki, T. (2004). Is there any "free" choice? *Psychological Science, 15*(8), 527–533. doi:10.1111/j.0956-7976.2004.00714.x

Kitayama, S., & Tompson, S. (2010). Envisioning the future of cultural neuroscience. *Asian Journal of Social Psychology, 13*(2), 92–101.

Kitayama, S., Yanagisawa, K., Ito, A., Ueda, R., Uchida, Y., & Abe, N. (2017). Reduced orbitofrontal cortical volume is associated with interdependent self-construal. *Proceedings of the National Academy of Sciences of the United States of America, 114*(30), 7969–7974. http://doi.org/10.1073/pnas.1704831114

Kuhn, M. H., & McPartland, T. S. (1954). An empirical investigation of self-attitudes. *American Sociological Review, 19*(1), 68. doi:10.2307/2088175

Kühnen, U., & Oyserman, D. (2002). Thinking about the self influences thinking in general: Cognitive consequences of salient self-concept. *Journal of Experimental Social Psychology, 38*(5), 492–499. doi:10.1016/s0022-1031(02)00011-2

Lau, A. S., Fung, J., Wang, S., & Kang, S. (2009). Explaining elevated social anxiety among Asian Americans: Emotional attunement and a cultural double bind. *Cultural Diversity and Ethnic Minority Psychology, 15*(1), 77–85. doi:10.1037/a0012819

Lewis, R. S., Goto, S. G., & Kong, L. L. (2008). Culture and context: East Asian American and European American differences in P3 event-related potentials and self-construal. *Personality and Social Psychology Bulletin, 34*(5), 623–634. http://doi.org/10.1177/0146167207313731

Li, L. M. W., Luo, S., Ma, J., Lin, Y., Fan, L., Zhong, S., Yang, J., Huang, Y., Gu, L., Fan, L, Dai, Z., & Wu, X. (2018). Functional connectivity pattern underlies individual differences in independent self-construal. *Social Cognitive and Affective Neuroscience, 13*(3), 269–280. http://doi.org/10.1093/scan/nsy008

Lin, Z., Lin, Y., & Han, S. (2008). Self-construal priming modulates visual activity underlying global/local perception. *Biological Psychology, 77*(1), 93–97. http://doi.org/10.1016/j.biopsycho.2007.08.002

Luo, S., & Han, S. (2014). The association between an oxytocin receptor gene polymorphism and cultural orientations. *Culture and Brain, 2*(1), 89–107.

Luo, S., Ma, Y., Liu, Y., Li, B., Wang, C., Shi, Z., Li, Xx., Zhang, W., & Han, S (2015). Interaction between oxytocin receptor polymorphism and interdependent culture values on human empathy. *Social Cognitive and Affective Neuroscience, 10*(9), 1273–1281. http://doi.org/10.1093/scan/nsv019

Ma, Y., Bang, D., Wang, C., Allen, M., Frith, C., Roepstorff, A., & Han, S. (2014). Sociocultural patterning of neural activity during self-reflection. *Social Cognitive and Affective Neuroscience, 9*(1), 73–80.

Ma, Y., Wang, C., Li, B., Zhang, W., Rao, Y., & Han, S. (2013). Does self-construal predict activity in the social brain network? A genetic moderation effect. *Social Cognitive and Affective Neuroscience, 9(9)*, 1360–1367. doi.org/10.1093/scan/nst125

Maguire, E. A., Gadian, D. G., Johnsrude, I. S., Good, C. D., Ashburner, J., Frackowiak, R. S., & Frith, C. D. (2000). Navigation-related structural change in the hippocampi of taxi drivers. *Proceedings of the National Academy of Sciences, 97*(8), 4398–4403.

Markus, H. R., & Kitayama, S. (1991). Culture and the self: Implications for cognition, emotion, and motivation. *Psychological Review, 98*(2), 224–253. doi:10.1037/0033-295x.98.2.224

Markus, H. R., & Kitayama, S. (2010). Cultures and selves. *Perspectives on Psychological Science, 5*(4), 420–430. doi:10.1177/1745691610375557

Masuda, T., & Nisbett, R. E. (2006). Culture and change blindness. *Cognitive Science, 30*(2), 381–399. doi:10.1207/s15516709cog0000_63

Mitchell, J. P., Banaji, M. R., & Macrae, C. N. (2005). General and specific contributions of the medial prefrontal cortex to knowledge about mental states. *NeuroImage, 28*(4), 757–762. http://doi.org/10.1016/j.neuroimage.2005.03.011

Morris, M. W., & Peng, K. (1994). Culture and cause: American and Chinese attributions for social and physical events. *Journal of Personality and Social Psychology, 67*(6), 949–971. doi:10.1037//0022-3514.67.6.949

Na, J., & Kitayama, S. (2011). Spontaneous trait inference is culture-specific. *Psychological Science: A Journal of the American Psychological Society / APS, 22*(8), 1025–1032. http://doi.org/10.1177/0956797611414727

Ng, S. H., Han, S., Mao, L., & Lai, J. C. L. (2010). Dynamic bicultural brains: fMRI study of their flexible neural representation of self and significant others in response to culture primes. *Asian Journal of Social Psychology, 13*(2), 83–91. http://doi.org/10.1111/j.1467-839X.2010.01303.x

Nisbett, R. E., Peng, K., Choi, I., & Norenzayan, A. (2001). Culture and systems of thought: Holistic versus analytic cognition. *Psychological Review, 108*(2), 291.

Northoff, G., Heinzel, A., de Greck, M., Bermpohl, F., Dobrowolny, H., & Panksepp, J. (2006). Self-referential processing in our brain—A meta-analysis of imaging studies on the self. *NeuroImage, 31*(1), 440–457. http://doi.org/10.1016/j.neuroimage.2005.12.002

Oyserman, D., Coon, H. M., & Kemmelmeier, M. (2002). Rethinking individualism and collectivism: Evaluation of theoretical assumptions and meta-analyses. *Psychological Bulletin, 128*(1), 3–72. doi:10.1037//0033-2909.128.1.3

Oyserman, D., & Lee, S. W. (2008). Does culture influence what and how we think? Effects of priming individualism and collectivism. *Psychological bulletin, 134*(2), 311.

Packer, D. J., Kesek, A., & Cunningham, W. A. (2011). Self-regulation and evaluative processing. In A. Todorov, S. T. Fiske, & D. A. Prentice (Eds.), *Social neuroscience: Toward understanding the underpinnings of the social mind* (pp. 147–159). Oxford University Press.

Park, G., Lewis, R. S., Wang, Y. C., Cho, H. J., & Goto, S. G. (2018). Are you mad at me? Social anxiety and early visual processing of anger and gaze among Asian American biculturals. *Culture and Brain*, 1–20. http://doi.org/10.1007/s40167-018-0067-1

Price, J. L., & Drevets, W. C. (2012). Neural circuits underlying the pathophysiology of mood disorders. *Trends in Cognitive Sciences*, 16(1), 61–71. http://doi.org/10.1016/j.tics.2011.12.011

Saxe, R., & Kanwisher, N. (2003). People thinking about thinking people: The role of the temporo-parietal junction in "theory of mind." *NeuroImage*, 19(4), 1835–1842. http://doi.org/10.1016/S1053-8119(03)00230-1

Shea, M., & Yeh, C. (2008). Asian American students' cultural values, stigma, and relational self-construal: Correlates of attitudes toward professional help seeking. *Journal of Mental Health Counseling*, 30(2), 157–172.

Singelis, T. M. (1994). The measurement of independent and interdependent self-construals. *Personality and Social Psychology Bulletin*, 20(5), 580–591. doi:10.1177/0146167294205014

Sui, J., & Han, S. (2007). Self-construal priming modulates neural substrates of self-awareness. *Psychological Science: A Journal of the American Psychological Society / APS*, 18(10), 861–866. http://doi.org/10.1111/j.1467-9280.2007.01992.x

Tang, Y., Zhang, W., Chen, K., Feng, S., Ji, Y., Shen, J., Reiman, E. M., & Liu, Y (2006). Arithmetic processing in the brain shaped by cultures. *Proceedings of the National Academy of Sciences of the United States of America*, 103(28), 10775–10780. http://doi.org/10.1073/pnas.0604416103

Trafimow, D., Triandis, H. C., & Goto, S. G. (1991). Some tests of the distinction between the private self and the collective self. *Journal of Personality and Social Psychology*, 60(5), 649–655. doi:10.1037/0022-3514.60.5.649

Triandis, H. C. (1989). The self and social behavior in differing cultural contexts. *Psychological Review*, 96(3), 506–520. doi:10.1037//0033-295x.96.3.506

Triandis, H. C., Bontempo, R., Villareal, M. J., Asai, M., & Lucca, N. (1988). Individualism and collectivism: Cross-cultural perspectives on self-ingroup relationships. *Journal of personality and Social Psychology*, 54(2), 323.

Triandis, H. C., & Gelfand, M. J. (1998). Converging measurement of horizontal and vertical individualism and collectivism. *Journal of Personality and Social Psychology*, 74(1), 118–128. doi:10.1037//0022-3514.74.1.118.

Triandis, H. C., McCusker, C., & Hui, C. H. (1990). Multimethod probes of individualism and collectivism. *Journal of Personality and Social Psychology*, 59(5), 1006–1020. doi:10.1037/0022-3514.59.5.1006

Varnum, M. E. W., Shi, Z., Chen, A., Qiu, J., & Han, S. (2014). When "Your" reward is the same as "My" reward: Self-construal priming shifts neural responses to own vs. friends' rewards. *NeuroImage*, 87(C), 164–169. http://doi.org/10.1016/j.neuroimage.2013.10.042

Wang, C., Ma, Y., & Han, S. (2014). Self-construal priming modulates pain perception: Event-related potential evidence. *Cognitive Neuroscience*, 5(1), 3–9. http://doi.org/10.1080/17588928.2013.797388

Wang, C., Oyserman, D., Liu, Q., Li, H., & Han, S. (2013). Accessible cultural mind-set modulates default mode activity: Evidence for the culturally situated brain. *Social Neuroscience*, 8(3), 203–216. http://doi.org/10.1080/17470919.2013.775966

Wang, F., Peng, K., Chechlacz, M., Humphreys, G. W., & Sui, J. (2017). The neural basis of independence versus interdependence orientations: A voxel-based morphometric analysis of brain volume. *Psychological Science: A Journal of the American Psychological Society / APS*, 28(4), 519–529. http://doi.org/10.1177/0956797616689079

Wang, C., Wu, B., Liu, Y., Wu, X., & Han, S. (2015). Challenging emotional prejudice by changing self-concept: priming independent self-construal reduces racial in-group bias in neural responses to other's pain. *Social cognitive and affective neuroscience*, 10(9), 1195–1201.

Woollett, K., & Maguire, E. A. (2011). Acquiring "the Knowledge" of London's layout drives structural brain changes. *Current Biology*, 21(24), 2109–2114. http://doi.org/10.1016/j.cub.2011.11.018

Yamaguchi, S., Kuhlman, D. M., & Sugimori, S. (1995). Personality correlates of allocentric tendencies in individualist and collectivist cultures. *Journal of cross-cultural psychology*, 26(6), 658–672.

Zhu, Y., Zhang, L., Fan, J., & Han, S. (2007). Neural basis of cultural influence on self-representation. *NeuroImage*, 34(3), 1310–1316. http://doi.org/10.1016/j.neuroimage.2006.08.047

Culture Shapes Face Processing

Caroline Blais *and* Roberto Caldara

Abstract

Cross-cultural studies have revealed striking differences in visual perception. Recent research has shown that even processes that have long been assumed to be universal, such as face processing, are in part shaped by the cultural environment in which one has grown up. This chapter gives an overview of the main findings with regard to the impact of culture on the visual processes involved in face identification and facial expression recognition. The chapter also discusses neurological conditions affecting face perception and how culture may interact with these conditions to modulate visual perception.

Key Words: culture, face recognition, facial expressions, visual perception, eye movements, psychophysics

Introduction

As with globalization multiculturalism increases in our contemporary societies, we are confronted with the ethical responsibility of developing a health system that should ideally take into account all sorts of variations across human beings. Some of these individual differences are obvious. For instance, it is well established that gender influences the response to some medications (e.g., Bergiannaki & Kostaras, 2016; Ohlsen & Pilowsky, 2007). Culture and ethnicity also play a critical role in modulating health issues (e.g., Yuan et al., 2005). However, what is much less obvious is the impact of culture on how individuals perceive their world, and how this may affect not only their approach to health (e.g., Gupta, 2010), pain (e.g., Edwards et al., 2001; Hsieh et al., 2010) and the health system in general (e.g., Pavlish et al., 2010; Sheikh & Furnham, 2000), but also the effectiveness and appropriateness of the treatments they receive (Fiscella et al., 2000).

Research in psychology has revealed that one's perception of the world is deeply influenced by cultural learning. Evidence of cultural influences span from complex, high-level psychological processes, such as how one interprets someone else's behavior (Choi et al., 1999; Morris & Peng, 1994) or makes important life decisions (Levine et al., 1995), to basic perceptual processes, such as the visual information on which one relies to process faces (Blais et al., 2008; Caldara et al., 2010; Tardif et al., 2017; for a review see Caldara,

2017), objects (Gutchess et al., 2006; Kelly et al., 2010; Paige et al., 2017), or simple visual arrays (Ueda et al., 2018).

With regard to face perception, research has so far focused on characterizing the cultural differences in the behavior and brain processes of normal individuals. However, deficits of face perception are observed in many neurological conditions, and how culture interacts with these conditions to modulate visual perception remains unknown. The present chapter will first provide an overview of the research on cultural differences in visual perception in general, and face perception in particular, as well as the potential sources for these differences. Then we will review some neurological conditions affecting face processing for which knowledge gathered so far suggests that treatments may benefit from being tailored to the individual's culture.

Cultural Differences in Visual Perception

The last few decades of research have led to evidence supporting the idea that the same visual stimulation is not perceived in the same way by all observers; in particular, culture has been shown to deeply affect visual processes (Caldara, 2017; Chen & Jack, 2017; Nisbett et al., 2001). A large part of the studies assessing the impact of culture on visual perception has compared individuals from East Asia (mainly from China, South Korea and Japan) with Westerners. This may be explained by a methodological issue: to assess the universality of a process, it is necessary to compare very different populations with regard to culture while controlling for the level of education, because the latter may affect the interpretation of instructions (Heine, 2015). Easterners and Westerners adhere to very different systems of values (Hofstede, 1991; Nisbett et al., 2001) but have similar systems of education. Thus, the present chapter will mostly focus on face processing studies comparing Easterners and Westerners, research in other populations is still cruelly lacking.

The cultural differences highlighted so far in visual perception may be grouped around three main categories of findings: (a) when processing a visual scene, Easterners attend to the context/background more than Westerners, and Westerners attend more to the focal objects of the scene than Easterners (Chua et al., 2005; Masuda et al., 2008; Masuda & Nisbett, 2001; but see Miellet et al., 2010); (b) Easterners process visual stimulations in a more global manner than Westerners (McKone et al., 2010; Nisbett & Miyamoto, 2005); and (c) Easterners deploy their visual attention over a larger area of their visual field than Westerners (Boduroglu et al., 2009; Boduroglu & Shah, 2017; Miellet et al., 2013; Tardif et al., 2017).

Attention to Context Versus Focal Objects

A seminal study by Masuda and Nisbett (2001) has revealed that when asked to describe a visual scene, Easterners describe more of the background than Westerners. Most interestingly, when presented with focal objects of the previously viewed scenes, the ability of Easterners to remember these objects depended on the background on which they were presented. More specifically, their performance dropped when the objects were presented over a new background. Crucially, this drop in performance was not observed for Westerner observers. The authors of that study concluded that Easterners encode focal objects in memory by binding them to the context in which they were perceived, whereas Westerners encode objects in memory separately from their context.

This conclusion was later extended by showing that not only memory-encoding processes are affected by culture, but also the final percept per se (Masuda et al., 2008). In fact, when Easterners have to judge the facial expression of a focal individual surrounded by other expressive individuals, their affective evaluation is more affected by the expression of the surrounding individuals than the Westerners. Interestingly, only ocular fixations occurring later than 1 second after stimulus onset differed in both cultural groups, which led the authors to conclude that the differences observed reflected late decisional processes rather than early perceptual processes. However, the ocular fixation pattern was averaged over 1-second periods, which decreased the temporal resolution of the results. In contrast, a study assessing the ocular fixations of Easterners and Westerners while they viewed natural visual scenes revealed cultural differences as early as 420 ms (Chua et al., 2005). Moreover, as will be discussed in more detail in the section "Cultural Differences in Face Identification", eye movements alone do not provide a complete picture of visual information processing. In fact, differences in late ocular fixation patterns may reflect earlier differences in covert attention (Estéphan et al., 2018; Tardif et al., 2017). Thus, the processing stage at which the background affects the foreground perception in Easterners is worth further investigation.

A higher tendency for Easterners than for Westerners to bind the background with focal objects was also observed with simpler visual stimulation. For instance, in the Rod and Frame test (Witkin et al., 1954), in which one has to judge the orientation of a "rod" (depicted as a line) independently of the frame (depicted as a square) in which it appears, Easterners are more affected than Westerners by the frame's orientation (Ji et al., 2000). In a similar vein, Easterners show more difficulty at inhibiting the context in the absolute version of the Frame-Line test (Kitayama et al., 2003; but see Zhou et al., 2008). The absolute version of that test consists in adjusting the length of a line inside a square such that it is of equal length with a previously viewed line appearing inside a square of different size. To perform accurately in such a task, one needs to process the line independently from the square in which it appears. Thus, evidence so far suggests that Easterners and Westerners differ in the degree to which they attend to the context of a visual scene and integrate this context with the objects it contains. Further evidence for such cultural perceptual bias has been recently found for a famous visual search problem parametrically varying in difficulty: *Where's Waldo* (Lüthold et al., 2018). East Asian observers were significantly much more impaired than Western Caucasian observers for finding Waldo, despite all observers having a comparable level of familiarity with the vignettes. Interestingly, Easterners showed a peculiar and systematic eye movement strategy consisting in returning more often to previously visited locations compared to Westerners. This suboptimal eye movement strategy in the Easterners might arise from their perceptual bias in using more extra-foveal information, which impaired the visual search for Waldo. Overall, this subtle perceptual difference shows that the processing of active visual search in scenes is modulated by the culture of the observer.

Global Versus Local Processing of Information

In addition to the differences observed in the processing of relations between objects and the context in which they appear, some have proposed that Easterners and Westerners differ in the degree to which they rely on global versus local processes. Using hierarchical letters (i.e., large letters composed of smaller ones, for instance, large H composed of small Es), it was shown that Easterners show a larger global advantage than Westerners (McKone et al., 2010). With hierarchical letters, a global advantage consists in being better at detecting a target letter when it is displayed as the large (global) letter than when it is displayed as the small (local) letters composing it. Using electrophysiology, Lao et al. (2013) showed that the higher tuning toward global than local information occurred in earlier processing stages for Easterners than for Westerners. Adding further support to the idea that Easterners process information in a more global manner than Westerners, it was also shown that they have a stronger tendency than Westerners at perceiving a face in Arcimboldo paintings (paintings depicting faces composed of objects such as fruits or vegetables; Rozin et al., 2016).

Nevertheless, not all studies assessing cultural differences on global versus local perceptual bias have found a larger global bias for Easterners than Westerners. In the aforementioned study by Lao and colleagues, although they found cultural differences in brain activity, they did not replicate the finding of a larger global advantage for Easterners than Westerners at the behavioral level. Another study using similar stimuli (hierarchical geometrical shapes) but a different task (visual similarity judgments instead of a target detection) obtained a larger global bias for British than for Japanese individuals (Oishi et al., 2014). Thus, although many studies point toward cultural differences in the global or local perceptual bias, findings are not systematic across studies. Note, however, that a study has shown that hierarchical letters and hierarchical shapes tap into different aspects of global/local processes (Dale & Arnell, 2013), which may explain the discrepancies observed across the studies described previously.

Breadth of Attentional Deployment

The third category of findings suggests that Easterners deploy their visual attention over a broader area of their visual field than Westerners. For instance, in a change detection task, Easterners have been shown to perform better than Westerners when the changes occur in more peripheral locations, whereas Westerners perform best when the changes occur in more central locations (Boduroglu et al., 2009). Moreover, it was recently shown that the spatial resolution with which Easterners process a simple visual scene is lower than that of Westerners (Boduroglu & Shah, 2017), a finding that would be expected following a broader allocation of attention (Balz & Hock, 1997; Goto et al., 2001). In fact, the findings of a global perceptual bias and of a broader deployment of attention by Easterners and Westerners may represent the same perceptual mechanism: it was shown that attending to the global versus local structure of an object affects the resolution with which it is processed (Shulman & Wilson, 1987). More specifically, attending to the global structure, which usually spans a larger area of the visual field, facilitates the processing of lower spatial frequencies, which code for coarser visual information. In contrast, attending to the local structure, which usually spans a smaller area of the visual field, facilitates the processing of higher spatial frequencies, which code for finer visual information. Cultural differences in the visual processing of objects have recently been supported by brain-level analyses: simple objects involve distinct multivoxel representations in the visual cortex of Easterners and Westerners (Ksander et al., 2018). Most interestingly, the authors of that study reported supplemental analysis suggesting that these distinct representations may be associated with the processing of distinct spatial frequencies (i.e., lower spatial frequencies for Easterners than Westerners). This finding coincides very well with the finding of cultural differences in the spatial frequencies used during face processing (Estéphan et al., 2018; Tardif et al., 2017), which will be described in more detail in the section "Cultural Differences in Face Identification".

Attentional Processes and System of Values

The findings of a different use of the relation between objects and their context, of different perceptual biases, and of different attentional breadth have for the most part been related to a dominant theory in the field proposing that exposition to an individualistic versus collectivistic system of values led to the development of different perceptual strategies (Nisbett et al., 2001). More specifically, according to this theory, exposition to collectivistic values prioritizing the group over the individual would shape cognitive and perceptual processes such that one tends to attend more to the relation between events and objects and deploy their attention across a broader area of the visual field. In contrast, exposition to individualistic values, prioritizing the individual over the group, would shape cognitive and perceptual processes such that one tends to attend more to focal objects located in a specific/local area of their visual field.

Another account that has recently gained support by studies measuring the global versus local perceptual bias in a remote African population, the Himba (Caparos et al., 2012; Linnell et al., 2013), proposes that many of the findings described earlier are attributable to the kind of physical environment to which one is exposed (Masuda & Nisbett, 2006). More specifically, exposition to a dense visual environment would lead to perceptual strategies favoring the processing of the background and the deployment of attention over broader areas, thus facilitating a global perceptual bias. The fact that Easterners show a larger global perceptual bias than Westerners, who themselves show a larger global perceptual bias than traditional Himba people, is congruent with the visual density to which each of these populations is exposed (Caparos et al., 2012).

Although more work is necessary to understand the source of cultural differences highlighted previously, evidence so far reveals a relatively systematic pattern of findings whereby culture modulates the way in which attention is deployed over the visual field. As will be described in the next section, this pattern of findings has also been observed in face perception studies.

Cultural Differences in Face Identification

In 2008, we published the first study revealing cultural differences in the visual strategies underlying face processing (Blais et al., 2008). We revealed that when encoding or recognizing the identity of a face and when categorizing the ethnicity of a face, Easterners and Westerners displayed different eye fixation patterns. Easterners fixated more the central area of a face than Westerners, whereas Westerners fixated more the eye and mouth areas than Easterners. Interestingly, these different eye fixation patterns were deployed despite the fact that the same facial areas, namely the eyes and the mouth, were used by both groups. In fact, the latter conclusion was reached in a following study where Caldara et al. (2010) used a gaze-contingent paradigm in which the size of the window through which the stimulus was visible was manipulated. When the size of the window was reduced, Easterners adopted a fixation pattern similar to that of Westerners, whereby they directly fixated the eye and mouth areas. Thus, this suggested that Easterners, just like Westerners, rely on the eye and mouth areas to recognize faces. However, Westerners spend more time than Easterners foveating these areas during visual information extraction. In contrast, Easterners spend more time than Westerners processing these areas in more peripheral locations of their retina. Interestingly, when using an inverse parametric gaze-contingent technique consisting in dynamically masking central vision – the *Blindspot* – Westerners progressively shifted the eye movements towards the typical Eastern central fixation pattern (Miellet, et al, 2012). This later observation confirmed the robustness of a fixation bias in a *focal* (i.e., Western) versus *peripheral* (i.e., Eastern) visual information sampling across cultures.

The different patterns of eye fixations during face processing corroborate well the findings described previously, consisting in a more global/larger attentional breadth in Easterners than Westerners. In fact, to process the features of a face while fixating on a more central location, one has to deploy their attention more broadly. Accordingly, Miellet et al. (2013) developed a computational model to estimate the breadth of attention in Easterners and Westerners during face processing and to estimate the resolution, in terms of spatial frequencies, with which they process visual information. Based on their model, they proposed that Easterners' attentional breadth is larger than Westerners', and that the former rely less than the latter on higher spatial frequencies. Also consistent with the reliance on a more global perceptual strategy, at least two studies have found a higher reliance on holistic/configural processing during face processing (Miyamoto et al., 2011; Rozin et al., 2016).

Nevertheless, the conclusion of different visual strategies and of a reliance on different granularities of visual information in Easterners and Westerners was challenged in a study by Or et al. (2015). These authors did not find cultural differences in early ocular fixations during face processing. Yet, early fixations have been shown to be sufficient for face recognition (Hsiao & Cottrell, 2008), thereby leading to questioning of whether the cultural differences observed in later ocular fixations are truly associated with face processing per se. In fact, Or and colleagues proposed that they most likely reflected norm-based cultural differences in the appropriateness of fixating someone else in the eyes, instead of differences in the perceptual strategies per se. However, this view has been challenged by the eye movement strategy deployed during the recognition of the facial expressions of emotion. East Asian observers deploy more fixations toward the eye region than toward the mouth region to decode facial expressions; this contrasts with the Western Caucasians' strategy whereby the fixations are evenly distributed on the eyes and mouth area (Geangu et al., 2016; Jack et al., 2009; see section "Cultural Differences in Facial Expression Processing"). Therefore, East Asian observers directly gaze at the eyes when this is task relevant. Social gaze avoidance as a potential explanation for the cultural contrast in face recognition also is not supported by the persistent central fixations directed toward nonface objects (i.e., Greebles) and nonhuman faces (i.e., sheep faces) by Easterners during recognition (Kelly et al., 2010). Or et al. (2015) study involved a face-matching task, while all our previous study used an old/new face recognition task. In addition, the methodological peculiarities adopted in the eye movement experiment conducted by Or et al. (2015) elicited the use of only a few fixations and did not prevent for anticipatory strategies. As such, those factors and differences across studies seem to be at the root of the absence of cultural differences observed in their study.

Further supporting the idea that culture impacts early processes in face identification, two recent studies have shown cultural differences in low-level visual information extraction occurring at early processing stages (Estéphan et al., 2018; Tardif et al., 2017). More specifically, using spatial frequency Bubbles (Willenbockel et al., 2010), a psychophysical classification image method, Tardif et al. (2017) showed that during two different face-processing tasks (face identification and face familiarity), Easterners use more of the lower spatial frequencies than Westerners, and Westerners used more of the higher spatial frequencies than Easterners. This pattern of results was replicated by Estéphan and colleagues, who further showed that the reliance on different spatial frequencies by both cultural groups started as early as 35 ms after stimulus onset. This makes very unlikely the conclusion that Easterners and Westerners differ only in late perceptual stages reflecting cultural norms in the appropriateness of looking someone else in the eye. Moreover, the pattern of spatial frequency utilization closely reflects what was expected based on the eye fixation pattern (i.e., when not considering the temporal dimension). Thus, this may indicate that even later ocular fixations reflect cultural differences in early covert attention.

So far, the source of these cultural differences in face processing remains unknown. The pattern, since it suggests a larger attentional breadth in Easterners than in Westerners, is consistent with both of the accounts mentioned in the section "Attentional Processes and System of Values". In fact, the theory proposing that exposure to different systems of values may shape perceptual processes predicts a larger attentional breadth in Easterners, who are exposed to more collectivistic values, than in Westerners, who are exposed to more individualistic values. A study by Kelly et al. (2011) has attempted to verify if the eye movement pattern of British-born Chinese was correlated with the degree to which they adhere to collectivistic values and failed to reveal a significant relation. The sample size was, however, relatively small, so the relation between visual strategies and adherence to collectivistic or individualistic values remains worth investigating.

Similarly, the theory proposing that exposure to dense visual environments leads to the adoption of a larger attentional breadth and a global perceptual bias is also consistent with the pattern of findings obtained in face processing. Testing a rural African population would help disambiguate between the two potential explanations. In fact, as explained earlier, traditional Himba people have been shown to be more local than British and Japanese individuals in two visual processing tasks that did not involve face stimuli (Caparos et al., 2012). In contrast, the system-of-values theory would have predicted a larger global bias for Himba than for British people, as the former adhere to more collectivistic values than the latter. Thus, although the system-of-values theory would predict a pattern of ocular fixations and a spatial frequency tuning closer to the one observed with Easterners in rural African populations, the visual environment hypothesis would predict rather a higher reliance on high spatial frequency and denser ocular fixations on the main facial features in rural Africans than in Westerners.

Another possibility is that the pattern of findings observed with faces reflects a different mechanism than the one underlying the findings in visual tasks involving nonsocial stimuli. In fact, Han and Ma (2014) have shown that different neural networks are associated with cultural differences during the processing of social and nonsocial visual stimuli. Perhaps one potential explanation lies in the frequency of exposure to face stimuli during early infancy and the preferred distance at which infants view faces across cultures. It was recently shown that Western infants younger than 3 months have front-view faces in their visual field almost three times more often than toddlers of 18 months (Jayaraman et al., 2017). Moreover, this high exposure to faces during young infancy is crucial for the development of face-processing mechanisms. In fact, young infants deprived of such exposure because of congenital cataracts show deficits in configural face processing even after having the cataracts removed and having been exposed to faces for many years (Le Grand et al., 2001). Nevertheless, although cultural differences in the frequency of face-to-face interactions have been observed (Keller, 2007), cultural differences in the developmental trajectory of this phenomenon have not been investigated so far. Most importantly, the distance at which infants from different cultures view faces most frequently may affect the degree to which they learn to rely on lower versus higher spatial frequencies. In fact, as the distance increases between someone's eyes and the face to be processed, the availability of higher spatial frequencies decreases (F. W. Smith & Schyns, 2009). Interestingly, a study comparing infant–mother interactions in Japan and the United States has shown that during face-to-face interactions, American mothers stand closer to their child (Fogel et al., 1988). This finding may be consistent with the Westerners tuning toward higher spatial frequencies. In any case, a systematic investigation of the frequency and distance at which infants of different cultures are exposed to faces may represent an interesting avenue for understanding the findings described in the present chapter with faces.

Cultural Differences in Facial Expression Processing

The field of emotion studies has witnessed a long-standing debate regarding the universality or cultural specificity of facial expressions of emotion and their recognition. The seminal work of Ekman and colleagues (Ekman et al., 1969; Ekman & Friesen, 1971) has argued in favor of the universality of a subset of emotions, called basic emotions (i.e., anger, disgust, fear, happiness, sadness, and surprise). A large part of the argument was first based on the discovery that a remote, isolated culture in New Guinea had the capacity to recognize, with a performance higher than chance, the emotions expressed by North Americans (Ekman & Friesen, 1971). The reverse was also true—that is, North Americans displayed a performance higher than chance at recognizing facial expressions displayed by Papua individuals. Thus, the authors suggested that enough signal was shared among the North Americans' and Papuasians' expressions to conclude that they were biologically determined and universal.

However, despite being able to recognize the expressions emitted by the other culture, both groups were impaired in comparison with their performance at recognizing their own-group expressions. In fact, a meta-analysis revealed a systematic impairment, across studies, at recognizing facial expressions of basic emotions when they are emitted by another cultural group than the observer (Elfenbein & Ambady, 2002). Interestingly, such an impairment can even be observed when observers come from a different region, but from the same country, than the emitter (Elfenbein & Ambady, 2002). Although an impairment at recognizing other-group expressions does not preclude the possibility that these expressions are universal, it suggests that culture at least nuances their appearance.

Revealing those nuances, however, is not trivial. For instance, one method consists in capturing spontaneous expressions in emotion-inducing situations. Using such a method, it is difficult to make sure that the situation used to induce emotions is interpreted in the same way across cultures and effectively induces the same emotion across cultures. An alternative to this method has been proposed in a series of studies using reverse correlation (Jack, Caldara, & Schyns, 2012; Jack, Garrod, et al., 2012; Jack et al., 2016). The traditional version of the reverse correlation method (Ahumada & Lovell, 1971; Eckstein & Ahumada, 2002; Mangini & Biederman, 2004) consists in embedding a stimulus in visual noise, such that the noise alters the stimulus appearance. On each trial, the noise is different, therefore changing the stimulus's appearance, and the participants are asked to make a decision about the stimulus presented. For instance, the noise properties, when added over a neutral face, may create stimuli that appear closer to someone's representation of anger, sadness, disgust, etc. After many such trials, it is possible to infer which noise properties led the participant to perceive each of these expressions; the method thus allows accessing the participant's mental representation of each expression. Using that method, Jack, Caldara, and Schyns (2012) showed that Easterners and Westerners build different representations of facial expressions of basic emotions. In fact, whereas expressions of Westerners include facial features located around the mouth, eye, and eyebrow areas, expressions of Easterners are mostly represented by changes in the eye area.

Building on this work, Jack and colleagues (2016) used a method developed by Yu et al. (2012) that combines dynamic structural face computer graphics with reverse correlation to extract the facial movements (i.e., more specifically, the Facial Action Units, based on Ekman and colleagues' work; Ekman & Friesen, 1978) representative of each facial expression of emotion in Chinese and British participants. In a very elegant study, they modeled over 60 culturally valid expressions of emotions in these two cultures and showed that they share four different patterns of facial movements. Based on these results, they suggested the existence of four, rather than six, emotions shared across cultures. Moreover, they showed that these basic patterns are nuanced by what they called "accents" and that those accents differed across cultures (for a similar proposition, see also Elfenbein, 2013). The observation, on the one hand, of cultural commonalities, and, on the other hand, of cultural accents to facial expressions was further supported by a recent study using a completely different method (Cordaro et al., 2018).

Slight differences in the appearance of facial expressions, like the ones observed across cultures, are likely to be associated with the development of different visual strategies during decoding. However, although many studies have investigated the visual strategies used by Westerners to recognize facial expressions of emotions (e.g., Adolphs et al., 2005; Blais et al., 2012, 2017; Calvo et al., 2014; Eisenbarth & Alpers, 2011; M. L. Smith et al., 2005), only a few have investigated if and how these strategies are modulated by culture (Jack et al., 2009; Mai et al., 2011). Jack and colleagues (2009) have shown that when categorizing the six basic facial expressions of emotions, Westerners' ocular fixations are mostly directed on the mouth and eye areas, whereas Easterners fixate mostly the eye area. This finding was congruent with those described earlier, showing that Easterners mostly represent the six basic facial expressions using variations in the eye area, whereas Westerners represent the basic expressions using featural variations in the eye, eyebrow, and mouth areas (Jack, Caldara, & Schyns, 2012). Consistently with these results, a study showed that the Chinese participants who perform better in a fake smile detection task are the ones who rely the most on the eye area (Mai et al., 2011). Although these studies are informative with regard to the areas typically fixated by Easterners and Westerners, more research is needed to compare different cultures on their utilization of low-level visual information, for instance, spatial frequencies, during facial expression recognition. More recently, Geangu et al. (2016) reported that such cultural differences are already present in 7-month-old infants. Altogether, these findings demonstrate that from an early stage in life, culture shapes the visual sampling strategies used to decode facial expressions of emotion.

Future Directions

As pointed out in the introduction, deficits at processing faces are observed in many neurological conditions or mental health disorders. For instance, impairments in recognizing facial expressions are observed in autism (Baron-Cohen et al., 2001; Humphreys et al., 2007; Wallace et al., 2008), schizophrenia (Kohler et al., 2009; Mandal et al., 1998), and social anxiety (Montagne et al., 2006). Moreover, profound impairments in processing the identity of a face are found in congenital (Behrmann & Avidan, 2005; Duchaine, 2000) and acquired (Rossion, 2014) prosopagnosia, conditions that are actually defined by that deficit. Several studies have looked into the visual strategies that may be associated with these perceptual deficits. However, whether culture interacts with these conditions in determining the type of visual strategies used during face perception remains unknown.

Interestingly, research has shown that certain genes interact with culture such that reverse behaviors may be observed in individuals with a similar genetic predisposition but different cultures (Kim & Sasaki, 2014). For instance, Kim et al. (2009) investigated the link between a serotonin receptor gene and the locus of attention, namely whether individuals reported paying more attention to focal objects or to the background of a scene. They found that the same genotype (homozygous on the G allele of the 5-HTR1A gene) was associated with inverse strategies as a function of culture: while Westerners with this genotype reported paying more attention to focal objects than to the background, Easterners with the same genotype instead reported paying more attention to the background than to focal objects. This finding is fascinating, as it suggests that individuals with similar biological constitutions may develop different perceptual strategies because of the way they might react and adapt to cultural forces. It also raises the question of whether similar neurological conditions may be associated with different perceptual deficits. In fact, on the one hand, cultural forces may interact with similar neurological alterations to create different behavioral manifestations. On the other hand, the studies presented in this chapter highlight striking differences in the visual perception of normal individuals of different cultures. Thus, it is highly plausible that an acquired neurological condition, such as prosopagnosia following a cerebral lesion, as well as developmental conditions, such as congenital prosopagnosia or autism, will be associated with different visual strategies in different cultures.

Take, for instance, the case of prosopagnosia. This condition has been associated, in Westerner populations, with an alteration at fixating (de Xivry et al., 2008) and processing (Bukach et al., 2008; Caldara et al., 2005) the eye area during the recognition of face identities. Moreover, it has been suggested that this condition is associated with a smaller perceptual window (Van Belle et al., 2015). No study has so far verified the visual strategies used by non-Western populations suffering from this condition. As explained in the section "Cultural Differences in Face Identification", during face recognition, Easterners fixate less the eye area, deploy their attention more broadly, and are tuned toward lower spatial frequencies than Westerners. What would be the functional consequence of a lesion leading to prosopagnosia in Easterners? Since they already make few fixations to the eye area because of their larger attentional breadth, would prosopagnosia lead to changes in fixations to the eye area? Would it be associated with a change in the spatial frequency tuning? Similarly, prosopagnosia is associated, in Westerners, with a deficit in recognizing facial expressions of emotion (Bowers et al., 1985; De Gelder et al., 2000) and with a decrease in the ocular fixations directed to the eye area, as well as a decreased processing of the visual information conveyed by that area (Fiset et al., 2017). As explained in the section "Cultural Differences in Facial Expressions Processing", Easterners rely mostly on the eye area during emotion categorization, making few fixations to the mouth area, compared with Westerners. Thus, would Easterner prosopagnosics be even more impaired than Westerner prosopagnosics at recognizing emotions? Would they show the same impairment in processing the eye area? Similar questions may be raised with regard to autism. In fact, Western individuals with autism have been shown to fixate (Spezio et al., 2007a) and process (Spezio et al., 2007b) less information conveyed by the eye area during the processing of faces (both identity and expressions). Since Easterners use this information less during the processing of identity but rely mostly on that information during the processing of emotion, would the same differences in perceptual strategies between neurotypical and autistic individuals be observed in East Asia?

Conclusion

In recent years, an important trend in research on face processing has been to characterize as precisely as possible the visual strategies underlying this biological skill, as well as the ones underlying deficits in this ability, to gather the necessary information to develop interventions that may help improve face-processing abilities (Caldara et al., 2005; Fiset et al., 2017; Nusseck et al., 2008; Peterson & Eckstein, 2012; Richoz et al., 2015; Royer et al., 2018; M. L. Smith et al., 2005; Tardif et al., 2019; Yovel & Duchaine, 2006). Cross-cultural studies have revealed striking differences in the visual strategies underlying the processing of faces, but the evolutionary, social, and biological forces rooting such effects are not well understood. In addition, as pointed out by Kitayama and Salvador (2017), we acknowledge that the field needs to expand the span of populations compared and whenever possible study other cultures. The question of whether the cultural differences reported here are genuinely related to culture or related to other environmental or biological forces remains to be validated, as these factors have been confounded in the large majority of cross-cultural studies.

Finally, whether and how these strategies are altered in different neurological and mental health conditions in non-Western populations remains unknown. Such knowledge, coupled with functional neuroimaging studies in the healthy population, will be very important to gather in the next years to develop interventions that are adapted to the culture, and thus to the nature of the visual deficit, of the patients.

References

Adolphs, R., Gosselin, F., Buchanan, T. W., Tranel, D., Schyns, P., & Damasio, A. R. (2005). A mechanism for impaired fear recognition after amygdala damage. *Nature, 433*(7021), 68.

Ahumada Jr., A., & Lovell, J. (1971). Stimulus features in signal detection. *Journal of the Acoustical Society of America, 49*(6B), 1751–1756.

Balz, G. W., & Hock, H. S. (1997). The effect of attentional spread on spatial resolution. *Vision Research, 37*(11), 1499–1510.

Baron-Cohen, S., Wheelwright, S., Hill, J., Raste, Y., & Plumb, I. (2001). The "Reading the Mind in the Eyes" test revised version: A study with normal adults, and adults with Asperger syndrome or high-functioning autism. *Journal of Child Psychology and Psychiatry, 42*(2), 241–251.

Behrmann, M., & Avidan, G. (2005). Congenital prosopagnosia: Face-blind from birth. *Trends in Cognitive Sciences, 9*(4), 180–187.

Bergiannaki, J. D., & Kostaras, P. (2016). Pharmacokinetic and pharmacodynamic effects of psychotropic medications: Differences between sexes. *Psychiatriki, 27*(2), 118–126.

Blais, C., Fiset, D., Roy, C., Saumure Régimbald, C., & Gosselin, F. (2017). Eye fixation patterns for categorizing static and dynamic facial expressions. *Emotion, 17*(7), 1107.

Blais, C., Jack, R. E., Scheepers, C., Fiset, D., & Caldara, R. (2008). Culture shapes how we look at faces. *PloS One, 3*(8), e3022.

Blais, C., Roy, C., Fiset, D., Arguin, M., & Gosselin, F. (2012). The eyes are not the window to basic emotions. *Neuropsychologia, 50*(12), 2830–2838.

Boduroglu, A., & Shah, P. (2017). Cultural differences in attentional breadth and resolution. *Culture and Brain, 5*(2), 169–181.

Boduroglu, A., Shah, P., & Nisbett, R. E. (2009). Cultural differences in allocation of attention in visual information processing. *Journal of Cross-Cultural Psychology, 40*(3), 349–360.

Bowers, D., Bauer, R. M., Coslett, H. B., & Heilman, K. M. (1985). Processing of faces by patients with unilateral hemisphere lesions: I. Dissociation between judgments of facial affect and facial identity. *Brain and Cognition, 4*(3), 258–272.

Bukach, C. M., Le Grand, R., Kaiser, M. D., Bub, D. N., & Tanaka, J. W. (2008). Preservation of mouth region processing in two cases of prosopagnosia. *Journal of Neuropsychology, 2*(1), 227–244.

Caldara, R. (2017). Culture reveals a flexible system for face processing. *Current Directions in Psychological Science, 26*(3), 249–255.

Caldara, R., Schyns, P., Mayer, E., Smith, M. L., Gosselin, F., & Rossion, B. (2005). Does prosopagnosia take the eyes out of face representations? Evidence for a defect in representing diagnostic facial information following brain damage. *Journal of Cognitive Neuroscience, 17*(10), 1652–1666.

Caldara, R., Zhou, X., & Miellet, S. (2010). Putting culture under the 'spotlight' reveals universal information use for face recognition. *PLoS One, 5*(3), e9708.

Calvo, M. G., Fernández-Martín, A., & Nummenmaa, L. (2014). Facial expression recognition in peripheral versus central vision: Role of the eyes and the mouth. *Psychological Research, 78*(2), 180–195.

Caparos, S., Ahmed, L., Bremner, A. J., de Fockert, J. W., Linnell, K. J., & Davidoff, J. (2012). Exposure to an urban environment alters the local bias of a remote culture. *Cognition, 122*(1), 80–85.

Chen, C., & Jack, R. E. (2017). Discovering cultural differences (and similarities) in facial expressions of emotion. *Current Opinion in Psychology, 17*, 61–66.

Choi, I., Nisbett, R. E., & Norenzayan, A. (1999). Causal attribution across cultures: Variation and universality. *Psychological Bulletin, 125*(1), 47.

Chua, H. F., Boland, J. E., & Nisbett, R. E. (2005). Cultural variation in eye movements during scene perception. *Proceedings of the National Academy of Sciences, 102*(35), 12629–12633.

Cordaro, D. T., Sun, R., Keltner, D., Kamble, S., Huddar, N., & McNeil, G. (2018). Universals and cultural variations in 22 emotional expressions across five cultures. *Emotion, 18*(1), 75–93.

Dale, G., & Arnell, K. M. (2013). Investigating the stability of and relationships among global/local processing measures. *Attention, Perception, & Psychophysics, 75*(3), 394–406.

De Gelder, B., Pourtois, G., Vroomen, J., & Bachoud-Lévi, A. C. (2000). Covert processing of faces in prosopagnosia is restricted to facial expressions: Evidence from cross-modal bias. *Brain and Cognition, 44*(3), 425–444.

de Xivry, J. J. O., Ramon, M., Lefèvre, P., & Rossion, B. (2008). Reduced fixation on the upper area of personally familiar faces following acquired prosopagnosia. *Journal of Neuropsychology, 2*(1), 245–268.

Duchaine, B. C. (2000). Developmental prosopagnosia with normal configural processing. *Neuroreport, 11*(1), 79–83.

Eckstein, M. P., & Ahumada, A. J. (2002). Classification images: A tool to analyze visual strategies. Journal of Vision, 2(1), doi: https://doi.org/10.1167/2.1.i.

Edwards, C. L., Fillingim, R. B., & Keefe, F. (2001). Race, ethnicity and pain. *Pain, 94*(2), 133–137.

Eisenbarth, H., & Alpers, G. W. (2011). Happy mouth and sad eyes: Scanning emotional facial expressions. *Emotion, 11*(4), 860.

Ekman, P., Sorenson, E. R., & Friesen, W. V. (1969). Pan-cultural elements in facial displays of emotion. Science, 164(3875), 86–88.

Ekman, P., & Friesen, W. V. (1971). Constants across cultures in the face and emotion. *Journal of Personality and Social Psychology, 17*(2), 124.

Ekman, P., & Friesen, W. V. (1978). *Facial action coding system: Investigator's guide.* Consulting Psychologists Press.

Elfenbein, H. A. (2013). Nonverbal dialects and accents in facial expressions of emotion. *Emotion Review, 5*(1), 90–96.

Elfenbein, H. A., & Ambady, N. (2002). On the universality and cultural specificity of emotion recognition: A meta-analysis. *Psychological Bulletin, 128*(2), 203.

Estéphan, A., Fiset, D., Saumure, C., Plouffe-Demers, M. P., Zhang, Y., Sun, D., & Blais, C. (2018). Time course of cultural differences in spatial frequency use for face identification. *Scientific Reports, 8*(1), 1816.

Fiscella, K., Franks, P., Gold, M. R., & Clancy, C. M. (2000). Inequality in quality: Addressing socioeconomic, racial, and ethnic disparities in health care. *Jama, 283*(19), 2579–2584.

Fiset, D., Blais, C., Royer, J., Richoz, A. R., Dugas, G., & Caldara, R. (2017). Mapping the impairment in decoding static facial expressions of emotion in prosopagnosia. *Social Cognitive and Affective Neuroscience, 12*(8), 1334–1341.

Fogel, A., Toda, S., & Kawai, M. (1988). Mother-infant face-to-face interaction in Japan and the United States: A laboratory comparison using 3-month-old infants. *Developmental Psychology, 24*(3), 398.

Geangu, E., Ichikawa, H., Lao, J., Kanazawa, S., Yamaguchi, M. K., Caldara, R., & Turati, C. (2016). Culture shapes 7-month-olds' perceptual strategies in discriminating facial expressions of emotion. *Current Biology, 26*(14), R663–R664.

Goto, M., Toriu, T., & Tanahashi, J. I. (2001). Effect of size of attended area on contrast sensitivity function. *Vision Research, 41*(12), 1483–1487.

Gupta, V. B. (2010). Impact of culture on healthcare seeking behavior of Asian Indians. *Journal of Cultural Diversity, 17*(1), 13–19.

Gutchess, A. H., Welsh, R. C., Boduroğlu, A., & Park, D. C. (2006). Cultural differences in neural function associated with object processing. *Cognitive, Affective, & Behavioral Neuroscience, 6*(2), 102–109.

Han, S., & Ma, Y. (2014). Cultural differences in human brain activity: A quantitative meta-analysis. *NeuroImage, 99*, 293–300.

Heine, S. J. (2015). *Cultural psychology* (3rd International Student ed.). WW Norton & Company.

Hofstede, G. (1991). *Cultures and organizations: Intercultural cooperation and its importance for survival: Software of the mind.* McGraw-Hill.

Hsiao, J. H. W., & Cottrell, G. (2008). Two fixations suffice in face recognition. *Psychological Science, 19*(10), 998–1006.

Hsieh, A. Y., Tripp, D. A., Ji, L. J., & Sullivan, M. J. (2010). Comparisons of catastrophizing, pain attitudes, and cold-pressor pain experience between Chinese and European Canadian young adults. *Journal of Pain*, *11*(11), 1187–1194.

Humphreys, K., Minshew, N., Leonard, G. L., & Behrmann, M. (2007). A fine-grained analysis of facial expression processing in high-functioning adults with autism. *Neuropsychologia*, *45*(4), 685–695.

Jack, R. E., Blais, C., Scheepers, C., Schyns, P. G., & Caldara, R. (2009). Cultural confusions show that facial expressions are not universal. *Current Biology*, *19*(18), 1543–1548.

Jack, R. E., Caldara, R., & Schyns, P. G. (2012). Internal representations reveal cultural diversity in expectations of facial expressions of emotion. *Journal of Experimental Psychology: General*, *141*(1), 19.

Jack, R. E., Garrod, O. G., Yu, H., Caldara, R., & Schyns, P. G. (2012). Facial expressions of emotion are not culturally universal. *Proceedings of the National Academy of Sciences*, *109*(19), 7241–7244.

Jack, R. E., Sun, W., Delis, I., Garrod, O. G., & Schyns, P. G. (2016). Four not six: Revealing culturally common facial expressions of emotion. *Journal of Experimental Psychology: General*, *145*(6), 708.

Jayaraman, S., Fausey, C. M., & Smith, L. B. (2017). Why are faces denser in the visual experiences of younger than older infants?. *Developmental Psychology*, *53*(1), 38.

Ji, L. J., Peng, K., & Nisbett, R. E. (2000). Culture, control, and perception of relationships in the environment. *Journal of Personality and Social Psychology*, *78*(5), 943.

Keller, H. (2007). *Cultures of infancy*. Erlbaum.

Kelly, D. J., Jack, R. E., Miellet, S., De Luca, E., Foreman, K., & Caldara, R. (2011). Social experience does not abolish cultural diversity in eye movements. *Frontiers in Psychology*, *2*, 95.

Kelly, D. J., Miellet, S., & Caldara, R. (2010). Culture shapes eye movements for visually homogeneous objects. *Frontiers in Psychology*, *1*, 6.

Kim, H. S., & Sasaki, J. Y. (2014). Cultural neuroscience: Biology of the mind in cultural contexts. *Annual Review of Psychology*, *65*, 487–514.

Kim, H. S., Sherman, D. K., Taylor, S. E., Sasaki, J. Y., Chu, T. Q., Ryu, C., Suh, E. M., & Xu, J. (2009). Culture, serotonin receptor polymorphism and locus of attention. *Social Cognitive and Affective Neuroscience*, *5*(2–3), 212–218.

Kitayama, S., Duffy, S., Kawamura, T., & Larsen, J. T. (2003). Perceiving an object and its context in different cultures: A cultural look at new look. *Psychological Science*, *14*(3), 201–206.

Kitayama, S., & Salvador, C. E. (2017). Culture embrained: Going beyond the nature-nurture dichotomy. *Perspectives on Psychological Science*, *12*(5), 841–854.

Kohler, C. G., Walker, J. B., Martin, E. A., Healey, K. M., & Moberg, P. J. (2009). Facial emotion perception in schizophrenia: A meta-analytic review. *Schizophrenia Bulletin*, *36*(5), 1009–1019.

Ksander, J. C., Paige, L. E., Johndro, H. A., & Gutchess, A. H. (2018). Cultural specialization of visual cortex. *Social Cognitive and Affective Neuroscience*, *13*(7), 709–718.

Lao, J., Vizioli, L., & Caldara, R. (2013). Culture modulates the temporal dynamics of global/local processing. *Culture and Brain*, *1*(2–4), 158–174.

Le Grand, R., Mondloch, C. J., Maurer, D., & Brent, H. P. (2001). Neuroperception: Early visual experience and face processing. *Nature*, *410*(6831), 890.

Levine, R., Sato, S., Hashimoto, T., & Verma, J. (1995). Love and marriage in eleven cultures. *Journal of Cross Cultural Psychology*, *26*, 554–571.

Linnell, K. J., Caparos, S., de Fockert, J. W., & Davidoff, J. (2013). Urbanization decreases attentional engagement. *Journal of Experimental Psychology: Human Perception and Performance*, *39*(5), 1232.

Lüthold, P., Lao, J., He, L., Zhou, X., & Caldara, R. (2018). Waldo reveals cultural differences in return fixations. Visual Cognition, 26(10), 817–830.

Mai, X., Ge, Y., Tao, L., Tang, H., Liu, C., & Luo, Y. J. (2011). Eyes are windows to the Chinese soul: Evidence from the detection of real and fake smiles. *PloS One*, *6*(5), e19903.

Mandal, M. K., Pandey, R., & Prasad, A. B. (1998). Facial expressions of emotions and schizophrenia: A review. *Schizophrenia Bulletin*, *24*(3), 399–412.

Mangini, M. C., & Biederman, I. (2004). Making the ineffable explicit: Estimating the information employed for face classifications. *Cognitive Science*, *28*(2), 209–226.

Masuda, T., Ellsworth, P. C., Mesquita, B., Leu, J., Tanida, S., & Van de Veerdonk, E. (2008). Placing the face in context: Cultural differences in the perception of facial emotion. *Journal of Personality and Social Psychology*, *94*(3), 365.

Masuda, T., & Nisbett, R. E. (2001). Attending holistically versus analytically: Comparing the context sensitivity of Japanese and Americans. *Journal of Personality and Social Psychology, 81*(5), 922.

Masuda, T., & Nisbett, R. E. (2006). Culture and change blindness. *Cognitive Science, 30*(2), 381–399.

McKone, E., Davies, A. A., Fernando, D., Aalders, R., Leung, H., Wickramariyaratne, T., & Platow, M. J. (2010). Asia has the global advantage: Race and visual attention. *Vision Research, 50*(16), 1540–1549.

Miellet, S., Zhou, X., He, L., Rodger, H., & Caldara, R. (2010). Investigating cultural diversity for extrafoveal information use in visual scenes. *Journal of Vision. 10*(6), 1–18.

Miellet, S., He, L., Zhou, X., Lao, J. & Caldara, R. (2012). When East meets West: gaze-contingent Blindspots abolish cultural diversity in eye movements for faces. *Journal of Eye Movement Research, 5*(2), 1–12.

Miellet, S., Vizioli, L., He, L., Zhou, X., & Caldara, R. (2013). Mapping face recognition information use across cultures. *Frontiers in Psychology, 4*, 34.

Miyamoto, Y., Yoshikawa, S., & Kitayama, S. (2011). Feature and configuration in face processing: Japanese are more configural than Americans. *Cognitive Science, 35*(3), 563–574.

Montagne, B., Schutters, S., Westenberg, H. G., van Honk, J., Kessels, R. P., & de Haan, E. H. (2006). Reduced sensitivity in the recognition of anger and disgust in social anxiety disorder. *Cognitive Neuropsychiatry, 11*(4), 389–401.

Morris, M. W., & Peng, K. (1994). Culture and cause: American and Chinese attributions for social and physical events. *Journal of Personality and Social Psychology, 67*(6), 949.

Nisbett, R. E., Peng, K., Choi, I., & Norenzayan, A. (2001). Culture and systems of thought: Holistic versus analytic cognition. *Psychological Review, 108*(2), 291.

Nisbett, R. E., & Miyamoto, Y. (2005). The influence of culture: Holistic versus analytic perception. *Trends in Cognitive Sciences, 9*(10), 467–473.

Nusseck, M., Cunningham, D. W., Wallraven, C., & Bülthoff, H. H. (2008). The contribution of different facial regions to the recognition of conversational expressions. Journal of Vision, 8(8), doi: https://doi.org/10.1167/8.8.1

Ohlsen, R. I., & Pilowsky, L. S. (2007). Gender and psychopharmacology. In M. Nasser, K. Baistow, & J. Treasure (Eds.), *The female body in mind: The interface between the female body and mental health* (pp. 238–252). Routledge/Taylor & Francis Group.

Oishi, S., Jaswal, V. K., Lillard, A. S., Mizokawa, A., Hitokoto, H., & Tsutsui, Y. (2014). Cultural variations in global versus local processing: A developmental perspective. *Developmental Psychology, 50*(12), 2654.

Or, C. C. F., Peterson, M. F., & Eckstein, M. P. (2015). Initial eye movements during face identification are optimal and similar across cultures. Journal of Vision, 15(13). doi: https://doi.org/10.1167/15.13.12

Paige, L. E., Ksander, J. C., Johndro, H. A., & Gutchess, A. H. (2017). Cross-cultural differences in the neural correlates of specific and general recognition. *Cortex, 91*, 250–261.

Pavlish, C. L., Noor, S., & Brandt, J. (2010). Somali immigrant women and the American health care system: Discordant beliefs, divergent expectations, and silent worries. *Social Science & Medicine, 71*(2), 353–361.

Peterson, M. F., & Eckstein, M. P. (2012). Looking just below the eyes is optimal across face recognition tasks. *Proceedings of the National Academy of Sciences, 109*(48), E3314–E3323.

Richoz, A. R., Jack, R. E., Garrod, O. G., Schyns, P. G., & Caldara, R. (2015). Reconstructing dynamic mental models of facial expressions in prosopagnosia reveals distinct representations for identity and expression. *Cortex, 65*, 50–64.

Rossion, B. (2014). Understanding face perception by means of prosopagnosia and neuroimaging. *Frontiers in Bioscience (Elite Edition), 6*, 308–317.

Royer, J., Blais, C., Charbonneau, I., Déry, K., Tardif, J., Duchaine, B., Gosselin, F., & Fiset, D. (2018). Greater reliance on the eye region predicts better face recognition ability. *Cognition, 181*, 12–20.

Rozin, P., Moscovitch, M., & Imada, S. (2016). Right: Left: East: West. Evidence that individuals from East Asian and South Asian cultures emphasize right hemisphere functions in comparison to Euro-American cultures. *Neuropsychologia, 90*, 3–11.

Sheikh, S., & Furnham, A. (2000). A cross-cultural study of mental health beliefs and attitudes towards seeking professional help. *Social Psychiatry and Psychiatric Epidemiology, 35*(7), 326–334.

Shulman, G. L., & Wilson, J. (1987). Spatial frequency and selective attention to local and global information. *Perception, 16*(1), 89–101.

Smith, F. W., & Schyns, P. G. (2009). Smile through your fear and sadness: Transmitting and identifying facial expression signals over a range of viewing distances. *Psychological Science, 20*(10), 1202–1208.

Smith, M. L., Cottrell, G. W., Gosselin, F., & Schyns, P. G. (2005). Transmitting and decoding facial expressions. *Psychological Science, 16*(3), 184–189.

Spezio, M. L., Adolphs, R., Hurley, R. S., & Piven, J. (2007a). Analysis of face gaze in autism using "Bubbles." *Neuropsychologia, 45*(1), 144–151.

Spezio, M. L., Adolphs, R., Hurley, R. S., & Piven, J. (2007b). Abnormal use of facial information in high-functioning autism. *Journal of Autism and Developmental Disorders, 37*(5), 929–939.

Tardif, J., Fiset, D., Zhang, Y., Estéphan, A., Cai, Q., Luo, C., Sun, D., Gosselin, F., & Blais, C. (2017). Culture shapes spatial frequency tuning for face identification. *Journal of Experimental Psychology: Human Perception and Performance, 43*(2), 294.

Tardif, J., Morin-Duchesne, X., Cohan, S., Royer, J., Blais, C., Fiset, D., Duchaine, B., & Gosselin, F. (2019). Use of face information varies systematically from developmental prosopagnosics to super-recognizers. *Psychological Science, 30*(2), 300–308.

Ueda, Y., Chen, L., Kopecky, J., Cramer, E. S., Rensink, R. A., Meyer, D. E., Kitayama, S., & Saiki, J. (2018). Cultural differences in visual search for geometric figures. *Cognitive Science, 42*(1), 286–310.

Van Belle, G., Lefèvre, P., & Rossion, B. (2015). Face inversion and acquired prosopagnosia reduce the size of the perceptual field of view. *Cognition, 136*, 403–408.

Wallace, S., Coleman, M., & Bailey, A. (2008). An investigation of basic facial expression recognition in autism spectrum disorders. *Cognition and Emotion, 22*(7), 1353–1380.

Willenbockel, V., Fiset, D., Chauvin, A., Blais, C., Arguin, M., Tanaka, J. W., Bub, D. N., & Gosselin, F. (2010). Does face inversion change spatial frequency tuning? *Journal of Experimental Psychology: Human Perception and Performance, 36*(1), 122.

Witkin, H. A., Lewis, H. B., Hertzman, M., Machover, K., Meissner, P. B., & Wapner, S. (1954). *Personality through perception: An experimental and clinical study.* Harper.

Yovel, G., & Duchaine, B. (2006). Specialized face perception mechanisms extract both part and spacing information: Evidence from developmental prosopagnosia. *Journal of Cognitive Neuroscience, 18*(4), 580–593.

Yu, H., Garrod, O. G., & Schyns, P. G. (2012). Perception-driven facial expression synthesis. *Computers & Graphics, 36*(3), 152–162.

Yuan, H. Y., Chen, J. J., Lee, M. M., Wung, J. C., Chen, Y. F., Charng, M. J., Lu, M. J., Hung, C. R., Wei, C. Y., Chen, C. H., Wu, J. Y., & Chen, Y. T. (2005). A novel functional VKORC1 promoter polymorphism is associated with inter-individual and inter-ethnic differences in warfarin sensitivity. *Human Molecular Genetics, 14*(13), 1745–1751.

Zhou, J., Gotch, C., Zhou, Y., & Liu, Z. (2008). Perceiving an object in its context—Is the context cultural or perceptual? Journal of Vision, 8(12), doi:https://doi.org/10.1167/8.12.2.

The Neuroscience of Cultural Imitative Learning and Connections to Global Mental Health

Morgan Gianola *and* Elizabeth A. Reynolds Losin

Abstract
Cultural learning via imitation is one of the primary means through which cultural behaviors are acquired, transmitted, and built upon over time. This chapters utilizes an interdisciplinary perspective to (a) outline the core cognitive processes of cultural learning as described in the psychological anthropology and social psychology literature, (b) propose an update of the model of the neural systems underlying cultural learning relating to these core cognitive processes, (c) review the nonhuman primate and human literatures supporting each neural system in the model, and (d) discuss mental health disorders that can affect the core cognitive and neural processes involved in cultural learning and their implications for understanding the interactions between cultural learning and mental health.

Key Words: cultural acquisition, cultural plasticity, imitation, theory of mind, reward, mirror system

Introduction: Studying Brain Mechanisms of Cultural Acquisition

The relationship between human culture and the human brain is reciprocal. The structure and function of the brain influence how we acquire our cultural beliefs and practices. At the same time, cultural information affects the way we think and behave, which, over time, can shape the structure and function of the brain (Han, 2015; Losin et al., 2010). The growing field of cultural neuroscience has focused primarily on one direction of this culture–brain relationship: the way in which cultural experience can shape the brain, which we refer to here as *cultural plasticity*. These cultural neuroscience studies typically compare groups of people from different cultural contexts, aiming to characterize neural similarities and differences. The other direction of this culture–brain relationship in which the brain enables the acquisition of cultural beliefs and practices, referred to here as *cultural acquisition,* is an arguably more fundamental process, as cultural acquisition is a necessary prerequisite for the brain to be shaped by cultural content (Losin et al., 2009).

A rich theoretical and empirical literature in psychological anthropology and social psychology has described behavioral and cognitive mechanisms related to cultural acquisition (Henrich & McElreath, 2003; Tomasello, 2016). Methods used in these endeavors include laboratory simulations of cultural transmission in evolutionary psychology (e.g., the transmission chain and closed group methods; Mesoudi & Whiten, 2008), laboratory simulations of observational learning in social psychology (e.g., the work of Alfred Bandura; Bandura & Kupers, 1964; Bandura et al., 1961), observational and experimental studies in wild and captive populations of nonhuman primates (e.g., (Horner et al., 2010; O'Malley et al., 2012), and evidence from ethnographic fieldwork in both small-scale and industrialized societies (e.g., Henrich & Broesch, 2011; Mace & Jordan, 2011). Over the past two decades, a growing body of literature in sociocultural, cognitive, and affective neuroscience has begun to reveal brain mechanisms that may support these behavioral and cognitive accounts of cultural learning (Losin et al., 2009). Brain mechanisms of cultural learning have been investigated with techniques ranging from experimental manipulations of brain function in animal models (e.g., rodents and nonhuman primates; Petrosini, 2007; Rizzolatti & Craighero, 2004; Rizzolatti & Fogassi, 2014) to experimental and observational studies using human neuroimaging (Gazzola, van der Worp, et al., 2007; Likowski et al., 2012). Thus, to fully understand the neural mechanisms of cultural learning, we must use an interdisciplinary approach that integrates biological and social scientific methods.

In this chapter, we will utilize this interdisciplinary perspective to (a) outline the core cognitive processes of cultural learning as described in the psychological anthropology and social psychology literature, (b) propose an update of our model of the neural systems underlying cultural learning relating to these core cognitive processes, (c) review nonhuman primate and human literature supporting each neural system in our model, and (d) discuss mental health disorders that can affect the cognitive and neural processes involved in cultural learning as well as their implications for understanding the interactions between cultural learning and mental health.

What Is Cultural Learning?

Cultural learning constitutes the primary means of cultural acquisition in humans and is defined by Tomasello et al. (1993) as a type of social learning in which perspective taking plays a key role in both the transmission of information and the stored cognitive representation. Cultural learning (unique to humans) can be distinguished from other types of social learning (in humans and animals) in that noncultural forms of social learning occur *because of* or *from* other individuals (e.g., from the results of their actions), as in location or stimulus enhancement (Whiten & van de Waal, 2016). In contrast, humans learn *through* other individuals by taking the other's perspective, gleaning the strategies needed to obtain specific results in particular situations.

According to the theory of cultural learning outlined in Tomasello et al. (1993) and recently updated in Tomasello (2016), cultural learning comprises three types of learning: imitative, instructed, and collaborative. These types of cultural learning emerge at successive developmental stages of perspective taking (theory of mind [ToM]). Humans' sophisticated ToM abilities in turn allow for faithful copying of both the means and intentions of others' actions and innovations, which further allows for their modification and improvement over time. Tomasello (1999) refers to this process of accumulating cultural change over generations as a "ratchet effect," which may set human cultural learning apart from that of other animals.

Core Cognitive Processes of Cultural Learning

Imitation

Imitation is at the core of human cultural learning, as it emerges first during development and continues to play an important role in cultural acquisition throughout life (Legare & Nielsen, 2015; Tomasello, 2016). Therefore, cultural learning via imitation will be the main focus of this chapter. Although the definition of imitation has been debated in the literature due to the high number of closely related mimetic processes (Chalmeau & Gallo, 1993), true imitation has been defined as a form of observational learning in which both the means and goal of an action are faithfully copied. Two other kinds of observational learning that share features with true imitation are mimicry, in which only the means of an action are copied, as seen in human neonates, and emulation, in which a goal is copied using different means (Tomasello, 1990; Whiten & van de Waal, 2016; Zentall, 2006). As well as defining imitation, extensive theoretical and empirical work has addressed the development of imitative behavior and the questions of how, what, and whom we imitate, each of which we will address in turn.

Even as newborns, children are able to imitate adult facial expressions, discriminate various actions (e.g., mouth open from tongue protrusion; Anisfeld et al., 1979; Meltzoff & Moore, 1983, 1992), monitor their own body, and detect equivalent movements in others (Grèzes et al., 1999; Petrosini et al., 2003). While newborns imitate rather indiscriminately to build up their movement repertoire, by 12 (Bellagamba & Tomasello, 1999) or 18 months (Meltzoff, 1995), infants can reproduce the goal of an adult actor's failed attempt without imitating the exact actions, demonstrating a recognition of goals as separate from the behavioral means employed to achieve them (Tomasello, 2016). However, high-fidelity imitative learning remains a primary means of acquiring new behaviors throughout much of childhood. For example, children as young as 3 years old can imitate to complete complex instrumental tasks or novel tool use, while innovation to achieve the same goal does not emerge until age 9 or 10 (Legare & Nielsen, 2015).

There are two opposing theories that describe the neurocognitive mechanisms of imitation: the ideomotor framework and the associative sequence learning model. The ideomotor framework is based on the idea that imitation is enabled by shared neural representations between action perception and action production (Prinz, 2005). In the associative sequence learning model, in contrast, separate neural systems underlie action perception and production and their functions are joined to enable imitation through the process of Hebbian learning (the strengthening of neural connections through repeated coincident firing; Heyes, 2005).

In terms of what we imitate during cultural learning, Legare and Nielsen (2015) have proposed two categories of information: instrumental skills and social conventions. Legare and Nielsen (2015) posit that the high-fidelity transmission of both types of information is necessary for human cumulative culture. Instrumental skills enable the use of specific tools and the awareness of when and why to use them, serving as the "technical toolkit of a cultural group" and providing opportunities for cultural innovation (Legare & Nielsen, 2015). In contrast, cultural conventions such as rituals, customs, and etiquette are group-specific, socially shared actions (Durkheim, 1915; Henrich, 2009; Whitehouse, 2012) that function to promote social cohesion within cultural groups (Fragaszy & Perry, 2003; Legare & Nielsen, 2015). Unlike instrumental skills, cultural conventions rarely present clear causal relationships between the actions performed and the desired outcome, meaning such conventions require high-fidelity copying with less room for innovation (Legare & Herrmann, 2013; Legare & Souza, 2012, 2014; Whitehouse, 2011).

The final question about imitation that we will address is that of who is imitated during cultural learning. Cultural learning theories from psychological anthropology (Henrich & McElreath, 2003) and social learning theories from social psychology (e.g., Alfred Bandura's social learning theory; Bandura, 1977) suggest that we preferentially imitate those who are prestigious, successful, and similar to us. It has been postulated that these model-based cultural learning biases are adaptive mechanisms that serve to increase the efficiency of cultural learning by increasing the chances of learning high-quality (prestige and success biases) and self-relevant (similarity bias) information (Henrich & McElreath, 2003). Therefore, we will discuss model-based learning biases relevant to each of the other cognitive components of cultural learning in the sections that follow.

Theory of Mind

ToM and its engagement, often referred to as mental state attribution or mentalizing, involves the recognition of others as intentional mental agents with mental states that differ from one's own (Saxe et al., 2004). ToM is a key component of cultural learning via imitation that allows imitators to understand the intentions behind the behaviors they are imitating (Tomasello, 2016; Tomasello et al., 1993). The ability to encode not only the means but also the intentions of others' actions during imitative learning enables the learner to modify learned behaviors with the model's original intent in mind. The iterative process of imitation with innovation allows for the progression of cultural change characteristic of human culture (i.e., Tomasello's "ratchet effect").

The first stage of ToM emerges around 9 to 12 months, when infants begin to show joint attention (triadic interactions) as they focus on the person or object to which an adult directs their attention. This engagement in joint attention shows the implicit recognition that, unlike objects, other people have feelings and intentions, allowing children to learn how others' minds respond to environmental events (Carpenter et al., 1998). By age 4, children can recognize a model's intent to teach, showing awareness that others have mental states that differ from their own. Recognition of others' didactic intentions facilitates the transmission and application of cultural knowledge and tendencies through explicit instruction. Finally, at 5 years, about 90% of children (and all children by age 6) are able to correctly predict how a false belief held by another person will affect their behavior (Frith & Frith, 2003). This developmental milestone shows cross-cultural consistency and instantiates the ability to think about another person as they reflect on the mental states of a third person outside of the direct social interaction (Avis & Harris, 1991). Thus, by 5 to 6 years old, children show explicit understanding of others' mental states and intentions and recognize when culturally relevant information is being transmitted, enabling increasingly sophisticated cultural learning.

Reward

The final core cognitive component of cultural learning discussed in this review is the reinforcement learning supported by the reward system. Rewards may play a special role in cultural learning, as it has been argued that cultural learning is intrinsically rewarding (Tomasello et al., 1993). Research into reward processing has suggested that rewards function to (a) induce learning, (b) promote approach behavior for the reward itself, and (c) increase positive feelings associated with the reward and rewarded behavior (Schultz, 2006). Rewards used to reinforce learned behaviors can be primary (unlearned and culturally invariant), including food and positive sensory experiences (Schultz, 2000), or secondary reinforcers (conditioned and culturally specific), such as money or desirable items (Basten et al., 2010; Prévost et al., 2010).

Vital for cultural learning, social stimuli, such as smiling or good reputation, can also serve as potent primary reinforcers (Izuma et al., 2008). During cultural learning, social rewards (e.g., conformity, group inclusion) can be a key factor driving children to imitate others. Children will emulate the goals of cultural actors, even though these goals are frequently causally opaque. Furthermore, Tomasello et al. (2005) suggest that the inherent social context of human cultural learning is itself a primary reinforcer with intrinsic reward value, a trend not seen in other primates. Social rewards such as collaborative environments can lead children to work harder and longer on tasks (Butler & Walton, 2013) and enforce conformity of normative conventions onto ingroup members (Schmidt et al., 2011). These and similar primary social rewards serve to develop positive associations with learned behaviors, promoting their imitative reproduction in the process of cultural learning.

A Neural Model of Cultural Learning in Humans

Based on the core cognitive capacities involved in cultural learning (imitation, ToM, and reinforcement learning), we have previously proposed a tentative neural model of cultural learning involving brain systems associated with these key functions (Losin et al., 2009). This model includes the human mirror system subserving imitation and intention understanding based on physical cues; the ToM network subserving mentalizing and intention understanding from an inferential perspective; and the reward system, which allows for flexible reinforcement of learned behaviors. The model also includes the roles of each of these systems in model-based learning biases as these biases engage all of the other core cognitive capacities involved in cultural learning.

Over the intervening decade since we first proposed this model (Losin et al., 2009), both our work and that of others in social, cognitive, and affective neuroscience have provided increasing support for the participation of these neural systems in sociocultural learning (Cross et al., 2013; Likowski et al., 2012; Losin et al., 2013, 2015; Losin, Iacoboni, Martin, & Dapretto, 2012; Sirigu & Duhamel, 2016; Spunt & Adolphs, 2014; Yang et al., 2015; Zhang et al., 2016). Furthermore, these findings have allowed us to refine our neural model (see Figure 17.1) and discuss the specific role(s) the different regions within each system may play in cultural learning. In the sections that follow we first describe basic cellular mechanisms of cultural learning. We then outline the literature describing the functions of the mirror system, ToM network, and reward system in

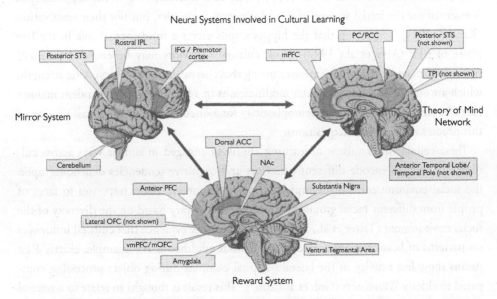

Figure 17.1. Neural model of cultural learning, with systems involved in imitation, mentalizing, and reinforcement learning. ACC: anterior cingulate cortex, IFG: inferior frontal gyrus, IPL: inferior parietal lobule, mPFC: medial prefrontal cortex, NAc: nucleus accumbens, OFC: orbitofrontal cortex, PC/PCC: precuneus/posterior cingulate cortex, PFC; prefrontal cortex, STS: superior temporal sulcus, TPJ: temporoparietal junction, vmPFC/mOFC: ventromedial prefrontal cortex/medial orbitofrontal cortex.

various aspects of human cultural learning as well as these systems' roles in social learning among nonhuman primates.

Cellular and Molecular Mechanisms of Cultural Learning

Empirical studies specifically directed at the cellular and molecular mechanisms of cultural learning through imitation have yet to be conducted. However, the same processes governing learning and memory more broadly are likely conserved for the encoding of cultural information (Chiao, 2018). The genetic processes underlying cultural learning are beyond the scope of this chapter (see Chapter 7 for a discussion of cultural genomics). At the neural level, culturally adaptive behaviors are learned and integrated into the neural landscape through processes of "Hebbian learning," that is, correlated activations between neurons that lead to long-term structural and functional synaptic modifications (Bi & Poo, 2001; Hebb, 1949). The precise timing of this correlated activity plays a major role in determining whether a synapse experiences long-term potentiation (LTP) or long-term depression (LTD)—long-lasting activity-dependent increases or decreases in synaptic strength, respectively (Levy & Steward, 1983; Malenka & Nicoll, 1999). The early stages of LTP, involved in short-term memory, result in local activation of enzymes, alterations of synaptic proteins, and strengthening of synaptic connections; conversely, the late phase of LTP, associated with long-term memory, requires changes in gene expression, new protein synthesis, and the formation of new synaptic connections throughout the excited neurons (Kandel, 2001; Milner et al., 1998; Teyler & DiScenna, 1987). The hippocampus is essential for the initial storage of these long-term memories, but not their reactivation (Kandel, 2001), suggesting that the hippocampus serves a fundamental role in the late phase of LTP (Abel et al., 1997). Thus, cultural behaviors may be encoded (learned) through associative neural activations causing short-term alterations in synaptic strength, which are engrained via intracellular modifications in a hippocampus-dependent manner (see Chapter 21 on culture and neuroplasticity for a discussion of the direct association of this process with cultural acquisition).

These cellular mechanisms of learning are likely engaged in similar ways across cultures but used to encode different behaviors and cognitive tendencies depending upon the social environment. For example, during development, brain responses to faces of people from different racial groups have been found to vary based on the diversity of the social environment (Telzer et al., 2013). There is further evidence that cultural influences on patterns of brain responses extend throughout adulthood. For example, elderly East Asians show less activity in the lateral occipital complex during object processing compared to elderly Westerners (Goh et al., 2007). This result is thought to relate to a general cultural pattern of holistic thinking among East Asians, in contrast to more analytic (e.g., object-focused) thinking among Westerners (Chiao, 2018). These brief examples illustrate how the cellular mechanisms of learning can produce divergent neural responses based on the cultural environment one experiences over the lifetime (see Chapter 19 for a discussion of cultural developmental neuroscience).

The Mirror System and Cultural Imitative Learning

In this section, we first discuss the initial discovery of mirror neurons in nonhuman primates, their associated neural structures, and their role in primate social learning. We go on to describe the putative human homologs of this mirror system and the cultural learning functions they support, promoting the inclusion of the mirror system in our neural model of cultural learning.

The Mirror Neuron System in Nonhuman Primate Social Learning

Neurons in the premotor cortex, which activate during both the execution of specific motor acts and the observation of the same acts performed by another, were first observed in the macaque monkey (Gallese et al., 1996). Subsequent neurophysiological studies in macaques have described these "mirror neurons" in the interconnected inferior parietal lobule (abbreviated PF in macaques) and ventral premotor (F5) cortex (Petrosini, 2007; Rizzolatti & Craighero, 2004; Rizzolatti & Fogassi, 2014). Also connected with the PF is the superior temporal sulcus (STS), which contains visual neurons responsive to body movements (Perrett et al., 1990). The ability of these frontal, parietal, and temporal regions, collectively termed the mirror neuron system (MNS), to link perception and action has led to the proposal that they may make up a "core circuit of imitation" (Iacoboni, 2005), wherein the STS provides a high-level visual account of observed actions, the PF encodes their motor aspects, and frontal activity relays the goal of the actions to be imitated (Iacoboni & Dapretto, 2006).

Neurophysiological studies in nonhuman primates also suggest that the functional properties of the MNS enable the second critical component of cultural learning, intention understanding, by encoding others' actions in the frame of one's own motor system (Whiten & van de Waal, 2016). Intention understanding via the MNS is also facilitated by the response properties of mirror neurons themselves. Some mirror neurons, termed "broadly congruent", discharge any time the goals of observed and executed motor acts are similar (e.g., observing hand grasp to eat and executing foot grasp to eat), whereas other "strictly congruent" mirror neurons only fire when the goal *and* method of observed and performed motor acts are identical (e.g., same goal and effector; Fabbri-Destro & Rizzolatti, 2008). Broadly and strictly congruent mirror neurons have been observed in the parietal component of the MNS (Cattaneo et al., 2007). This means and goal sensitivity of certain mirror neurons may facilitate high-fidelity copying in nonhuman primate social learning, as exemplified by the transmission of techniques to open food canisters with specific body parts among vervet monkey social groups (van de Waal & Whiten, 2012). In humans, these mirror neuron properties likely enable the true imitation required for human cultural learning, particularly in the acquisition of cultural conventions, when the causal relationship between actions and outcomes is unclear (Legare & Nielsen, 2015).

These functional characterizations of mirror neurons and the regions containing them in nonhuman primates demonstrate the ability of the MNS to link observed and performed actions and respond selectively to the goals of those actions. This literature provides support for the inclusion of the MNS as a central component of our neural model of cultural learning.

The Human Mirror System in Cultural Imitative Learning

Human neuroimaging studies have suggested that a homologous system to the macaque MNS exists in humans. The inferior frontal gyrus (IFG) pars opercularis (homolog of macaque F5) and inferior parietal lobule (IPL, homolog of macaque PF), thought to constitute the core frontoparietal components of the human mirror system, are active during both perception and performance of basic actions, just as in macaques (Kilner et al., 2009; Oosterhof et al., 2010). Importantly, the human mirror system is also thought to support more sophisticated social activities, including true imitation (Iacoboni et al., 1999), intention understanding (Iacoboni et al., 2005), and self-representation (Uddin et al., 2005), making the mirror system a core component of cultural learning via imitation. For example, in humans, complex imitative tasks consistently activate premotor and parietal cortices, as shown via meta-analysis, though activation of the inferior frontal cortex during imitation is less consistent (Molenberghs et al., 2009). During action observation, humans also show more even distribution of activity across prefrontal, inferior parietal, and inferotemporal areas than do chimpanzees, in whom activity is more biased toward frontal regions including the ventrolateral prefrontal cortex (PFC), as demonstrated via functional magnetic resonance imaging (fMRI; Hecht et al., 2013). This greater cortical integration during action observation in humans may promote the implicit (rather than goal-directed) translation of others' behaviors into a personal reference frame (Hecht et al., 2013), facilitating cultural learning.

Although a substantial body of evidence has provided support for the existence of a human mirror system (e.g., Likowski et al., 2012; Ocampo et al., 2011; Oosterhof et al., 2010), there is some controversy surrounding the degree to which the human mirror system is truly analogous to that of macaques as well as what functions it serves (Jeon & Lee, 2018). However, the alternative explanations of human mirror system function do not detract from the proposed role of this system in cultural learning and in some cases even add further support for it. One controversy surrounding human mirror system function has arisen due to the engagement of mirror system regions during complementary acts and other nonmirroring behaviors (Newman-Norlund et al., 2007). These findings have led some critics to hypothesize that purported human "mirror neuron" activity actually represents contributions from separable sensory and motor neural populations (Heyes, 2014), as described in the associative sequence learning model (Heyes, 2005).

Another related controversy stems from the reliance on neuroimaging (e.g., fMRI) to describe the mirror system, a technique that cannot measure the behavior of single neurons. However, one single-cell recording study in humans has revealed neurons showing mirror properties in response to hand and facial actions within the supplementary motor area (SMA) as well as in and near the hippocampus (Mukamel et al., 2010). Notably, such studies are not able to test for mirror neuron activity within the core mirror system areas (e.g., IFG, IPL), as these regions are not typically where electrodes are placed for the detection of seizure foci, the medical procedure permitting such single-neuron recordings in humans (Mukamel et al., 2010). However, regardless of whether responses of human mirror system regions stem from a single or multiple populations of neurons encoding perception and action, the engagement of mirror system regions during complementary actions only increases the utility of this system in supporting social and cultural learning, in which complementary actions and copying with innovation play a central role (Legare & Nielsen, 2015).

A number of other brain regions interact with the core frontoparietal mirror system to support imitative learning and cultural acquisition (see Figure 17.2). For example, the observation of imitable actions has been found to engage the bilateral dorsal visual stream, premotor cortex, and right cerebellum, while further activity in the SMA and orbitofrontal cortex distinguishes whether or not these actions are meaningful (Grèzes, 1998). Parallel lesion and virtual lesion (repeated transcranial magnetic stimulation [rTMS]) studies of imitative learning in rats and humans, respectively, have further elucidated the roles of the cerebellum and PFC in imitative learning (Petrosini, 2007). Petrosini (2007) found that cerebellar lesions in rats and rTMS in humans before observational training

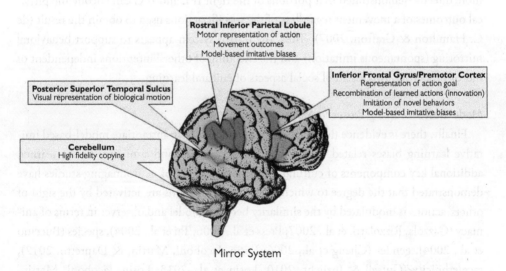

Figure 17.2. Neural structures contributing to the behavioral mirroring components of imitative learning and their proposed roles during cultural learning.

on a Morris water maze or pattern drawing task, respectively, impair imitative learning. In contrast, prefrontal rTMS in humans before observational training interfered with both drawing newly trained patterns and drawing different patterns observed before rTMS. These findings suggest that the cerebellum may encode actions to be imitated during observation, whereas the dorsolateral PFC may contribute to assembling the components of observed actions into new arrangements (innovation). These neural regions that complement mirror system activity may thus serve roles in the high-fidelity reproduction of cultural behaviors (cerebellum) and the innovative ratchet effect of cultural evolution (dorsolateral PFC).

As in nonhuman primates, the human literature offers evidence that the mirror system plays an important role in the social aspects of imitation and mirroring, providing further support for this system as a core neural substrate of cultural learning. For example, there is evidence that the mirror system contributes to the spontaneous behavioral mirroring often seen in naturalistic social interactions (Likowski et al., 2012) as well as the instructed imitation typically performed in neuroimaging studies (Lieberman, 2007). Importantly, implicit mimicry and imitation are likely more representative of real-world cultural learning scenarios compared to instructed, explicit imitation. This spontaneous mirroring may promote cultural learning by integrating the intentions of imitated acts, inferred from their visual properties (typically supported by the mirror system), with inferences about the model's intentions, gained by directly reflecting on them (typically supported by the ToM network; de Lange et al., 2008). Additional evidence of mirroring models' intentions rather than the visual properties of their actions comes from the observation of mirror system activity in aplasics (patients without arms or hands) in response to viewing hand movements (Gazzola, van der Worp, et al., 2007). Other studies have also more directly demonstrated that portions of the right IPL and IFG can encode the physical outcomes of a movement regardless of the specific actions used to obtain the result (de C. Hamilton & Grafton, 2007). Thus, the mirror system appears to support behavioral mirroring (spontaneous imitation) and the encoding of others' intentions independent of motor properties, two essential social aspects of cultural learning.

Model-Based Learning Biases in Mirror System Activity

Finally, there is evidence that the mirror system may help instantiate model-based imitative learning biases related to the model's social status and similarity to the learner, additional key components of cultural learning. A number of neuroimaging studies have demonstrated that the degree to which mirror system regions are activated by the sight of others' actions is modulated by the similarity between model and observer in terms of animacy (Gazzola, Rizzolatti, et al., 2007; Press et al., 2006; Tai et al., 2004), species (Buccino et al., 2004), gender (Cheng et al., 2006; Losin, Iacoboni, Martin, & Dapretto, 2012), race/ethnicity (Gutsell & Inzlicht, 2010; Losin et al., 2013; Losin, Iacoboni, Martin, Cross, & Dapretto, 2012; Molnar-Szakacs et al., 2007), and even culturally created social groups (Molenberghs et al., 2013). For example, in a study using assigned social groups (a minimal group paradigm), participants who showed greater ingroup bias exhibited increased IPL activity when observing the actions of ingroup relative to outgroup members (Molenberghs et al., 2013). Similar results emerge among demographic groups, as Gutsell and Inzlicht (2010) found that Caucasian participants expressed greater electroencephalogram (EEG) mu suppression (interpreted as greater mirroring) when viewing ingroup (Caucasian) compared to outgroup (African Canadian, East Asian, and South Asian) individuals performing various actions.

Interestingly, although the mirror system seems to encode models' characteristics during imitation (in addition to action observation), there is evidence that the direction of this effect may be reversed. For example, we previously found more activity in the IFG and IPL when White participants imitated the actions of White compared to African American models (Losin, Iacoboni, Martin, Cross, & Dapretto, 2012). However, in a subsequent study, African American participants exhibited the same pattern of activity as White participants, with heightened activity in mirror system regions paralleling participants' ratings of the social status they associated with each ethnic/racial group rather than the similarity they felt toward the models (Losin et al., 2013). Thus, the mirror system may be more active when observing those whom one is more likely to imitate in daily life (e.g., those who are self-similar), perhaps due to increased attention to these individuals, but also more active during imitation of those whom one is less likely to imitate in daily life (e.g., those one perceives as lower in social status), possibly due to the increased difficulty of doing so (Losin et al., 2013). Together, these findings demonstrate that in addition to matching action perception and performance and encoding an action's intentions, the mirror system also carries information about the imitated model, potentially underlying the model-based imitative biases that shape cultural learning.

The Theory of Mind Network in Cultural Imitative Learning

In this section we begin with a treatment of precursors to ToM in nonhuman species, noting similarities to certain human capacities. We then discuss the more sophisticated expression of ToM in humans, highlighting the neural structures associated with ToM and their relationship to imitative acquisition of cultural behaviors as support for this network's inclusion in our neural model.

Self-Awareness and Theory of Mind in Nonhuman Animals

While ToM is a primary hallmark of human sociality, it has been argued to be a byproduct of more basic social cognitive abilities like self-awareness (Gallup, 1982), which may represent precursors to human ToM (Gallese & Goldman, 1998; Keenan et al., 2000). These ToM precursors have been investigated in various social species, particularly higher primates. To characterize self-recognition abilities in animals, several research groups have relied on the mirror test, in which an animal is exposed to a mirror in its home environment before being covertly marked on a part of its body that is only visible in the mirror; reflection-guided, mark-directed touching then serves as an indication of self-recognition. Given prior mirror exposure, chimpanzees (Gallup, 1970; Povinelli et al., 1997) and orangutans (Suárez & Gallup, 1981) will touch this covert mark on their face after noticing it in their reflection, whereas few gorillas (Suárez & Gallup, 1981) and no monkeys demonstrate such behavior (Suarez & Gallup, 1986). Other social species including dolphins (Reiss & Marino, 2001), elephants (Plotnik et al., 2006), and magpies (Prior et al., 2008) also pass this test. This recognition of oneself as distinct from other social actors indicates a form of self-awareness and appears necessary for the ability to model one's own mental state (Gallup, 1970).

Another precursor to ToM that has been investigated in nonhuman primates is a basic ability to recognize the intentions of others. A potential neural correlate of intention recognition has been identified in macaques using single-cell recordings. Jellema et al. (2000) identified a subset of cells in macaque STS that are responsive to viewing others' limb movements and modulated by their focus of attention, which the authors suggest may underlie the detection of intentional behaviors.

The social intelligence hypothesis proposes a connection between ToM precursors, like self-recognition and intention recognition, and the cultural sophistication seen in humans (Humphrey, 1976; Whiten & van de Waal, 2016). Specifically, this hypothesis posits that expanding social networks were a catalyst for the evolutionarily recent enlargement of primate brains, which then facilitated social learning and the subsequent acceleration of cultural transmission in early hominids (Humphrey, 1976; Whiten & van de Waal, 2016).

The Human Theory of Mind Network in Cultural Learning

Imitative learning and modification of cultural behaviors in humans are made possible by humans' ability to understand the mental states of those being imitated (i.e., ToM; Braadbaart et al., 2014; Brass et al., 2009; Saxe & Wexler, 2005; Wang & Hamilton, 2012). Several neural regions are thought to underlie human ToM abilities and to interact with networks related to imitation and intention understanding during social learning. For these reasons the ToM network is the second major component of our neural model of cultural learning.

The neural systems involved in ToM have been studied primarily using neuroimaging during a variety of behavioral tasks thought to employ mentalizing. ToM tasks include those which require the understanding of false beliefs (e.g., the Sally-Anne Test; Baron-Cohen et al., 1985) or others' emotions (e.g., the "Reading the Mind in the Eyes" task; Baron-Cohen et al., 2001), and tasks in which inanimate objects behave in an animate fashion, such as the Heider and Simmel animation (Heider & Simmel, 1944). A recent meta-analysis of studies using these different ToM tasks has revealed a network of brain regions including the medial prefrontal cortex (mPFC), precuneus/posterior cingulate (PC/PCC), anterior temporal lobe/temporal pole, temporoparietal junction (TPJ), and posterior STS that are active across these tasks (Yang et al., 2015). Although only a subset of these brain regions are typically active during a given ToM task, a more recently developed task, requiring participants to think about how or why observed actions were performed, has been found to engage all of these ToM-associated brain regions simultaneously (Spunt & Adolphs, 2014), reinforcing the notion of a coherent ToM network (see Figure 17.3). In a separate literature using functional connectivity analyses to understand brain mechanisms during rest, a similar network of brain regions, termed the default mode network (DMN), has been identified (see Raichle, 2015, for a review). One explanation for the similarity of the ToM network and DMN is that they represent the same or overlapping systems, as during rest, humans are thought to reflect on personal and general information about the mental states of self and others by default (Greicius et al., 2003).

The developmental stages of ToM, described earlier, from individual perspective taking to instructed learning to mutual collaboration (Tomasello, 2016; Tomasello et al., 1993), suggest that ToM and its associated neural network may be composed of two distinct components (Saxe et al., 2004). These ToM components emerge in successive stages of development and may contribute to unique aspects of cultural learning via imitation. The early developing ToM system is thought to be used for reasoning about others' goals, beliefs, and emotions. For example, early recognition of biological motion and the intentionality of movements is associated with the posterior STS (Allison et al., 2000; Jellema et al., 2000). Also part of the early developing system, the mPFC has been implicated in the inhibition of imitative responses, which may be related to the perception of whether a model's goals are compatible with one's own (Brass et al., 2005, 2009; Cross et al., 2013).

The later-developing ToM system is thought to be involved in representing the content of others' beliefs. This system may help the cultural learner innovate based on a detailed understanding of the model's original beliefs and intentions related to a given action

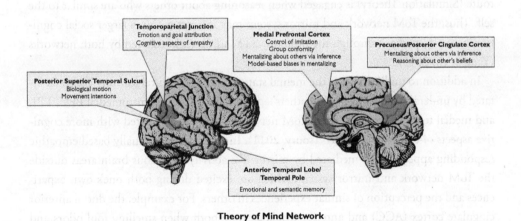

Figure 17.3. Brain regions involved in theory of mind and mentalizing processes and their proposed roles during cultural learning.

or object. For example, activity in the dorsomedial PFC, which continues to develop throughout adolescence (Blakemore, 2012), is implicated in overt thinking about others' mental states (Frith & Frith, 2003). Similarly, the right TPJ, also showing functional alterations throughout the teenage years (Güroğlu et al., 2011), is involved in attributing emotions or goals to others to explain or predict their actions (Saxe & Wexler, 2005). Reasoning about another's mental state further requires inhibiting one's own experiences to take the other's perspective, a process engaging the ventrolateral PFC (Samson et al., 2005; Vogeley et al., 2001). The late development of these prefrontal areas involved in the more complex aspects of ToM helps to explain young children's tendency to overimitate (i.e., copy irrelevant parts of an observed act) during cultural learning (Horner & Whiten, 2005; Lyons et al., 2007).

Importantly for our neural model of cultural learning, both behavioral (Apperly, 2008) and neural accounts (de Lange et al., 2008; Van Overwalle & Baetens, 2009) of ToM suggest that the ToM network and the mirror system interact. Within the behavioral literature, two theories have been proposed to explain the cognitive mechanisms underlying ToM: Theory Theory and Simulation Theory (see Apperly, 2008, for a review). Theory Theory suggests that a set of folk psychological rules are used to relate external states and behaviors to internal beliefs and desires. This inferential route to ToM is thought to engage the ToM network. In contrast, Simulation Theory posits that others' mental states are understood directly using the same mental mechanisms as if one were experiencing the state themselves. The simulation route to intention understanding is thought to rely on the mirror system and related neural structures. While these theories were originally considered mutually exclusive, several hybrid accounts of ToM have since been proposed (e.g., Asakura & İnui, 2016; Carruthers & Smith, 1996; Nichols & Stich, 2003), suggesting that an inferential route (Theory Theory) to intention understanding may be engaged when reasoning about others perceived to be dissimilar to the self, whereas a simulation route (Simulation Theory) is engaged when reasoning about others who are similar to the self. Thus, the ToM network and mirror system may interact within a larger social cognition network, perhaps through the posterior STS, a hub region shared by both networks (Yang et al., 2015).

In addition to understanding the mental states of others, cultural learning is also facilitated by understanding and sharing others' emotional states. The ventromedial PFC, TPJ, and medial temporal regions in the ToM network have been associated with more cognitive aspects of empathy (Shamay-Tsoory, 2011). In contrast, perceptually based empathic responding appears to be mediated by mirror-like activity in various brain areas outside the ToM network and mirror system, which are excited during both one's own experiences and the perception of similar experiences in others. For example, the dorsal anterior cingulate cortex (ACC) and anterior insula activate both when smelling foul odors and watching others smell the same odors (Wicker et al., 2003), as well as when experiencing pain and viewing another in pain (Botvinick et al., 2005; Jackson et al., 2005; Lamm et al., 2011; Lloyd et al., 2004; Singer et al., 2004); the strength of this other-driven activity correlates with self-reported empathy (Singer et al., 2004). Furthermore, a measure of empathic capacity, the empathy quotient, has been found to correlate with activity in the PFC and predict accuracy during imitation of facial expressions (Braadbaart et al., 2014). Taken together, these findings suggest that empathic neural responding may facilitate mentalizing during imitative behaviors via the dorsal ACC and anterior insula, similar to the mirroring and cognitive ToM processes that rely on lateral and medial frontoparietal structures.

Model-Based Learning Biases in the Theory of Mind Network

There is evidence that the ToM network and brain regions involved in empathy may help instantiate model-based cultural learning biases. For example, a number of studies have found that the mPFC, which has been associated with mentalizing about the self, is also engaged when mentalizing about self-similar others (Mitchell et al., 2005, 2006; Zhu et al., 2007), and that the amount of mPFC activation increases as perceived self-similarity of the target increases (Mitchell et al., 2005). We previously conducted a study specifically focused on measuring the effects of the nonperceptual aspects of self-similarity (i.e., political ideology) on imitative learning and its neural correlates (Losin et al., 2015). We found that participants were more accurate when imitating models who shared their political ideology and that this effect was mediated by brain regions associated with imitation and its control (precentral and inferior frontal gyri), as well as mentalizing (dorsomedial PFC). These brain regions were more active when participants imitated those who did not share their political views, a condition showing lower accuracy (Losin et al., 2015). These findings provide support for the idea that increased dorsomedial PFC activity during imitation of those perceived to be different from the self stems from the increased difficulty of imitating dissimilar others. Furthermore, these results are in line with the predictions of simulation theory and cultural learning biases to learn from those who are self-similar.

The perceptual perspective taking associated with empathy and accompanying activity within the ACC and anterior insula also appears to vary based on perceived self-similarity of the target. Heightened empathic responses and heightened ACC and anterior insula activity when empathizing with ingroup compared to outgroup members is a broad phenomenon observed for gender, race, political affiliation, and artificial group assignments (see Molenberghs, 2013, for a review). In one representative study, both Chinese and Caucasian participants showed greater empathy-related ACC activations when viewing ingroup members experiencing pain compared to seeing pain in outgroup members (Xu et al., 2009). Together, findings of studies on self-similarity biases in mentalizing, empathy, and their associated neural components support a potential role for the ToM network in instantiating model-based biases during the intention understanding associated with cultural learning.

Reinforcement and the Reward System in Cultural Imitative Learning

This section begins with a treatment of the circuitry of reward learning in nonhuman primates with a focus on the role of reinforcement in the expression of nonhuman primate emulation. The subsequent section goes on to describe the brain areas contributing to reward learning in humans and their activity within social and imitative contexts, which is a key component of our neural model.

Reinforcement Learning in Nonhuman Primates

The neural structures of reinforcement learning have been characterized through numerous cellular recording studies in nonhuman primates. These reward-related structures include subcortical dopaminergic nuclei (i.e., striatum, substantia nigra, amygdala, internal globus pallidus, ventral tegmental area) and prefrontal cortical structures such as the ACC, orbitofrontal cortex (OFC), and ventromedial prefrontal cortex (vmPFC; Sirigu & Duhamel, 2016). Single-cell recording approaches have been used to further clarify the specific reward-related functions coordinated by these various brain regions. For example, striatal neurons in nonhuman primates have been found to respond to both the anticipation and delivery of food rewards (Schultz, 2000). A portion of the ventral striatum, the nucleus accumbens (NAc), also encodes information about reward availability, value, and context, and is critical for the acquisition of Pavlovian stimulus–reward associations (see Day & Carelli, 2007, for a review). Comparable neural recording investigations have highlighted that, broadly speaking, activity within the ACC reflects the value of both potential and received rewards and monitors alterations in behavioral decisions (e.g., changes in target selection; Hayden et al., 2009). The dorsal ACC has been specifically associated with social aspects of reward tracking and decision making (e.g., choosing to share or hoard rewards; Reardon, 2014). Similarly, the amygdala and hypothalamus have been implicated in "liking" of specific food rewards, and the OFC has been linked to associative learning of changes in the reward significance of predictive cues (Rolls, 2000). Additionally, with extensive descending projections to the NAc (Zahm, 2000), the OFC may further serve to regulate subcortical positive affective responses (Berridge, 2003). Together, these core neural components of reward processing enable the types of reinforcement learning characteristic of nonhuman primates.

While the neural recording literature has typically relied on primary (i.e., food) rewards to investigate reinforcement learning, the social aspects of reinforcement learning most likely to be tied to social and cultural learning in humans have primarily been described through observational studies. Such studies have shown that social emulative learning in nonhuman primates is influenced both by the physical rewards linked to the observed behavior and by the social relationship between the observer and the model. As an example of the former, free-ranging capuchins will selectively attend to the most proficient nut-cracking adult models (Ottoni et al., 2005), showing that the potential for a food reward produces more sustained social attention (Whiten & van de Waal, 2016). However, in chimpanzees the strength of this attention is seen to vary by gender, with juvenile females spending more time watching their mothers use stem tools to extract food from termite mounds, enabling them to master this skill a full year before their male counterparts (Lonsdorf et al., 2004). Juvenile female chimpanzees also show closer matching of their tool use to that of their mothers' (e.g., length of stem, depth of probing), demonstrating that the social relation of the observer and model can refine subsequent emulative behaviors. This bias to initially learn from one's mother is also observed in vervet monkeys, implying that, beyond physical rewards, social motivations to behave like the models with which a primate feels closest can guide attention and shape emulative responses (van de Waal et al., 2013). These findings suggest that emulative social learning is sensitive to both the rewards inherent in learned behaviors and the relationship between the model and observer, representing potential precursors to human model-based learning biases.

The Human Reward System in Cultural Imitative Learning

Human reward processing has been shown to recruit a core cortical-basal ganglia circuit comprising many regions analogous to those involved in reward learning in nonhuman primates, including the ventral striatum (Hein et al., 2010), ACC, OFC, midbrain dopamine neurons (e.g., substantia nigra, ventral tegmental area), and ventral pallidum (Haber & Knutson, 2010). This core network is regulated in turn by a number of extensive prefrontal and subcortical structures (see Figure 17.4), which neuroimaging research increasingly finds to relate to those regions highlighted by nonhuman primate cellular recording approaches and neuroanatomical studies (see Haber & Knutson, 2010, for a review). While the NAc and other basal ganglia structures receiving convergent input from prefrontal, insular, and cingulate cortices make up a major part of this reward system (Haber & Knutson, 2010), much of the human imaging research has centered on cortical

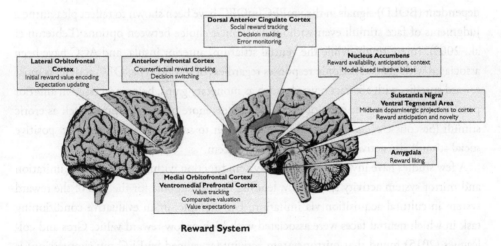

Figure 17.4. Neural structures implicated in reward processing and reinforcement learning and their proposed roles during cultural learning.

responses during reward processing. Our present discussion will therefore focus on a few key prefrontal and cortical components of the reward system that are thought to regulate lower-order structures (Berridge, 2003; Haber & Knutson, 2010) in a process that may aid the imitative acquisition of cultural behaviors.

In humans, the major cortical components of reward-guided learning and decision making include the lateral OFC, vmPFC and adjacent medial OFC (mOFC), ACC, and anterior PFC (Rushworth et al., 2011). Among these regions, the vmPFC/mOFC appear to track comparative reward value during decision making and reinforcement (Basten et al., 2010; Kable & Glimcher, 2007; Prévost et al., 2010; Sescousse et al., 2010; Tanaka et al., 2004; Tom et al., 2007), signaling both aversive and rewarding value expectations (Plassmann et al., 2010; Tom et al., 2007). In broad terms, the lateral OFC encodes the initial reward value of a single option and the positive or negative outcomes of behavioral decisions (O'Doherty et al., 2001; Walton et al., 2010). Anterior PFC activity has been found to reflect the reward value of unchosen choices, being predictive of the decision to switch between different rewarded behaviors (Boorman et al., 2009). Finally, the ACC appears to serve a role in both value encoding and error monitoring (Quilodran et al., 2008). Together, the reward processing within these regions promotes cultural learning by allowing humans to compare the subjective value of potential behaviors, select actions with the greatest associated reward, and alter such decisions in response to reinforcement feedback.

While many human imaging experiments utilize monetary reinforcers (Basten et al., 2010; Prévost et al., 2010; Tom et al., 2007) to study reward processing, positive social cues also recruit activity within this reward system, providing further evidence for its significance in cultural learning. For example, Izuma and colleagues (2008) found that the acquisition of good reputation activated many of the same brain regions responsive to obtaining monetary rewards, including the striatum. Similarly, blood oxygen level–dependent (BOLD) signals in the vmPFC/mOFC have been shown to reflect pleasantness judgments of face stimuli even without an explicit choice between options (Lebreton et al., 2009). Interestingly, while the ventral striatum, anterior insula, and ACC have been associated with general hedonic responses regardless of reward type, OFC activity is more reward specific, with abstract rewards, such as monetary gains, being processed in anterior portions, while posterior parts of the OFC process more primary rewards, such as erotic stimuli (Sescousse et al., 2010). Thus, in addition to secondary reinforcement, positive social stimuli also activate the human reward system.

A few studies have investigated reward system function within the context of imitation and mirror system activity specifically, lending further support for the role of the reward system in cultural acquisition via imitation. For example, in an evaluative conditioning task in which neutral faces were associated with high or low reward value, Gros and colleagues (2015) found that mirror system activity (as gauged by EEG mu suppression) is modulated by the reward value of social stimuli. In terms of imitation, Zhang et al. (2016)

found that the error detection functions of the ACC may serve to track imitative accuracy to make real-time corrections. Specifically, activity in the ACC and posterior cingulate was shown to increase during performance feedback while performing imitative finger gestures (Zhang et al., 2016). Reward processing also plays a role for the person being imitated, as recognition of being imitated as compared to not being imitated produces more positive affect and greater activity in the mOFC/vmPFC (Kühn et al., 2010). During periods of imitative recognition, these prefrontal structures also showed greater effective connectivity with the striatum and midposterior insula (Kühn et al., 2010), potentially corroborating the mOFC/vmPFC's function as regulators of downstream hedonic centers. Taken together, the reward system's role in reinforcement learning in general and social learning and imitation in particular provide support for the inclusion of the reward system as a key component in our neural model of cultural learning.

Model-Based Biases in Reinforcement of Imitative Behaviors

As with the mirror system and ToM network, there is some theoretical and empirical evidence that the reward system may play a role in instantiating model-based imitative learning biases during cultural learning. Foremost in terms of theoretical work is the social learning theory of Alfred Bandura; this theory was informed by studies in which participants who were told they shared some qualities (e.g., background, preferences, personality) with a model were more inclined to imitate new responses of that model as compared to participants told they shared no common characteristics with the model (see Bandura, 1969, for a review). These and other findings suggested to Bandura that people may assume that those with features similar to one's own also experience similar outcomes ("reinforcement contingencies") when performing specific behaviors, thus promoting biases to imitate people one views as similar to oneself (1969). Building on this theory, Bussey and Perry (1976) showed that young children are more accurate in imitating models who they believe are subject to the same reinforcement contingencies as them (i.e., the child and model will be rewarded for the same behavior). The authors concluded that this belief in shared reward outcomes serves to mediate the relationship between perceived similarity and imitative accuracy described in other studies (Bussey & Perry, 1976). In this way, theoretical accounts have sought to characterize how reward learning contributes to similarity biases in imitation.

In more recent years, observations of such similarity biases have been extended to the neural responses of the reward system as well. In one study, participants exhibited increased feelings of similarity and ventral striatum activity when viewing models who behave in a socially desirable manner win a monetary reward, as compared to models expressing undesirable behaviors (Mobbs et al., 2009). Furthermore, when contrasting trials in which the model being rewarded was socially desirable compared to undesirable, feelings of similarity were shown to correlate with activity in the vmPFC and ventral ACC as well as with connectivity between the ventral striatum and ventral ACC (Mobbs et al., 2009). Regarding physical aspects of model–imitator similarity, we previously conducted an fMRI study aimed at characterizing the neural mechanisms underlying model-based imitative biases related to perceived gender. During imitation of own- as compared to other-gender models, participants showed greater activity in reward system regions, including the dorsal and ventral striatum (NAc), OFC, and amygdala (Losin, Iacoboni, Martin, & Dapretto, 2012). These results suggested that imitation of self-similar others is accompanied by intrinsic reinforcement, which may in turn facilitate the acquisition of cultural practices relating to the shared characteristic (e.g., gender norms; Losin, Iacoboni, Martin, & Dapretto, 2012). Based on this work, the reward system appears to play an integral role in shaping the similarity biases observed in the imitative acquisition of cultural behaviors.

Imitation Impairments, Mental Health, and the Role of Cultural Learning

A number of mental health disorders have been associated with alterations to the core behavioral, cognitive, and neural systems related to cultural learning: imitation, intention understanding, and reinforcement learning. We first focus on autism, the most common and well-described disorder involving imitative deficits. We discuss the behavioral manifestations of the imitative deficits seen in autism, their purported neural basis, and the role of cultural context in the expression and treatment of autism. Next we provide a brief overview of William's syndrome and schizophrenia, as these disorders also involve pathological alterations in imitative learning capacities. We conclude with an evaluation of the potential effects of the cultural environment on the development and management of schizophrenia within a global context.

Dysfunctional Imitation in Autism Spectrum Disorder

Although the cultural environment plays an important role in the expression of many mental health disorders, general imitative deficits are a widely recognized symptom of autism spectrum disorder (ASD). Difficulty with imitation is frequently a first sign of ASD, while dysfunctions relating to ToM begin to express themselves later in development (Rogers & Pennington, 1991). Behavioral and neural evidence suggests that the imitative deficits seen in ASD do not represent a complete inability to imitate, but rather reduced imitative control, affecting the decision to imitate or to inhibit imitative responses (de C. Hamilton, 2015). Behavioral symptoms of ASD such as echolalia or echopraxia (i.e., meaningless repetition of words or actions, respectively) may implicate abnormal functional development of prefrontal structures that typically inhibit the mirror system (de C. Hamilton, 2015; Williams et al., 2001). This reduced inhibitory control may help explain why those with ASD express hyperactivity of the pars opercularis of the IFG (a component of the mirror system) during observation of human motion (Martineau et al., 2010). Similarly, EEG studies demonstrate that while observing motor acts, children with ASD do not suppress mu rhythms, an index of motor resonance, as much as typically developing (TD) children (Martineau et al., 2008; Oberman et al., 2005). Finally, the severity of ASD symptoms is inversely related to IFG activity during an imitative task (i.e., greater behavioral deficits associated with reduced IFG activity; Dapretto et al., 2006), potentially further signaling reduced control of this frontal element of the mirror system. Thus, while children and adults with ASD are cognitively able to imitate observed behaviors, the deficits they express involve controlling imitative responses and selecting which intentional actions to imitate (Tomasello, 1999).

This recognition of reduced inhibitory control of imitation in ASD has led to the "broken mirror hypothesis," which suggests that patients with ASD do not process observed actions in the same way as TD individuals (Ramachandran & Oberman, 2006). Rather than seeing composite behaviors as a whole to gauge their instrumental or conventional purpose, it is posited that individuals with ASD break the action into separate motor components, which they then struggle to assemble into complex unitary acts (Cattaneo et al., 2007). For instance, Cattaneo et al. (2007) found that TD children exhibit muscle activations corresponding to the end goal of an observed behavior even at the start of the action, whereas this activation is absent in children with ASD. This finding suggests that TD individuals have a motor representation of the entire observed action before it is executed, enabling them to directly understand the goals of the action, while those with ASD may not. This lack of movement integration for complex actions may be a key factor underlying deficits in intention understanding in ASD, potentially resulting from deficient or absent internal replicas of the observed behaviors (Rizzolatti & Fabbri-Destro, 2010).

Relevant research also helps to clarify why goal-directed imitation is largely intact in ASD while social imitation tends to be stunted. Given that individuals with ASD have trouble understanding others as intentional agents (Tomasello, 1999), explicit cues to the end goal of another's actions may help those with ASD to correctly assemble motor units of an act without needing to model the act's intention. Such strategies that circumvent ToM-dependent learning may in turn promote the communicative deficits and lack of social insight often seen in ASD (Castelli et al., 2002). Additionally, an inability to perceive others' intentions may produce the diminished social motivation typical of individuals with ASD (see Chevallier et al., 2012, for a review), conceivably manifesting into reduced motivation to engage in the inherently social act of imitation. Taken together, these described impairments in intention processing and social imitation may impede various aspects of cultural learning in individuals with ASD.

The Role of Cultural Context in the Expression and Treatment of Autism

Relatively little is understood about how cultural contexts may influence the recognition and treatment of autism (Daley, 2002). Some researchers have proposed that wide international recognition of diagnostic criteria for autism (e.g., *Diagnostic and Statistical Manual of Mental Disorders* [DSM]) implies reliable symptom expression across cultures and thus reflects a consistent underlying biology (D. J. Cohen & Volkmar, 1997).

Conversely, it is also argued that some forms of autism may present themselves across the globe while still being susceptible to cultural influences in their development, identification, and treatment (Daley, 2002). After surveying children with autism in Africa, Lotter noted that social isolation as a central expression of ASD requires greater cross-cultural study since local expectations about what constitutes "normal" social behavior can vary dramatically (Lotter, 1980). Across cultures, there is wide variability in the terms applied and stigmas tied to disordered behaviors. Whereas in Senegal children with ASD symptoms are referred to as "*nit-ku-bon*" or "marvelous children," in rural Laos a term with more negative connotations, "*samqng uan*," is used to describe any children with delayed learning and difficulty getting along with others (Daley, 2002). In prior decades, misunderstanding about ASD among Indian and Sri Lankan families were documented, with some parents attributing ASD symptoms to primitive instincts, spiritual causes, or altered rates of socio-cognitive development (see Daley, 2002, for a review). In one cross-national survey of families with children with ASD in Brazil, Italy, Greece, and Germany, it was found that, across the sample, health-related cognitions were most improved by "coherence" between parents about the process of living with ASD in the family (Probst, 1998). In this way, similar ASD symptomatology can be interpreted differentially across communities, which can be of profound importance when determining if and how ASD is treated within specific cultures.

In addition to variability in the identification and contextualization of autism across cultures, various aspects of the disorder can manifest differentially within distinct contexts. One of the earliest examples of such a phenomenon came when Lotter (1980) compared expression of ASD in nine English-speaking African countries to that observed in Britain. He noted that stereotyped movements known to be characteristic of ASD in the United States and Britain were less pervasive among his sample of children with ASD in Africa (Lotter, 1980). Specifically, the movement peculiarities of African children with ASD tended to be more indicative of repetitive play with objects as compared to the flapping, self-aggression, and elaborate ritual play that characterized the British ASD sample (Lotter, 1978). These findings suggested that the imitative deficits typically observed in autism may be accentuated or attenuated through specific culturally learned behaviors.

Even among developed countries, differences in symptom expression have been seen to emerge across domains of nonverbal socialization, verbal communication, insistence of sameness (i.e., dislike of change and compulsion for consistency), and restricted interests (Matson et al., 2011). Using the Autism Spectrum Disorder-Diagnostic for Children (ASD-DC) to examine symptoms among children with ASD in Israel, South Korea, the United Kingdom, and the United States, Matson and colleagues (2011) found that children in the United Kingdom scored highest on all four subscales, while those in Israel scored the lowest; multivariate analysis of covariance (MANCOVA) revealed that this pattern was not due to age or gender differences across groups. Moreover, endorsement of some specific items varied dramatically across the samples: "saying words and phrases repetitively" was expressed by only 34% of Israeli children, compared to 70% in South Korea and the United States, and 59% in the United Kingdom; "repetitive movements for no reason" were seen in only 50% of the Israeli sample, compared to 65% in South Korea, 80% in the United States, and 88.9% in the United Kingdom (Matson et al., 2011). These disparate expressions of ASD symptoms suggest that the cultural context in which such behaviors are learned has a substantial influence on the frequency of their manifestation. As a condition affecting communication, language usage may also shape the expression of ASD symptoms and could be used within paradigms for testing ToM (Daley, 2002). One multilingual teenager with ASD in India was observed to automatically speak the language of an interaction partner in spite of other social deficits (Daley, 2002), demonstrating a contextually learned social awareness that is typically lacking among other patients with ASD. While these findings do not suggest that autistic imitative deficits are entirely culture driven, they do imply that the manifestation of disordered behavior is sensitive to learning within the cultural environment.

Beyond these differences in the expression of autistic symptoms, there is also considerable variability in time to diagnosis and treatment approaches for ASD across various cultures. For instance, some ultra-orthodox communities in Israel may not seek treatment programs for children with autism, rather engaging in a form of facilitated communication whereby the children are used to receive messages from God; these messages are believed to bypass the body and make direct contact with the pure soul of a child with ASD (Bilu & Goodman, 1997). In this view, the more mentally and physically impaired the child is, the more receptive they are to these morally colored messages (Bilu & Goodman, 1997); thus, alleviation of symptoms may be less emphasized in these communities. Furthermore, in India, different beliefs about what constitutes "normal" development may lead to significant delays in the diagnosis of ASD. Historically, many Indian professionals followed guidelines that speech is not delayed until a child is 3 years old (Kumar, 1988), contributing to first identification of problem behaviors occurring an average of 7 months later than typical first recognition in the United States (Hackett & Hackett, 1999). Due to language delays not being seen as specific to autism and a lack of consensus about their causes, many families in South India reported not recognizing autistic symptoms as anything other than normal misbehavior until a researcher pointed it out as ASD (Daley, 2002; Hackett & Hackett, 1999). However, more recently the Indian Academy of Pediatrics has worked to formulate new national consensus guidelines which emphasize that intervention should begin as early as possible whether or not the diagnosis is completely definitive (Dalwai et al., 2017). Moreover, even when ASD is correctly identified, there is huge variation in treatment approaches, which range from traditional Western therapies to allopathy, Unani traditions, and Ayurvedic homeopathy (Daley, 2002). In one sample of Indian autistic children, three-quarters had taken and 42% were presently using some form of pharmacological treatment, despite a lack of demonstrated efficacy for relieving ASD symptoms (Daley, 2002). Similarly, over half the sample used either or both

Ayurvedic and homeopathic treatments, while smaller portions had tried treatments such as pranic healing, astrology, vitamin therapy, reflexology, yoga, acupressure, or behavior therapy (Daley, 2002). However, this tendency to rely on untested treatments is not unique to India. One study found that nonscientifically supported ASD treatments (e.g., facilitated communication, music therapy, antifungal medications) received four times as much positive commentary in media coverage in the United States as compared to negative comments (Schreck et al., 2013). More study across a greater diversity of national samples is needed to understand the true extent of the influence of cultural environments on the diagnosis and treatment of autism. This literature highlights that cultural forces can influence how autistic symptoms are expressed, when they are detected, and what approaches are used in addressing them, emphasizing the need for cultural diversity in the implementation of international aid programs focused on ASD.

Imitative Learning in Other Clinical Disorders

Another disorder with implications for imitation and cultural learning is William's syndrome (WS), a genetic condition associated with a highly social personality as well as an array of medical (e.g., gastrointestinal, kidney, bladder, and cardiovascular disorders) and developmental (e.g., learning disabilities) impairments (Williams Syndrome Association, 2018). An example of the hypersociality characteristic of WS can be seen in a study using the yummy–yucky task in which a researcher expresses liking and disgust for two different foods, then asks the child to offer the food item that the researcher will want (Fidler et al., 2007). In this task, children with WS display heightened affective imitation (i.e., mimicking facial reactions) compared to matched children with nonspecific developmental disabilities. Despite increased emotional imitation in WS, appropriate social decision making within the yummy–yucky task is not improved, as children with WS spend more time than controls trying to convince the model that the researcher's unliked food is actually desirable (Fidler et al., 2007). While affective imitation may be intact or enhanced in WS, children and adults with WS show performance equivalent to typical 5-year-old controls on elicited verbal imitation tasks (Grant et al., 2002), demonstrating that the preservation or enhancement of initiative abilities in WS is only present for a specific subset of social imitative behaviors. Along similar lines, imitation of instrumental acts with a tangible end goal is comparable for children with WS and ASD, but unlike ASD, increased social engagement with the model promotes attention and imitative learning in WS (Vivanti et al., 2016). Thus, while social forms of imitation are intact or enhanced in WS, imitative behaviors relying on more cognitive capacities are delayed or stunted. The divergent pattern of impairments in social imitation between WS and ASD could imply that differential functions of ToM-related neural structures may differentiate these conditions and lead to distinct cultural learning deficits.

More prevalent than WS, the mental health disorder schizophrenia is also associated with impairments in multiple components of the neural systems involved in cultural learning via imitation as described in this chapter. To begin, signals generated in the mirror system can produce echopraxia (excessive and uncontrolled imitation), a symptom commonly seen in schizophrenia; this occurs when internal representations of observed behaviors, processed in the IFG, connected anterior cingulate, and motor cortex, are interpreted as potential movements (Pridmore et al., 2008). These potential actions are then more readily executed in individuals with schizophrenia due to reduced behavioral inhibition and increased general arousal, both prevalent in this population (Pridmore et al., 2008). Moreover, this lack of behavioral control is frequently accompanied by cognitive deficits in ToM and self-awareness. Similar to behaviors seen in individuals with ASD, those with schizophrenia often exhibit impaired mirror self-recognition, responding as if in the presence of another person (Gallup et al., 2003). Impaired self-recognition in schizophrenia can be accompanied by symptoms of passivity phenomena (e.g., illusory alien control), which are associated with hyperactivation in the right IPL (supramarginal gyrus), a parietal component of the mirror system (Spence et al., 1997) implicated in self-referential processing and own-body representation (Uddin et al., 2005). Together the reduced inhibitory control and impaired attribution of mental and physical states to self and others may contribute to impaired cultural learning in individuals with schizophrenia.

Taken as a whole, findings of impaired cognitive and neural systems involved in cultural learning via imitation in ASD, WS, and schizophrenia demonstrate that the impacts of mental health disorders are not limited to deficits in socioemotional functioning but may also influence cultural learning and cultural integration. More research focusing on the connections between mental health disorders and their cultural consequences is needed to fully understand these relationships and inform interventions aimed at addressing any impairments in sociocultural functioning. As little research has been conducted addressing how the cultural environment shapes expression of and treatment for WS, the following discussion of the impact of the cultural environment in influencing perceptions and approaches to mental illness will be specifically focused on schizophrenia.

The Role of Cultural Context in the Expression and Treatment of Schizophrenia

Views about the consequences of schizophrenia and the social stigmas tied to this disorder can vary widely across cultures. One cross-cultural study found that Japanese participants, due to societal taboos about mental illness, viewed schizophrenics as more abnormal and dangerous compared to a British sample who expressed more concern about the rights of schizophrenics and the need for individual care, as opposed to society-level change (Furnham & Murao, 2000). Similarly, British people tended to emphasize more psychological and biological beliefs about the causes and treatment of schizophrenia when contrasted against a Chinese sample, which held more negative attitudes as well as superstitions and religious beliefs about the forces causing schizophrenia (Furnham & Wong, 2007). Terminology may also contribute to negative attitudes about schizophrenia. For example, "jing-shen-fen-lie-zheng" ("mind-split-disease") is used to refer to schizophrenia in many areas utilizing the Chinese writing system, where "*jing-shen*" is often associated with the stereotype of insanity (Chung & Chan, 2004). A newer term, "*si-jue-shi-diao*" ("thought-perception dysregulation"), began to be implemented in Hong Kong in 2001 with the hope of reducing negative stigmas, making it more likely for schizophrenics to accept their diagnosis and seek treatment (Furnham & Wong, 2007). However, the use of this new term was not seen to reduce negative attitudes about the disorder among a student sample in Hong Kong (Chung & Chan, 2004). Thus, the ingrained cultural learning of attitudes about schizophrenia appears to extend beyond the terms applied to this disorder in this specific Chinese example, suggesting that a more systemic cultural approach may be required to reduce negative stereotypes about schizophrenia (see Chapter 20 for a discussion of cultural change). In these ways, cultural viewpoints about the causes and effects of schizophrenia show extensive variability across cultural contexts, potentially affecting regional diagnosis and willingness of patients to seek out treatment for this disorder.

There is further evidence to indicate that the expression and treatment of schizophrenia are also sensitive to cultural contexts. According to a systematic review of studies by Saha et al. (2005), rates of schizophrenia do not differ across urban and rural sites or by gender, but schizophrenia is more common among migrants (1.8 times native-born prevalence) and homeless populations (see Bhugra, 2005, for a summary of these results). However, it is difficult to verify whether such situational factors make individuals more susceptible to schizophrenia or if schizophrenics are more likely to become homeless or tend to migrate as a result of the disorder (i.e., whether increased prevalence is a cause or an effect of these situational factors). Moreover, prevalence is reported to be greater in developed and emerging nations as compared to developing countries (Bhugra, 2005), though again, this difference could result either from lower prevalence or less treatment seeking and fewer national surveys of prevalence within developing nations. Along with general prevalence, expression of specific symptoms also varies across national contexts, as catatonia (the tendency to remain in a fixed stuporous state for long periods) was observed in 10% of schizophrenic cases in developing countries (e.g., India, Nigeria, USSR) as compared to only 1% of cases in developed nations (e.g., Denmark, United States, United Kingdom; Jablensky et al., 1992). This cross-national discrepancy in rates of catatonia may reflect a culturally learned process of avoiding catatonic states, more consistent external stimulation, or other contextual factors that vary across these countries. At the same time, the proportion of schizophrenic cases with acute onset was twice as high in developing compared to developed countries (A. Cohen, 1992), possibly reflecting either cross-cultural divergence in disease manifestation or a lack of immediate diagnosis in less developed nations (see Bhugra, 2005, for a review).

Traditional medicine is frequently used in place of or concurrently with Western mental health care in treating schizophrenia, with these non-Western health practices consistently emphasized in developing nations in a manner similar to the treatment of autism across cultures. For example, Jablensky et al. (1992), in a study conducted across 10 developed and developing countries, note that while 39% of the schizophrenic cases in their nearly 1,400 participant sample first sought help with a psychiatrist, at least 200 cases of schizophrenia would have been missed if traditional practitioners had not been contacted. As an example of non-Western treatments, China's Hebei hospital began using acupuncture, a highly culturally salient medical practice, as a treatment for schizophrenia in 1956, claiming to have an 84% success rate in alleviating symptoms (Han-Kuang, 1957). Furthermore, culturally acquired social stigmas about mental illness led many Chinese families to be more likely to hide schizophrenic relatives and less likely to make friends with schizophrenics compared to a British sample (Furnham & Wong, 2007). Thus, culturally learned views and social contexts can produce profound impacts on the behavioral expression and treatments of schizophrenia across regions, stressing the need for culturally sensitive educational efforts to better diagnose, encourage treatment seeking in, and improve care for those suffering from this mental health disorder.

Future Directions in Research on Cultural Learning via Imitation

The neural model of cultural acquisition through cultural imitative learning presented in this chapter (see Figure 17.1) represents a foundation that is still being built upon through ongoing research. Several research questions not addressed in the current chapter represent promising directions for future investigations into the neurobiological mechanisms underlying cultural learning, which will in turn further refine our neural model.

First, the extent to which the neural mechanisms of cultural learning proposed here operate in real-world sociocultural contexts needs to be determined. Many neuroimaging studies of imitation and other cognitive components of cultural learning rely on highly simplified tasks due to the constraints of the fMRI environment. Thus, some researchers have posited that the social and goal-directed imitation characteristic of most natural cultural learning may require brain processes beyond those currently described in the neuroimaging literature (de C. Hamilton, 2015). We have previously tried to increase the ecological validity of studies addressing imitation through the development of a novel video imitation stimulus set that included more complex hand gestures and the body and face of the person being imitated (e.g., Losin, Iacoboni, Martin, & Dapretto, 2012). Importantly, however, these stimuli remain far less complex than those common to naturalistic environments and few others have adopted this more ecologically valid approach. Thus, studies that investigate brain mechanisms underlying cultural learning in more naturalistic contexts are needed to further refine our understanding of this process.

Second, although in this chapter we sought to describe ostensibly universal aspects of human cultural imitative learning, it remains unclear whether the process of cultural learning, rather than just the content and circumstances of such learning, varies appreciably across cultures (Tomasello, 2016). In the cultural neuroscience literature there is already some evidence that there may indeed be variability in the core cognitive components of cultural learning and their neural underpinnings. For example, several studies have demonstrated differences in the function of neural regions within the ToM network when East Asian versus Western individuals engage in mentalizing tasks (Cheon et al., 2013; Kobayashi et al., 2006; Zhu et al., 2007). Therefore, more cross-cultural research on cognitive and neural mechanisms underlying cultural learning is needed to characterize global variation in these processes.

Finally, although many mental health disorders include deficits in the core cognitive components of cultural learning, the clinical neuroscience literature typically does not consider these disorders' impacts on cultural functioning. As discussed in the mental health section of this chapter, the potential impairments in the acquisition of cultural norms, beliefs, and practices associated with certain mental health disorders such as ASD, schizophrenia, and WS may be substantial. These cultural learning deficits as well as cultural variation in perceptions about and treatments for these disorders may in turn lead to deficits in sociocultural integration for individuals with these and other mental health disorders. For this reason, more research into cultural learning deficits and cross-cultural variability in the prevalence, expression, and treatment of various mental health disorders is needed to inform interventions aimed at improving sociocultural functioning within the context of global mental health.

Conclusions

Cultural learning via imitation is one of the primary means through which cultural behaviors are acquired, transmitted, and built upon over time. In this chapter, we reviewed human and nonhuman primate research over the past several decades that has begun to reveal the cognitive and brain mechanisms underlying these cultural learning processes. These mechanisms include imitative learning supported by the human mirror system, mentalizing supported by the ToM network, and reinforcement learning supported by the reward system. We also presented clinical research on mental health disorders in which cultural learning via imitation and its associated neural mechanisms have gone awry, including ASD, WS, and schizophrenia. We further discussed how the cultural context surrounding mental health disorders can have profound impacts for their expression and treatment. We used this literature as a basis to propose an updated and extended model of the neural systems involved in cultural learning via imitation, which we first proposed nearly a decade ago.

The bulk of research in the growing field of cultural neuroscience and cultural psychiatry has focused on ways in which cultural experience shapes the brain, that is, *cultural plasticity*. The brain mechanisms that enable *cultural acquisition* explored in this chapter represent an equally important component of the larger system of cognitive and neural mechanisms enabling the complexity of human cultural capacities. As such, we hope this chapter serves to aggregate relevant literatures on cultural acquisition from nonhuman primate research and human cultural psychology, psychological anthropology, and sociocultural and cognitive neuroscience, which are often isolated by disciplinary boundaries. Additionally, we hope this chapter helps to stimulate future cross-disciplinary research on the process of cultural acquisition and its interplay with mental health.

Acknowledgments

This work was supported by start-up funds from the University of Miami College of Arts and Sciences (EARL).

References

Abel, T., Nguyen, P. V., Barad, M., Deuel, T. A., Kandel, E. R., & Bourtchouladze, R. (1997). Genetic demonstration of a role for PKA in the late phase of LTP and in hippocampus-based long-term memory. *Cell, 88*(5), 615–626.

Allison, T., Puce, A., & McCarthy, G. (2000). Social perception from visual cues: Role of the STS region. *Trends in cognitive sciences, 4*(7), 267–278.

Anisfeld, M., Masters, J. C., Jacobson, S. W., Kagan, J., Meltzoff, A. N., & Moore, M. K. (1979). Interpreting "imitative" responses in early infancy. *Science, 205*(4402), 214–219. https://doi.org/10.1126/science.451593

Apperly, I. A. (2008). Beyond simulation-theory and theory-theory: Why social cognitive neuroscience should use its own concepts to study "theory of mind." *Cognition, 107*(1), 266–283. doi:10.1016/j.cognition.2007.07.019

Asakura, N., & Inui, T. (2016). A Bayesian framework for false belief reasoning in children: A rational integration of theory-theory and simulation theory. *Frontiers in Psychology, 7*, 2019.

Avis, J., & Harris, P. L. (1991). Belief-desire reasoning among Baka children: Evidence for a universal conception of mind. *Child Development, 62*(3), 460–467.

Bandura, A. (1969). Social-learning theory of identificatory processes. In D. A. Goslin (Ed.), *Handbook of socialization theory and research* (pp. 213–262). Rand McNally and Company.

Bandura, A. (1977). *Social learning theory*. Prentice-Hall.

Bandura, A., & Kupers, C. J. (1964). Transmission of patterns of self-reinforcement through modeling. *Journal of Abnormal and Social Psychology, 69*(1), 1.

Bandura, A., Ross, D., & Ross, S. A. (1961). Transmission of aggression through imitation of aggressive models. *Journal of Abnormal and Social Psychology, 63*(3), 575–582.

Baron-Cohen, S., Leslie, A. M., & Frith, U. (1985). Does the autistic child have a "theory of mind"? *Cognition, 21*(1), 37–46.

Baron-Cohen, S., Wheelwright, S., Hill, J., Raste, Y., & Plumb, I. (2001). The "Reading the Mind in the Eyes" Test revised version: A study with normal adults, and adults with Asperger syndrome or high-functioning autism. *Journal of Child Psychology and Psychiatry and Allied Disciplines, 42*(2), 241–251.

Basten, U., Biele, G., Heekeren, H. R., & Fiebach, C. J. (2010). How the brain integrates costs and benefits during decision making. *Proceedings of the National Academy of Sciences, 107*(50), 21767–21772.

Bellagamba, F., & Tomasello, M. (1999). Re-enacting intended acts: Comparing 12-and 18-month-olds. *Infant Behavior and Development, 22*(2), 277–282.

Berridge, K. C. (2003). Pleasures of the brain. *Brain and Cognition, 52*(1), 106–128.

Bhugra, D. (2005). The global prevalence of schizophrenia. *PLoS Medicine, 2*(5), e151.

Bi, G.-q., & Poo, M.-m. (2001). Synaptic modification by correlated activity: Hebb's postulate revisited. *Annual Review of Neuroscience, 24*(1), 139–166.

Bilu, Y., & Goodman, Y. C. (1997). What does the soul say?: Metaphysical uses of facilitated communication in the Jewish ultraorthodox community. *Ethos, 25*(4), 375–407.

Blakemore, S.-J. (2012). Imaging brain development: The adolescent brain. *Neuroimage, 61*(2), 397–406.

Boorman, E. D., Behrens, T. E., Woolrich, M. W., & Rushworth, M. F. (2009). How green is the grass on the other side? Frontopolar cortex and the evidence in favor of alternative courses of action. *Neuron, 62*(5), 733–743.

Botvinick, M., Jha, A. P., Bylsma, L. M., Fabian, S. A., Solomon, P. E., & Prkachin, K. M. (2005). Viewing facial expressions of pain engages cortical areas involved in the direct experience of pain. *Neuroimage, 25*(1), 312–319.

Braadbaart, L., De Grauw, H., Perrett, D., Waiter, G. D., & Williams, J. (2014). The shared neural basis of empathy and facial imitation accuracy. *Neuroimage, 84,* 367–375.

Brass, M., Derrfuss, J., & von Cramon, D. Y. (2005). The inhibition of imitative and overlearned responses: A functional double dissociation. *Neuropsychologia, 43*(1), 89–98.

Brass, M., Ruby, P., & Spengler, S. (2009). Inhibition of imitative behaviour and social cognition. *Philosophical Transactions of the Royal Society of London B: Biological Sciences, 364*(1528), 2359–2367.

Buccino, G., Lui, F., Canessa, N., Patteri, I., Lagravinese, G., Benuzzi, F., Porro, C., & Rizzolatti, G. (2004). Neural circuits involved in the recognition of actions performed by nonconspecifics: An fMRI study. *Journal of Cognitive Neuroscience, 16*(1), 114–126.

Bussey, K., & Perry, D. G. (1976). Sharing reinforcement contingencies with a model: A social-learning analysis of similarity effects in imitation research. *Journal of Personality and Social Psychology, 34*(6), 1168.

Butler, L. P., & Walton, G. M. (2013). The opportunity to collaborate increases preschoolers' motivation for challenging tasks. *Journal of Experimental Child Psychology, 116*(4), 953–961.

Carpenter, M., Nagell, K., Tomasello, M., Butterworth, G., & Moore, C. (1998). Social cognition, joint attention, and communicative competence from 9 to 15 months of age. *Monographs of the Society for Research in Child Development, 63*(4), i–174.

Carruthers, P., & Smith, P. K. (1996). *Theories of theories of mind.* Cambridge University Press.

Castelli, F., Frith, C., Happé, F., & Frith, U. (2002). Autism, Asperger syndrome and brain mechanisms for the attribution of mental states to animated shapes. *Brain, 125*(8), 1839–1849.

Cattaneo, L., Fabbri-Destro, M., Boria, S., Pieraccini, C., Monti, A., Cossu, G., & Rizzolatti, G. (2007). Impairment of actions chains in autism and its possible role in intention understanding. *Proceedings of the National Academy of Sciences, 104*(45), 17825–17830.

Chalmeau, R., & Gallo, A. (1993). Social transmission among nonhuman-primates. *Annals of Psychology, 93*(3), 427–439.

Cheng, Y. W., Tzeng, O. J. L., Decety, J., Imada, T., & Hsieh, J. C. (2006). Gender differences in the human mirror system: A magnetoencephalography study. *Neuroreport, 17*(11), 1115.

Cheon, B. K., Im, D.-M., Harada, T., Kim, J.-S., Mathur, V. A., Scimeca, J. M., . . . Chiao, J. Y. (2013). Cultural modulation of the neural correlates of emotional pain perception: The role of other-focusedness. *Neuropsychologia, 51*(7), 1177–1186.

Chevallier, C., Kohls, G., Troiani, V., Brodkin, E. S., & Schultz, R. T. (2012). The social motivation theory of autism. *Trends in Cognitive Sciences, 16*(4), 231–239.

Chiao, J. Y. (2018). Developmental aspects in cultural neuroscience. *Developmental Review, 50,* 77–89.

Chung, K. F., & Chan, J. H. (2004). Can a less pejorative Chinese translation for schizophrenia reduce stigma? A study of adolescents' attitudes toward people with schizophrenia. *Psychiatry and Clinical Neurosciences, 58*(5), 507–515.

Cohen, A. (1992). Prognosis for schizophrenia in the Third World: A reevaluation of cross-cultural research. *Culture, Medicine and Psychiatry, 16*(1), 53–75.

Cohen, D. J., & Volkmar, F. (1997). Conceptualizations of autism and intervention practices: International perspectives. In D. J. Cohen & F. R. Volkmar (Eds.), *Handbook of autism and pervasive developmental disorders* (pp. 947–950). Wiley.

Cross, K. A., Torrisi, S., Reynolds Losin, E. A., & Iacoboni, M. (2013). Controlling automatic imitative tendencies: Interactions between mirror neuron and cognitive control systems. *Neuroimage, 83,* 493–504. doi:10.1016/j.neuroimage.2013.06.060

Daley, T. C. (2002). The need for cross-cultural research on the pervasive developmental disorders. *Transcultural Psychiatry, 39*(4), 531–550.

Dalwai, S., Ahmed, S., Udani, V., Mundkur, N., Kamath, S. S., & Nair, M. K. C. (2017). Consensus statement of the Indian academy of pediatrics on evaluation and management of autism spectrum disorder. *Indian pediatrics, 54*(5), 385–393.

Dapretto, M., Davies, M. S., Pfeifer, J. H., Scott, A. A., Sigman, M., Bookheimer, S. Y., & Iacoboni, M. (2006). Understanding emotions in others: Mirror neuron dysfunction in children with autism spectrum disorders. *Nature Neuroscience, 9*(1), 28–30. doi:10.1038/nn1611

Day, J. J., & Carelli, R. M. (2007). The nucleus accumbens and Pavlovian reward learning. *The Neuroscientist, 13*(2), 148–159.

de C. Hamilton, A. F. (2015). The neurocognitive mechanisms of imitation. *Current Opinion in Behavioral Sciences, 3*, 63–67.

de C. Hamilton, A. F., & Grafton, S. T. (2007). Action outcomes are represented in human inferior frontoparietal cortex. *Cerebral Cortex, 18*(5), 1160–1168.

de Lange, F. P., Spronk, M., Willems, R. M., Toni, I., & Bekkering, H. (2008). Complementary systems for understanding action intentions. *Current Biology, 18*(6), 454–457. doi:10.1016/j.cub.2008.02.057

Durkheim, E. (1915). *The elementary forms of the religious life* (Joseph Ward Swain, Trans.). Dover Publications, Inc.

Fabbri-Destro, M., & Rizzolatti, G. (2008). Mirror neurons and mirror systems in monkeys and humans. *Physiology (Bethesda), 23*, 171–179. doi:10.1152/physiol.00004.2008

Fidler, D. J., Hepburn, S. L., Most, D. E., Philofsky, A., & Rogers, S. J. (2007). Emotional responsivity in young children with Williams syndrome. *American Journal on Mental Retardation, 112*(3), 194–206.

Fragaszy, D. M., & Perry, S. (2003). Towards a biology of traditions. In D. M. Fragaszy & S. Perry (Eds.), *The biology of traditions: Models and evidence* (pp. 1–32). Cambridge University Press.

Frith, U., & Frith, C. D. (2003). Development and neurophysiology of mentalizing. *Philosophical Transactions of the Royal Society of London B: Biological Sciences, 358*(1431), 459–473. doi:10.1098/rstb.2002.1218

Furnham, A., & Igboaka, A. (2007). Young people's recognition and understanding of schizophrenia: A cross-cultural study of young people from Britain and Nigeria. *International Journal of Social Psychiatry, 53*(5), 430–446.

Furnham, A., & Murao, M. (2000). A cross-cultural comparison of British and Japanese lay theories of schizophrenia. *International Journal of Social Psychiatry, 46*(1), 4–20.

Furnham, A., & Wong, L. (2007). A cross-cultural comparison of British and Chinese beliefs about the causes, behaviour manifestations and treatment of schizophrenia. *Psychiatry Research, 151*(1–2), 123–138.

Gallese, V., Fadiga, L., Fogassi, L., & Rizzolatti, G. (1996). Action recognition in the premotor cortex. *Brain, 119*(2), 593.

Gallese, V., & Goldman, A. (1998). Mirror neurons and the simulation theory of mind-reading. *Trends in Cognitive Sciences, 2*(12), 493–501. doi:10.1016/S1364-6613(98)01262-5

Gallup, G. G. (1970). Chimpanzees: Self-recognition. *Science, 167*(3914), 86–87.

Gallup, G. G. (1982). Self-awareness and the emergence of mind in primates. *American Journal of Primatology, 2*(3), 237–248.

Gallup, G. G., Anderson, J. R., & Platek, S. M. (2003). Self-awareness, social intelligence and schizophrenia. In T. Kircher & A. David (Eds.), *The self in neuroscience and psychiatry* (pp. 147–165). Cambridge University Press.

Gazzola, V., Rizzolatti, G., Wicker, B., & Keysers, C. (2007). The anthropomorphic brain: The mirror neuron system responds to human and robotic actions. *Neuroimage, 35*(4), 1674–1684. doi:10.1016/j.neuroimage.2007.02.003

Gazzola, V., van der Worp, H., Mulder, T., Wicker, B., Rizzolatti, G., & Keysers, C. (2007). Aplasics born without hands mirror the goal of hand actions with their feet. *Current Biology, 17*(14), 1235–1240. doi:10.1016/j.cub.2007.06.045

Goh, J. O., Chee, M. W., Tan, J. C., Venkatraman, V., Hebrank, A., Leshikar, E. D., . . . Park, D. C. (2007). Age and culture modulate object processing and object—scene binding in the ventral visual area. *Cognitive, Affective, & Behavioral Neuroscience, 7*(1), 44–52.

Grant, J., Valian, V., & Karmiloff-Smith, A. (2002). A study of relative clauses in Williams syndrome. *Journal of Child Language, 29*(2), 403–416.

Greicius, M. D., Krasnow, B., Reiss, A. L., & Menon, V. (2003). Functional connectivity in the resting brain: A network analysis of the default mode hypothesis. *Proceedings of the National Academy of Sciences, 100*(1), 253–258.

Grèzes, J. (1998). Top down effect of strategy on the perception of human biological motion: A PET investigation. *Cognitive Neuropsychology, 15*(6–8), 553–582.

Grèzes, J., Costes, N., & Decety, J. (1999). The effects of learning and intention on the neural network involved in the perception of meaningless actions. *Brain, 122* (Pt 10), 1875–1887.

Gros, I. T., Panasiti, M. S., & Chakrabarti, B. (2015). The plasticity of the mirror system: How reward learning modulates cortical motor simulation of others. *Neuropsychologia, 70*, 255–262.

Güroğlu, B., van den Bos, W., van Dijk, E., Rombouts, S. A., & Crone, E. A. (2011). Dissociable brain networks involved in development of fairness considerations: Understanding intentionality behind unfairness. *Neuroimage, 57*(2), 634–641.

Gutsell, J. N., & Inzlicht, M. (2010). Empathy constrained: Prejudice predicts reduced mental simulation of actions during observation of outgroups. *Journal of Experimental Social Psychology, 6*, 841–845.

Haber, S. N., & Knutson, B. (2010). The reward circuit: Linking primate anatomy and human imaging. *Neuropsychopharmacology, 35*(1), 4.

Hackett, R., & Hackett, L. (1999). Child psychiatry across cultures. *International Review of Psychiatry, 11*(2–3), 225–235.

Han, S. (2015). Understanding cultural differences in human behavior: A cultural neuroscience approach. *Current Opinion in Behavioral Sciences, 3*, 68–72. doi:10.1016/j.cobeha.2015.01.013

Han-Kuang, T. (1957). A preliminary report on the acupuncture treatment of 53 cases of mental illness. *Journal of New Chinese Medicine, 11*, 923–928.

Hayden, B. Y., Pearson, J. M., & Platt, M. L. (2009). Fictive reward signals in the anterior cingulate cortex. *Science, 324*(5929), 948–950.

Hebb, D. O. (1949). *The organization of behavior*. Wiley.

Hecht, E. E., Murphy, L. E., Gutman, D. A., Votaw, J. R., Schuster, D. M., Preuss, T. M., . . . Parr, L. A. (2013). Differences in neural activation for object-directed grasping in chimpanzees and humans. *Journal of Neuroscience, 33*(35), 14117–14134.

Heider, F., & Simmel, M. (1944). An experimental study of apparent behavior. *American Journal of Psychology, 57*(2), 243–259.

Hein, G., Silani, G., Preuschoff, K., Batson, C. D., & Singer, T. (2010). Neural responses to ingroup and outgroup members' suffering predict individual differences in costly helping. *Neuron, 68*(1), 149–160. doi:10.1016/j.neuron.2010.09.003

Henrich, J. (2009). The evolution of costly displays, cooperation and religion. *Evolution and Human Behavior, 30*(4), 244–260.

Henrich, J., & Broesch, J. (2011). On the nature of cultural transmission networks: Evidence from Fijian villages for adaptive learning biases. *Philosophical Transactions of the Royal Society B: Biological Sciences, 366*(1567), 1139–1148.

Henrich, J., & McElreath, R. (2003). The evolution of cultural evolution. *Evolutionary Anthropology, 12*(3), 123–135. doi:10.1002/evan.10110

Heyes, C. (2005). Imitation by association. In S. Hurley & N. Chater (Eds.), *Perspectives on imitation: From neuroscience to social science* (pp. 157–176). MIT Press.

Heyes, C. (2014). Tinbergen on mirror neurons. *Philosophical Transactions of the Royal Society B: Biological Sciences, 369*(1644), 20130180.

Horner, V., Proctor, D., Bonnie, K. E., Whiten, A., & de Waal, F. B. (2010). Prestige affects cultural learning in chimpanzees. *PLoS One, 5*(5), e10625.

Horner, V., & Whiten, A. (2005). Causal knowledge and imitation/emulation switching in chimpanzees (Pan troglodytes) and children (Homo sapiens). *Animal Cognition, 8*(3), 164–181.

Humphrey, N. K. (1976). The social function of intellect. In P. P. G. Bateson & R. A. Hinde (Eds.), *Growing points in ethology* (pp. 303–317). Cambridge University Press.

Iacoboni, M. (2005). Neural mechanisms of imitation. *Current Opinion in Neurobiology, 15*(6), 632–637. doi:10.1016/j.conb.2005.10.010

Iacoboni, M., & Dapretto, M. (2006). The mirror neuron system and the consequences of its dysfunction. *Nature Reviews Neuroscience, 7*(12), 942–951. doi:10.1038/nrn2024

Iacoboni, M., Molnar-Szakacs, I., Gallese, V., Buccino, G., Mazziotta, J. C., & Rizzolatti, G. (2005). Grasping the intentions of others with one's own mirror neuron system. *PLoS Biology, 3*(3), e79. doi:10.1371/journal.pbio.0030079

Iacoboni, M., Woods, R. P., Brass, M., Bekkering, H., Mazziotta, J. C., & Rizzolatti, G. (1999). Cortical mechanisms of human imitation. *Science, 286*(5449), 2526–2528.

Izuma, K., Saito, D. N., & Sadato, N. (2008). Processing of social and monetary rewards in the human striatum. *Neuron, 58*(2), 284–294.

Jablensky, A., Sartorius, N., Ernberg, G., Anker, M., Korten, A., Cooper, J. E., . . . Bertelsen, A. (1992). Schizophrenia: Manifestations, incidence and course in different cultures: A World Health Organization ten-country study. *Psychological Medicine Monograph Supplement, 20*, 1–97.

Jackson, P. L., Meltzoff, A. N., & Decety, J. (2005). How do we perceive the pain of others? A window into the neural processes involved in empathy. *Neuroimage, 24*(3), 771–779.

Jellema, T., Baker, C., Wicker, B., & Perrett, D. (2000). Neural representation for the perception of the intentionality of actions. *Brain and Cognition, 44*(2), 280–302.

Jeon, H., & Lee, S.-H. (2018). From neurons to social beings: Short review of the mirror neuron system research and its socio-psychological and psychiatric implications. *Clinical Psychopharmacology and Neuroscience, 16*(1), 18.

Kable, J. W., & Glimcher, P. W. (2007). The neural correlates of subjective value during intertemporal choice. *Nature Neuroscience, 10*(12), 1625.

Kandel, E. R. (2001). The molecular biology of memory storage: A dialogue between genes and synapses. *Science, 294*(5544), 1030–1038.

Keenan, J. P., Wheeler, M. A., Gallup, G. G., Jr., & Pascual-Leone, A. (2000). Self-recognition and the right prefrontal cortex. *Trends in Cognitive Science, 4*(9), 338–344.

Kilner, J. M., Neal, A., Weiskopf, N., Friston, K. J., & Frith, C. D. (2009). Evidence of mirror neurons in human inferior frontal gyrus. *Journal of Neuroscience, 29*(32), 10153–10159.

Kobayashi, C., Glover, G. H., & Temple, E. (2006). Cultural and linguistic influence on neural bases of 'Theory of Mind': An fMRI study with Japanese bilinguals. *Brain and Language, 98*(2), 210–220. doi:10.1016/j.bandl.2006.04.013

Kühn, S., Müller, B. C., van Baaren, R. B., Wietzker, A., Dijksterhuis, A., & Brass, M. (2010). Why do I like you when you behave like me? Neural mechanisms mediating positive consequences of observing someone being imitated. *Social Neuroscience, 5*(4), 384–392.

Kumar, R. (1988). *Child development in India (health, welfare and management)* (Vol. I). Ashish Publishing House.

Lamm, C., Decety, J., & Singer, T. (2011). Meta-analytic evidence for common and distinct neural networks associated with directly experienced pain and empathy for pain. *Neuroimage, 54*(3), 2492–2502. doi:10.1016/j.neuroimage.2010.10.014

Lebreton, M., Jorge, S., Michel, V., Thirion, B., & Pessiglione, M. (2009). An automatic valuation system in the human brain: Evidence from functional neuroimaging. *Neuron, 64*(3), 431–439.

Legare, C. H., & Herrmann, P. A. (2013). Cognitive consequences and constraints on reasoning about ritual. *Religion, Brain & Behavior, 3*(1), 63–65.

Legare, C. H., & Nielsen, M. (2015). Imitation and innovation: The dual engines of cultural learning. *Trends in Cognitive Sciences, 19*(11), 688–699.

Legare, C. H., & Souza, A. L. (2012). Evaluating ritual efficacy: Evidence from the supernatural. *Cognition, 124*(1), 1–15.

Legare, C. H., & Souza, A. L. (2014). Searching for control: Priming randomness increases the evaluation of ritual efficacy. *Cognitive Science, 38*(1), 152–161.

Levy, W., & Steward, O. (1983). Temporal contiguity requirements for long-term associative potentiation/depression in the hippocampus. *Neuroscience, 8*(4), 791–797.

Lieberman, M. D. (2007). Social cognitive neuroscience: A review of core processes. *Annual Review of Psychology, 58*, 259–289.

Likowski, K. U., Mühlberger, A., Gerdes, A., Wieser, M. J., Pauli, P., & Weyers, P. (2012). Facial mimicry and the mirror neuron system: Simultaneous acquisition of facial electromyography and functional magnetic resonance imaging. *Frontiers in Human Neuroscience, 6*, 214.

Lloyd, D., Di Pellegrino, G., & Roberts, N. (2004). Vicarious responses to pain in anterior cingulate cortex: Is empathy a multisensory issue? *Cognitive, Affective, & Behavioral Neuroscience, 4*(2), 270–278.

Lonsdorf, E. V., Eberly, L. E., & Pusey, A. E. (2004). Sex differences in learning in chimpanzees. *Nature, 428*(6984), 715–716.

Losin, E. A., Dapretto, M., & Iacoboni, M. (2009). Culture in the mind's mirror: How anthropology and neuroscience can inform a model of the neural substrate for cultural imitative learning. *Progress in Brain Research, 178*, 175–190. doi:10.1016/S0079-6123(09)17812-3

Losin, E. A., Dapretto, M., & Iacoboni, M. (2010). Culture and neuroscience: Additive or synergistic? *Social Cognitive Affective Neuroscience, 5*(2–3), 148–158. doi:10.1093/scan/nsp058

Losin, E. A. R., Cross, K. A., Iacoboni, M., & Dapretto, M. (2013). Neural processing of race during imitation: Self-similarity versus social status. *Human Brain Mapping, 35*, 1723–1739. doi:10.1002/hbm.22287

Losin, E. A. R., Iacoboni, M., Martin, A., Cross, K. A., & Dapretto, M. (2012). Race modulates neural activity during imitation. *Neuroimage, 59*(4), 3594–3603. doi:10.1016/j.neuroimage.2011.10.074

Losin, E. A. R., Iacoboni, M., Martin, A., & Dapretto, M. (2012). Own-gender imitation activates the brain's reward circuitry. *Social Cognitive Affective Neuroscience, 7*(7), 804–810. doi:10.1093/scan/nsr055

Losin, E. A. R., Woo, C.-W., Krishnan, A., Wager, T. D., Iacoboni, M., & Dapretto, M. (2015). Brain and psychological mediators of imitation: Sociocultural versus physical traits. *Culture and Brain, 3,* 93–111. doi:10.1007/s40167-015-0029-9

Lotter, V. (1978). Childhood autism in Africa. *Journal of Child Psychology and Psychiatry, 19*(3), 231–244.

Lotter, V. (1980). Cross cultural perspectives on childhood autism. *Journal of Tropical Pediatrics, 26*(4), 131–133.

Lyons, D. E., Young, A. G., & Keil, F. C. (2007). The hidden structure of overimitation. *Proceedings of the National Academy of Sciences, 104*(50), 19751–19756.

Mace, R., & Jordan, F. M. (2011). Macro-evolutionary studies of cultural diversity: A review of empirical studies of cultural transmission and cultural adaptation. *Philosophical Transactions of the Royal Society B: Biological Sciences, 366*(1563), 402–411.

Malenka, R. C., & Nicoll, R. A. (1999). Long-term potentiation—A decade of progress? *Science, 285*(5435), 1870–1874.

Martineau, J., Andersson, F., Barthélémy, C., Cottier, J.-P., & Destrieux, C. (2010). Atypical activation of the mirror neuron system during perception of hand motion in autism. *Brain Research, 1320,* 168–175.

Martineau, J., Cochin, S., Magne, R., & Barthelemy, C. (2008). Impaired cortical activation in autistic children: Is the mirror neuron system involved? *International Journal of Psychophysiology, 68*(1), 35–40.

Matson, J. L., Worley, J. A., Fodstad, J. C., Chung, K.-M., Suh, D., Jhin, H. K., . . . Furniss, F. (2011). A multinational study examining the cross cultural differences in reported symptoms of autism spectrum disorders: Israel, South Korea, the United Kingdom, and the United States of America. *Research in Autism Spectrum Disorders, 5*(4), 1598–1604.

Meltzoff, A. N. (1995). Understanding the intentions of others: Re-enactment of intended acts by 18-month-old children. *Developmental Psychology, 31*(5), 838.

Meltzoff, A. N., & Moore, M. K. (1983). Newborn infants imitate adult facial gestures. *Child Development, 54*(3), 702–709.

Meltzoff, A. N., & Moore, M. K. (1992). Early imitation within a functional framework: The importance of person identity, movement, and development. *Infant Behavior and Development, 15*(4), 479–505.

Mesoudi, A., & Whiten, A. (2008). The multiple roles of cultural transmission experiments in understanding human cultural evolution. *Philosophical Transactions of the Royal Society B: Biological Sciences, 363*(1509), 3489–3501. doi:10.1098/rstb.2008.0129

Milner, B., Squire, L. R., & Kandel, E. R. (1998). Cognitive neuroscience and the study of memory. *Neuron, 20*(3), 445–468.

Mitchell, J. P., Banaji, M. R., & Macrae, C. N. (2005). The link between social cognition and self-referential thought in the medial prefrontal cortex. *Journal of Cognitive Neuroscience, 17*(8), 1306–1315. doi:10.1162/0898929055002418

Mitchell, J. P., Macrae, C. N., & Banaji, M. R. (2006). Dissociable medial prefrontal contributions to judgments of similar and dissimilar others. *Neuron, 50*(4), 655–663. doi:10.1016/j.neuron.2006.03.040

Mobbs, D., Yu, R., Meyer, M., Passamonti, L., Seymour, B., Calder, A. J., . . . Dalgleish, T. (2009). A key role for similarity in vicarious reward. *Science, 324*(5929), 900–900.

Molenberghs, P. (2013). The neuroscience of in-group bias. *Neuroscience & Biobehavioral Reviews, 37*(8), 1530–1536.

Molenberghs, P., Cunnington, R., & Mattingley, J. B. (2009). Is the mirror neuron system involved in imitation? A short review and meta-analysis. *Neuroscience & Biobehavioral Reviews, 33*(7), 975–980.

Molenberghs, P., Halász, V., Mattingley, J. B., Vanman, E. J., & Cunnington, R. (2013). Seeing is believing: Neural mechanisms of action–perception are biased by team membership. *Human Brain Mapping, 34*(9), 2055–2068.

Molnar-Szakacs, I., Wu, A. D., Robles, F. J., & Iacoboni, M. (2007). Do you see what I mean? Corticospinal excitability during observation of culture-specific gestures. *PLoS One, 2*(7), e626. doi:10.1371/journal.pone.0000626

Mukamel, R., Ekstrom, A. D., Kaplan, J., Iacoboni, M., & Fried, I. (2010). Single-neuron responses in humans during execution and observation of actions. *Current Biology, 20*(8), 750–756. doi:10.1016/j.cub.2010.02.045

Newman-Norlund, R. D., van Schie, H. T., van Zuijlen, A. M., & Bekkering, H. (2007). The mirror neuron system is more active during complementary compared with imitative action. *Nature Neuroscience, 10*(7), 817.

Nichols, S., & Stich, S. P. (2003). *Mindreading: An integrated account of pretence, self-awareness, and understanding other minds*: Clarendon Press/Oxford University Press.

O'Doherty, J., Kringelbach, M. L., Rolls, E. T., Hornak, J., & Andrews, C. (2001). Abstract reward and punishment representations in the human orbitofrontal cortex. *Nature Neuroscience, 4*(1), 95.

O'Malley, R. C., Wallauer, W., Murray, C. M., & Goodall, J. (2012). The appearance and spread of ant fishing among the Kasekela chimpanzees of Gombe: A possible case of intercommunity cultural transmission. *Current Anthropology, 53*(5), 650–663.

Oberman, L. M., Hubbard, E. M., McCleery, J. P., Altschuler, E. L., Ramachandran, V. S., & Pineda, J. A. (2005). EEG evidence for mirror neuron dysfunction in autism spectrum disorders. *Cognitive Brain Research, 24*(2), 190–198. doi:10.1016/j.cogbrainres.2005.01.014

Ocampo, B., Kritikos, A., & Cunnington, R. (2011). How frontoparietal brain regions mediate imitative and complementary actions: An fMRI study. *PLoS One, 6*(10), e26945.

Oosterhof, N. N., Wiggett, A. J., Diedrichsen, J., Tipper, S. P., & Downing, P. E. (2010). Surface-based information mapping reveals crossmodal vision–action representations in human parietal and occipitotemporal cortex. *Journal of Neurophysiology, 104*(2), 1077–1089.

Ottoni, E. B., de Resende, B. D., & Izar, P. (2005). Watching the best nutcrackers: What capuchin monkeys (Cebus apella) know about others' tool-using skills. *Animal Cognition, 8*(4), 215–219.

Park, B., Tsai, J. L., Chim, L., Blevins, E., & Knutson, B. (2015). Neural evidence for cultural differences in the valuation of positive facial expressions. *Social Cognitive and Affective Neuroscience, 11*(2), 243–252.

Perrett, D., Mistlin, A., Harries, M., & Chitty, A. (1990). Understanding the visual appearance and consequence of hand actions. In M. A. Goodale (Ed.), *Vision and action: The control of grasping* (pp. 163–342). ABLEX Publishing corporation.

Petrosini, L. (2007). "Do what I do" and "do how I do": Different components of imitative learning are mediated by different neural structures. *The Neuroscientist, 13*(4), 335–348.

Petrosini, L., Graziano, A., Mandolesi, L., Neri, P., Molinari, M., & Leggio, M. G. (2003). Watch how to do it! New advances in learning by observation. *Brain Research Reviews, 42*(3), 252–264.

Plassmann, H., O'Doherty, J. P., & Rangel, A. (2010). Appetitive and aversive goal values are encoded in the medial orbitofrontal cortex at the time of decision making. *Journal of Neuroscience, 30*(32), 10799–10808.

Plotnik, J. M., De Waal, F. B., & Reiss, D. (2006). Self-recognition in an Asian elephant. *Proceedings of the National Academy of Sciences, 103*(45), 17053–17057.

Povinelli, D. J., Gordon, G., Gallup, J., Eddy, T. J., Bierschwale, D., Engstrom, M. C., Perilloux, H. K., & Toxopeus, I. B. (1997). Chimpanzees recognize themselves in mirrors. *Animal Behaviour, 53*(5), 1083–1088.

Press, C., Gillmeister, H., & Heyes, C. (2006). Bottom-up, not top-down, modulation of imitation by human and robotic models. *European Journal of Neuroscience, 24*(8), 2415–2419. doi:10.1111/j.1460-9568.2006.05115.x

Prévost, C., Pessiglione, M., Météreau, E., Cléry-Melin, M.-L., & Dreher, J.-C. (2010). Separate valuation subsystems for delay and effort decision costs. *Journal of Neuroscience, 30*(42), 14080–14090.

Pridmore, S., Brüne, M., Ahmadi, J., & Dale, J. (2008). Echopraxia in schizophrenia: Possible mechanisms. *Australian & New Zealand Journal of Psychiatry, 42*(7), 565–571.

Prinz, W. (2005). An ideomotor approach to imitation. In *Perspectives on imitation: From neuroscience to social science* (Vol. 1, pp. 141–156). MIT Press.

Prior, H., Schwarz, A., & Güntürkün, O. (2008). Mirror-induced behavior in the magpie (Pica pica): Evidence of self-recognition. *PLoS Biology, 6*(8), e202.

Probst, P. (1998). Child health related cognitions of parents with autistic children: A cross-national exploratory study. In U. P. Gielen & A. L. Communian (Eds.), *Family and family therapy in international perspective* (pp. 461–483).

Quilodran, R., Rothe, M., & Procyk, E. (2008). Behavioral shifts and action valuation in the anterior cingulate cortex. *Neuron, 57*(2), 314–325.

Raichle, M. E. (2015). The brain's default mode network. *Annual Review of Neuroscience, 38*, 433–447.

Ramachandran, V. S., & Oberman, L. M. (2006). Broken mirrors: A theory of autism. *Scientific American, 295*(5), 62–69.

Reardon, S. (2014). *Monkey brains wired to share.* Macmillan Publishers.

Reiss, D., & Marino, L. (2001). Mirror self-recognition in the bottlenose dolphin: A case of cognitive convergence. *Proceedings of the National Academy of Sciences, 98*(10), 5937–5942.

Rizzolatti, G., & Craighero, L. (2004). The mirror-neuron system. *Annual Review of Neuroscience, 27,* 169–192. doi:10.1146/annurev.neuro.27.070203.144230

Rizzolatti, G., & Fabbri-Destro, M. (2010). Mirror neurons: From discovery to autism. *Experimental Brain Research, 200*(3–4), 223–237.

Rizzolatti, G., & Fogassi, L. (2014). The mirror mechanism: Recent findings and perspectives. *Philosophical Transactions of the Royal Society B: Biological Sciences, 369*(1644), 20130420.

Rogers, S. J., & Pennington, B. F. (1991). A theoretical approach to the deficits in infantile autism. *Development and Psychopathology, 3*(2), 137–162.

Rolls, E. T. (2000). The orbitofrontal cortex and reward. *Cerebral Cortex, 10*(3), 284–294.

Rushworth, M. F., Noonan, M. P., Boorman, E. D., Walton, M. E., & Behrens, T. E. (2011). Frontal cortex and reward-guided learning and decision-making. *Neuron, 70*(6), 1054–1069.

Saha, S., Chant, D., Welham, J., & McGrath, J. (2005). A systematic review of the prevalence of schizophrenia. *PLoS Medicine, 2*(5), e141.

Samson, D., Apperly, I. A., Kathirgamanathan, U., & Humphreys, G. W. (2005). Seeing it my way: A case of a selective deficit in inhibiting self-perspective. *Brain, 128*(5), 1102–1111.

Saxe, R., Carey, S., & Kanwisher, N. (2004). Understanding other minds: Linking developmental psychology and functional neuroimaging. *Annual Review of Psychology, 55,* 87–124. doi:10.1146/annurev.psych.55.090902.142044

Saxe, R., & Wexler, A. (2005). Making sense of another mind: The role of the right temporo-parietal junction. *Neuropsychologia, 43*(10), 1391–1399. doi:10.1016/j.neuropsychologia.2005.02.013

Schmidt, M. F., Rakoczy, H., & Tomasello, M. (2011). Young children attribute normativity to novel actions without pedagogy or normative language. *Developmental Science, 14*(3), 530–539.

Schreck, K. A., Russell, M., & Vargas, L. A. (2013). Autism treatments in print: Media's coverage of scientifically supported and alternative treatments. *Behavioral Interventions, 28*(4), 299–321.

Schultz, W. (2000). Multiple reward signals in the brain. *Nature Reviews Neuroscience, 1*(3), 199.

Schultz, W. (2006). Behavioral theories and the neurophysiology of reward. *Annual Review of Psychology, 57,* 87–115.

Sescousse, G., Redouté, J., & Dreher, J.-C. (2010). The architecture of reward value coding in the human orbitofrontal cortex. *Journal of Neuroscience, 30*(39), 13095–13104.

Shamay-Tsoory, S. G. (2011). The neural bases for empathy. *The Neuroscientist, 17*(1), 18–24.

Singer, T., Seymour, B., O'Doherty, J., Kaube, H., Dolan, R. J., & Frith, C. D. (2004). Empathy for pain involves the affective but not sensory components of pain. *Science, 303*(5661), 1157–1162.

Sirigu, A., & Duhamel, J.-R. (2016). Reward and decision processes in the brains of humans and nonhuman primates. *Dialogues in Clinical Neuroscience, 18*(1), 45.

Spence, S. A., Brooks, D. J., Hirsch, S. R., Liddle, P. F., Meehan, J., & Grasby, P. M. (1997). A PET study of voluntary movement in schizophrenic patients experiencing passivity phenomena (delusions of alien control). *Brain: A Journal of Neurology, 120*(11), 1997–2011.

Spunt, R. P., & Adolphs, R. (2014). Validating the why/how contrast for functional MRI studies of theory of mind. *Neuroimage, 99,* 301–311.

Suarez, S. D., & Gallup, G. G. (1986). Social responding to mirrors in rhesus macaques (Macaca mulatta): Effects of changing mirror location. *American Journal of Primatology, 11*(3), 239–244.

Suárez, S. D., & Gallup Jr., G. G. (1981). Self-recognition in chimpanzees and orangutans, but not gorillas. *Journal of Human Evolution, 10*(2), 175–188.

Tai, Y. F., Scherfler, C., Brooks, D. J., Sawamoto, N., & Castiello, U. (2004). The human premotor cortex is 'mirror' only for biological actions. *Current Biology, 14*(2), 117–120.

Tanaka, S. C., Doya, K., Okada, G., Ueda, K., Okamoto, Y., & Yamawaki, S. (2004). Prediction of immediate and future rewards differentially recruits cortico-basal ganglia loops. *Nature Neuroscience, 7*(8), 887.

Telzer, E. H., Humphreys, K. L., Shapiro, M., & Tottenham, N. (2013). Amygdala sensitivity to race is not present in childhood but emerges over adolescence. *Journal of Cognitive Neuroscience, 25*(2), 234–244.

Teyler, T. J., & DiScenna, P. (1987). Long-term potentiation. *Annual Review of Neuroscience, 10*(1), 131–161.

Tom, S. M., Fox, C. R., Trepel, C., & Poldrack, R. A. (2007). The neural basis of loss aversion in decision-making under risk. *Science, 315*(5811), 515–518.

Tomasello, M. (1990). Cultural transmission in the tool use and communicatory signaling of chimpanzees? In S. T. Parker & K. R. Gibson (Eds.), *"Language" and intelligence in monkeys and apes: Comparative developmental perspectives* (pp. 274–311). Cambridge University Press. doi:10.1017/CBO9780511665486.012

Tomasello, M. (1999). The human adaptation for culture. *Annual Review of Anthropology, 28*, 509–529.

Tomasello, M. (2016). Cultural learning redux. *Child Development, 87*(3), 643–653.

Tomasello, M., Carpenter, M., Call, J., Behne, T., & Moll, H. (2005). Understanding and sharing intentions: The origins of cultural cognition. *Behavioral and Brain Sciences, 28*(5), 675–691; discussion 691–735.

Tomasello, M., Kruger, A. C., & Ratner, H. H. (1993). Cultural learning. *Behavioral and Brain Sciences, 16*(3), 495–511.

Uddin, L. Q., Kaplan, J. T., Molnar-Szakacs, I., Zaidel, E., & Iacoboni, M. (2005). Self-face recognition activates a frontoparietal "mirror" network in the right hemisphere: An event-related fMRI study. *Neuroimage, 25*(3), 926–935. doi:10.1016/j.neuroimage.2004.12.018

van de Waal, E., Borgeaud, C., & Whiten, A. (2013). Potent social learning and conformity shape a wild primate's foraging decisions. *Science, 340*(6131), 483–485.

van de Waal, E., & Whiten, A. (2012). Spontaneous emergence, imitation and spread of alternative foraging techniques among groups of vervet monkeys. *PLoS One, 7*(10), e47008.

Van Overwalle, F., & Baetens, K. (2009). Understanding others' actions and goals by mirror and mentalizing systems: A meta-analysis. *Neuroimage, 48*(3), 564–584. doi:10.1016/j.neuroimage.2009.06.009

Vivanti, G., Hocking, D. R., Fanning, P., & Dissanayake, C. (2016). Social affiliation motives modulate spontaneous learning in Williams syndrome but not in autism. *Molecular Autism, 7*(1), 40.

Vogeley, K., Bussfeld, P., Newen, A., Herrmann, S., Happé, F., Falkai, P., . . . Zilles, K. (2001). Mind reading: Neural mechanisms of theory of mind and self-perspective. *Neuroimage, 14*(1 Pt 1), 170–181. doi:10.1006/nimg.2001.0789

Walton, M. E., Behrens, T. E., Buckley, M. J., Rudebeck, P. H., & Rushworth, M. F. (2010). Separable learning systems in the macaque brain and the role of orbitofrontal cortex in contingent learning. *Neuron, 65*(6), 927–939.

Wang, Y., & Hamilton, A. F. d. C. (2012). Social top-down response modulation (STORM): A model of the control of mimicry in social interaction. *Frontiers in Human Neuroscience, 6*.

Whitehouse, H. (2011). The coexistence problem in psychology, anthropology, and evolutionary theory. *Human Development, 54*(3), 191–199.

Whitehouse, H. (2012). Ritual, cognition, and evolution. In R. Sun (Ed.), *Grounding social sciences in cognitive sciences* (p. 265). MIT Press.

Whiten, A., & van de Waal, E. (2016). Social learning, culture and the 'socio-cultural brain' of human and non-human primates. *Neuroscience & Biobehavioral Reviews, 82*, 58–75.

Wicker, B., Keysers, C., Plailly, J., Royet, J.-P., Gallese, V., & Rizzolatti, G. (2003). Both of us disgusted in my insula: The common neural basis of seeing and feeling disgust. *Neuron, 40*(3), 655–664.

Williams, J. H., Whiten, A., Suddendorf, T., & Perrett, D. I. (2001). Imitation, mirror neurons and autism. *Neuroscience & Biobehavioral Reviews, 25*(4), 287–295.

Williams Syndrome Association. (2018). What is William's syndrome? https://williams-syndrome.org/what-is-ws

Xu, X., Zuo, X., Wang, X., & Han, S. (2009). Do you feel my pain? Racial group membership modulates empathic neural responses. *Journal of Neuroscience, 29*(26), 8525–8529. doi:10.1523/JNEUROSCI.2418-09.2009

Yang, D. Y., Rosenblau, G., Keifer, C., & Pelphrey, K. A. (2015). An integrative neural model of social perception, action observation, and theory of mind. *Neuroscience and Biobehavioral Reviews, 51*, 263–275. doi:10.1016/j.neubiorev.2015.01.020

Zahm, D. S. (2000). An integrative neuroanatomical perspective on some subcortical substrates of adaptive responding with emphasis on the nucleus accumbens. *Neuroscience & Biobehavioral Reviews, 24*(1), 85–105.

Zentall, T. R. (2006). Imitation: Definitions, evidence, and mechanisms. *Animal Cognition, 9*(4), 335–353. doi:10.1007/s10071-006-0039-2

Zhang, K., Wang, H., Dong, G., Wang, M., Zhang, J., Zhang, H., . . . Du, X. (2016). Neural activation during imitation with or without performance feedback: An fMRI study. *Neuroscience Letters, 629*, 202–207.

Zhu, Y., Zhang, L., Fan, J., & Han, S. (2007). Neural basis of cultural influence on self-representation. *Neuroimage, 34*(3), 1310–1316. doi:10.1016/j.neuroimage.2006.08.047

Culture and Dehumanization: A Case Study of the Doctor–Patient Paradigm and Implications for Global Health

Emily P. Sands *and* Lasana T. Harris

Abstract

Dehumanization manifests itself in people's everyday lives. Through a dehumanization lens, one can deconstruct and comprehend many aggressive behavioral trends that are not always overt expressions of bias but rather continuous and pervasive cultural and societal tendencies. However, dehumanization may also have benefits, facilitating pro-social behaviors in medical contexts. This chapter will explore how dehumanization manifests in intergroup, objectifying, and dietary contexts, comparing these to the doctor-patient relationship. It then reviews emerging research in the medical context where dehumanization may be beneficial, contrasting it with the more notorious aforementioned instances. Since dehumanization manifests itself constantly and ubiquitously in modern society, pulling apart such intricacies allows one to identify, understand, and intervene with the intention of highlighting the beneficial and detrimental effects dehumanization has on global health. Importantly, this chapter will evaluate and explore dehumanization from a cultural neuroscience perspective rather than from a social processing viewpoint, with the intention of demystifying the functionality of the fundamental cognitive practices that generate the behaviors seen in dehumanization practices.

Key Words: dehumanization, infrahumanization, cultural neuroscience, doctor–patient relationship, interspecies prejudice, objectification, flexible social cognition, global mental health

Introduction

Dehumanization is often conceptualized as an overt discriminatory act against another person or group of people with the intent of denying them varying opportunities, experiences, political rights, and basic human needs (Fiske, 2013a). This renunciation comes in the form of a distorted belief system in which those who are dehumanized are denied mental states, a prerequisite for humanness, and therefore are excluded from moral protection (Harris, 2017). In other words, people *essentialize* the dehumanized, reserving the human "essence" for those who are humanized (those who are attributed an inner life or mind). This creates a distinction between self and other, where "human" represents the self. Importantly, dehumanization serves several self regulatory functions within social interactions; it facilitates behavior reserved for nonhuman entities (Bandura et al., 1996; Bar-Tal, 1998; Opotow, 1990), it regulates emotional responses and intrusive thoughts that could harm goal pursuit (Cameron et al., 2015; Shaw et al., 1994), or it provides a post hoc justification for immoral behavior (Castano & Giner-Sorrolla, 2006). Moreover, dehumanization can be manifested explicitly or subtly (Harris & Fiske, 2006, 2009; Kteily et al., 2015; Leyens et al., 2001, 2003). It is this latter form of dehumanization that we intend to explore and analyze, since it pertains to a social interaction rife with dehumanization: the doctor–patient relationship.

The doctor–patient relationship is complex in nature, paternalistic, and asymmetrical. Doctors are expected to be authoritative while also taking on the roles of teachers, caregivers, and empathetic listeners. This extremely complex and precarious relationship forms a continuous balance of cognitions, emotions, and behaviors for the physician; it requires a conscious and involved compartmentalization and deployment of cognitions and emotions, as well as a disengagement or suppression of cognitions and emotions, particularly when medical interventions require behavior atypical of generic social interactions. The problem solving and beneficial compulsion of mechanization (imagining patients as mechanical organisms made up of interacting parts) is a necessity when operating surgically, designing treatment plans, and accepting the body's limitations (Haque & Waytz, 2012). Therefore, dehumanization in these instances may allow a vital therapeutic disengagement from the patient's internal states, complicating and highlighting the cognitive, behavioral, and social complexities of dehumanization.

Dehumanization has broad implications for global mental health. How does dehumanization manifest itself in our daily lives broadly, and the medical context specifically? What are the effects on global health and safety? How do professionals, when possible, identify, prevent, and intervene? To consider these questions, we will begin by reviewing three functions of dehumanization within distinct contexts: post hoc justification motivating infrahumanization of social groups, bodies as a means to an end during sexual objectification, and proactive emotion regulation employed to facilitate meat consumption. Specifically, we begin by deconstructing the literature on infrahumanization, comparing symbolic versus real threats to outline the psychological conditions that lead to distorted cognition, affect, and behavior in group settings. A cross-cultural analysis of Eastern and Western cultures will provide a framework for a case study on immigration and asylum seekers with the intent of highlighting the underlying behaviors and outcomes of infrahumanization, and its role in post hoc justification of attitudes toward and policy against immigrants. Secondly, we will review dehumanization manifesting as objectification by deconstructing the literature on sexual and self-objectification (Fiske, 2005; Qingqing et al., 2013). We will use the example of pornography (Western and explicit) in juxtaposition to culturally sanctioned sexual harassment (pervasive and implicit) in varying societal contexts. We will then conceptualize objectification as a tool used in systems of dominance and oppression. Next, we will review research on meat consumption as a manifestation of dehumanization. We will use an interspecies model of prejudice to examine religious and cultural practices in relation to meat consumption. Specifically, we will review literature on meat consumption trends and examine the differences between carnivorous and vegetarian practices, and the potential of these contrasts to cast light on larger societal dehumanizing trends. Finally, we will juxtapose the discussion of dehumanization thus far with dehumanization in medical contexts, looking specifically at the doctor–patient relationship. Through this lens, we will conclude that dehumanization can serve as a proactive emotion regulatory strategy in medical contexts, rather than as a means to an end or post hoc justification.

There is no denying that the complexities and challenges of understanding the psychological mechanisms of dehumanization are daunting at best. However, the goal of this chapter is to clarify and streamline research and findings with the intent of highlighting literature that helps delineate and separate the stages and manifestations of dehumanization within the medical context. Our aim is to not only highlight important research across disciplines but also stimulate conversation about the implicit behaviors, affects, and cognitions that create, maintain, and propagate dehumanization trends in our everyday lives, and the broader implications dehumanization has on global health.

Infrahumanization as Post Hoc Justification

Infrahumanization research stems from a well-known theory and intellectual tradition of social identity (Tajfel, 1974). People intellectualize their identities through the personification of their group membership. This perspective argues that stereotyping is a normal cognitive process, allowing us to rationalize and understand our identity and social group memberships. This results in an us-versus-them mentality. The desire to categorize and separate socially often leads to an exaggeration of group differences and similarities. Infrahumanization research demonstrates that we associate more uniquely secondary human emotions to our ingroup and deny these complex emotions to those outside of our group, while attributing primary emotions equally to both ingroups and outgroups (Viki & Abrams, 2003, Leyens et al., 2001, 2007). Secondary emotions can only be attributed to human beings because they require the perceiver to infer the mental states of the target, while basic emotions can be attributed to human and nonhuman animals because they lack this requirement (Viki & Abrams, 2003).

Neuroscience research on dehumanization supports the mental state inference hypothesis; it characterizes dehumanization as a form of flexible social cognition (mental state inference) where one suppresses or fails to engage social cognitive processing in the presence of another human being (see Harris & Fiske, 2009, for a review). In the brain, parts of the neocortex, including the medial prefrontal cortex (mPFC), precuneus, and temporoparietal junction (TPJ) extending along the superior temporal sulcus (STS) to the anterior temporal pole (ATP) and posterior cingulate cortex (PCC), trigger social perception and awareness (see Fourie et al., 2014; Mars et al., 2012; Van Overwalle, 2011). These brain regions are less engaged during dehumanization, providing physiological evidence for this phenomenon (Harris & Fiske, 2006, 2007, 2011). Social contexts, group dynamics, goals, and other socially derived individual personifications determine whether the social cognition brain network is engaged to a dehumanized target (Harris & Fiske, 2007).

Therefore, we can conceptualize infrahumanization as an act of disconnecting what are considered uniquely human traits from people outside of our social and cultural connections. These disconnects can come in the form of physical features associated with being human, or the denial of attributes associated with human nature such as higher emotions, religiosity, and intellect (Bain et al., 2009). As such, infrahumanization may be used to legitimize war and violence; warring factions often minimize their enemy's human emotions through animal epithets, a psychological technique that helps rationalize violent acts by reducing responsibility, regulating conflicting emotions, and rationalizing the ingroup's superiority over the enemy (Bain, et al., 2009).

Research has examined the rationalization of violence towards others by studying how the perception of violence, (direct or indirect) effects the magnitude of infrahumanization on outgroup members (Castano & Giner-Sorolla, 2006; Motyl et al., 2010). In one study, researchers described violent transgressions of Americans of European descent against Native Americans, then explored the attribution of emotions to Native Americans by modern American participants of predominantly European descent. The violent transgressions were described either directly through acts of genocide or indirectly through disease. The results concluded that infrahumanization of Native Americans was stronger in the case of genocidal acts than disease, consequently supporting the hypothesis that denying full human status to victims allows perpetrators to disengage from collective responsibility of genocidal acts generationally (Castano & Giner-Sorolla, 2006).

Importantly, infrahumanization is not just an issue of the past, but continues today. To conceptualize how infrahumanization may lead to dehumanizing behaviors, we must first analyze the underlying causes of our judgments of others and our grouping mentality (Ibanez et al., 2009). Researchers of social cognition, evolution, personality psychology, neuroscience, and sociology have all debated and theorized about prejudicial manifestations among groups. Early theorists tended to emphasize the significance of direct and explicit practices of prejudice (e.g., Adorno, 1950; Dollard et al., 1939, Sherif, 1961), while modern theorists often emphasize indirect and implicit (benevolent and ambivalent) forms of prejudicial behavior (Glick & Fiske,1996; Dovidio et al., 2009; Fiske et al., 2019; Sherman et al., 2005; Pettigrew & Meertens, 2005). Recent research highlights the interplay of these two concepts, particularly how judgments of others can be extremely paradoxical in nature and do not operate in isolation, but rather in tandem with both attitudes and behavior. The important marrying of two opposing theories allows for a more holistic and complete picture of the complexities surrounding infrahumanization and intergroup relations.

Social dominance theory (SDT; Sidanius & Pratto,1999), which identifies the underlying cognitive and behavioral mechanisms that create and maintain group-based inequalities, is one of the main pillars of the Leyens et al. (2001) theory of infrahumanization. SDT postulates that the use of force and discrimination among groups can be disguised or made acceptable by cultural ideologies termed *legitimizing myths*. These myths are widely accepted beliefs (stereotypes) and emotional responses (prejudices) that become the doctrine in maintaining the ingroup and outgroup hierarchical structure (Fiske, 2013b). Infrahumanization delineates further from *legitimizing myths* into realistic threats (threats to the existence or well-being of the ingroup) and symbolic threats (related to the differences between groups in terms of beliefs, morals, and standards, challenging the ingroup's worldview; Leyens et al., 2001). Both materialize in explicit and implicit prejudices, forming the underlying justifications for dehumanizing outgroup members.

To conceptualize infrahumanization in a global context, one can consider the current political climate between the West and Middle East. Western allies currently are using the legitimizing myths of security, counterterrorism, and freedom fighters, in conjunction with the stereotypical contrasting views of their enemies as brutal and barbaric, to justify war, close borders to refugees, and politicize isolationist policies (Álvarez-Gálvez & Salvador-Carulla, 2013). For example, research on the effects of dehumanization and Islamophobia attempted to establish the degree to which infrahumanization and explicit dehumanization of Syrian refugees within a Spanish population existed (Gómez-Martínez & Moral-Jiménez, 2018). Researchers postulated that those who believed that the Syrian refugees were victims would have lower scores on both implicit and explicit dehumanization measures compared with those who viewed the refugees as a threat to Europe. Researchers were also interested in the relationship between Islamophobia and dehumanization and predicted that people who scored higher on racism measures would also score higher on infrahumanization and dehumanization measures. The results indicated that the mean attribution score of positive feelings toward the Syrian refugees was much lower than the mean score of positive feelings attributed to the control ingroup. This difference in the ingroup and outgroup scores highlights the lack of empathy toward Syrian refugees regarding their vulnerability and need for humanitarian care. The findings draw attention to the detrimental social and political effects that implicit forms of infrahumanization can have on vulnerable populations.

What can be established from this example is that the potential long-term effects on political and social stability are problematic if we consider the outcome of this study and others like it (Motyl et al., 2010). It is in some respects fair to make the leap that infrahumanization and dehumanization are currently changing the global, political, and social climate through examples such as Brexit, walling off the Mexican border, repealing the Dream Act in the United States, and continued disagreements about refugees and immigrants throughout Europe. This study and others like it (Falomir-Pichastor & Frederic, 2013), uncover the cognitive and social mechanisms that foster and dictate the cycle of prejudicial behavior, resulting in the inevitable questions concerning the propensities of human nature. Predominantly, there is a pendulum effect of our social and psychological inclinations and the modern predicaments that test our ability to identify, regulate, and control these evolutionary misgivings. Juxtaposing the detrimental effects of dehumanization to its potential evolutionary benefits, (a proactive emotion regulatory strategy in medical contexts, for example) should not be overlooked but rather recognized as a significant factor in understanding the entirety of its cognitive and behavioral functionality, particularly in relation to the repercussions on global mental health.

Objectification as a Means to an End

Research on sexual objectification has been colored with political, social, and cultural clashes within the feminist, scientific, and political community. Depending on the point of view of the theorist, pornography lies on a scale in relation to its detrimental outcomes. Radical feminist and theorist Russell (1993) sees pornography as "material that combines sex . . . the exposure of genitals with abuse or degradation in the manner that appears to endorse or encourage such behavior" (p. 3). Radical feminists Mackinnon & Dworkin (1998) similarly conceptualize pornography as "the sexually explicit subordination of women, graphically depicted, whether in pictures or words" (p. 512). Contradictorily, liberal feminists define pornography as multifaceted and note that it cannot be simply portrayed as male domination versus female subordination but rather a part of a complex political, social, and power structure that is individually defined (McElroy, 2008).

The use of pornography is consistent with objectification theory (Fredrickson & Roberts, 1997), defined as the stripping away of a person's humanity, mind, and morality, equating a person to an inanimate object. At its core, objectification of others is a socially sanctioned dehumanizing process that denies an individual autonomy, agency, and subjectivity, often with the intent to reduce a person to a body part (Fredrickson & Roberts, 1997). Objectification is multidimensional in nature, and all humans, (men, women, and children) are objectified in varied ways across cultures with distinct consequences. In this section, we will examine dehumanization as a strategy to treat people as a means to an end and discuss the detrimental effects objectification has on societies at interpersonal, political, and cultural levels, before relating it to dehumanization in the medical context.

Sexual objectification research helps us to understand how contextual factors impact women's lives, specifically how their bodies can be used as a tool of oppression by those who wish to control and legitimize patriarchal ideologies (Dworkin, 1999; MacKinnon, 1987, 1989, 2006). The discussion surrounding the effects of pornography as an explicit form of sexual objectification has been a topic of discussion in law and in the feminist arena for decades. There is ample research that pornography is linked to physical and emotional crimes committed against women (Dworkin, 1999; MacKinnon, 1987, 1989, 2006). However, pornography is a billion-dollar industry that persists throughout the world. Its effects are not only explicit in nature but also an important link and clue to the pervasive and implicit forms of sexually sanctioned objectification that occurs in the daily lives of women across the globe, exposing how macro-aggressions (sex industries, human trafficking, pornography, women in advertising) can function as a precondition to micro-aggressions (implicit bias, body shaming, victim blaming, sexist language, and sexual harassment, to name a few). This highlights the complex feedback loop that maintains objectification patterns within Western societies through the legitimization of behaviors that diminish women physically and mentally.

From a cognitive and behavioral perspective rather than a philosophical one, pornography is an antisocial behavior that is publicly permitted, making its dehumanizing attributes acceptable, appropriate, and justified. Many scholars conceptualize pornography as a threatening but legally sanctioned tool used in systems of dominance and oppression. For example, pornography's violent images of women have been linked to the violent sexual behavior of men (Berger, 1977). Feminist and theorist Russell (1993) vividly depicts a perpetrator's justification for forcing oral sex onto his victim through socially sanctioned and commercialized media: "I had seen far-out stuff in movies and thought it would be fun to mentally and physically torture a woman" (p. 214). This type dehumanized socialization exemplifies how pornography is not just fantasy, but rather a reflection of how patriarchal ideologies fetishize and conceptualize women's bodies, minds, roles, and functions within Western societies. Radical feminist Mackinnon (1997) clearly describes this phenomenon as follows: "Men treat women as whom they see women to be and porn constructs this image" (p. 197).

Recent research on image and objectification of females took the rationalization and legitimization of overtly discriminatory behavior further by analyzing local versus global processing in cognition in relation to sexual objectification practices (Gervais et al., 2012). The study tested the hypothesis of a bias in sexual body part recognition by showing participants male and female sexualized body parts, in isolation and in the context of the entire body. Results confirmed the sexual body part recognition bias; women's sexualized body parts, when presented in isolation, were more easily identified, while men's sexual body parts were more recognizable in the context of the entire body (Gervais et al., 2012). Interestingly, the effects were not gender specific; both men and women objectified women's bodies to sexual parts, highlighting the power of social influences, the potential for self-objectification, and the perpetuation of male stereotypes consistent with pornography (Mackinnon, 1998). The detriments to mental health linked with objectification through imagery such as pornography illustrates how a macro-aggression reflects societal expectations, becomes a sanctioned form of infrahumanization, and thus leads to dehumanization of the self and others on an immense scale. Objectification theory synthesizes the vast amount of research on objectification, obliterating the political and social justifications for blaming female-related mental illnesses on women by substantiating with evidence that extreme and pervasive tendencies to equate women with their bodies can have dangerous consequences for women's mental health (Fredrickson & Roberts, 1997).

Macro-aggressions and micro-aggressions are complex and interlinked, working to construct and maintain the status quo, minimizing the status of women in their daily lives while also maximizing its desired effect and control through larger avenues of influence. By these means dehumanization can facilitate the processing of people as a means to an end. Many academics believe that the most effective form of dehumanization is the covert micro-aggressions that are systematically deployed through daily degradation and oppression to the individual, eventually converting the minds of those oppressed (Zurbriggen, 2013). To demonstrate this concept, we can look to the pivotal work on ambivalent sexism and the complex patterns of explicit and implicit prejudicial beliefs that lead to discriminatory behaviors at an intergroup level (Glick & Fiske, 1996, 2001; Viki & Abrams 2003). Sexist attitudes come in two forms: hostile sexism and benevolent sexism. Hostile sexism is defined as expressing overt hostility toward women who specifically challenge male power, while by contrast benevolent sexism refers to attitudes that are seemingly supportive in nature and harmless (Glick & Fiske, 1996, 2001). For example, benevolent sexism would take the form of an apparent compliment having the implication that women are fragile and need protection, that they are only nurturers of children, and that they represent kindness and understanding (Glick & Fiske, 1996, 2001). These seemingly benign and ambivalent judgments on the inherited traits of women bind them to conventional gender roles by encouraging the admiration of women and men who conform to these ideals and contempt for those who challenge them. In other words, one's membership within the group and secondary humanizing characteristics are questioned and often stripped from one's identity if one challenges the symbolic identifying features of the group. This illustration shows the danger of benevolent prejudice through its covert behaviors and its ability to create conforming reactions without drawing notice, thus forming, maintaining, and generating antipathy between groups (Glick & Fiske 1996, 2001).

The term *self-objectification* encompasses this phenomenon, where the oppressed internalize societal expectations by conforming, policing, and even acting against those within their group who do not conform. A categorical system created by psychologists is often used as a tool to help identify the stages of self-objectification as a means for victims to regain a chosen sense of self through the identification of their oppression. The stages include the observer perspective, negative beliefs about self and own group, negative actions against own group, and identification with the aggressor (Zurbriggen, 2013). Self-objectification is behaviorally and psychologically complex because the woman is both the perpetrator and the victim. By maintaining and propagating patriarchal ideals and norms, women are inadvertently negatively impacting their cognitive functions and behaviors including body shaming, appearance anxiety, disordered eating, depression, and sexual dysfunction (Calogero et al., 2011; Qingqing et al., 2013).

Although this is only a brief overview of sexual objectification, it illustrates the complexity of the problem at every structural level. The need for continued interdisciplinary research particularly in institutionally sanctioned oppression and its generational effects, is an area of great importance and concern. Research on oppression needs to extend beyond theory and become applicable to public officials, educators, and medical professionals who can initiate local and global change.

The Meat Paradox as Proactive Emotion Regulation

One argument about the roots of human prejudices against outgroups stems from our belief about the human–animal divide, which normally includes the assumption that humans are superior to animals (Allen et al., 2000). This concept originates from the *interspecies model of prejudice*, which hypothesizes that the greater the human–animal divide within a culture, the more likely we are to dehumanize each other, particularly those outside of our ingroup, increasing our prejudices and representing outsiders as "animal-like" (Allen et al., 2000). The root of this argument is that if we legitimize animals by making them equal, we will be unable to use them as markers for social worth in human-to-human interactions. Recent research has shown that individuals who demonstrate higher levels of prejudicial beliefs toward humans are more willing to show exploitative behavior towards animals, and vice versa (Dhont et al., 2014).

Theorists believe that humans who view themselves superior to animals rationalize and legitimize their behaviors because of their ideological belief systems. Ideologies can be conflicting in nature, contradictory, and easily distorted. For example, in one instance a person is volunteering to save the elephants from poachers while happily consuming meat. Researchers coin this concept the "meat paradox." Although most humans care for animals and do not want to see them harmed, this concern is conditional, allowing mistreatment if it is beneficial to humans, particularly in relation to consumption. In this section, the moral paradox of dehumanization manifesting as meat consumption will be explored by analyzing the contradictions, manifestations, and repercussions of our choices, before relating them to the medical context.

Animal categories are artificially and culturally bound. The treatment of animals can be categorized into three basic classifications that are cross-cultural: pets, wild animals, and farm animals (Allen et al., 2000). The closer the animal is in relation to the human within a cultural framework, the better the treatment of that animal. For instance, in many Western cultures, dogs are pets and are intimate parts of families, whereas cows are farm animals, disconnected from the home and therefore ranked lower on the human–animal divide, and are seen as food. Cultures in Eastern and Western Asia treat dogs in some instances as food (China), street animals (India), and unclean pests (Saudi Arabia), while cows may be considered sacred (India). Thus, the animal–human divide is arbitrary and culturally dependent (Dhont et al., 2014). Such divides permeate our moral ideologies, allowing us to disengage and emotionally regulate consumption choices as being perfectly acceptable because they are culturally sanctioned.

To better understand how the animal–human divide manifests and is culturally bound, researchers in New Zealand compared the values and beliefs of vegetarians and carnivores, hypothesizing that meat consumption habits correlate directly with our political and social ideologies (Allen & Ng, 2003). Results validated the hypothesis; carnivores were more likely to endorse principles associated with hierarchal social structures and dominating political ideologies, while also placing less importance on emotion and feelings (Allen & Ng, 2003). Those who leaned toward conscious food consumption, (vegans and vegetarians) were more concerned with emotions and less connected to hierarchal structures and dominance-related ideologies (Allen & Ng, 2003). Research conducted in the United States replicated this finding by demonstrating that right-wing political supporters consumed more meat and exploited animals more frequently than their liberal counterparts (Dhont & Hodson, 2014). The researchers highlighted two findings: (a) right-wing supporters are threatened by and push back against vegetarianism and veganism due to their traditions and cultural beliefs, and (b) they showed a stronger and more significant distinction between humans and animals, viewing themselves superior, consistent with their ideologies, beliefs, and attitudes (Dhont & Hodson, 2014). These findings suggest that dehumanization may facilitate meat consumption by reducing negative emotional experiences that result from viewing animals as similar to humans.

Current empirical research shows promising support of the interspecies model of prejudice. Specifically, it reveals how human value systems, symbolism, and an individual's endorsements and adherence to certain ideologies indicates the development of dehumanization tendencies towards species (Allen et al., 2000). A recent study analyzed this concept further, identifying specific human traits linked to dehumanizing behaviors via the social dominance orientation (SDO) spectrum and Universal Orientation scale (UOS; Costello & Hodson, 2009). Those who scored higher on the SDO and lower on the UOS were more likely to reject human-to-animal similarities and more likely to dehumanize immigrants, reiterating the significance of the animal–human divide (Costello & Hodson, 2009).

The implications of these studies are meaningful in that we can potentially identify characteristics, ideologies, and attitudes that are connected to dehumanization. However, the philosophical questions surrounding meat consumption, the validity of these studies, and the direct links to dehumanization are still debatable. Although dehumanization and meat consumption appear to be correlated, there is not necessarily a direct causation as many confounding variables might be associated with this connection. Meat eating is also an inherent part of the human diet across history and cultures. Many cultures and societies did not and still do not have the luxury of choice when nutrients are needed for survival.

Nevertheless, the research points out that those whose views exacerbate the difference between humans and animals do indeed dehumanize outgroup members more often (Costello & Hodson, 2009). The reasoning behind this is still highly contested but none the less still important to consider. An important connection can be made with the role of proactive emotional regulation as a cognitive consequence of dehumanization, which is shared with the doctor–patient paradigm. People who consume meat may actively engage in resolving moral conflicts through restructuring and rationalizing their cognitive dissonance, in the same way that doctors rationalize "hurting" a patient (surgery, for example) to help a patient (healing). They are, in effect, partaking in a similar cognitive operation that allows them to act in ways that would normally conflict with their moral and ideological framework.

Nevertheless, as will be shown with the doctor–patient illustration, it is important to acknowledge how the cognitive mechanism associated with the positive effects of dehumanization as a cognitive coping function can have negative societal outcomes. Education is at the root of change when it comes to understanding when and how dehumanization can be used as a pro social tool (such as a doctor using cognitive dissociation to cope with surgery), rather than a negative consequence of a prejudicial justification. Recent research (and ordinary human experience over millennia) has shown that values may be changed by early education; such education or "recategorization" via reconnecting the humanness of the outgroup member to the ingroup created more empathetic feelings and positive connections (Costello & Hodson, 2009). Malleability goes in both directions, highlighting the ease with which humans can be manipulated and controlled without conscious awareness as an important implication within itself, and more research in this area is needed. The cognitive mechanisms through which beliefs in human superiority develop, how these mechanisms affect our behaviors toward animals and humans, and how ideologies mold our cognitive perceptions of reality are important in the continued growth of how cognition is affected by context.

Doctor–Patient Paradigm

Dehumanization in virtually all cases enables people to experience fewer moral concerns by reducing empathy. As illustrated by the case studies of infrahumanization, objectification, and the meat paradox, the reduction of empathy (a negative emotional experience) leads to behavior that has detrimental individual and societal implications, whether assessed from a systemic or mental health perspective. This prejudicial behavior is legitimized and perpetuated by the ingroup's ideologies and cultural and societal norms, making dehumanization and its fallout difficult to identify and prevent. However, in juxtaposition to these models, dehumanization may have evolutionary functionality, principally to regulate emotion and to compartmentalize conflicting moral dilemmas with the purpose of alleviating cognitive dissonance. Medical practice and the doctor–patient paradigm provide quintessential examples of how dehumanization can function as a beneficial cognitive and behavioral tool, not resulting from malevolent intent but rather working as an integral function of medicine, a necessity for both problem solving and emotional regulation. Here we will discuss dehumanization as a functional cognitive and behavioral strategy in the doctor–patient paradigm, conceptually analyzing dehumanization through mechanization, empathy reduction, and moral disengagement (Haque & Waltz, 2012).

Mechanization is the act of considering a human as a mechanical system made up of interacting parts rather than an emotional being (Haslam, 2006, 2007). This concept closely resembles objectification but differs because of its intent and functionality. Doctors conceptualize humans as body parts to become better doctors. For example, when operating (surgery) and when problem solving (treatment plans, medical procedures, diagnosis), if doctors are concerned with the emotional aspect of the patient rather than the mechanical, the outcome could be less than ideal due to the moral dilemma of hurting and healing. In this example, compartmentalization of emotional activation allows a disengagement that is beneficial to the physician and the patient (Haque & Waltz, 2012). Medical problem solving often necessitates focusing on the human as a system, understanding how pharmacological factors interplay and work within this system, testing and probing, and planning and preparing what can often be uncomfortable or painful treatments (Haque & Waltz, 2012). Although one can make the argument, and many do, that doctors need to treat the entire patient, not just the parts, there are functional and legitimizing reasons to dehumanize patients in many circumstances (Haque & Waltz, 2012).

Diminishing the patient to mechanical parts requires the physician to engage in empathy reduction. Recent research in neuroscience examined pain empathy in physicians who practice acupuncture (Decety et al., 2010). The physicians watched films depicting body parts being pricked with needles and conversely being touched with cotton swabs. The study found that physicians showed significantly less brain activation over prefrontal cortex areas associated with empathy for pain than their civilian counterparts. Importantly, the physicians also showed significantly greater activation in areas involved in executive control and self-regulation, suggesting that they adjusted their emotional response due to the demands of their profession and the normalization of repetitive medical procedures (Decety et al., 2010).

Once again, the previous example shows that neural mechanisms are an intricate and essential aspect of dehumanization. This study furthers the evidence that the prefrontal cortex affects both our innate ability and our learned ability to dehumanize. With the potential for the prefrontal cortex to change and evolve as antisocial behaviors become more normalized, there is evidence that dehumanization may be more malleable then originally assumed. If it is a behavior that is both innate and affected by the environment, more research in perceptual processes could uncover important findings for outcomes in global mental health. This research also suggests that continued activation of the prefrontal cortex is what leads to reduced emotional engagement, which leads to more cognitive resources and thus the enhancement of executive functions and problem-solving abilities, an interesting phenomenon and potentially positive effect of the neurological processes of dehumanization.

Importantly, medical training encourages the regulation of negative emotional responses for this precise reason via a "hidden curriculum." If a physician is cognitively taxed with continuous empathetic concern for their patient, limited cognitive resources remain available for executive functions such as problem solving. Before entrance into medical school, medical students report higher-than-normal levels of empathy compared with the general student population and continue to feel higher-than-normal levels of empathy through the initial experience of medical school (Hojat et al., 2009). However, there is a drastic decline in empathy as soon as students have contact with patients during their training. This decline continues throughout training and into practice, showing how education and context can change emotional regulation practices (Neumann et al., 2011).

Recent research proposes that the brain networks involved in both social and nonsocial problem-solving strategies are inverse, indicating that there is a trade-off that occurs (Whitfield-Gabrieli et al., 2009). In addition to neuroscientific evidence, behaviorally and psychologically there seems to be evidence that executive functioning and problem solving during complex medical examinations and procedures inherently diminish empathy and increase dehumanization. This may be beneficial when the need to deliver effective care is essential and humanizing patients increases stress and decreases objectivity (Di Bernardo et al., 2011). It is clear that in the medical context dehumanizing patients is a useful behavior for physicians when they need to cope with stress and discomfort, especially when the stakes can be life or death. Moral disengagement, just like empathy reduction, is a cognitive coping mechanism that allows doctors to perform medical procedures. Physicians constantly find themselves in contradictory contexts where they are often inflicting pain that is required for treatment purposes and healing. Dehumanization can be a functional and powerful tool, allowing the physician to partake in routine procedures neutrally and empirically (Vaes & Muratore, 2011).

Notably, dehumanization in the physician–patient paradigm can also have serious negative consequences for the patient and the physician. Diminished agency of the patient is a common issue in the doctor–patient relationship. Because they are physically, mentally, or psychologically impaired, patients may lose a sense of self and thus the ability to function and plan. This impairment decreases their agency and overall humanness, which in many cases increases the chances for dehumanization to occur between the physician and the patient (Haslam, 2006). A second common cause of dehumanization in the doctor–patient paradigm is the asymmetrical relationship between the physician and the patient, from a humanistic and medicalization perspective. Patients are inherently ill and therefore are seemingly different from the stereotypical ideal human, making them less human by default due to their illness. The cognitive and behavioral mechanisms of dehumanization are most active when we perceive extreme differences between self and other, and the nature of illness is often dehumanizing. Doctors are also seen as authoritative and patients as subordinate. Power relations can directly increase the likelihood for dehumanization to occur (Gruenfeld et al., 2008). In one study, participants were given hypothetical medical roles of either a surgeon or a nurse. Participants in the surgical role were found to describe patients using a dehumanizing vocabulary and were more willing to give painful procedures than those assigned to the low-power nursing role (Lammers & Stapel, 2010). This research highlights how power dynamics operate even in cases where there is no malevolent intent, facilitating dehumanization (Lammers & Stapel, 2010). As we have shown, the doctor–patient paradigm in relation to dehumanization is complex and not without negative aspects. However, dehumanization with its ability to be used as a regulatory emotional strategy is useful in the doctor–patient paradigm, demonstrating the important interconnectivity between context, cognition, and behavior.

Conclusion/Future Directions: New Areas of Interest, Implications for Global Mental Health

The scope and intensity of global mental illness is at an all-time high. According to a report from the World Health Organization (WHO, 2013), behavioral health disorders are on course to surpass physical diseases as a major cause of disability by 2020 (WHO, 2013). Each year approximately $2.5 trillion is lost in the global economy to mental illness, which is projected to increase by $6 trillion over the next decade (WHO, 2013). Approximately one in four people suffers from a mental illness, and in the current political and social environment, the global mental health crisis is increasing, not diminishing (WHO, 2013). When we consider how to confront this growing dilemma, it can seem impossible. Breaking down the issues that directly affect global mental health is complex and paradoxical, particularly when it comes to protecting vulnerable populations who often are seen as burdensome to the relevant ingroup, who control how public funds are spent and how social resources are distributed. The basic underlying societal mechanisms (prejudicial beliefs, racism, oppression, and sexism, to name a few) that create these stark and divergent groupings need to be adequately addressed across cultures and backed by empirical research and data.

The negative consequences of oppression and prejudice have been highlighted by the WHO as being a top priority, an exciting and unprecedented move. The 2013–2020 Mental Health Action Plan specifically discusses low-income regions, citing the strong correlation between mental illness and poverty. More specifically, this plan mentions how poor populations have inadequate access to health care and treatment and receive little or no protection against discrimination, reiterating cross-culturally the social and political impact of dehumanization and its detrimental effects on human development across the globe.

As we unpack the science behind dehumanization, it is important that we continue to study the underlying cognitive and behavioral mechanisms within cultural contexts, across demographics, and within a local and global framework. If we do not understand how dehumanization manifests itself in our daily lives, in both explicit and implicit ways, it will continue to be difficult to understand the covert perpetuation of oppression and its ideological framework, or to find interventions and trends that curb actions associated with societies that are built to create and maintain hierarchal structures of oppression that further exacerbate mental health disparities within and among cultures.

Past research surrounding dehumanization describes issues retroactively, attempting to explain why a phenomenon has occurred, rather than proactively hypothesizing what may occur in the future. Recently, dehumanization and its onset have been studied in children and adolescents, an evolving area of interest in relation to education and prevention for global mental health. Research investigated children's perceptions of racial prejudices by examining how they perceived uniquely human emotions and traits when shown pictures of Black and White children (Costello & Hodson, 2012). This study revealed that children associated more human-like attributes with the White children, in the same manner as adults do, substantiating the use of attribute-based dehumanization measures among children (Costello & Hodson, 2012). Researchers (Costello & Hodson, 2012) indirectly linked the children's dehumanizing techniques to their parents, furthering the evidence that suggests there may be a genetic component involved in our preferences towards inequality and ideological beliefs (Kandler, Bleidorn, & Riemann, 2012). Costello & Hodson conclude that future research should consider the relationship between the psychological and genetic transmission of group dominance norms (Costello & Hodson, 2012).

Interventions should be considered as a first resort, not last. Prevention through education should be our goal to improve mental health in relation to dehumanization. Recent research studied whether imagined intergroup contact among Italian fourth graders would increase positive attributes to outgroup members via a 3-week-long intervention. The children were asked to imagine meeting an unknown immigrant child in various settings. The results established that there was an indirect effect of imagined contact on behavioral intentions as well as an increase in attributing uniquely human emotions to the outgroup members (Vezzali et al., 2011). This study showed that education can curtail the negative outcomes associated with infrahumanization, if undertaken correctly and early (Vezzali et al. 2011). If we can prevent and intervene on an educational level, is it possible to intervene more globally?

Researchers, political scientists, and activists are studying early intervention methods that reflect on larger cultural and social effects particularly how meritocratic and egalitarian norms foster infrahumanization attitudes and behaviors. Recent research analyzed the relationship between the degrees of humanity and discrimination, specifically in regard to how normative contexts moderate the role of symbolic threats (Pereira et al., 2009). The norms of egalitarianism (equality, social justice) versus meritocracy (competition, merit, hierarchy) were studied in relation to dehumanizing societal norms. The research concluded that infrahumanization elicits both perceived symbolic threats and discrimination

(Pereira et al., 2009). However, both normative contexts (egalitarian or meritocratic threat) can be used to dehumanize the outgroup either directly (meritocratic) or passively (egalitarian). The difference in context provided justification to dehumanize the outgroup for any basis in societal ideology.

Another important area to consider is how dehumanization is affected by advancements in technology. The rapid pace of technological advancements makes it difficult to analyze the potential consequences to individuals and societies from a social cognition perspective, making conjectural and abstract research imperative in predicting outcomes to interpret future intervention approaches. The focus of research surrounding violent video games and the negative repercussions of this technological advancement are well documented in behavioral and psychological research, exposing the association between cyber violence and increased aggression. Researchers have found that violent video games diminish perceptions of human qualities in the self and others in real-life settings and elicit a dehumanizing brain response (Weber et al., 2006). Virtual environments desensitize the repercussions of violence, allowing the player to morally disengage, normalizing violent behavior (Bastian et al., 2012. Cyber-violence can reduce attribution of humanity in both the player and their victims; engaging in violent acts in virtual settings increased aggression, decreased empathy, and increased dehumanizing behaviors toward self and others (Bastian et al., 2012).

Engaging in what seems like harmless imagination appears to be an authentic simulation of real life and sufficient enough contextually to stimulate the cognitive processes that normalize dehumanizing behavior. The societal effects of violent video games are only theoretical, and violent events such as mass shootings and other antisocial behavior in young men are only now being understood and connected to scientific findings. The important application of these findings to global mental health is astonishing and could possibly be the key to successful societal interventions.

Social media networks provide another cyber platform for implicit violence against people, an anonymous platform for adolescents to bully one another. Unlike traditional intimidation, which involves a face-to-face interaction, cyber victims may never know their harassers, and aggressors can morally disengage effortlessly due to the physical distance, the protection of anonymity, and lack of supervision (Wang et al., 2011). In a recent study, a group of 7,508 adolescents in 6th through 10th grade was surveyed about their experiences with cyber-bullying. The students were questioned about their experiences with both traditional and cyber-bullying to better understand the underlying differences in psychological consequences (Wang et al., 2011). The study found that with traditional bullying, both the victim and abuser had similar experiences with depression. However, with cyber-bullying, the victim was more likely to report feelings of depression, while the perpetrators did not show signs of depression to a similar degree (Wang et al., 2011). Researchers concluded that those who experienced cyber-bullying in comparison to traditional bullying felt more isolated, dehumanized, and helpless due to the anonymity created by the virtual environment. The findings suggest that the association between cyber-bullying and depression is distant from traditional bullying, emphasizing the importance for further research in the area of mental health and intervention techniques specific to cyber settings (Wang et al., 2011). Dehumanization among children and adolescents is a new and evolving area of interest. Whether it be how technology affects interactions between our youth, creating new outlets to dehumanize, or when prejudicial beliefs are formed, studying how and when children are affected by parental and societal ideologies is an emerging area of interest (Noorden et al., 2013).

There appears to be no single reason that humans across cultures and contexts dehumanize one another. What the multitude of research and findings show is that there is a complex matrix of social, cultural, cognitive, and behavioral factors that interplay in dehumanization. Evidence also suggests that dehumanization can play a useful functional role, as shown in the doctor–patient paradigm: dehumanization can be a successful cognitive tool for emotional regulation. However, controversial this idea may be, dehumanization is not directly linked to morality. It is a complex cognitive function that can be activated rightfully or wrongfully in situations of cognitive dissonance. If we want to curb the harmful effects of dehumanization on global mental health, we must better understand the neurological systems that activate dehumanizing emotional regulatory measures in relation to context and ideology, and what interventions will work best to prevent their onset.

References

Adorno, T. W. (1950). *The Authoritarian personality.* New York: Harper & Row.

Allen, M. W., & Ng, S. H. (2003). Human values, utilitarian benefits and identification: The case of meat. *European Journal of Social Psychology,* (1).

Allen, M. W., Wilson, M., Ng, S. H., & Dunne, M. (2000). Values and beliefs of vegetarians and omnivores. *Journal of Social Psychology,* (4).

Alvarez-Galvez, J., & Salvador-Carulla, L. (2013). Perceived discrimination and self-rated health in Europe: Evidence from the European Social Survey (2010). *PLoS One, 8*(9). doi:10.1371/journal.pone.0074252

Bain, P., Park, J., Kwok, C., & Haslam, N. (2009). Attributing human uniqueness and human nature to cultural groups: Distinct forms of subtle dehumanization. *Group Processes & Intergroup Relations, 12*(6), 789–805. doi:10.1177/1368430209340415

Bandura, A., Barbaranelli, C., Caprara, G. V., & Pastorelli, C. (1996). Mechanisms of moral disengagement in the exercise of moral agency. *Personality and Social Psychology, 71*(2), 364–374.

Bar-Tal, D. (1998). Societal beliefs in times of intractable conflict: The Israeli case. *International Journal of Conflict Management, 9*(1), 22–50. doi:10.1108/eb022803

Bastian, B., Jetten, J., & Radke, H. R. (2012). Cyber-dehumanization: Violent video game play diminishes our humanity. *Journal of Experimental Social Psychology, 48*(2), 486–491. doi:10.1016/j.jesp.2011.10.009

Berger, F. R. (1977). Pornography, sex, and censorship. *Social Theory and Practice, 4*(2), 183–209. doi:10.5840/soctheorpract19774216

Calogero, R. M., Tantleff-Dunn, S., & Thompson, J. K. (2011). *Self-objectification in women: Causes, consequences, and counteractions.* American Psychology Association.

Cameron, C. D., Harris, L. T., & Payne, B. K. (2015). The emotional cost of humanity. *Social Psychological and Personality Science, 7*(2), 105–112. doi:10.1177/1948550615604453

Castano, E., & Giner-Sorolla, R. (2006). Not quite human: Infrahumanization in response to collective responsibility for intergroup killing. *Journal of Personality and Social Psychology, 90*(5), 804–818. doi:10.1037/0022-3514.90.5.804

Costello, K., & Hodson, G. (2009). Exploring the roots of dehumanization: The role of animal—human similarity in promoting immigrant humanization. *Group Processes & Intergroup Relations, 13*(1), 3–22. doi:10.1177/1368430209347725.

Costello, K., & Hodson, G. (2012). Explaining dehumanization among children: The interspecies model of prejudice. *British Journal of Social Psychology,* (1):175–197. doi: 10.1111/bjso.12016.

Decety, J., Yang, C., & Cheng, Y. (2010). Physicians down-regulate their pain empathy response: An event-related brain potential study. *NeuroImage, 50*(4), 1676–1682. doi:10.1016/j.neuroimage.2010.01.025

Dhont, K., & Hodson, G. (2014). Why do right-wing adherents engage in more animal exploitation and meat consumption? *Personality and Individual Differences, 64,* 12–17. doi:10.1016/j.paid.2014.02.002.

Dhont, K., Hodson, G., Costello, K., & Macinnis, C. C. (2014). Social dominance orientation connects prejudicial human–human and human–animal relations. *Personality and Individual Differences, 61,* 105–108.

Di Bernardo, G. A., Visintin, E. P., Dazzi, C., Capozza, D. (2011, January 28). Patients' dehumanization in health contexts. Poster presented at the 12th Annual Meeting of the Society for Personality and Social Psychology, San Antonio, TX.

Dollard, J., Miller, N. E., Doob, L. W., Mowrer, O. H., & Sears, R. R. (1939). *Frustration and aggression.* Yale University Press. https://doi.org/10.1037/10022-000

Dovidio, J. F., Gaertner, S. L., & Saguy, T. (2009). Commonality and the Complexity of "We": Social Attitudes and Social Change. *Personality and Social Psychology Review,13*(1), 3–20. doi:10.1177/1088868308326751

Dworkin, A. (1999). *Pornography: Men possessing women.* Women's Press.

MacKinnon, C. A., & Dworkin, A. (1998). *In harms way: The pornography civil rights hearings.* Cambridge, MA: Harvard University Press.

Falomir-Pichastor, J. M., & Frederic, N. S. (2013). The dark side of heterogeneous ingroup identities: National identification, perceived threat, and prejudice against immigrants. *Journal of Experimental Social Psychology, 49*(1), 72–79.

Fiske, S. T. (2013a). A millennial challenge: Extremism in uncertain times. *Journal of Social Issues, 69*(3), 605–613. doi:10.1111/josi.12031

Fiske, S. T. (2013b). Varieties of (de) humanization: Divided by competition and status. *Nebraska Symposium on Motivation Objectification and (De)Humanization, 60,* 53–71. doi:10.1007/978-1-4614-6959-9_3

Fiske, S. T. (2005). *Social Cognition and the Normality of Prejudgment.* In J. F. Dovidio, P. Glick, & L. A. Rudman (Eds.), *On the nature of prejudice: Fifty years after Allport* (pp. 36–53). Blackwell Publishing. https://doi.org/10.1002/9780470773963.ch3

Fiske, S. T., Cuddy, A. J., Peter, G., & Xu, J. (2019). "A model of (often mixed) stereotype content: Competence and warmth respectively follow from perceived status and competition": Correction to Fiske et al. (2002). *Journal of Personality and Social Psychology.* doi:10.1037/pspa0000163

Fourie, M. M., Thomas, K. G., Amodio, D. M., Warton, C. M., & Meintjes, E. M. (2014). Neural correlates of experienced moral emotion: An fMRI investigation of emotion in response to prejudice feedback. *Social Neuroscience,9*(2), 203–218. doi:10.1080/17470919.2013.878750

Fredrickson, B. L., & Roberts, T.-A. (1997). Objectification Theory: Toward Understanding Women's Lived Experiences and Mental Health Risks. *Psychology of Women Quarterly, 21*(2), 173–206. https://doi.org/10.1111/j.1471-6402.1997.tb00108.x

Gervais, S. J., Vescio, T. K., Forster, J., Maass, A., & Suitner, C. (2012). Seeing women as objects: The sexual body part recognition bias. *European Journal of Social Psychology, 42*(6), 743–753. doi:10.1002/ejsp.1934

Glick, P., & Fiske, S. T. (1996). The ambivalent sexism inventory: Differentiating hostile and benevolent sexism. *Journal of Personality and Social Psychology, 70*(3), 491–512. doi:10.1037//0022-3514.70.3.491

Glick, P., & Fiske, S. T. (2001). An ambivalent alliance: Hostile and benevolent sexism as complementary justifications for gender inequality. *Beyond Prejudice, 70–88.* doi:10.1017/cbo9781139022736.005

Gómez-Martínez, C., & Moral-Jiménez, M. D. (2018). Dehumanization and Islamophobia: Attitudes towards the Syrian refugee crisis [Deshumanización e islamofobia: Actitudes ante la crisis de los refugiados sirios]. *Revista De Psicología Social, 33*(2), 215–239. doi:10.1080/02134748.2018.1435218

Gruenfeld, D. H., Inesi, M. E., Magee, J. C., & Galinsky, A. D. (2008). Power and the objectification of social targets. *Journal of Personality and Social Psychology, 95*(1), 111–127. doi:10.1037/0022-3514.95.1.111

Haque, O. S., & Waytz, A. (2012). Dehumanization in medicine. *Perspectives on Psychological Science, 7*(2), 176–186. doi:10.1177/1745691611429706

Harris, L. T. (2017). *Invisible mind: Flexible social cognition and dehumanization.* MIT Press.

Harris, L. T., & Fiske, S. T. (2006). Dehumanizing the lowest of the low. *Psychological Science, 17*(10), 847–853. doi:10.1111/j.1467-9280.2006.01793.x

Harris, L. T., & Fiske, S. T. (2007). Social groups that elicit disgust are differentially processed in mPFC. *Social Cognitive and Affective Neuroscience, 2*(1), 45–51. doi:10.1093/scan/nsl037

Harris, L. T., & Fiske, S. T. (2009). Social neuroscience evidence for dehumanised perception. *European Review of Social Psychology, 20*(1), 192–231. doi:10.1080/10463280902954988

Harris, L. T., & Fiske, S. T. (2011). Dehumanized Perception. *Zeitschrift Für Psychologie, 219*(3), 175–181. doi:10.1027/2151-2604/a000065

Haslam, N. (2006). Dehumanization: An integrative review. *Personality and Social Psychology Review, 10,* 252–264.

Haslam, N. (2007). Humanising medical practice: The role of empathy. *Medical Journal of Australia, 187,* 381–382.

Hojat, M., Vergare, M. J., Maxwell, K., Brainard, G., Herrine, S. K., Isenberg, G. A., . . . & Gonnella, J. S. (2009). The devil is in the third year: a longitudinal study of erosion of empathy in medical school. *Academic Medicine, 84*(9), 1182–1191.

Ibanez, A., Haye, A., Gonzalez, R., Hurtado, E., & Henriquez, R. (2009). Multi-level analysis of cultural phenomena. *Theory of Social Behaviour, 39,* 81–110.

Kandler, C., Bleidorn, W., & Riemann, R. (2012). Left or right? Sources of political orientation: The roles of genetic factors, cultural transmission, assortative mating, and personality. *Journal of Personality and Social Psychology, 102,* 633–645. doi:10.1037/a0025560

Kteily, N., Bruneau, E., Waytz, A., & Cotterill, S. (2015). The ascent of man: Theoretical and empirical evidence for blatant dehumanization. *Journal of personality and social psychology, 109*(5), 901.

Lammers, J., & Stapel, D. A. (2010). Power increases dehumanization. *Group Processes & Intergroup Relations, 14*(1), 113–126. doi:10.1177/1368430210370042

Leyens, J., Cortes, B., Demoulin, S., Dovidio, J. F., Fiske, S. T., Gaunt, R., . . . Vaes, J. (2003). Emotional prejudice, essentialism, and nationalism: The 2002 Tajfel lecture. *European Journal of Social Psychology, 33*(6), 703–717. doi:10.1002/ejsp.170

Leyens, J., Demoulin, S., Vaes, J., Gaunt, R., & Paladino, M. P. (2007). Infra-humanization: The wall of group differences. *Social Issues and Policy Review, 1*(1), 139–172. doi:10.1111/j.1751-2409.2007.00006.x

Leyens, J., Rodriguez-Perez, A., Rodriguez-Torres, R., Gaunt, R., Paladino, M., Vaes, J., & Demoulin, S. (2001). Psychological essentialism and the differential attribution of uniquely human emotions to ingroups and outgroups. *European Journal of Social Psychology, 31*(4), 395–411. doi:10.1002/ejsp.50

MacKinnon, C. A. (1987). *Feminism unmodified discourses on life and law.* Cambridge, Mass.: Harvard Univ. Pr.

MacKinnon, C. A. (1989). *Toward a feminist theory of the state.* Cambridge, MA: Harvard Univ. Press.

MacKinnon, C. A. (2006). *Are women human?: And other international dialogues.* Cambridge, MA: Belknap Press of Harvard University Press.

Mars, R. B., Neubert, F., Noonan, M. P., Sallet, J., Toni, I., & Rushworth, M. F. (2012). On the relationship between the "default mode network" and the "social brain". *Frontiers in Human Neuroscience, 6.* doi:10.3389/fnhum.2012.00189

McElroy, Wendy (2008). "Feminism and Women's Rights". *The Encyclopedia of Libertarianism* (pp. 173–176). doi:10.4135/9781412965811.n106.

Motyl, M., Hart, J., & Pyszczynski, T. (2010). When animals attack: The effects of mortality salience, infrahumanization of violence, and authoritarianism on support for war. *Journal of Experimental Social Psychology, 46*(1), 200–203. doi:10.1016/j.jesp.2009.08.012

Neumann, M., Edelhäuser, F., Tauschel, D., Fischer, M. R., Wirtz, M., Woopen, C., . . . Scheffer, C. (2011). Empathy decline and its reasons: A systematic review of studies with medical students and residents. *Academic Medicine, 86*(8), 996–1009. doi:10.1097/acm.0b013e318221e615

Van Noorden, T. H., Haselager, G. J., Cillessen, A. H., & Bukowski, W. M. (2014). Dehumanization in children: The link with moral disengagement in bullying and victimization. *Aggressive behavior, 40*(4), 320–328.

Opotow, S. (1990). Moral exclusion and injustice: An introduction. *Journal of Social Issues, 46*(1), 1–20. doi:10.1111/j.1540-4560.1990.tb00268.x

Overwalle, F. V. (2011). A dissociation between social mentalizing and general reasoning. *NeuroImage, 54*(2), 1589–1599. doi:10.1016/j.neuroimage.2010.09.043

Pereira, C., Vala, J., & Leyens, J. P. (2009). From infra-humanization to discrimination: The mediation of symbolic threat needs egalitarian norms. *Journal of experimental social psychology, 45*(2), 336–344.

Pettigrew, T. F., & Tropp, L. R. (2008). How does intergroup contact reduce prejudice? Meta-analytic tests of three mediators. *European Journal of Social Psychology, 38*(6), 922–934. doi:10.1002/ejsp.504

Russell, D. E. (1993). Making violence sexy: feminist views on pornography//Review. *Canadian Woman Studies, 14*(3), 120.

Shaw, L. L., Batson, C. D., & Todd, R. M. (1994). Empathy avoidance: Forestalling feeling for another in order to escape the motivational consequences. *Journal of Personality and Social Psychology, 67*(5), 879–887. doi:10.1037//0022-3514.67.5.879

Sherman, D., Hogg, M., Maitner, A., & Moffitt, G. (2005). Uncertainty and intergroup perception: Relations among entitativity, identification, and attitude polarization. *PsycEXTRA Dataset.* doi:10.1037/e529412014-204

Sherif, M. (1961). Conformity-deviation, norms, and group relations. *Conformity and Deviation,* 159–198. doi:10.1037/11122-006

Sidanius, J., & Pratto, F. (1999). *Social dominance: An intergroup theory of social hierarchy and oppression.* Cambridge University Press.

Tajfel, H. (1974). Social identity and intergroup behaviour. *Social Science Information, 13*(2), 65–93. doi:10.1177/053901847401300204

Vaes, J., & Muratore, M. (2011, July). Defensive dehumanization in the medical practice: The effects of humanizing patients' suffering on physicians' burnout. Symposium conducted at the 16th general meeting of the European Association for Social Psychology, Stockholm, Sweden.

Vezzali, L., Capozza, D., Giovannini, D., & Stathi, S. (2011). Improving implicit and explicit intergroup attitudes using imagined contact: An experimental intervention with elementary school children. *Group Processes & Intergroup Relations, 15*(2), 203–212. doi:10.1177/1368430211424920

Wang, J., Nansel, T. R., & Iannotti, R. J. (2011). Cyber and traditional bullying: Differential association with depression. *Journal of Adolescent Health, 48*(4), 415–417. doi:10.1016/j.jadohealth.2010.07.012

Weber, R., Ritterfeld, U., & Mathiak, K. (2006). Does Playing Violent Video Games Induce Aggression? Empirical Evidence of a Functional Magnetic Resonance Imaging Study. *Media Psychology, 8*(1), 39–60. doi:10.1207/s1532785xmep0801_4

World Health Organization (WHO). (2013). *Mental health action plan 2013–2020* (Rep.). WHO Document Publication Services.

Zurbriggen, E. L. (2013). Objectification, Self-Objectification, and Societal Change. *Journal of Social and Political Psychology, 1*(1), 188–215. https://doi.org/10.5964/jspp.v1i1.94

PART III

Prevention and Early Interventions in Global Mental Health

Cultural Changes in Neural Structure and Function

Michael E. W. Varnum *and* Ryan S. Hampton

Abstract

Human cultures are not static. An emerging body of research has documented cultural changes in a wide variety of behaviors, psychological tendencies, and cultural products. Increasingly, this field has also begun to test hypotheses regarding the causes of these changes and to create forecasts for future patterns of change. Yet to date, the question of how our brains may change as a function of systematic changes in our environments has received relatively little attention and scant empirical testing. This chapter begins by reviewing the literature on cultural change, including Varnum and Grossmann's program of research using a behavioral ecology framework to understand patterns of cultural change. Next the chapter offers some initial predictions for changes in neural structure and function that may occur in the coming decades and discusses implications for global mental health. Finally, the chapter offers some ideas about how empirical tests of these predictions might be conducted and discusses challenges and opportunities for extending the study of cultural change to neuroscience.

Key Words: cultural change, cultural evolution, behavioral ecology, cultural neuroscience, cultural psychology

How and why do human cultures change? In recent years social psychologists have developed increasingly sophisticated methods to document changes over time in human behavior and psychological tendencies and to test theories regarding the causes of these shifts (Greenfield, 2016; Kashima, 2014; Varnum & Grossmann, 2017a). However, to date, this work has focused largely on changes in cultural products, attitudes and values, performance on psychological tests, and behavior. In this chapter we attempt to envision a framework to study cultural changes using neural methods. In doing so we draw on a diverse set of theoretical perspectives including cultural psychology, cultural neuroscience, behavioral ecology, and evolutionary psychology.

First, we summarize extant research documenting cultural changes in a wide variety of phenomena ranging from individualism/collectivism to life history strategies. We also discuss evidence regarding the causes of many of these changes, which appear to be linked to adaptive responses to key dimensions of ecology. Next, we offer a set of tentative predictions for changes that may be occurring in neural structure and function as a result of changes in ecology (i.e., increased population density and mobility), changes in technology (i.e., the advent of online social networks and widespread use of GPS-based navigation), and changes in the prevalence of mental health issues (i.e., increasing levels of anxiety and depression). We also discuss the implications of these changes for changes in the prevalence of a number of mental health problems in a global context. We then address methods that would allow these predictions to be tested, providing a possible roadmap for large-scale neuroscience studies of cultural change and highlighting key methodological issues that would likely be encountered in such an enterprise. Finally, we end by discussing both the promises and challenges of a future neuroscience of cultural change.

Cultural Change Individualism

Perhaps the most studied phenomenon in research on cultural change has been individualism/collectivism, which can be broadly thought of as an emphasis on the individual self and a view of the self as separate from others versus an emphasis on relationships and a view of the self as fundamentally intertwined and interconnected with others (Markus & Kitayama, 1991; Nisbett et al., 2001; Triandis, 1995; Varnum et al., 2010). Levels of individualism have risen dramatically over the past several decades (and even over the past two centuries) in the United States as indicated by increasing use of words reflecting individualist values (Greenfield, 2013; Grossmann & Varnum, 2015; Twenge et al., 2014) as well as first-person singular pronouns (Twenge et al., 2013) in American books. Other indicators of individualism show the same effect, including increasing frequency of relatively unique names (Grossmann & Varnum, 2015; Twenge, Abebe, & Campbell, 2010), higher rates of divorce (Grossmann & Varnum, 2015), and increasing endorsement of individualistic values (Santos et al., 2017). Similar effects have been observed in the United States (Greenfield, 2013), China (Cai et al., 2018; Hamamura & Xu, 2015; Zeng & Greenfield, 2015), and Japan (Hamamura, 2012; Ogihara, 2018). These shifts are not confined to a handful of countries, and in fact individualism appears to have increased (at least over the past 50 years) in the majority of societies around the globe including countries as diverse as Chile, India, Nigeria, Russia, and Turkey (Santos et al., 2017). In a similar vein, levels of conformity, a phenomenon linked to collectivism, also appear to have declined over time (Bond & Smith, 1996).

Self-Esteem and Narcissism

Another major area of inquiry has been whether levels of self-esteem and related variables have changed from the 1960s to the present. In one study, Twenge and Campbell (2001) found that American children's average levels of self-esteem declined from 1965 to 1979 and increased from 1980 to 1993. In a similar vein, several studies have documented increases in narcissism from the 1950s to the 1990s among American college students (Roberts & Helson, 1997; Twenge & Foster, 2008; Twenge et al., 2008). Other evidence suggests that beliefs in illusory superiority have also increased among American college students from the 1960s to the 2000s (Twenge et al., 2012a). However, other researchers have found that levels of narcissism and self-enhancement among American college and high school students remained fairly stable from the 1980s to the mid-2000s (Trzesniewski et al., 2008a, 2008b). The claim that narcissism has continued to rise has been challenged by researchers who have demonstrated a lack of measurement equivalence over time on a commonly used narcissism inventory and found that, controlling for measurement inequivalence, there has in fact been a decline in narcissism among U.S. college students from the 1990s to the 2010s (Wetzel et al., 2017). Further, a recent cross-temporal meta-analysis of studies measuring self-esteem among Australians shows a slight decline in levels of self-esteem from the 1970s to the 2010s (Hamamura & Septarini, 2017). Thus, at present the evidence is mixed regarding shifts in self-esteem and related variables over the past several decades.

Well-Being and Emotions

Are people becoming more or less happy over time? A number of converging lines of evidence suggest that Americans at least are becoming less happy. The percentage of positive versus negative language used in American books and a leading national newspaper has declined substantially from 1800 to present (Iliev et al., 2016). Further, self-reported subjective well-being declined from the 1970s to the late 2000s according to data from the General Social Survey (Oishi et al., 2011). The prevalence of depressive and anxious symptoms has increased markedly from the 1930s to the 2000s (Twenge, Gentile, et al., 2010) according to a cross-temporal meta-analysis of studies using the Minnesota Multiphasic Personality Inventory. Further, nationally representative data from U.S. high school students shows an increase in self-reported symptoms related to mood disorders from 1982 to 2013 (Twenge, 2015). Further analysis of Centers of Disease Control and Prevention (CDC) data shows an increase in suicide rates in nearly all U.S. states between 1999 and 2016 (Stone et al., 2018). Interestingly, as Americans have become less happy, they also appear to have become less contemptuous. Varnum and Grossmann (2017b) analyzed the frequency of contempt-related language in American books and movies and found a dramatic decrease over time from the early 20th century to the mid-2000s. More recently, research has linked increasing use of new media (i.e., social media, smartphones) to increasing rates of mental health issues among American adolescents (Twenge et al., 2018). Thus, Americans appear to have become markedly less happy over time. However, this trend does not appear to be universal. In fact, according to data from the World Values Survey, most societies have become happier from the 1980s to the present (Roser & Ortiz-Ospina, 2017).

Social Capital and Gender Equality

Researchers have also assessed changes in the way societies are organized in terms of relationships to institutions, attitudes regarding how society should be structured, and related social norms and practices. In a set of seminal studies on cultural change, the political scientist Robert Putnam documented a set of changes in American society from the 1950s to the 1990s that he dubbed a decline in social capital (Putnam, 1995, 2000). During this time period Putnam found a decline in civic participation, membership in voluntary organizations, and levels of general trust. More recently, Twenge and colleagues found that trust in others and confidence in a wide variety of institutions declined among American adults and adolescents over a 40-year period from 1972 to 2012 (Twenge et al., 2014). Interestingly, this pattern was not observed in a study examining levels of trust in 34 European societies, with trust remaining fairly stable from 2002 to 2012 (Olivera, 2015).

Another area of marked change has been in the arena of gender equality. Survey data shows a sizeable increase in the United States in support for policies favoring equality among the sexes from the 1960s to the 2000s (Thornton & Young-DeMarco, 2001). Complementary evidence was found from a cross-temporal meta-analysis of studies using the Attitudes Toward Women scale, which found greater support for feminism among men and women from the 1970s to the 1990s (Twenge, 1997), and from an analysis of cultural products, which found greater parity in the use of female and male pronouns in American books (Twenge et al., 2012b). More recently, Varnum and Grossmann (2016) constructed an index of gender inequality using a combination of indicators including male:female wage ratio, male:female pronoun use in books, female political representation, and sexist work attitudes. From the 1950s to the 2010s, this index showed a dramatic decline in the United States, and from the 1940s to the 2010s, a similar index showed the same effect in the United Kingdom.

Relationship With the Natural World

Other work has explored shifts in how societies think about and engage with the natural world. In their analysis of references to nature in cultural products, Kesebir and Kesebir (2017) report a decline in nature-related language (i.e., references to birds, trees, flowers, seasons, etc.) in American and British fiction, popular song lyrics from Anglophone countries, and storylines from Anglophone films from the mid-20th century onward. Interestingly, though, mentions of nature in fiction appear to have increased somewhat from 1900 to 1950 and to have declined thereafter.

Although an emphasis on the natural world appears to be on the decline in cultural products, recent work suggests that climate change may increase the amount of time people spend outdoors in much of the United States. Using data from 2002 to 2012, Obradovich and Fowler (2017) find that recreational physical activity is linked to fluctuations in temperature and other climatic factors, and that projections for effects of climate change suggest that in large swaths of the North, Midwest, and Pacific Northwest, levels of outdoor physical activity should increase over the 21st century, whereas they are likely to decrease in parts of the Southwest and South.

Preference for Complexity

Cultural changes have also been observed in preference for complexity. Cultural products, such as songs, television shows, visual art, literature, and political speeches, vary in terms of the complexity of the ideas or information presented. Although some have argued that such cultural products show evidence of increasing average complexity in recent years (i.e., Johnson, 2005), only more recently has this proposal been subjected to empirical tests. In an analysis of song lyrics from over 14,000 songs entering the Billboard charts from 1958 to 2016, Varnum and colleagues (2021) found that lyrics of popular songs have become increasingly repetitive. Further, forecasts using auto-ARIMA suggest that this trend will continue for the next several decades and that this effect is driven in part by greater amounts of music being produced in a given year. This preference for reduced complexity is also evident in the language used by successful American politicians, namely American presidents. Pennebaker and Jordan (2018) show that over the past century, speeches by American presidents show diminishing levels of analytic language, suggesting a trend toward preference for leaders with simpler styles of expression.

Intelligence

Intelligence has also been a key topic in the study of cultural change. In several countries large increases in fluid and crystallized intelligence have been documented from the 1930s into the late 20th century. This phenomenon is dubbed the Flynn effect (Flynn, 1987) and has also been observed in several cross-temporal meta-analyses, including studies extending the effect into the 2010s (Pietschnig & Voracek, 2015; Raven, 2000; Trahan et al., 2014). Further, as some have argued that there are multiple flavors or types of intelligence beyond cognitive capacities that have typically been studied (Gardner, 2011; Sternberg, 1985), it is interesting to note that athletic performance in a wide variety of sports has increased considerably during the past century (Kaufman, 2013).

Life History Strategies

Finally, there is also evidence in the United States and many other societies of a shift toward slower life history strategies. Life history strategy refers to a suit of physiological and behavioral dimensions related to the timing of reproduction, delay of gratification, and orientation toward future or present, which have been found to vary across species and among groups and individuals within species, including humans (Charnov, 1993; Del Giudice et al., 2015; Kenrick & Griskevicius, 2015; Sng et al., 2018; Stearns, 1992). Fast life history strategies involve early reproduction, greater number of offspring, greater risk taking, reduced delay of gratification, and shorter life expectancies, whereas slower life history strategies involve delayed reproduction, fewer offspring, greater investment in offspring, delay of gratification, investment in long-term outcomes, and longer lifespans. Sociologists and demographers have long noted a demographic transition in which life expectancies have increased and birth rates have decreased (i.e., Lesthaeghe, 2015). Further, recent studies have found declining rates of teen pregnancy in the United States and United Kingdom (Varnum & Grossman, 2016) and evidence of a shift toward slower life history behaviors among American adolescents over the past four decades (i.e., reduced sexual activity, less participation in the workforce, and decreased prevalence of adult activities; Twenge & Campbell, 2018; Twenge & Park, 2017). In fact globally fertility rates have declined over the past 6 decades in virtually every society for which there is data (Rotella et al., 2021).

Why Do Cultures Change?

Modernization Theories

Modernization theories argue that a variety of recent changes in human societies can be understood as the results of economic development. With greater economic development, according to these accounts, a cluster of changes have occurred in values and practices that are linked to institutional changes and a broad range of other phenomena (Inglehart, 1997; Inglehart & Welzel, 2005), including more emphasis on individual autonomy and freedoms, greater tolerance, and democratic institutions. In this view, as greater numbers of people in a society become able to meet basic needs, their goals and values shift in the direction of individualism, self-expression, freedom, and tolerance. Such preferences and beliefs reflect more abstract concerns, which people can afford to attend to once they have sufficient food, shelter, security, etc.

In a similar vein, Greenfield's theory of cultural change and human development holds that a host of changes have occurred simultaneously in the past couple centuries, such as urbanization, industrialization, and loosening of family ties, which has led to rising individualism as well as other cultural shifts such as greater innovation, more abstract reasoning, and greater tolerance (Greenfield, 2013, 2016, 2017). In this view, modern urban living in market economies pushes individuals toward greater focus on their own goals and outcomes, weakens traditional social bonds, and encourages modes of reasoning and values that are more conducive to success in these changed social conditions.

Although these theories have been highly influential, in some regards the answers they provide can be seen as theoretically shallow. Typically research in this tradition is not grounded in evolutionary logic, nor does it tend to assess the relative importance of various factors that are theoretically orthogonal to the changes these theories seek to explain. In addition, these frameworks offer somewhat intermediate as opposed to ultimate explanations for observed cultural changes and often do not conceptually or empirically assess which variables in these models are endogenous versus exogenous. Such theories also tend to view all observed societal changes that have occurred in recent decades or centuries as part of the same broader process. However, this research in many ways provided an excellent starting point for more recent work on cultural change by documenting a variety of cultural changes and by pointing to structural changes that might be linked to them.

Ecological Theories

Other theories regarding the causes of cultural change emphasize the role of ecology. Some of these studies explicitly adopt a behavioral ecological framework, emphasizing how variations across and changes within human societies may be understood as driven by evoked adaptive responses to recurring environmental threats and affordances, such as infectious diseases, population density, resource availability, mortality threat, and relatedness, originally derived from research on other species (Sng et al., 2018; Varnum & Grossmann, 2017a). To this list of key ecological factors, we might also add climatic stress (Van de Vliert, 2013) and income inequality, which is arguably a proxy for resource patchiness in modern human societies (Sng et al., 2018). In a long-running collaboration, Igor Grossmann and I have used this framework to assess the causes of a variety of cultural changes.

We have done so by simultaneously testing the unique contribution of multiple ecological dimensions and by using techniques like cross-correlation function analysis and Granger causality analysis to assess temporal precedence, and more recently auto-ARIMA modeling and Tiokhin-Hruschka (2017) null distribution methods for correcting significance thresholds to assess whether these relationships hold while accounting for temporal autocorrelation observed in the time series (Rotella et al., 2021; Varnum et al., 2021). We have found that shifts in individualism are most strongly linked to changes in markers of resource availability, with greater levels of white-collar jobs, education, and income emerging as stronger and more consistent predictors of increasing individualism than other ecological dimensions (Grossmann & Varnum, 2015; Santos et al., 2017). We also found that indicators of resource levels were the best predictor of changes in expressions of contempt over time (Varnum & Grossmann, 2017b). Further, we recently examined the relationship between innovation and gross domestic product per capita in the United States and United Kingdom during the first and second industrial revolution and into the present. We find evidence in both countries (after using first-order detrending) that there appear to be bidirectional lagged relationships between rising resource levels and innovation (i.e., patents, trademarks, unique book publications), suggesting that as societies become more materially secure, their members are more willing to generate novel ideas, and vice versa (Varnum & Grossmann, 2019). These results are generally consistent with the predictions of modernization theory as well as those of behavioral ecology. However, we also observed some relationship between declining pathogens and rising levels of individualism and declining contempt, as well as contributions by markers of increasing population density to rising individualism, and some evidence of an interaction between climatic stress and resource levels predicting levels of individualism over time (Grossmann & Varnum, 2015; Varnum & Grossmann, 2017b; Santos et al., 2017). The strongest predictor of increases in gender equality appears to be declines in rates of infectious disease, an effect partially mediated by a shift toward slower life history strategies among women as indexed by teen birth rates (Varnum & Grossmann, 2016). Further, this line of research found empirical evidence that changes in resource levels temporally precede changes in individualism and that changes in pathogen levels temporally precede changes in gender equality (Grossmann & Varnum, 2015; Santos et al., 2017; Varnum & Grossmann, 2016). This work suggests that cultural change on varied dimensions is not monolithic, but rather that specific changes appear driven by specific ecological shifts. In a similar vein, recent work by Twenge and Park (2017) found links between markers of resource availability and pathogen levels and changes in the prevalence of adult activities among American adolescents, such that increases in markers of resource abundance and decreases in pathogen prevalence are linked to declines in the frequency of adult activities, which is indicative of a shift toward slower life history strategies. However, more recently, Rotella and colleagues (2021) have shown that declines in fertility around the world (an indicator of shifts toward slower strategies) appear to be largely driven by increasing population density.

Other research has also found links between ecological factors and cultural changes without adopting an explicitly behavioral ecological framework. For example, declining levels of subjective well-being appear linked to measures of income inequality (Oishi et al., 2011), and reductions in linguistic positivity bias appear linked to levels of unemployment and inflation (Iliev et al., 2016). Similarly, Bianchi (2016) found strong links between unemployment levels and cultural shifts in individualism. Other research has linked levels of income inequality to changes in levels of social capital (Twenge et al., 2014). Finally, a series of studies by Obradovich suggests that changes in climate (increasing maximum temperatures and average precipitation) are linked to a variety of cultural phenomena ranging from electoral turnover (Obradovich, 2017) to rising levels of mental health difficulties (Obradovich et al., 2018) and that continuing climate change is likely to accelerate these social shifts in the decades to come. Taken together, these lines of research suggest that changes in basic dimensions of our physical and social ecologies may be key to understanding and predicting patterns of cultural change.

Finally, in recent work my colleagues and I have begun to consider other aspects of the ecology that speak to information or choices available in the environment. We find, for example, that increases in preference for lyrically simple popular music over time appear to be driven by increases in the amount of novel musical choices available in a given year, an effect that holds when controlling for standard behavioral ecological dimensions as well as immigration, residential mobility, population size, and when controlling for temporal autocorrelation (Varnum et al., 2021). Others have proposed that the Flynn effect on intelligence might be due to increasingly stimulating environments, including greater exposure to more complex visual media, modern technology, and more stimulating work environments (Flynn, 2007). Taken together, this work suggests that it may be useful to expand an ecological framework to encompass environmental features of the informational landscape. It also suggests potential links between a behavioral ecological approach to cultural change and cultural evolutionary frameworks (see Muthukrishna & Uchiyama, this volume), which tend to focus on transmitted culture and the features of information and human information processing biases, which also adaptively shape culture over time (for a more detailed discussion of the differences between these approaches and potential synergies see Varnum & Grossmann, 2017a).

How Have/Will Our Brains Change?

At the core of cultural neuroscience is a set of premises: that the human brain is plastic and shaped by repeated experiences, that cultural contexts can provide systematically different sets of experiences, and that to the extent that such contexts provide different sets of experiences we should expect corresponding differences across cultural groups in neural function and structure (Chiao & Blizinsky, 2016; Han, 2013; Kitayama & Uskul, 2011). For a more in-depth discussion of culture and neuroplasticity, see Goh (this volume), and for a more in-depth discussion of the philosophical meaning of cultural differences in neural structure and function, see Northoff (this volume). Consistent with these ideas, in the past decade, dozens of studies have indeed found differences in neural function and structure across cultural groups (Hampton & Varnum, 2018a; Han & Ma, 2014; Kim & Sasaki, 2014; Kitayama et al., 2019). For example, recent event-related potential (ERP) studies have found that European Americans show evidence of an implicit positivity bias for the self, whereas Chinese do not appear to show this bias (Hampton & Varnum, 2018b), and that European Americans (and those from Mexican cultural backgrounds) are better able to intentionally up-regulate neural affective responses than people from East Asian cultural backgrounds (Hampton et al., 2021; Varnum & Hampton, 2017). Further, research using functional magnetic resonance imaging (fMRI) has found that the neural substrates involved in processing self-relevance appear culturally influenced; Chinese show comparable activation in the medial prefrontal cortex (mPFC) when making judgments regarding the relevance of adjectives to the self and one's mother, whereas Westerners show greater activation in this region for self- versus mother-relevant judgments (Zhu et al., 2007). Other research suggests that there may be structural correlates of different modes of construing the self, with interdependent self-construal—a view of the self as overlapping and interconnected with close others that is more predominant in East Asian cultures (Markus & Kitayama, 1991; Varnum et al., 2010)—being linked to reduced volume in the orbitofrontal cortex (Kitayama et al., 2017). These findings represent only a small portion of the broad and expanding empirical literature documenting cultural influences on neural responses and neural structure. Taken together, this work suggests that culture does indeed have a measurable effect on how the human brain is structured and how it functions.

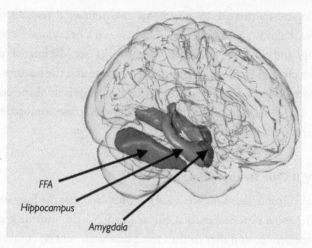

FFA

Hippocampus

Amygdala

Figure 19.1. Brain areas for which we predict changes in average volume or connectivity over time. Images created using the Human Brainnetome Atlas template (Fan et al., 2016) and the Scalable Brain Atlas software program, (Bakker, Tiesinga, & Kötter, 2015).

This body of literature has implications not only for understanding how brains may differ across cultural groups but also for predicting how brains may change over time as changes occur within a cultural context. In this section we outline a set of predictions for neural changes at the population level in many societies that may occur due to shifts in ecology, use of novel technologies, and other cultural changes (see Figure 19.1 for relevant neural structures). This set of predictions applies broadly across societies as the trends that we believe will lead to neural changes are happening in a fairly global fashion. However, to the extent that societies vary in these exogenous trends, we would also predict variation in the degree to which we observe the predicted neural changes. And if there are reversals in the exogenous trends, then we would expect corresponding reversals in the predicted neural changes.

Changes in Fusiform Face Area Volume

In the past several decades (and centuries in many cases), most societies have experienced dramatic shifts in the distribution of their populations due to migration from rural to urban areas, as well as population growth, leading to increased population density (Roser & Ortiz-Ospina, 2017; United Nations, 2014). Further, migration has increased (Martin et al., 2014; United Nations, 2013) and travel has become more common (Schuttenhelm, 2016). In addition, the past decade has seen the development and widespread adoption of online social networks and video chat services. We suspect that as a result of these developments, people in most societies have exposure to a greater number of individuals than in past. Thus, we propose that these changes should enhance the neural circuitry involved in people's ability to detect, differentiate, and identify human faces, in particular the fusiform face area (FFA). The FFA is a region of the fusiform gyrus that research suggests is devoted to facial processing (Gauthier et al., 2000; Kanwisher et al., 1997; Kanwisher & Yovel, 2006; Sergent et al., 1992). Thus, to the extent that trends like urbanization, mobility, and use of online social networks continue to increase within a given society, we would predict that we should observe increases in average volume of the FFA among members of that society.

Changes in Hippocampal Volume

Another marked change in many societies has occurred in the past decade: the widespread adoption of accurate hand-held artificial navigation technology. A key region involved in spatial navigation is the hippocampus (Ghaem et al., 1997; Maguire et al., 1998), and importantly, individuals who develop high levels of expertise in spatial navigation (such as London taxi drivers) show greater hippocampal volume, suggesting plasticity in this region as a function of experience among adults (Maguire et al., 2000). However, with the advent and widespread adoption of technologies such as mobile map apps, GPS, and other applications that provide step-by-step real-time directions, one would expect that in many societies individuals should show reductions in nonassisted navigational abilities. Hence, to the extent that artificial navigation technologies are increasingly used in a society, we should observe decreases in average volume of the hippocampus among its members.

Changes in Amygdala Reactivity

As noted earlier in this chapter, levels of well-being appear to have declined substantially in the United States over the past century, with evidence of increases in the prevalence of anxiety and depressive symptoms. Recent work suggests that declines in the amount of time people spend engaged in deep real-world social interactions (vs. online) and increases in the unpleasantness of weather (more heat, more rain) have led and will continue to lead to greater prevalence of mental health problems (Obradovich et al., 2018; Twenge et al., 2018). What changes might we see in the brain as a result? Heightened reactivity of the amygdala to negative emotional stimuli has been associated with trait anxiety and neuroticism (Stein et al., 2007), social anxiety disorder (Bergman et al., 2014; Etkin & Wager, 2007), and depression (Canli et al., 2005; Gaffrey et al., 2011; Redlich et al., 2018; Siegle et al., 2007). Thus, to the extent that depression and anxiety become more prevalent in a society over time (due to changes in the social and physical environment), we would predict that we should see neural changes associated with these symptoms, particularly increased average reactivity of the amygdala to negative emotional stimuli.

Implications for Mental Health

Although our predictions regarding changes in average amygdala reactivity have fairly clear implications for anxiety and depression, it may also be the case that the structural changes we predict for the hippocampus and FFA might also be relevant for making predictions regarding prevalence of a variety of mental health problems. In this section we speculate about potential impacts of such changes on a variety of mental illnesses, drawing predictions based on associations observed in previous literature between these regions and these conditions, and we also discuss how such changes may play out in a global context.

If average hippocampal volume does indeed decrease in a given population, it is possible we might also expect an increase in the incidence of depression, schizophrenia, and bipolar disorder, as previous research has linked atrophy in these regions to these conditions (Campbell & Macqueen, 2004). Further, the hippocampus is implicated in memory, and some have speculated that certain memory impairments observed among people suffering major depressive disorder may be linked to changes in hippocampal structure or function (Campbell & Macqueen, 2004).

Further, if FFA volume increases as a result of experience corresponding to increased activation in this neural structure in response to faces, it may have implications for the prevalence of autism. Research suggests that reduced activation in the FFA is associated with autism spectrum disorder (ASD; Schultz, 2005; Schultz et al., 2003), a finding confirmed by a recent meta-analysis (Patriquin et al., 2016). Thus, it may be that the changes we forecast for this region may suggest that the prevalence of ASD may begin to decline in societies in which such changes occur. However, it is worth noting that some evidence has suggested that the FFA may be abnormally enlarged among those with ASD due to deficient neural pruning (see Schultz, 2005, for a review). Thus, implications for changes in FFA volume for ASD prevalence rates are somewhat ambiguous.

Further, given that societies in the developing world are beginning to experience changes in their social and technological landscapes that parallel those that have recently occurred in more affluent societies like the United States, United Kingdom, and Japan, we might expect increases (or decreases as the case may be) in the prevalence of mental health problems along these lines, and in many cases such changes in the prevalence of various symptoms may be more pronounced in these societies in the coming years as they begin to catch up with richer societies. This may pose unique challenges as in many developing countries mental illness is associated with greater stigma and there tends to be more limited access to mental health treatment. That said, we regard these predictions as even more speculative than our main predictions for cultural-level neural changes.

How Can We Study Cultural Change at the Neural Level?

In this section we attempt to envision what a neuroscience of cultural change might look like. The logistical challenges such an endeavor would entail are nontrivial but potentially surmountable given sufficient funding and motivation. Such an enterprise would also have to address other issues common to time-series research (i.e. temporal autocorrelation). Finally, as with other time-series research using more traditional methods, for truly satisfying tests of hypotheses regarding cultural changes in neural structure and function, it is necessary to develop models not only to explain past patterns of temporal change but also to forecast future patterns.

Sampling

Assessing cultural change at the neural level will require coordinated data collection at a fairly unprecedented scale for research using magnetic resonance imaging (MRI) or fMRI (with the IMAGEN project providing a notable exception). To have confidence that the data gathered for each time point are reasonably representative of the overall state of the society, minimum sample sizes will likely need to be at least comparable to those used in large-scale survey research (i.e., $N > 1,000$) and selected so that they are demographically representative. Data will also need to be gathered yearly for a minimum of several decades to have a chance of capturing meaningful patterns of cultural fluctuations or shifts in neural structure and function. Given the high cost and other logistical hurdles involved in data collection on this scale, it might seem tempting to instead sample individuals at a single time point from different birth cohorts; however, this approach would make it difficult to rule out developmental factors as alternative explanations for any effects observed. Alternatively, one might opt for a cross-temporal meta-analysis design (for details of this approach see Gentile et al., 2014). This approach, although initially appealing, is limited by the fact that MRI/fMRI studies tend to have fairly small Ns and by an important set of challenges in pooling data across MRI scanners. This latter issue is discussed in more detail in the next section of this chapter. Thus, in envisioning a future neuroscience of cultural change, the gold standard would likely involve yearly structural and functional scans from large representative samples of a given society conducted on the same scanner or same set of scanners (and even this would involve tests for comparability of the data gathered on the same scanners over time) over the span of at least five decades and preferably over a much longer time span.

Comparisons Across Scanners/Testing Sites

For the scale of data acquisition necessary to assess cultural change, the use of similar scanners across different sites or the use of the same scanners over time presents substantial challenges in controlling for variance due to the machines used to acquire the data. The blood level oxygen–dependent (BOLD) signal used in fMRI studies makes up a relatively small percentage of the overall signal acquired by a scanner, with random noise originating from both physical artifacts caused by the participant and fluctuations by the scanner (Liu, 2016; Matthews, 2001). Testing for and tracking the latter is critical in determining image stability across time on the same scanner and across scanners. Assessing this stability is done primarily by characterizing the temporal signal-to-noise ratio (tSNR), defined as the mean amplitude divided by the standard deviation of noise over time (for a more in-depth definition see Liu, 2016).

The methods for testing scanner stability using the tSNR range from relatively simple approaches, such as plotting the tSNR as a function of the size of region of interest (ROI; Weisskoff, 1996), to more complex modeling of the signal. Previous large-scale fMRI initiatives such as the Human Connectome Project (Marcus et al., 2013) using multiple scanning sites across time have employed the use of quality assurance tools such as the agar phantom (Friedman & Glover, 2006). This process uses a "phantom" plastic sphere filled with a doped agar gel to act as a static source of relative electrical silence (i.e., no areas are "activating") that mimics the conductivity of brain tissue. The phantom is scanned using the parameters meant for human data acquisition across all sites and time points and fed into a freely available quality assurance (QA) tool (fmriqa_phantomqa.pl[1]). This tool gives indices of tSNR, percent signal fluctuation and drift, smoothness, scanner stability, and intensity of ghosting, or the presence of spontaneously large signals in certain ROIs. Recommendations for determining how much variance in tSNR and other QA measures warrants concern about system differences can be found in Simmons et al. (1999).

Measuring Putative Exogenous Causes

An important step in rigorous cultural change research is to empirically test putative causes of patterns of cultural change. In the case of the predictions we have outlined so far, this would likely mean gathering time-series data on population density, use of online social networks (and average size of such networks), use of GPS or computer-assisted navigation, and rates of anxiety and depressive symptoms. It would also be wise to gather data on other factors previously linked to cultural change, including markers of resource levels and infectious disease prevalence. Population-level data on these variables may be easier to come by than population-level neural time-series data, but for many variables the span for which data are extant is limited. Thus, providing tests of the causes of any observed neural changes will likely involve prospective studies.

Common Issues in Time-Series Research

Perhaps the most vexing problem in research using time-series data is ruling out spurious associations. This is especially true if two time series being assessed contain high degrees of autocorrelation (Tiokhin & Hruschka, 2017; Vigen, 2015): two variables may appear to have a strong relationship when in fact the relationship is spurious and due simply to the fact that both exhibit a strong degree of autocorrelation. Some of the more humorous examples include correlations between marriages in Kentucky and fishing-related deaths (Vigen, 2015) and mentions of Jennifer Lawrence in news media and the performance of the Dow Jones Index (Fawcett, 2015). In research on cultural change, the time-series datasets we tend to be interested in are interesting precisely *because* they exhibit secular trends.

---

[1] https://xwiki.nbirn.org:8443/xwiki/bin/view/Function-BIRN/AutomatedQA

So how can researchers be confident that the relationships they observe are not spurious? There are several approaches to this problem. One is simply to remove linear trends from the data using a method such as first-differences detrending (e.g., Tiokhin & Hruschka, 2017; Varnum & Grossmann, 2019). Similarly, one may assess associations between two time series controlling for year (or other unit of time) using partial correlation analysis (e.g., Bianchi, 2016; Varnum et al., 2021), or controlling for time in multi-level models (e.g. Santos et al., 2017; Rotella et al., in press) . However, the argument can be made that these approaches cause important information to be lost, especially as from a theoretical standpoint most cultural change researchers are interested in long-term trends rather than short-term fluctuations, and as the indicators we tend to use in this research may contain a degree of noise or error. Alternative approaches include using Granger causality tests (e.g., Grossmann & Varnum, 2015; Jackson et al., 2019); correcting significance thresholds by simulating bootstrapped null distributions with datasets containing the same number of data points and the same degrees of first-order autocorrelation observed in the actual time series, a method devised by Tiokhin and Hruschka (2017; Varnum et al., 2021); or using advanced forecasting methods like auto-ARIMA, an algorithm developed by Hyndman and Khandakar (2008; e.g., Rotella, et al., in press; Varnum, 2018; Varnum et al., 2021).

Auto-ARIMA is an algorithm that generates the optimal forecasting model based on error residual reduction. It assesses the extent to which a variety of models, including autoregressive components of the respective time series, moving averages, and various types of differencing, fit the data and assesses the contribution made by theorized exogenous factors above and beyond the contributions made by autoregressive components of the time series. If the optimal model includes the exogenous variable, then researchers can have confidence that the relationship between two time series is not likely spurious even in the presence of a high degree of temporal autocorrelation among both time series. Auto-ARIMA also generates forecasts for future values, and this technique can be used to assess the validity of these models by comparing them with real future observations. If relationships between two highly autocorrelated time series hold when using a combination of these approaches to deal with autocorrelation, we suggest that researchers should have confidence that these relationships are not likely to be spurious. Thus, we highly recommend that researchers use at least one of these methods if a high degree of temporal autocorrelation is present in at least one of their time series to improve confidence in the conclusions they draw.

Controlling for Alternative Explanations and Forecasting the Future

We also have some recommendations for ensuring rigor in a neuroscience of cultural change, and in cultural change research more broadly. First, we recommend that researchers demonstrate that their models are robust. In the simplest sense this involves demonstrating that a proposed association between an exogenous factor (i.e., changes in gross domestic product, pathogen prevalence, climate, inequality, etc.) and dependent variables holds when controlling for other factors that might plausibly explain the effect. Unfortunately, this is not yet common in cultural change research, though it is standard in other types of correlational research in psychology and related disciplines. In our view it also involves dealing empirically with the possibility of spurious associations due to temporal autocorrelation using one or more of the methods we outlined in the previous section. Finally, we recommend that researchers studying cultural change, whether using neuroscience methods or not, publish forecasts for future trends based on their hypothesized models in addition to demonstrating relationships in past data (Varnum & Grossmann, 2017a). Whether future observations fit the predictions of these models derived from past observations should in our view be the gold standard for assessing their validity. In truth, the promise of a science of cultural change has more to do with predicting the future than explaining the past.

Summary and Conclusion

We began this chapter by noting that human cultures are not static and provided evidence of changes in a wide variety of mental and behavioral phenomena over the past several decades and centuries in a number of societies. We suspect that the structure and function of our brains may have also changed during this time and may continue to do so in the decades and centuries to come. We generated several predictions for how changes in our social, physical, and technological environments may be reshaping our brains and provided a broad outline for how such hypotheses may be tested in the future. Although others have speculated about ways in which recent developments may be affecting our brains, the present chapter, to our knowledge, represents the first roadmap for a rigorous and systematic study of this question and provides the first concrete predictions for what types of neural changes we might expect to see in the coming years.

These changes may have important implications for forecasting trends in mental health in the coming decades and may broaden our understanding of how environmental features may affect the risk for developing various forms of mental illness. Further, to the extent that relevant ecological changes occur at different rates around the globe, the risk of a variety of mental health problems may increase more dramatically in developing societies, which face greater challenges in providing treatment for these illnesses. Governments, policymakers, nongovernmental organizations, and clinicians may want to consider these issues when devising plans to improve mental health in the developing world.

We believe that there is now an exciting, though daunting, opportunity to create a field devoted to the study of how changes in the environment and society lead to changes in our brains at the scale of whole cultural groups. This would be an ambitious endeavor, but one that could be very fruitful. For the first time we have the capability to track how changes in our societies are impacting the way our brains are structured and function. This new field also represents an opportunity to build bridges across a variety of disciplines, including social psychology, clinical psychology, evolutionary psychology, economics, political science, and cultural neuroscience, and to connect theories and methods in a way that may produce a more complete understanding of human social dynamics than has previously been possible.

References

Bakker, R., Tiesinga, P., & Kötter, R. (2015). The scalable brain atlas: Instant web-based access to public brain atlases and related content. *Neuroinformatics*, *13*(3), 353–366.

Bergman, O., Åhs, F., Furmark, T., Appel, L., Linnman, C., Faria, V., Bani, M., cih, E. M., Bettica, P., Hennigsson, S., Manuck, S. B., Ferrell., R. E., Nikolova, Y. S., Hariri, A. R., Fredikson, M., Westberg, L., & Eriksson, E. (2014). Association between amygdala reactivity and a dopamine transporter gene polymorphism. *Translational Psychiatry*, *4*, e420. http://doi.org/10.1038/tp.2014.50

Bianchi, E. C. (2016). American individualism rises and falls with the economy: Cross-temporal evidence that individualism declines when the economy falters. *Journal of Personality and Social Psychology*, *111*(4), 567–584. http://doi.org/10.1037/pspp0000114

Bond, R., & Smith, P. B. (1996). Culture and conformity: A meta-analysis of studies using Asch's line judgment task. *Psychological Bulletin*, *119*(I), 111–137. http://doi.org/10.1037//0033-2909.119.1.111

Cai, H., Zou, X., Feng, Y., Liu, Y., & Jing, Y. (2018, May). Increasing need for uniqueness in contemporary China: Empirical evidence. *Frontiers in Psychology*, *9*, 1–7. http://doi.org/10.3389/fpsyg.2018.00554

Campbell, S., & Macqueen, G. (2004). The role of the hippocampus in the pathophysiology of major depression. *Journal of Psychiatry & Neuroscience: JPN*, *29*(6), 417–426.

Canli, T., Omura, K., Haas, B. W., Fallgatter, A., Constable, R. T., & Lesch, K. P. (2005). Beyond affect: A role for genetic variation of the serotonin transporter in neural activation during a cognitive attention task. *Proceedings of the National Academy of Sciences*, *102*(34), 12224–12229. http://doi.org/10.1073/pnas.0503880102

Charnov, E. L. (1993). *Life history invariants: Some explorations of symmetry in evolutionary ecology* (Vol. 6). Oxford University Press.

Chiao, J. Y., & Blizinsky, K. D. (2016). Cultural neuroscience: Bridging cultural and biological sciences. In E. Harmon-Jones & M. Inzlicht (Eds.), *Social neuroscience: Biological approaches to social psychology* (pp. 245–275). Taylor & Francis.

Del Giudice, M., Gangestad, S. W., & Kaplan, H. S. (2015). Life history theory and evolutionary psychology. In D. M. Buss (Ed.), *The handbook of evolutionary psychology*. Wiley.

Etkin, A., & Wager, T. D. (2007). Functional neuroimaging of anxiety: A meta-analysis of emotional processing in PTSD, social anxiety disorder, and specific phobia. *American Journal of Psychiatry*, *164*(10), 1476–1488. http://doi.org/10.1176/appi.ajp.2007.07030504

Fan, L., Li, H., Zhuo, J., Zhang, Y., Wang, J., Chen, L., . . . Jiang, T. (2016). The human brainnetome atlas: A new brain atlas based on connectional architecture. *Cerebral Cortex*, *26*, 3508–3526. http://doi.org/10.1093/cercor/bhw157

Fawcett, T. (2015, January 28). Avoiding common mistakes with time series [Blog post]. https://svds.com/avoiding-common-mistakes-with-time-series/

Flynn, J. R. (1987). Massive IQ gains in 14 nations: What IQ tests really measure. *Psychological Bulletin*, *101*(2), 171–191. http://doi.org/10.1037/0033-2909.101.2.171

Flynn, J. R. (2007). *What is intelligence? Beyond the Flynn effect*. Cambridge University Press.

Friedman, L., & Glover, G. H. (2006). Report on a multicenter fMRI quality assurance protocol. *Journal of Magnetic Resonance Imaging*, *23*(6), 827–839. http://doi.org/10.1002/jmri.20583

Gaffrey, M. S., Luby, J. L., Belden, A. C., Hirshberg, J. S., Volsch, J., & Barch, D. M. (2011). Association between depression severity and amygdala reactivity during sad face viewing in depressed preschoolers: An fMRI study. *Journal of Affective Disorders*, *129*(1–3), 364–370. http://doi.org/10.1016/j.jad.2010.08.031

Gardner, H. (2011). *Frames of mind: The theory of multiple intelligences*. Basic Books.

Gauthier, I., Tarr, M. J., Moylan, J., Skudlarski, P., Gore, J. C., & Anderson, A. W. (2000). The fusiform "face area" is part of a network that processes faces at the individual level. *Journal of Cognitive Neuroscience*, *12*(3), 495–504. http://doi.org/10.1162/089892900562165

Gentile, B., Campbell, W. K., & Twenge, J. M. (2014). Generational cultures. In A. B. Cohen (Ed.), *Culture reexamined: Broadening our understanding of social and evolutionary influences* (pp. 31–48). American Psychological Association.

Ghaem, O., Mellet, E., Crivello, F., Tzourio, N., Mazoyer, B., Berthoz, A., & Denis, M. (1997). Mental navigation along memorized routes activates the hippocampus, precuneus, and insula. *NeuroReport, 8*(3), 739–744. http://doi.org/10.1097/00001756-199702100-00032

Greenfield, P. M. (2013). The changing psychology of culture from 1800 through 2000. *Psychological Science, 24*(9), 1722–1731. http://doi.org/10.1177/0956797613479387

Greenfield, P. M. (2016). Social change, cultural evolution, and human development. *Current Opinion in Psychology, 8*, 84–92. http://doi.org/10.1016/j.copsyc.2015.10.012

Greenfield, P. M. (2017). Cultural change over time: Why replicability should not be the gold standard in psychological science. *Perspectives on Psychological Science, 12*(5), 762–771.

Grossmann, I., & Varnum, M. E. W. (2015). Social structures, infectious diseases, disasters, secularism and cultural change in America. *Psychological Science, 26*, 311–324. http://doi.org/10.1177/0956797614563765

Hamamura, T. (2012). Are cultures becoming individualistic? A cross-temporal comparison of individualism-collectivism in the United States and Japan. *Personality and Social Psychology Review, 16*(1), 3–24. http://doi.org/10.1177/1088868311411587

Hamamura, T., & Septarini, B. G. (2017). Culture and self-esteem over time: A cross-temporal meta-analysis among Australians, 1978–2014. *Social Psychological and Personality Science, 8*(8), 904–909. http://doi.org/10.1177/1948550617698205

Hamamura, T., & Xu, Y. (2015). Changes in Chinese culture as examined through changes in personal pronoun usage. *Journal of Cross-Cultural Psychology, 46*(7), 930–941. http://doi.org/10.1177/0022022115592968

Hampton, R. S., Kwon, J. Y., & Varnum, M. E. W. (2021). Variations in the regulation of affective neural responses across three cultures. *Emotion, 21*, 283–296.

Hampton, R. S., & Varnum, M. E. W. (2018a). The cultural neuroscience of emotion regulation. *Culture and Brain, 6*, 130–150.

Hampton, R. S., & Varnum, M. E. W. (2018b). Do cultures vary in self-enhancement? ERP, behavioral, and self-report evidence. *Social Neuroscience, 13*, 566–578.

Han, S. (2013). How to identify mechanisms of cultural influences on human brain functions. *Psychological Inquiry, 24*(1), 37–41. http://doi.org/10.1080/1047840X.2013.765755

Han, S., & Ma, Y. (2014). Cultural differences in human brain activity: A quantitative meta-analysis. *NeuroImage, 99*, 293–300. http://doi.org/10.1016/j.neuroimage.2014.05.062

Hyndman, R. J., & Khandakar, Y. (2008). Automatic time series forecasting: The forecast package for R. *Journal of Statistical Software, 27*(3), 1–22. http://doi.org/10.18637/jss.v027.i03

Iliev, R., Hoover, J., Dehghani, M., & Axelrod, R. (2016). Linguistic positivity in historical texts reflects dynamic environmental and psychological factors. *Proceedings of the National Academy of Sciences, 113*(49), E7871–E7879. http://doi.org/10.1073/pnas.1620120114

Inglehart, R. (1997). *Modernization and postmodernization: Cultural, economic, and political change in 43 societies*. Princeton University Press.

Inglehart, R., & Welzel, C. (2005). *Modernization, cultural change, and democracy: The human development sequence*. Cambridge University Press.

Jackson, J. C., Gelfand, M., De, S., & Fox, A. (2019). The loosening of American culture over 200 years is associated with a creativity–order trade-off. *Nature Human Behaviour, 3*(3), 244–250.

Johnson, S. (2005). *Everything bad is good for you: How popular culture is making us smarter*. Penguin.

Kanwisher, N., McDermott, J., & Chun, M. M. (1997). The fusiform face area: A module in human extrastriate cortex specialized for face perception. *Journal of Neuroscience, 17*(11), 4302–4311. http://doi.org/10.1098/Rstb.2006.1934

Kanwisher, N., & Yovel, G. (2006). The fusiform face area: A cortical region specialized for the perception of faces. *Philosophical Transactions of the Royal Society B: Biological Sciences, 361*(1476), 2109–2128. http://doi.org/10.1098/rstb.2006.1934

Kashima, Y. (2014). How can you capture cultural dynamics? *Frontiers in Psychology, 5*, 1–16. http://doi.org/10.3389/fpsyg.2014.00995

Kaufman, S. B. (2013). *The complexity of greatness: Beyond talent or practice*. Oxford University Press.

Kenrick, D. T., & Griskevicius, V. (2015). Life history, fundamental motives, and sexual competition. *Current Opinion in Psychology, 1*, 40–44.

Kesebir, S., & Kesebir, P. (2017). A growing disconnection from nature is evident in cultural products. *Perspectives on Psychological Science, 12*(2), 258–269.

Kim, H. S., & Sasaki, J. Y. (2014). Cultural neuroscience: Biology of the mind in cultural contexts. *Annual Review of Psychology, 65*, 487–514. http://doi.org/10.1146/annurev-psych-010213-115040

Kitayama, S., & Uskul, A. K. (2011). Culture, mind, and the brain: Current evidence and future directions. *Annual Review of Psychology, 62*, 419–449. http://doi.org/10.1146/annurev-psych-120709-145357

Kitayama, S., Varnum, M. E. W., & Salvador, C. (2019). Cultural neuroscience. In D. Cohen & S. Kitayama (Eds.), *Handbook of cultural psychology* (2nd ed.) (pp. 79–118). Guilford Press.

Kitayama, S., Yanagisawa, K., Ito, A., Ueda, R., Uchida, Y., & Abe, N. (2017). Reduced orbitofrontal cortical volume is associated with interdependent self-construal. *Proceedings of the National Academy of Sciences, 114*(30), 7969–7974.

Lesthaeghe, R. J. (2015). *The decline of Belgian fertility, 1800–1970*. Princeton University Press.

Liu, T. T. (2016). Noise contributions to the fMRI signal: An overview. *NeuroImage, 143*, 141–151. http://doi.org/10.1016/j.neuroimage.2016.09.008

Maguire, E. A., Burgess, N., Donnett, J. G., Frackowiak, R. S. J., Frith, C. D., & Okeefe, J. (1998). Knowing where and getting there. *Science, 280*(5365), 921–924.

Maguire, E. A., Gadian, D. G., Johnsrude, I. S., Good, C. D., Ashburner, J., Frackowiak, R. S. J., & Frith, C. D. (2000). Navigation-related structural change in the hippocampi of taxi drivers. *Proceedings of the National Academy of Sciences, 97*(8), 4398–4403. http://doi.org/10.1073/pnas.070039597

Marcus, D. S., Harms, M. P., Snyder, A. Z., Jenkinson, M., Wilson, J. A., Glasser, M. F., . . . Van Essen, D. C. (2013). Human Connectome Project informatics: Quality control, database services, and data visualization. *NeuroImage, 80*, 202–219. http://doi.org/10.1016/j.neuroimage.2013.05.077

Markus, H. R., & Kitayama, S. (1991). Culture and the self: Implications for cognition, emotion, and motivation. *Psychological Review, 98*(2), 224–253. http://doi.org/10.1037/0033-295X.98.2.224

Martin, S. F., Weerasinghe, S., & Taylor, A. (2014). *Humanitarian crises and migration: Causes, consequences and responses*. Routledge.

Matthews, P. M. (2001). An introduction to functional magnetic resonance imaging of the brain. In P. M. Jezzard, P. M. Matthews, & S. M. Smith (Eds.), *Functional MRI: An introduction to methods* (pp. 3–34). Oxford University Press.

Nisbett, R. E., Peng, K., Choi, I., & Norenzayan, A. (2001). Culture and systems of thought: Holistic versus analytic cognition. *Psychological Review, 108*(2), 291–310. http://doi.org/10.1037/0033-295X.108.2.291

Obradovich, N. (2017). Climate change may speed democratic turnover. *Climatic Change, 140*(2), 135–147.

Obradovich, N., & Fowler, J. H. (2017). Climate change may alter human physical activity patterns. *Nature Human Behaviour, 1*(5), 1–7. http://doi.org/10.1038/s41562-017-0097

Obradovich, N., Migliorini, R., Paulus, M. P., & Rahwan, I. (2018). Empirical evidence of mental health risks posed by climate change. *Proceedings of the National Academy of Sciences, 115*(43), 10953–10958.

Ogihara, Y. (2018). The rise in individualism in Japan: Temporal changes in family structure, 1947–2015. *Journal of Cross-Cultural Psychology, 49*, 1219–1226.

Oishi, S., Kesebir, S., & Diener, E. (2011). Income inequality and happiness. *Psychological Science, 22*(9), 1095–1100. http://doi.org/10.1177/0956797611417262

Olivera, J. (2015). Changes in inequality and generalized trust in Europe. *Social Indicators Research, 124*(1), 21–41. http://doi.org/10.1007/s11205-014-0777-5

Patriquin, M. A., DeRamus, T., Libero, L. E., Laird, A., & Kana, R. K. (2016). Neuroanatomical and neurofunctional markers of social cognition in autism spectrum disorder. *Human Brain Mapping, 37*(11), 3957–3978.

Pennebaker, J. W., & Jordan, K. (2018). *Cultural shifts in the presidents we choose*. Presented at the 19th annual meeting of the Society for Personality and Social Psychology, Atlanta, GA.

Pietschnig, J., & Voracek, M. (2015). One century of global IQ Gains: A formal meta-analysis of the Flynn effect (1909–2013). *Perspectives on Psychological Science, 10*(3), 282–306. http://doi.org/10.1177/1745691615577701

Putnam, R. D. (1995). Tuning in, tuning out: The strange disappearance of social capital in America. *PS: Political Science & Politics, 28*(4), 664–683.

Putnam, R. D. (2000). Bowling alone: America's declining social capital. In L. Crothers & C. Lockhart (Eds.), *Culture and politics: A reader* (pp. 223–234). Palgrave Macmillan. http://doi.org/10.1007/978-1-349-62397-6

Raven, J. (2000). The Raven's Progressive Matrices: Change and stability over culture and time. *Cognitive Psychology*, *41*(1), 1–48. http://doi.org/10.1006/cogp.1999.0735

Redlich, R., Opel, N., Bürger, C., Dohm, K., Grotegerd, D., Förster, K., . . . Dannlowski, U. (2018). The limbic system in youth depression: Brain structural and functional alterations in adolescent in-patients with severe depression. *Neuropsychopharmacology*, *43*(3), 546–554. http://doi.org/10.1038/npp.2017.246

Roberts, B. W., & Helson, R. (1997). Changes in culture, changes in personality: The influence of individualism in a longitudinal study of women. *Journal of Personality and Social Psychology*, *72*(3), 641–651. http://doi.org/10.1037/0022-3514.72.3.641

Roser, M., & Ortiz-Ospina, E. (2017). Global extreme poverty. *Our World in Data*, 1–38. https://ourworldindata.org/world-population-growth

Rotella, A., Varnum, M. E. W., Sng, O., & Grossmann, I. (in press). Increasing population densities predict decreasing fertility rates over time: A 174-nation investigation. *American Psychologist*.

Santos, H. C., Varnum, M. E. W., & Grossmann, I. (2017). Global increases in individualism. *Psychological Science, 28*, 1228–1239.

Schultz, R. T. (2005). Developmental deficits in social perception in autism: The role of the amygdala and fusiform face area. *International Journal of Developmental Neuroscience*, *23*(2–3), 125–141.

Schultz, R. T., Grelotti, D. J., Klin, A., Kleinman, J., Van der Gaag, C., Marois, R., & Skudlarski, P. (2003). The role of the fusiform face area in social cognition: Implications for the pathobiology of autism. *Philosophical Transactions of the Royal Society of London. Series B, Biological Sciences*, *358*(1430), 415–427.

Schuttenhelm, R. (2016). http://www.bitsofscience.org/graph-global-air-travel-increase-6848/

Sergent, J., Ohta, S., & MacDonald, B. (1992). Functional neuroanatomy of face and object processing: A positron emission tomography study. *Brain, 115*, 15–36.

Siegle, G. J., Thompson, W., Carter, C. S., Steinhauer, S. R., & Thase, M. E. (2007). Increased amygdala and decreased dorsolateral prefrontal BOLD responses in unipolar depression: Related and independent features. *Biological Psychiatry*, *61*(2), 198–209. http://doi.org/10.1016/j.biopsych.2006.05.048

Simmons, A., Moore, E., & Williams, S. C. (1999). Quality control for functional magnetic resonance imaging using automated data analysis and Shewhart charting. *Magnetic Resonance in Medicine*, *41*(6), 1274–1278.

Sng, O., Neuberg, S. L., Varnum, M. E. W., & Kenrick, D. T. (2018). The behavioral ecology of cultural variation. *Psychological Review, 125*, 714–745.

Stearns, S. C. (1992). *The evolution of life histories*. Oxford University Press.

Stein, M. B., Simmons, A. N., Feinstein, J. S., & Paulus, M. P. (2007). Increased amygdala and insula activation during emotion processing in anxiety-prone subjects. *American Journal of Psychiatry*, *164*(2), 318–327. http://doi.org/10.1176/ajp.2007.164.2.318

Sternberg, R. J. (1985). Implicit theories of intelligence, creativity, and wisdom. *Journal of Personality and Social Psychology*, *49*(3), 607–627. http://doi.org/10.1037/0022-3514.49.3.607

Stone, D. M., Simon, T. R., Fowler, K. A., Kegler, S. R., Yuan, K., & Holland, K. M. (2018). Vital signs: Trends in state suicide rates — United States, 1999 – 2016 and circumstances contributing to suicide — 27 States, 2015. *Morbidity and Mortality Weekly Report, 67*(22), 617–624. http://doi.org/10.15585/mmwr.mm6722a1

Thornton, A., & Young-DeMarco, L. (2001). Four decades of trends in attitudes toward family issues in the United States: The 1960s through the 1990s. *Journal of Marriage and Family*, *63*(4), 1009–1037. http://doi.org/10.1111/j.1741-3737.2001.01009.x

Tiokhin, L., & Hruschka, D. (2017). No evidence that an Ebola outbreak influenced voting preferences in the 2014 elections after controlling for time-series autocorrelation: A commentary on Beall, Hofer, and Schaller (2016). *Psychological Science*, *28*(9), 1358–1360.

Trahan, L., Stuebing, K. K., Hiscock, M. K., & Fletcher, J. M. (2014). The Flynn effect: A meta-analysis. *Psychological Bulletin*, *140*(5), 1332–1360. http://doi.org/10.1037/a0037173.The

Triandis, H. (1995). *Individualism & collectivism*. Westview Press.

Trzesniewski, K. H., Donnellan, M. B., & Robins, R. W. (2008a). Do today's young people really think they are so extraordinary. *Psychological Science*, *19*(2), 181–189. http://doi.org/10.1111/j.1467-9280.2008.02065.x

Trzesniewski, K. H., Donnellan, M. B., & Robins, R. W. (2008b). Is "Generation Me" really more narcissistic than previous generations? *Journal of Personality*, *76*(4), 903–918. http://doi.org/10.1111/j.1467-6494.2008.00508.x

Twenge, J. M. (1997). Attitudes toward women, 1970–1995. *Psychology of Women Quarterly*, *21*(1), 35–51.

Twenge, J. M. (2015). Time period and birth cohort differences in depressive symptoms in the U.S., 1982–2013. *Social Indicators Research*, *121*(2), 437–454. http://doi.org/10.1007/s11205-014-0647-1

Twenge, J. M., Abebe, E. M., & Campbell, W. K. (2010). Fitting in or standing out: Trends in American parents' choices for children's names, 1880–2007. *Social Psychological and Personality Science*, *1*(1), 19–25. http://doi.org/10.1177/1948550609349515

Twenge, J. M., & Campbell, W. K. (2001). Age and birth cohort differences in self-esteem: A cross-temporal meta-analysis. *Personality and Social Psychology Review*, *5*, 296–320. http://doi.org/10.1207/S15327957PSPR0504

Twenge, J. M., & Campbell, W. K. (2018). Cultural individualism is linked to later onset of adult-role responsibilities across time and regions. *Journal of Cross-Cultural Psychology*, *49*(4), 673–682.

Twenge, J. M., Campbell, W. K., & Carter, N. T. (2014). Declines in trust in others and confidence in institutions among American adults and late adolescents, 1972–2012. *Psychological Science*, *25*(10), 1914–1923. http://doi.org/10.1177/0956797614545133

Twenge, J. M., Campbell, W. K., & Gentile, B. (2012a). Increases in individualistic words and phrases in American books, 1960–2008. *PLoS One*, *7*(7). http://doi.org/10.1371/journal.pone.0040181

Twenge, J. M., Campbell, W. K., & Gentile, B. (2012b). Male and female pronoun use in U.S. books reflects women's status, 1900–2008. *Sex Roles*, *67*(9–10), 488–493. http://doi.org/10.1007/s11199-012-0194-7

Twenge, J. M., Campbell, W. K., & Gentile, B. (2013). Changes in pronoun use in American books and the rise of individualism, 1960–2008. *Journal of Cross-Cultural Psychology*, *44*(3), 406–415. http://doi.org/10.1177/0022022112455100

Twenge, J. M., & Foster, J. D. (2008). Mapping the scale of the narcissism epidemic: Increases in narcissism 2002–2007 within ethnic groups. *Journal of Research in Personality*, *42*(6), 1619–1622. http://doi.org/10.1016/j.jrp.2008.06.014

Twenge, J. M., Gentile, B., DeWall, C. N., Ma, D., Lacefield, K., & Schurtz, D. R. (2010). Birth cohort increases in psychopathology among young Americans, 1938–2007: A cross-temporal meta-analysis of the MMPI. *Clinical Psychology Review*, *30*(2), 145–154. http://doi.org/10.1016/j.cpr.2009.10.005

Twenge, J. M., Joiner, T. E., Rogers, M. L., & Martin, G. N. (2018). Increases in depressive symptoms, suicide-related outcomes, and suicide rates among US adolescents after 2010 and links to increased new media screen time. *Clinical Psychological Science*, *6*(1), 3–17.

Twenge, J. M., Konrath, S., Foster, J. D., Campbell, W. K., & Bushman, B. J. (2008). Further evidence of an increase in narcissism among college students. *Journal of Personality*, *76*(4), 919–928. http://doi.org/10.1111/j.1467-6494.2008.00509.x

Twenge, J. M., & Park, H. (2017). The decline in adult activities among U.S. adolescents, 1976–2016. *Child Development*, 1–17. http://doi.org/10.1111/cdev.12930

United Nations, Department of Economic and Social Affairs Population Division. (2013). *Trends in international migration*.

United Nations, Department of Economic and Social Affairs Population Division (2014). World urbanization prospects: The 2014 revision, highlights. *Demographic Research*. http://doi.org/10.4054/DemRes.2005.12.9

Van de Vliert, E. (2013). Climato-economic habitats support patterns of human needs, stresses, and freedoms. *Behavioral and Brain Sciences*, *36*(5), 465–480. http://doi.org/10.1017/S0140525X12002828

Varnum, M. E. W. (2018, March). *Making psycho-history a reality: The emerging science of cultural change*. Presented at the Advances in Cultural Psychology Preconference at the 19th annual meeting of the Society for Personality and Social Psychology, Atlanta, GA.

Varnum, M. E. W., & Grossmann, I. (2016). Pathogen prevalence is associated with cultural changes in gender equality. *Nature Human Behaviour*, *1*. http://doi.org/10.1038/s41562-016-0003

Varnum, M. E. W., & Grossmann, I. (2017a). Cultural change: The how and the why. *Perspectives on Psychological Science*, *12*(6), 956–972. http://doi.org/10.1177/1745691617699971

Varnum, M. E. W., & Grossmann, I. (2017b). Socio-ecological factors are linked to changes in prevalence of contempt over time. *Behavioral and Brain Sciences*, *40*, e250.

Varnum, M. E. W., & Grossmann, I. (2019). The wealth->life history->innovation account of the industrial revolution is largely inconsistent with empirical time series data. *Behavioral and Brain Sciences*, *42*, e212.

Varnum, M. E. W., Grossmann, I., Kitayama, S., & Nisbett, R. E. (2010). The origin of cultural differences in cognition: The social orientation hypothesis. *Current Directions in Psychological Science*, *19*(1), 9–13. http://doi.org/10.1177/0963721409359301

Varnum, M. E. W., & Hampton, R. S. (2017). Cultures differ in the ability to enhance affective neural responses. *Social Neuroscience, 12*, 594–603.

Varnum, M. E. W., Krems, J. A., Morris, C., Wormley, A. S., & Grossmann, I. (2021). People prefer simpler content when there are more choices: A time series analysis of lyrical complexity in six decades of American popular music. *PLOS ONE, 16, e0244576*

Vigen, T. (2015). *Spurious correlations*. Hachette Books.

Weisskoff, R. M. (1996). Simple measurement of scanner stability for functional NMR imaging of activation in the brain. *Magnetic Resonance in Medicine, 36*(4), 643–645. http://doi.org/10.1002/mrm.1910360422

Wetzel, E., Brown, A., Hill, P. L., Chung, J. M., Robins, R. W., & Roberts, B. W. (2017). The narcissism epidemic is dead: Long live the narcissism epidemic. *Psychological Science, 28*(12), 1833–1847. http://doi.org/10.1177/0956797617724208

Zeng, R., & Greenfield, P. M. (2015). Cultural evolution over the last 40 years in China: Using the Google Ngram viewer to study implications of social and political change for cultural values. *International Journal of Psychology, 50*(1), 47–55. http://doi.org/10.1002/ijop.12125

Zhu, Y., Zhang, L., Fan, J., & Han, S. (2007). Neural basis of cultural influence on self-representation. *Neuroimage, 34*(3), 1310–1316.

Acculturation by Plasticity and Stability in Neural Processes: Considerations for Global Mental Health Challenges

Joshua O. S. Goh

Abstract

The cultural environment can have significant influence on the brain. This is not surprising given that plasticity with respect to environmental stimulation defines neural morphological changes and functioning that instantiate cognitive operations in the brain. Nevertheless, certain aspects of neural structure and function such as neurophysiological regulatory mechanisms at the cellular level and neural processing of informational commonalities should also remain stable across different environments. This chapter considers how the interplay between neuroplasticity with stability might be a general principle for brain and behavioral acculturation such as in the processing of physical regularities, social mores, self-related information, causal inference, and biological homeostasis. Gleaning from work on prediction error processing, the chapter presents a framework that views stability and plasticity as neural mechanisms that habitualize behaviors or make them extinct, and also considers clinical implications when these mechanisms are dysregulated. From this, the presence of cultural differences in social interactions between people groups is suggested to reflect the brain's normative solution to solving the problem of dynamic environments. The chapter incorporates this perspective of brain acculturation into applications for global mental health challenges, particularly in light of the advancement in communication technology and globalization that has resulted in increased cultural interactions and cultural mixing.

Key Words: culture, mental health, cognition, social processing, prediction, prediction error, reward learning, neuroplasticity, neurostability

Motivation and Scope

People who grow up and live in different environments have different cultural experiences that shape their ways of thinking and behavior. People with different cultural backgrounds also have distinct experiences and viewpoints despite a given physical event being the same. Thus, while the environment influences the human mind, the human mind also maintains its biases when engaging with the environment. An issue that arises from such culturally specified mind–environment interactions pertains to the characterization of when these interactions are normative and when they reflect pathology. Like cultural influences, pathology in the human brain and mind is also associated with differences with which affected persons engage with and interpret the environment. Moreover, certain behaviors, while considered psychiatric in one culture, might be construed as exceptional but still normative in another (Kurihara et al., 2000). Also, cultural influences direct individuals to preferentially engage certain neural processing strategies when approaching even basic cognitive tasks (Goh et al., 2007; Hedden et al., 2008), which might be misdiagnosed as nonnormative if not accounted for in performance population norms. Indeed, recent consensus toward globally addressing current challenges in medical treatments and costs of mental, neurological, and substance use (MNS) disorders has considered the critical role culture occupies in clinical applications (Chiao et al., 2017; Collins et al., 2011). To this end, there is a need to more fundamentally apprehend the complex and varied manifestations of cultural and clinical influences on the mind and brain.

This chapter highlights the notion that both cultural and clinical influences operate and induce cognitive differences in the brain primarily via the plasticity of neural processes. Specifically, cultural differences in human cognition and behavior arise because neural processes have some level of plasticity as opposed to always remaining stable or rigid under different environmental influences. However, pathology sets in when neural dysregulation occurs such that there is either too much plasticity or too much stability with respect to the culturally dynamic environmental information being processed. Thus, while there are many challenges in developing culturally specific diagnostic and treatment approaches to MNS disorders, a framework based on neuroplasticity as a common neural processing principle for cultural and clinical phenomena might make the problem more tenable.

Consider that the dynamic exchange between the human mind and environment potentiates the formation of local human cultures as social solutions for local physical environmental problems. For instance, the quantification of physical length is of clear importance in many situations, and the communication and agreement of observed lengths are also paramount for effective social exchange. Human beings have thus developed scales to facilitate communication about different lengths. However, different groups of persons are used to different notions of scales of length (e.g., meter, foot, span, fathom) that were applied under specific geographical and historical contexts. Such an example of acculturation of the concept of length occurs because of the principle of locality in social transmission. We learned our own notions of units of length from our caretakers, peers, and educators. These specific notions of length, however, are not immutable and are subject to change as an individual interacts with other social groups over their lifetime. Moreover, a clinical case might arise in which an individual's notions of reality are not easily subject to normative change despite social interactions. Critically, the central mechanism for such culture-ability of the human brain to efficiently operate relies on neuroplasticity (and the complementary process, neurostability), which essentially describes how the brain carries out information processing.

Neuroplasticity and human cultural differences are both well-researched domains with their respective findings and principles reasonably established. As such, this chapter will not reiterate extant theory or data. Rather, the goal here is to make linkages between these research areas toward a conceptual integration of how neuroplasticity and cultural behavior both reflect the basic operation of the brain in processing information. The notion that neural operations reflect both updating and maintenance of cognitive representations in the brain as well as brief clinical implications has also been treated in another work by the author's group (Goh et al., 2020). As such, this chapter extends from there with more specific considerations at the level of neurobiological models such as long-term potentiation and long-term depression as accounts for brain and behavioral acculturation as well as mental health deviations.

To orientate the rest of this chapter, a limited operational definition of culture is given to make subsequent discussion more tractable. Then, a very brief review is provided on empirical evidence for differences in human brain structure and function associated with cultural differences in behavior. This is followed by a cursory introduction to some of the common neurobiological processes that are thought to underlie plasticity in brain function. Critically, a juxtaposition of the importance for stability in neurobiological operations and neural processing in tandem with plasticity is highlighted to reconcile the notion that the brain must simultaneously balance between objective physical stimuli and accompanying social biases in environmental information. From there, the argument is made that cultural differences in human behavior begin when there are differences between expected and experienced outcomes in interacting with the environment that consists of physical and social information. This experiential discrepancy results in prediction error signals that direct neuroplasticity in brain function toward cultural norms. Highlight is then made on the pathological dysregulation of neuroplasticity when appropriate prediction error signals are not generated or not integrated in environmental interactions. In this light, avenues are finally considered for clinical applications in definitions, assessments, and treatments for mental health in the diverse global arena.

Operational Definition of Culture

A limited but nevertheless working operationalization of the notion of culture must be stated to initiate practical discussion. By culture, it is broadly meant that there are groups of individuals who display a common set of ideological, social, and cognitive behaviors that is distinct from other groups. For instance, most East Asian individuals outwardly express behaviors that reflect an emphasis on the value of collectivism or interdependence. In concordance with this value, it is common and acceptable in East Asian cities to find adults of working age still living with their parents. By contrast, individuals who subscribe to more Western culture display emphasis on individualism and independence.

Using the same example, it is common and acceptable in Western culture to find working adults staying apart from their parents even if their residences are in close proximity. While the majority of studies have compared cultural differences between East Asians and Westerners, this is mostly due to experimental convenience and also perhaps due to historical, geopolitical, and economic factors. As such, the basic range of empirical works reviewed in this chapter will also focus on comparisons between East Asian and Western groups. Nevertheless, it is asserted that issues of cultural differences inclusively apply to other culture groups based on other forms of geopolitical or social boundaries. Cultural differences between different people groups other than East Asians and Westerners are by no means absent and are beginning to be explored as globalization progresses. Overall, as extant data reviewed later will show, the influences of differences in the social mores of East Asians and Westerners pervade even to the level of cognitive operations that may even be transparent to the individual.

A common characterization and evaluation of culture-related differences between East Asians and Westerners has already been extensively reviewed in past literature that stem from a consideration of ideological or philosophical differences (Nisbett, 2003; Nisbett et al., 2001; Nisbett & Miyamoto, 2005; Oyserman & Lee, 2008; Triandis, 1995; Triandis et al., 1988). In these works, it is suggested that many aspects of modern Western ideology may be traced back to Greek antiquity. This zeitgeist emphasized the parsing of physical phenomena from their more abstract sense in an individual's internal experience as well as the parsing of the component features of physical objects. Indeed, many empirical studies have noted that Western ideological pursuits tend to center around constructs that reflect independence, hedonism, and self-seeking motivations (Hofstede, 1980, 2001; Hofstede & Bond, 1984; Rohan, 2000; Schwartz, 1990, 1992; Schwartz & Bilsky, 1990). Such ideology and motivations are associated with cognitive styles that reflect analytic attention to features that define objects and traits that define persons. Implicit in such cognitive styles is the default and primary perspective that things should be considered independent from other things. By contrast, East Asian thought is considered to evince more dialectical arguments that attend more to how concepts and things are related or bound to each other rather than independent. A reflection of this mode of thinking might be seen in the East Asian emphasis on finding a middle ground to resolve conflicts and the sense that crimes or faults of an individual also implicate the family. Thus, under the same framework for ideological and motivational constructs, East Asian culture is characterized by a value for interdependence, harmony, and self-transcendence. In association with such a worldview, cognitive processing in East Asians is characterized as having a more holistic style as the default, attending more to the relationship of objects to other objects or the context in which an object is embedded.

Interestingly, it has also been suggested that such cultural differences associated with an individualism versus collectivism dimension, as seen between Westerners and East Asians, might also emerge due to differences in agricultural practices or other broad human socioenvironmental interactions (Talhelm et al., 2014). Specifically, the farming of wheat in Western cultures might encourage more individualistic communication strategies between farmers because wheat is more robust and requires less integration of resources. By contrast, rice farming in East Asian cultures requires more cooperation between persons due to the more complex infrastructure involved to adapt to the greater sensitivity of rice to minute environmental changes. Whether philosophical or socioenvironmental influences or both shaped East Asian and Western cultures, it is clear that these people groups evince behaviors that can be dissociated by mental constructs to do with individualism and collectivism. As can be seen in the consideration of neuroscientific findings next, there is evidence for this dichotomy in terms of neural computation as well.

Evidence for Cultural Differences in Neural Processes

With the accessibility of in vivo neuroimaging technology, an increasing corpus of findings have accumulated that reflect differences in brain gross structure and regional brain function across samples from different cultural backgrounds (Goh & Park, 2009; Goh & Huang, 2012; Goh et al., in press; Park & Huang, 2010). Specifically, myriad findings support mental and neural processing differences in East Asians and Westerners consistent with an individualistic–collectivistic dichotomy. In the domain of visual perception and attention, East Asians are more sensitive to visual information occurring in background scenes than objects in the foreground, whereas Westerners are more sensitive to object changes (Masuda & Nisbett, 2001, 2006). Such culture-related differences in perception and attention behavior extend to even fundamental judgments of simple physical quantities such as line length (Kitayama et al., 2003). In addition, East Asians evince eye movements that reflect a rapid overall scanning approach to naturalistic pictures consisting of focal objects embedded in scenes, whereas Westerners tend to focus more on central objects (Chua et al., 2005; Goh et al., 2009). In vivo functional brain imaging revealed that East Asians engage fewer neural resources when processing relative physical length judgments, whereas Westerners engage fewer neural resources for absolute length judgments (Goh et al., 2013; Hedden et al., 2008). A series of functional magnetic resonance imaging (fMRI) studies revealed that ventral visual functional responses in older East Asians also treat composite pictures with objects and background contexts as holistic scenes as a default viewing strategy compared to older Westerners, who parse the objects more distinctively from the background contexts (Chee et al., 2006; Goh et al., 2004, 2007).

In the domain of semantic judgments, we note that East Asians tend to regard words as related to each other more by function (e.g., cows eat grass), whereas Westerners regard word relations based more on featural categories (e.g., cows and chickens are both animals; Chiu, 1972). Developing from this, East Asians are shown to engage greater lateral occipital processing of object–scene incongruence compared to Westerners, although both groups showed similar processing of incongruence in the parahippocampal place area

(Jenkins et al., 2010). This pattern of neural responses suggests that violations of semantic associations engaged greater visual object computation in East Asians than Westerners, further suggesting that the scene was more important than the object. That is, the object was the out-of-place element in the picture and had to be resolved more so than the scene.

Finally, in the domain of social perception and processing of interpersonal values, there is evidence that East Asians show greater sensitivity to social norm violations compared to Westerners (Mu et al., 2015) and engage differential brain areas when processing moral judgments involving others (Han et al., 2014). Cultural differences in the attention to and neural engagement for faces and facial emotion expressions have also been consistently reported (Akechi et al., 2013; Blais et al., 2008; Chiao et al., 2008; Goh et al., 2010; Jack et al., 2009, 2016; Masuda et al., 2008; Tu et al., 2018), contrasting with the notion of universality face emotions (Darwin, 1872; Ekman et al., 1987; Ekman & Friesen, 1977; Izard, 1994). Such profound cultural differences in processing of social information might stem from differences in perceptions of social distance from the self and thus, perhaps, engage different senses of personal responsibility or relevance. Indeed, findings have shown that East Asians engage more relational neural responses treating close others as more similar to their self-concept compared to Westerners (Zhu et al., 2007). Also, several studies have evaluated how cultural behavioral and neural differences reflect differences in the perception of the self in relation to others (Chiao et al., 2010; Hitokoto et al., 2016; Hong et al., 2001; Kitayama & Park, 2010; Park & Kitayama, 2014).

Taking the aforementioned empirical findings together, it is clear that there are meaningful and quantifiable differences in the manner that East Asian and Westerner brains process environmental information at various levels of abstraction (from physical visual stimuli, to the self, to social morals), and that these differences have something to do with the notion of an individualism–collectivism dimension of motivation or mental bias. In addition, beneath the notions of historical ideological or social causes accounting for observed cultural differences in individualism and collectivism is the assumption that how the brain is acculturated centers around the influence of environmental forces on neural processes in the brain, the "goal" of the brain, and how the brain then acts on the environment. In this light, the following sections consider how these culture-related differences might arise due to basic computational operations that neuronal activity must natively have to perform their roles effectively in processing information about the environment and in promoting survival of the organism.

Argument for the Role of Neuroplasticity in Acculturation of the Brain

As mentioned, the notion that differences in environmental stimulation shape neural activity via neuroplasticity is neither novel nor controversial. Nevertheless, in considering how neuroplasticity might be associated with brain acculturation, it is helpful to first delineate a general goal for all neural processes and, therefore, the general computational goal of the brain itself. A reasonable premise is that the brain has a primary goal to promote the survival of the organism via integration of environmental information to select actions that meet that goal (Knill & Pouget, 2004; Parr & Friston, 2017). For instance, an organism's search for food might yield information that food can be found around trees and less around rocks. Subsequently, when the organism later moves to different locations, it might evince greater likelihood to choose locations with trees than locations with only rocks because it had experience that the former is generally better for its survival. A more general premise is that actions that meet the survival goal are actions that are based on appropriately represented information that lead to operations on the environment that yield predicted outcomes. Continuing the example, the organism's acquired bias to move toward locations with trees might be construed as reflecting an internal neural representation or mapping of the functional relationship between trees and food (perhaps a proposition that trees produce food). Finally, information about the environment is most appropriately represented when it reflects the truth about the environment most accurately (Friston et al., 2006, 2009; Goh et al., 2018; Lochmann & Deneve, 2011; Shams & Beierholm, 2010; Tenenbaum et al., 2011). In the example, to the extent that trees really do produce food, the neural representation in the organism that drives the behavior to select trees over rocks should result in the expected outcomes and thus the representation and action should persist. Applying these concepts at the neuronal level, then, neuronal activity subserving the sensation, computation, and subsequent transmission of information about stimuli within its receptive field should be driven to reflect the real local physical environment as closely as possible.

In this light, it is important to note that the physical environment and the information received by sensory receptors are by no means linear phenomena. Not only does environmental stimulation impinging on sensory receptors change at each instance, but also the functional associations between them changes. Consider the simple example that in one instance, the printed letter "A" occurs independently of other print, and in another instance within close proximity, it occurs bound by a "C" on the left and a "T" on the right. Both occurrences of physical light due to "A" should result in the same stimulation on the retina, subsequent visual neurons, and downstream processes. Yet, we all invariably and effortlessly mentally experience and interpret the first type of "A" as an article and the latter as part of a conceptual representation of an animal. To code stimuli with such contextual and associative contingencies, neuronal firing thus must have the ability to dynamically capture variations with respect to the changing stimuli as well as the changing associations between stimuli. The key mechanism for neuronal computation to adapt to such temporal environmental variation, then, is through functional plasticity. Specifically, at the neuronal level again, a neuron's outputs for given present stimuli input change in accordance with past input–output histories.

Extending these notions, consider that physical stimuli in our daily experiences are inextricably bound within social contexts. For instance, a child learns to read almost certainly by interacting with their caretaker, who might offer interpretations of the read material. In so doing, the caretaker might engage in the cultural transmission of ideas beyond the information conveyed by the physical stimuli. Moreover, interactions with the environment sans social validations might even be considered meaningless and uninteresting to the child. In addition, considerable work has investigated how human judgment of physical stimuli and even facts is often susceptible to peer or social pressure (Asch, 1956; Berns et al., 2005; Campbell-Meiklejohn et al., 2010; Izuma, 2013; Klucharev et al., 2009; Nook & Zaki, 2015; Zaki et al., 2011). Thus, neural processing of physical stimuli and the social contexts in which they are bound involves representing different physical as well as social stimuli associations that "distort" the physical information. Differential experiences with such physical-social associative information over time cumulatively shape the pattern of neuronal and neural network input–output functions and facilitates subsequent information processing in a manner that is then congruent with past experiences. Cultural environments, as specific sets of physical and social interactions over experience, then also imprint specific sets of physical-social stimuli associations represented in neural network computation patterns that effect corresponding biases in mental processes and behavior. Critically, this culture-specific neural network computation can only arise because neuronal function is plastic in nature rather than impervious to stimuli contingencies.

Neural Mechanisms of Neuroplasticity

General neurobiological mechanisms that drive functional plasticity in neural information processing are basic well-studied topics in the fields of experimental and computational neuroscience and neurobiology, and the interested reader is strongly encouraged to consult other sources for more in-depth coverage if needed (Andersen et al., 2017; Escobar & Derrick, 2007; Hebb, 1949; Kandel, 2001; Kandel et al., 2013). Here, only a brief introduction of the necessary knowledge is given for the purposes of facilitating subsequent broad discussion on neuroplasticity and acculturation. At the neuronal level, plasticity can be understood in terms of synaptic changes in the likelihood of generation of axonal action potentials (a sharp firing or depolarization of the neuronal cell membrane voltage potential constituting the neuronal detection of information), as well as specific patterns of firing activity in postsynaptic neurons in response to presynaptic neuronal signals. By contrast, a state of limited synaptic plasticity occurs when action potentials or firing patterns remain invariant over time. It is well known that presynaptic neuronal signals primarily come in the form of neurotransmitter molecules that are released by the presynaptic neuron into the synaptic cleft and that bind with receptor molecules on the cell membrane of the postsynaptic neuron. Note that postsynaptic receptors might be ligand-gated ion channels that have primary and fast operation in the scale of milliseconds. Such receptors respond directly to neurotransmitter binding, and these neurotransmitters are also rapidly removed. However, the influences of culture-related experiential information on the plasticity of neuronal activity are more likely due to secondary modulatory effects on direct ligand-gated ion channel neuronal responses that involve other types of receptor molecules and mechanisms. Specifically, these secondary effects are characterized by differential neurotransmitter–receptor-binding operations at the time scale of seconds or longer and that involve molecular signals that modulate subsequent likelihood of postsynaptic membrane depolarization (Kandel, 2001; Purves et al., 2004; Waxman, 2013; see also Plested, 2016, for a broad review of neurotransmitter–receptor mechanisms across species).

Critically, modulation of neuronal firing likelihood occurs as a function of incoming stimulation in relation to the neuron's own current state (and the states of the other neurons in synaptic connection with it) and is thus dynamically activity dependent. Specifically, whether a neuron is likely to generate a specific activity pattern depends on the afferent presynaptic activity pattern as well as the neuron's own prior likelihood to generate activity, which are determined by its neurobiological state, at that time. Biomolecular mechanisms suggested to jointly underlie such synaptic changes in likelihoods for action potential and neuronal activity pattern initiation can be dichotomized into two broad classes of short-term and long-term mechanisms.

Short-term neurobiological mechanisms of neural plasticity include changes such as presynaptic neurotransmitter and postsynaptic receptor availability or efficacy that involve modulation of primary ligand-gated ion channel receptor responses (which again occur within milliseconds) typically in the time scale of seconds to minutes. Specifically, over these time scales, the number of neurotransmitter molecules released or present in the synaptic cleft or the number of receptor molecules available for binding to neurotransmitters might be maintained or reduced. These scenarios might occur because other signaling molecules are generated in pre- or postsynaptic neurons to accelerate or dampen neurotransmitter reuptake from the synaptic cleft or neurotransmitter–receptor binding and release. Alternatively, multiple types of neurotransmitters or receptors might also be recruited at a given synapse to enhance or restrict postsynaptic neuronal depolarization. A neurobehavioral phenomenon that relies on such short-term synaptic response changes might be the reduction of neuronal activity (and enhancement of behavior) to recently repeated stimuli such as in the case of rapid repetition-related priming (Grill-Spector et al., 2006). Specifically, stimuli recently processed by a neuron seconds or minutes ago typically engage lower levels of neuronal activity. Importantly, such reduction in neuronal activity associated with the frequency of stimuli occurrence likely stems from the synaptic modulatory mechanisms mentioned earlier that involve short-term biomolecular changes in postsynaptic receptor sensitivity to neurotransmitters.

When stimuli and stimuli association occurrences are frequently encountered or are attached with particular salience, long-term plasticity neuronal mechanisms might then begin to operate. Specifically, regular repetitive patterns of the aforementioned activity-dependent synaptic processes contribute to raising the level of neuronal intracellular signals such as Ca^{2+} and cyclic nucleotides, among others (Purves et al., 2004; Waxman,

2013). These intracellular molecular signals lead to a cascade of events inside the neuron that include modulation of gene expression and synthesis of proteins that subsequently are involved in neuronal structural changes such as in dendritic morphology. Indeed, extensive repetitive stimulation alters the number of dendrites, dendritic arborization, dendritic spine formation and reinforcement, and synaptogenesis in postsynaptic neurons, at the very least. These dendritic functional and morphological changes ultimately result in either long-term potentiation (LTP) or long-term depression (LTD) of the likelihood of subsequent neuronal activity.

As the name suggests, LTP refers to neuronal changes that increase the likelihood of postsynaptic firing in response to regularly co-occurring presynaptic inputs. LTP is generally supported by increases in dendritic and synaptic density of excitatory connections, which enhance the sensitivity of postsynaptic neurons to presynaptic neurotransmitters. By contrast, LTD refers to neuronal changes that decrease the likelihood of postsynaptic firing. LTD might be supported by reductions in dendritic and synaptic density for excitatory connections or the enhancement of the contributions of synaptic connections that are inhibitory. LTP and LTD are two general models of plasticity in neuronal activity that likely operate together to maximize the selectivity of neural circuits to engage sparse coding in neural representations of information as well as to maintain a homeostatic level of neural activity (more later on homeostasis). Whereas LTP might enhance neural activity to stimuli occurrences, LTD prunes neural activity to only that which is necessary. It should be noted that these neurobiological mechanisms for LTP or LTD do not constitute an exhaustive list, and more candidate cellular pathways are currently still being discovered. In addition, studies on LTP and LTD have largely focused on the medial temporal area as the focus of associative memory processing. Thus, other broader forms of neuroplasticity, for instance, at the network computation level, should also be noted.

Beyond neuronal LTP and LTD in medial temporal areas, another broader form of plasticity in brain function is seen in how memories are consolidated and transferred from dependence on medial temporal to neocortical circuits (Eichenbaum, 2013; Laroche et al., 2000; Preston & Eichenbaum, 2013; Sekeres et al., 2018; Squire et al., 2004; Wiltgen et al., 2004). The classic example of patient H. M. demonstrates that while lesions of medial temporal structures are detrimental to the formation of new episodic memories, they have minimal effects on past established memories (Squire, 2009). That is, initial associative memories require medial temporal processes for integration and formation; however, with time, the core of these memory associations might migrate to frontal or other brain areas that are perhaps hierarchically deeper brain networks. In another example, the occipital lobe that is specifically responsive to visual stimuli in normal persons shows responses to auditory stimuli in blind persons (Bedny et al., 2015; Merabet et al., 2004; Poirier et al., 2006), reflecting again the functional plasticity of neural cortices across individual experiences. Thus, the whole-brain system, itself constituted by billions of neurons, can be construed as implementing plasticity in information representation and processing at the systemic network level.

In sum, several different mechanisms of neurobiological molecular and morphological changes as well as more systemic changes at the level of interregional brain networks make up the phenomenon of neuroplasticity. Such neural network dynamics are how information processing in the brain captures variability in frequencies and complex associations in environmental stimuli. It is this plasticity at all levels of neural processing from the molecular to the brain as a system that enables learning and also acculturation to the different sets of physical-social associations across cultural experiences. Critically, the aforementioned neurobiological mechanisms either strengthen or dampen the likelihood of specific stimuli resulting in particular patterns of neuronal responses in the brain. In this manner, neuronal response patterns are constantly modulated to the extent that there are changes encountered in environmental stimulation and made stronger by environmental associations that occur invariantly.

Importance of Stability in Neural Processes

It is now important to consider the flip side of the neuroplasticity story, as it were. While dynamism in physical and social associations is present in the environment, it is perhaps sometimes overlooked that there are also many regularities. Thus, while neuroplasticity allows encoding dynamic environmental associative changes and potentiates cultural differences in information processing, plasticity of neural processes must also grasp invariability in environmental associations where present. Importantly, this competing drive to code for stability as opposed to dynamism in environmental information is also part of the goal of the brain to represent the environment in a manner that is as close to the truth as possible. Indeed, only if neural networks also maintain some aspects of regularity can the mental phenomena of learning, memory, and expectation occur.

Support for the need for stability in neural processing can be seen in the many brain functions that are common across different individuals. Similarity across human individuals in brain structural and neural organization as well as molecular operations is not surprising considering that biological structures are certainly largely determined by genetic factors. Nevertheless, it is remarkable that brain functional responses are also generally similar across individuals in specific brain regions and processes, for which there is no clear genetic basis. For example, primary visual cortices evince topological orientation selectivity as part of their functional responses to changes in light information across mammals including humans (Hubel & Wiesel, 1962; Schmolesky et al., 2000; Sun et al., 2013). Also, the complexity of information managed in brain regions increases in abstraction in a similar manner across individuals from sensory to primary associative to secondary and tertiary associative cortices (Goh et al., 2004; Grill-Spector et al., 1998). Commonality of brain function modularity is also seen in the presence of the fusiform face area (Kanwisher et al., 1997; Kanwisher & Yovel, 2006), visual word form area (Bouhali et al., 2014; Dien,

2009; Vogel et al., 2014; although see Price & Devlin, 2003), lateral occipital complex (Grill-Spector et al., 2001; Malach et al., 1995), parahippocampal place area (Epstein & Kanwisher, 1998), lingual landmark area (Aguirre et al., 1998), and extrastriate body area (Downing et al., 2001; Ross et al., 2014) in largely the same brain loci in most individuals. Perhaps even more remarkable is that language processes are typically more predominant in the left hemisphere, classically in Wernicke's and Broca's areas, albeit language is by no means only localized to these regions (Fujii et al., 2016; Hagoort, 2014; Tremblay & Dick, 2016).

Another indication of the affinity of the brain for stability in information processing is seen in the formation of habits (Graybiel, 2008). Many motor actions are more difficult, involving extensive neural resources during initial acquisition, but require fewer neural computational resources when automatized over repetitive practice and the processes are made more invariable and thus reliable. Such automatization or habitualizing of motor behaviors include many common actions such as walking, riding a bicycle, playing a musical instrument, and even producing verbal utterances. Critically, habit learning in principle extends also to more purely mental processes such attentional biases, sensory perceptual heuristics, and social perceptual heuristics. Indeed, repeated stimuli tend to engage less neural processing perhaps to avoid the redundancy of processing the same information again by integrating the consistency of information over time (Grill-Spector et al., 2006). Thus, so long as environmental associations remain the same, engaging the same behavior or cognitive process in interacting with the environment should lead to the same expected outcome. As such, the brain will habitualize the input–output mapping so that fewer neural resources will be used up to achieve the desired goal.

As can be seen, neurostability and neuroplasticity in fact describe different aspects of neural processing in general. Thus, the same neurobiological mechanisms underlying neuroplasticity described earlier, including LTP, LTD, and systemic reorganization of neural functional networks, can also subserve neurostability. Environmental stimuli associations and internal states that are frequently and consistently encountered will lead to strengthening of specific neuronal synapses (LTP) as well as more efficient pruning of neural responses (LTD) such that specificity of the coded representation is further accentuated and less likely to dynamically change. Moreover, with extended experience of similar associations and states over time, information coded in neuronal connections via LTP and LTD might undergo network-level functional reorganization and become even more stable. Environmental stimuli associations and internal states that are less frequently experienced or that have overly variable contingencies (i.e., less stable) will thus prevent these neural processing operations from proceeding along a specific trajectory.

In summary, neural computation is characterized by simultaneously competing models of neuroplasticity and neurostability. Importantly, contention between these two mechanisms should be understood as distinct from neurostochasticity, which implies that certain aspects of observed neural activity patterns reflect inconsequential noise. Rather, the strong view of neuroplasticity and neurostability as dichotomous processes of neural computation is that no neural firing is noise. Indeed, all neural activities are weighted contributors to the final mental phenomena either to bias plasticity or stability, no matter how obscure the contribution. As the argument has been made about the role and importance of neuroplasticity in information processing of the brain, the role of neurostability in brain function is now considered.

Roles of Neurostability

Homeostasis

The brain is one of the most metabolically active organs in the body so that a key challenge for neurons is to maintain their homeostatic level of function, which involves maintaining a balance of energy utilization (Peters et al., 2004). Note that while there are many different energy-releasing metabolic processes in neurons, the main currency of energy is in the form of the adenosine triphosphate (ATP) molecule. Hydrolysis of ATP into its substrates releases energy, which is critical to do work for various neuronal functions. Energy is directly needed in the maintenance of the electrochemical potential differences between the intra- and extracellular fluid across the phospholipid membrane that is critical for the formation of action potentials. Energy is also required in molecular synthesis of structural proteins that maintain and alter cell morphology (such as in dendritic arborization or axonal projections). Energy is again needed for the generation of receptor, neurotransmitter, and other signaling molecules. Thus, chronically heightened engagement of action potentials, the generation of new synaptic connections (i.e., new dendrites or new receptors), and increased production of signaling molecules all consume sustained amounts of energy. Note also that neural cells have minimal energy storage so that much of the energy needed to maintain structure and function are thought to be stored in surrounding nonneural tissue (e.g., astrocytes; Bélanger et al., 2011). As such, neurons might signal neighboring astrocytes to release or store energy according to the metabolic requirement. Regardless, extended high levels of neuronal activity associated with high energy consumption renders the neural network metabolic state untenable and mechanisms must operate to lower neural metabolism.

Thus, neurons and the networks they are part of might adjust their synaptic connections to engage information processing in a manner that maintains metabolic homeostasis. When neural networks process novel information or information that is unexpected, there should in principle be high levels of synaptic activity in response to the stimuli. Specifically, to code the new information, more action potentials are generated, higher levels of neurotransmitters are produced, or new dendrites or synapses might be formed. As long as the information is persistently processed as novel (i.e., similarity or repetition with respect to past information is not coded), the neural network will have to maintain a high metabolic state, which cannot be sustained indefinitely. One solution to this is that the neural network might detect heightened metabolic states that drive morphological changes in reaction whenever possible. Specifically, the neural network might code that the current stimulus is similar or predictable based on past stimuli and can thus use more efficient coding schemes that require less energy while maintaining a base level of responsivity to novel stimuli associations when the need arises. For example, LTD might operate so that only a few neurons fire at the next instance of a repeat of the same or similar stimulus. In tandem, LTP might increase the signaling level of the fewer involved neurons, indicating greater certainty that a given stimulus is encountered. Thus, only consistent stimulus features evoke stronger neuronal activity with variable features less influential so that overall network stability is enhanced. In this manner, metabolic homeostasis of neural cells might play a role in endogenously stabilizing neuronal function and neural network connections vis-à-vis plasticity of neurobiological changes in response to unexpected or predictable stimuli. Returning to the role of culture, modes of neurocognitive processing and behaviors that are associated with less neural effort might be strengthened, whereas those that require higher metabolism might either be quickly integrated or extinguished.

Physical Regularities and Social Mores

Statistical regularities in physical and social information in environmental stimuli likely reflect certain realities in the environment, and neurocognitive processing of such regular information facilitates the goal of neural networks to capture true environmental associations (see earlier) and in so doing engage lower metabolism. Thus, neurocognitive processing of physical and social informational regularities provides an important impetus for stability in neural network computations. The common principle applies again in that physical and social stimuli associations frequently encountered in the environment modulate neural networks to strengthen informative connections and dampen noninformative ones. In so doing, neural processing of regular information occurs with greater ease, and fewer resources are needed when processing predictable stimuli. By contrast, processing novel or infrequent stimuli requires greater neural computational work and is more effortful.

Several examples demonstrate how regularities in physical phenomena selectively strengthen and stabilize neural processing of the specific phenomena (and not others) over time that is a part of basic cognition and behavioral interaction with the environment. Cats exposed only to vertical (or only horizontal) lines from birth show behavioral and neurodevelopmental abnormalities characteristic of the specific visual deprivation (Blakemore & Cooper, 1970; Hirsch & Spinelli, 1970; Leventhal & Hirsch, 1975; Tieman & Hirsch, 1982). Recovery from such extreme deprivation of visual stimulation is limited (Wiesel & Hubel, 1965). Also, less extreme alteration of visual input such as via refractive prisms results in difficulty interacting with the physical visual environment in owls (Knudsen & Knudsen, 1989), with primates and humans also showing behavioral errors, albeit being able to rapidly adapt (Harris, 1963, 1965; Held & Bossom, 1961).

Projecting to cultural differences in visual environments, it is noted that East Asian cities tend to contain more complex visual features than Western cities even after controlling for various levels of urbanization (Miyamoto et al., 2006). It can be extrapolated that the eye movements in East Asians and Westerners reviewed earlier thus reflect different default strategies to scan visual scenes, which stem from differences in culturally different environmental visual input to the brain processes acquired over experience. Specifically, East Asians might engage eye movements that rapidly shift focus between objects and contexts, in contrast to longer dwell times with fewer saccades in Westerners, because the former eye movement style is more consistent with experiences in more complex visual contextual environments containing physical visual information spread out over scenes. Thus, culture-specific eye movement patterns reflect default and stabilized neural network processes (via LTP, LTD, and systemic neural functional reorganization) that the individuals from respective cultures have acquired, which they then applied in a non-effortful way across different physical scene viewing situations.

In addition, regularities in social signals are also a factor that might drive stability in neural processes that are associated with specific behaviors. For instance, jumping onto the dining table during a meal is an unacceptable behavior in most modern-day family contexts. Such notions of "table manners" must be socially learned through observation of peer behavior in similar contexts as well as feedback signals of approval or disapproval (via verbal expressions, facial emotions, etc.) regarding the behavior. Importantly, social behaviors that are common in a culture group must be processed in the brain so that the involved actions are preferred over uncommon or unaccepted behaviors. Indeed, violations of preferred behaviors generally evoke greater neural processing involving medial and lateral prefrontal, anterior cingulate, insula, and ventral striatal areas, marking the relative difficulty in processing behaviors that have been negatively associated with social mores (Mu et al., 2015; Xiang et al., 2013; Zinchenko & Arsalidou, 2018). Also, using cultural differences in eye movements as an example again, East Asians tend to fixate mainly on the center of the face around the nose area, whereas Westerners' fixations center on the eyes and mouths of face photographs (Blais et al., 2008). Moreover, facial expressions in which there is direct eye contact relative to averted eye gazes elicit higher indications of anxiety and perceptions of aggression and anger in East Asians compared to Westerners (Akechi et al., 2013). As suggested in these studies, such patterns of eye movements to faces are consistent with the social more in East Asians that discourages direct eye contact since it might be construed as a challenge. Thus, in this case, social regularity has shaped and stabilized neural network processing of eye movements that are consistent with culturally specific social mores on eye contact, such that these eye movements are applied by default and less effortfully across different situations. Critically, socially learned norms stabilize how individuals engage cognitive interpretation and selection of behavioral responses as default approaches to neutral physical stimuli in the contexts of their cultural environments.

Self-Processing

Perhaps the most stable of all mental processes have to do with the self, which is present in all individual experiences of physical and social phenomena. Indeed, the most robust dissociation of neural network systems in the brain is between task-active processing brain regions and the default-mode network that is involved in self-related processing (Buckner et al., 2008; Gusnard et al., 2001). Specifically, the default-mode network is consistently observed to be more active during off-trial rest epochs, attributed to periods of introspection, compared to on-trial epochs in experimental tasks (Raichle et al., 2001). The default-mode network is also composed of the key functional hubs in terms of the connectivity of the brain at rest, again to do with introspection (Greicius et al., 2003). Critically, neural responses in the default-mode network vary according to different modulations of self-related processing in experimental tasks as well (Andrews-Hanna, Reidler, Huang, & Buckner, 2010; Andrews-Hanna, Reidler, Sepulcre, et al., 2010; Gusnard et al., 2001; Spreng et al., 2009). In addition, differences in self-construal across cultures, such as along the individualism–collectivism dimension, have also been related to differences in default-mode network activity (Chiao et al., 2009, 2010; Kitayama & Park, 2010; Zhu et al., 2007).

Consider that the notion of the self involves a set of mental representations that is always present across different physical and social experiences over the lifespan. Also, the self is hierarchically one of the deepest constructs characterizing a person's mental faculties that receives information about all exogenous sensory input and endogenous mental states and then generates attitudes, motivations, and behavioral actions. Thus, the set of computations engaged in this network of processes must integrate all the different contingencies of physical and social associations as well as endogenous neurobiological states to produce input–output mapping in a consistent manner. That is, self-processing as the agenda of the default-mode network must reconcile between the many different agreements and discrepancies in experiences over the lifespan and across different cultures so that a stable self-schema and worldview are maintained as the individual interacts with dynamic and culturally specific environments. Compromises to the consistency of the neural processing of these input–output mappings then implicate the stability of the self and the ability of the brain to accurately represent and appropriately interact with the environment.

Causal Inference

As mentioned earlier, one important impetus of brain function is to capture associations between exogenous physical and social stimuli and endogenous mental states in a manner that represents the truth as much as possible. An efficient way for the brain to model the true associations between these sources of information is to make causal inferences about the nature of influences between the phenomena experienced (Friston, 2010; Friston et al., 2006; Lochmann & Deneve, 2011; Shams & Beierholm, 2010; Tenenbaum et al., 2011). Take, for instance, an apple falling to the ground. Coding the statistical regularity that a red-colored object consistently moves from a higher to lower position when there are no intervening objects is sufficient for predicting that subsequent red-colored objects under similar contexts would proceed with the trajectory. However, such associative links are insufficient to generalize predictions regarding other or dissimilar non-red-colored objects, or what might happen under other variable contexts (e.g., trajectories under partially intervening barriers). Rather, coding that there is a proposition of a general gravitational force that will act on any object with a particular form of influence, a causal inference, will more likely afford significantly greater ease in subsequent predictions for variable objects under variable contexts.

A social example more relevant to cultural differences might also more critically convey the fundamental importance of causal inference for encoding sensory information during interpersonal interactions. For instance, a person might frequently observe that Alice tends not to smile. Normative reactions to such observations about a person would be to make causal inferences that she does so because she has a melancholic personality or her cultural background does not generally encourage outward emotional expressions. Such attributions of a person's outward behaviors are more useful than only making the shallow association that Alice's repertoire of facial expression does not include smiles. Critically, beliefs about causes for outward phenomena (e.g., one is living in an emotionally conservative culture) that more accurately model the truth lead to fewer discrepancies between predictions and outcomes and should therefore be more stable and thus more generative for future interactions with the environment (e.g., one should not display exaggerated emotional expressions). By contrast, beliefs that are inaccurate should frequently be met with outcomes that are in disagreement with predictions and are thus likely to be modified.

Mitigating Stability and Plasticity
The Role of Prediction Error Signals

Plasticity and stability in neural network operations are thus competing mechanisms that jointly mediate the goal of the brain to represent environmental information as accurately as possible. How might neural networks ascertain when neuronal connections and responses should show plasticity and when they should remain stable? As alluded to in several places previously, a key means for brain operations to determine whether neural computations yield desired results in interacting with the environment is the evaluation of prediction error (Schultz & Dickinson, 2000). The notion of prediction error assumes that the brain makes predictions about what to expect in the environment, and does so in a Bayesian manner based on past experiences and beliefs (Bar, 2011; Knill & Pouget, 2004; Ma & Jazayeri, 2014). When neural representations of the predictions about the environment are followed by expected outcomes, neural representations of the subsequent environmental information are in agreement with predictive representations and prediction error is minimal. In such cases, the predicted representations, which are based on prior beliefs, can be considered as relatively accurate and need not undergo much modification and may even be strengthened (i.e., stabilized). However, when outcomes are unexpected, neural representations of resulting environmental events are not consistent with predicted representations, resulting in greater prediction error. In this case, the prediction error signals neuronal operations to modify beliefs to better fit incoming experiences so that subsequent predictions might result in less prediction error. Critically, this cycle of prediction, prediction error, belief updating, and prediction again can be applied to all levels of neural computation, from the neurobiological to the brain as a complex neural network, to even social networks between persons and with the physical environment.

Neural mechanisms of prediction error signals in the brain might be seen in animal reinforcement learning studies as well as human value-based decision studies (Schultz, 2016; Steinberg et al., 2013; van der Schaaf et al., 2014). These studies implicate dopamine modulation as an important neurotransmitter involved in reward learning and predictive coding particularly in the ventral striatum, a key neural target of dopaminergic neurons from the ventral tegmental area. Specifically, increased dopaminergic activity in these and related brain areas typically signals unexpected rewards, whereas unexpected punishments are associated with activity suppression.

Another neurotransmitter that might be involved in prediction error is serotonin, which has been shown to modulate the ability to process delayed rewards (Beaudoin-Gobert et al., 2015; Cools et al., 2011; den Ouden et al., 2013; Miyazaki et al., 2012, 2014; Zhou et al., 2015). Further, findings in these studies suggest that dopaminergic and serotonergic systems act in a complementary manner to each other. Thus, the influence and interaction of at least two monoamine neurotransmitters are implicated in prediction error signaling in the brain with respect to modulating neural network expectations about the environment and integrating of actual outcome experiences. Indeed, evidence suggests that the level to which an individual is susceptible to cultural influences on cognition is associated with differences in dopamine-related genotypes (Kitayama et al., 2014). In addition, etiological considerations have also noted differences in the distribution of serotonin-related genotypes across people groups, suggesting a protective effect of collectivism for the genotype coding serotonin efficacy associated with increased risk of depression (Chiao & Blizinsky, 2010). Moreover, prediction error–like learning principles are also what enables dynamism and stability in many computational neural network algorithms being studied and applied in the fields of computer science and artificial intelligence (Chauvin & Rumelhart, 1995; LeCun et al., 2015; Lin et al., 2017; Rumelhart et al., 1986).

Social Behavioral Culture as the Neural Solution to the Environment

The previous sections have reviewed the evidence for cultural differences in behavior and neural processing in the way humans interact with each other and with the physical environment. The proposition is also made that one goal of neural computations in the brain is to implement a veridical model of the physical and social environment, or belief, based on the sensory information received as well as internal mental states. The mechanism underlying this broad function of the brain is neuroplasticity, which describes neurobiological and neurocomputational principles of *plasticity* as well as *stability* in the manner in which neuronal and neural systems respond to environmental stimuli over the human lifespan. Specifically, neural network activity in the brain instantiates predictions about the environment, integrates experienced real outcomes via prediction error signals, and updates prior beliefs so that subsequent prediction errors are reduced. Through this prediction–integration cycle of external and endogenous associative information, dynamism and regularities in physical and social environmental stimuli are captured in the learned input–output mappings in the neural networks of the brain. Under this rubric, culturally different behaviors and mental processes can then be construed as distinctive sets of learned input–output neural mappings that represent the brain's beliefs and predictions of the physical and social environment that it is embedded in. Simultaneously, differences in brain and behavior across people groups that are common between individuals in the groups thus reflect the local environmental and endogenous factors that define the cultural boundaries of individuals from the same culture.

At the societal level, this Bayesian process of dynamically predicting and integrating the culturally local environment over time culminates in shared culturally specific social behaviors. That is, a particular set of learned input–output neural mappings in an individual becomes more dominant or easier to maintain than other mappings because it is associated with less prediction error in interacting with things and other individuals in the local environment. Importantly, these neural mappings are shaped by generations of experiences and predictions over cohorts of societies living in similar environmental contexts and are passed down to progenies. Broadly, then, behavioral and mental commonalities across individual responses to the same environmental stimuli as well as cultural biases between social groups and between persons represent neural solutions modeling possible truths about the physical environment that perpetuate each specific set of behaviors.

It is certainly conceded that this line of reasoning is vast, is complex, and involves many qualifications that span different levels of scientific inquiry including neurobiology, neural systems, and individual and social behaviors. Nevertheless, the principles that can account for each of these different levels of investigation are remarkably similar and relatively straightforward, all things considered. Critically, despite the potentially unwieldy scale, understanding core principles of how human neural networks operate in dynamic and local environments is unavoidable if more effective implementations of policies and interventions are sought regarding mental health and other societal issues in the globalizing world.

Dysregulation of Plasticity and Stability in Neural Processing and Mental Health

As yet, plasticity and stability of neural operations in the brain have been framed as normative mechanisms for cultural influences on neurocognitive processing and behavior. Recall also that these neural mechanisms subserve the goal of brain neural computations to veridically represent the physical and social environment. Moreover, it is proposed that neural networks assess the consistency of their representations with reality based on prediction error signals and also use these signals to update their representations as needed. It is certainly possible, however, for these neural mechanisms to evince dysregulation. In the author's own work at least, there are substantial individual differences in older adults' brain engagement for value predictions and prediction error responses (Goh et al., 2016). Specifically, a double dissociative pattern of neural responses was observed in frontal, striatal, and medial temporal regions in older adults such that with increasing expected value of lottery stakes, risk averters increased activity in these brain areas, whereas risk takers decreased activity instead. Thus, while these findings were based on normative samples, they demonstrate that neural indicators of predictive processing have bearing on decision behaviors. Critically, extremely risky decision behaviors correspond with more exaggerated neural responses that reflect less veridical processing of true expected value.

Indeed, pathological behaviors associated with MNS disorders are likely due to neural responses that inadequately apply appropriate predictions about environmental realities and also inadequately integrate the prediction errors that ensue despite the generated behavioral actions leading to clearly unfavorable outcomes. For instance, the intake of illegal substances might be met with social disapproval signals in the family or some public contexts. This phenomenon of substance abuse behavior might be construed as occurring because the neural network connections in the abuser predict that the engagement of the behavior will lead to a valued outcome. Although the subjectively valued outcome is not consistent with real social values and negative social signals are encountered, this prediction error is not integrated into the neural network processes so that the given behavior might be dampened.

Using the neuroplasticity framework, neural network states that are inflexible to prediction error signals evince pathological stability in their synaptic connections. Specifically, LTP and LTD might typically modulate excitatory and inhibitory signaling to integrate new information in the brain. By contrast, in pathology, LTP operation might be insufficient to strengthen neuronal connections to social information in the environment that are discrepant to the existing neural network state. LTD operation might also be insufficient to dampen neuronal connections that potentiate pathological thoughts and behaviors. Consequently, unlike cultural influences on the brain that are adaptive, the neural networks in patients with MNS disorders evince dysregulated neuroplasticity and stability and violate the aforementioned principles of neural processing toward maximizing survival.

Directions for Applications in Global Mental Health Challenges

Modern advancement in medical technology as well as societal infrastructures such as in communication and economy has made basic health care largely available to the public. As a result, the average person in the current world population has lower risk for many fatal or debilitating diseases that affected the masses in the past. However, the majority of health care solutions available target bodily diseases, and understanding of diseases that affect the brain and mind is still in its infancy. Addressing mental illnesses presents a particular challenge because of the substantial individual differences in symptomology and response to drugs and treatment that likely stems from differences in life experiences and lifestyles—a person's cultural background. As such, it is necessary to understand the etiologies of mental diseases that are common across human individuals as well as the specific cultural influences on mental and brain operations for more complete, accurate, and targeted diagnoses and treatments for each person in context. To this end, considerations of the mechanisms of neuroplasticity that drive flexibility as well as stability in neural computations in interacting with the dynamic external environment provide an objective framework to characterize cultural influences on the brain and mental health. From this framework, commonalities and differences in mental health norms for assessment tools and treatment prognoses can be more precisely determined and linked to specific culture-related factors.

For instance, assessments of cognitive abilities and neural functions accounting for a person's cultural background might reduce the rate of misdiagnosis. Consider the examples showing that basic arithmetic operations of addition and multiplication engage different neural circuits in individuals who learned mathematics in Chinese or English or other languages (Imbo & LeFevre, 2009; Rodic et al., 2015; Tang et al., 2006; Tang & Liu, 2009). Also, semantic categorizations are approached differently in different cultures' experiences (i.e., categorizing based on function rather than features; Chiu, 1972). Clinical cognitive assessments commonly involve number manipulation as well as semantic access, such as the arithmetic, letter–number sequencing, digit-span, and word-paired association subtests in the Wechsler Adult Intelligence Scale (Wechsler, 1981). In these tests, reaction time and accuracy performance norms usually account for age, sex, and education. In current practice, however, cultural differences are generally not accounted for and approaches to address this issues involve either using limited tests with "culture fair" metrics, which typically mean tests do not require language processing (i.e., graphical tests), or translated versions with specific norms that apply only within the translated language/culture. With respect to cultural differences in number and semantic processing, behavioral differences between culture groups in these abilities are associated with neural processing differences so that clinical assessment might not reflect the same psychological constructs and are not equal measures of ability across cultures. In the author's own work, a failure to detect hippocampal response during binding memory in older adults might be construed as reduced medial temporal efficacy associated with age-related cognitive decline or a cultural bias to encode binding information' differently (Chee et al., 2006; Goh et al., 2004, 2006). Thus, there are real cultural variations in brain processes and behavioral responses to the same stimuli and tasks that might be independent of the mental abilities assessed using current metrics.

Integrating with the role of neuroplasticity in brain acculturation outlined earlier, the proposition is that a neurocognitive processing framework based on a common base metric of neural network computation, prediction error, can more appropriately and universally characterize cultural differences in processing strategies across different tasks across persons with different cultural backgrounds. The principles of neural processing of prediction error in response to cultural differences in physical and social environmental stimuli might afford a means to derive culturally contextualized assessment tools with more generalizable norms. Such metrics might incorporate the notion of individual differences in prediction error processing to help distinguish when a displayed behavior is culturally adaptive from when it reflects dysregulation of neuroplasticity. Pharmacological treatments targeting the specific neurobiological mechanisms of neuroplasticity reviewed in this chapter might thus also offer promising culture-specific and person-centered medical care for people with MNS disorders.

In summary, the findings reviewed in this chapter and the arguments presented highlight some key concerns and propositions that future work in global health care might consider. First, at present, we can only have limited confidence in assuming that perceptions, even about physical phenomena, are similar across culture. Second, we also have limited confidence that the same metric used in clinical diagnosis of mental illnesses applies equally in all cultures, even when using translated or language-independent measures. Finally, it is proposed that a framework that is based on prediction error given cultural differences in physical and social experiences might be a means to address the previous two issues, which stem from neuroplasticity as a fundamental mechanism of the brain. Indeed, an adequately integrative framework that is conceptualized around individual and cultural differences in the way the brain processes environmental information might itself provide new insight into therapeutic methods. Specifically, different responses across culture groups to a given mental disease might reflect different neural solutions to pathology, which if understood can be applied in health care. As health care seeks to be more precise in encompassing different mental health issues relevant to countries and world cultures, catering closer and closer to individual needs must necessarily integrate more precise knowledge about the individual's past psychological experience. Only then can what is normative and what is pathological mental processing be determined, and subsequently what is pathological might then be normalized.

References

Aguirre, G. K., Zarahn, E., & D'Esposito, M. (1998). An area within human ventral cortex sensitive to "building" stimuli: Evidence and implications. *Neuron, 21*(2), 373–383.

Akechi, H., Senju, A., Uibo, H., Kikuchi, Y., Hasegawa, T., & Hietanen, J. K. (2013). Attention to eye contact in the West and East: Autonomic responses and evaluative ratings. *Plos One, 8*(3), e59312. doi:10.1371/journal.pone.0059312

Andersen, N., Krauth, N., & Nabavi, S. (2017). Hebbian plasticity in vivo: Relevance and induction. *Current Opinion in Neurobiology, 45*, 188–192. doi:10.1016/j.conb.2017.06.001

Andrews-Hanna, J. R., Reidler, J. S., Huang, C., & Buckner, R. L. (2010). Evidence for the default network's role in spontaneous cognition. *Journal of Neurophysiology, 104*(1), 322–335. doi:10.1152/jn.00830.2009

Andrews-Hanna, J. R., Reidler, J. S., Sepulcre, J., Poulin, R., & Buckner, R. L. (2010). Functional-anatomic fractionation of the brain's default network. *Neuron, 65*(4), 550–562. doi:10.1016/j.neuron.2010.02.005

Asch, S. E. (1956). Studies of independence and conformity: I. A minority of one against a unanimous majority. *Psychological Monographs: General and Applied, 70*(9), 1.

Bar, M. (2011). *Predictions in the brain: Using our past to generate a future.* Oxford University Press.

Beaudoin-Gobert, M., Epinat, J., Météreau, E., Duperrier, S., Neumane, S., Ballanger, B., Lavenne, F., Liger, F., Tourvielle, C., Bonnefoi, F., Costest, N., Le Bars, D., Broussolle, E., Thobois, S., Tremblay, L, & Sgambato-Faure, V. (2015). Behavioural impact of a double dopaminergic and serotonergic lesion in the non-human primate. *Brain, 138*(Pt 9), 2632–2647. doi:10.1093/brain/awv183

Bedny, M., Richardson, H., & Saxe, R. (2015). "Visual" cortex responds to spoken language in blind children. *Journal of Neuroscience, 35*(33), 11674–11681. doi:10.1523/JNEUROSCI.0634-15.2015

Bélanger, M., Allaman, I., & Magistretti, P. J. (2011). Brain energy metabolism: Focus on astrocyte-neuron metabolic cooperation. *Cell Metabolism, 14*(6), 724–738. doi:10.1016/j.cmet.2011.08.016

Berns, G. S., Chappelow, J., Zink, C. F., Pagnoni, G., Martin-Skurski, M. E., & Richards, J. (2005). Neurobiological correlates of social conformity and independence during mental rotation. *Biological Psychiatry, 58*(3), 245–253. doi:10.1016/j.biopsych.2005.04.012

Blais, C., Jack, R. E., Scheepers, C., Fiset, D., & Caldara, R. (2008). Culture shapes how we look at faces. *Public Library of Science One, 3*(8), e3022.

Blakemore, C., & Cooper, G. F. (1970). Development of the brain depends on the visual environment. *Nature, 228*(5270), 477–478. doi:10.1038/228477a0

Bouhali, F., Thiebaut de Schotten, M., Pinel, P., Poupon, C., Mangin, J.-F., Dehaene, S., & Cohen, L. (2014). Anatomical connections of the visual word form area. *Journal of Neuroscience, 34*(46), 15402–15414. doi:10.1523/JNEUROSCI.4918-13.2014

Buckner, R. L., Andrews-Hanna, J. R., & Schacter, D. L. (2008). The brain's default network: Anatomy, function, and relevance to disease. *Annals of the New York Academy of Sciences, 1124*, 1–38. doi:10.1196/annals.1440.011

Campbell-Meiklejohn, D. K., Bach, D. R., Roepstorff, A., Dolan, R. J., & Frith, C. D. (2010). How the opinion of others affects our valuation of objects. *Current Biology, 20*(13), 1165–1170. doi:10.1016/j.cub.2010.04.055

Chauvin, Y., & Rumelhart, D. E. (1995). *Backpropagation: Theory, architectures, and applications.* Psychology Press.

Chee, M. W. L., Goh, J. O. S., Venkatraman, V., Tan, J. C., Gutchess, A., Sutton, B., Hebrank, A., Leshikar, E., & Park, D. (2006). Age-related changes in object processing and contextual binding revealed using fMR adaptation. *Journal of Cognitive Neuroscience, 18*(4), 495–507. doi:10.1162/jocn.2006.18.4.495

Chiao, J. Y., & Blizinsky, K. D. (2010). Culture-gene coevolution of individualism-collectivism and the serotonin transporter gene. *Proceedings of the Royal Society B: Biological Sciences, 277*(1681), 529–537. doi:10.1098/rspb.2009.1650

Chiao, J. Y., Harada, T., Komeda, H., Li, Z., Mano, Y., Saito, D., Parrish, T. B., Sadato, N., & Iidaka, T. (2009). Neural basis of individualistic and collectivistic views of self. *Human Brain Mapping, 30*(9), 2813–2820. doi:10.1002/hbm.20707

Chiao, J. Y., Harada, T., Komeda, H., Li, Z., Mano, Y., Saito, D., Parrish, T. B., Sadato, N., & Iidaka, T. (2010). Dynamic cultural influences on neural representations of the self. *Journal of Cognitive Neuroscience, 22*(1), 1–11. doi:10.1162/jocn.2009.21192

Chiao, J. Y., Iidaka, T., Gordon, H. L., Nogawa, J., Bar, M., Aminoff, E., Sadato, N., & Ambady, N. (2008). Cultural specificity in amygdala response to fear faces. *Journal of Cognitive Neuroscience, 20*(12), 2167–2174. doi:10.1162/jocn.2008.20151

Chiao, J. Y., Li, S.-C., Turner, R., Lee-Tauler, S. Y., & Pringle, B. A. (2017). Cultural neuroscience and global mental health: Addressing grand challenges. *Culture and Brain, 5*(1), 4–13.

Chiu, L. H. (1972). A cross-cultural comparison of cognitive styles in Chinese and American children. *International Journal of Psychology, 7*(4), 235–242.

Chua, H. F., Boland, J. E., & Nisbett, R. E. (2005). Cultural variation in eye movements during scene perception. *Proceedings of the National Academy of Sciences USA, 102*(35), 12629–12633.

Collins, P. Y., Patel, V., Joestl, S. S., March, D., Insel, T. R., Daar, A. S., Scientific Advisory Board and the Executive Committee of the Grand Challenges on Global Mental Health, Anderson, W., Dhansay, M. A., Phillips, A., Shurin, S., Walport, M., Ewart, W., Savill, S. J., Bordin, I. A., Costello, E. J., Durkin, M., Fairburn, C., Glass, R. I., Hall, W., . . . Stein, D. J. (2011). Grand challenges in global mental health. *Nature, 475*(7354), 27–30.

Cools, R., Nakamura, K., & Daw, N. D. (2011). Serotonin and dopamine: Unifying affective, activational, and decision functions. *Neuropsychopharmacology, 36*(1), 98–113. doi:10.1038/npp.2010.121

Darwin, C. (1872). *The expression of the emotions in man and animals* (J. M. Londres, Ed.). Printed by William Clowes and Sons, Stamford Street, and Charing Cross. doi:10.1017/CBO9780511694110

den Ouden, H. E. M., Daw, N. D., Fernandez, G., Elshout, J. A., Rijpkema, M., Hoogman, M., Franke, B., & Cools, R. (2013). Dissociable effects of dopamine and serotonin on reversal learning. *Neuron, 80*(4), 1090–1100. doi:10.1016/j.neuron.2013.08.030

Dien, J. (2009). A tale of two recognition systems: Implications of the fusiform face area and the visual word form area for lateralized object recognition models. *Neuropsychologia, 47*(1), 1–16. doi:10.1016/j.neuropsychologia.2008.08.024

Downing, P. E., Jiang, Y., Shuman, M., & Kanwisher, N. (2001). A cortical area selective for visual processing of the human body. *Science, 293*(5539), 2470–2473. doi:10.1126/science.1063414

Eichenbaum, H. (2013). What H.M. taught us. *Journal of Cognitive Neuroscience, 25*(1), 14–21. doi:10.1162/jocn_a_00285

Ekman, P., & Friesen, W. V. (1977). *Facial Action Coding System.* Consulting Psychologists Press.

Ekman, P., Friesen, W. V., O'Sullivan, M., Chan, A., Diacoyanni-Tarlatzis, I., Heider, K., Krause, R., LeCompte, W. A., Pitcairn, T., Ricci-Bitti, P. E., Scherer, K., Tomita, M., & Tzavaras, A. (1987). Universals and cultural differences in the judgments of facial expressions of emotion. *Journal of Personality and Social Psychology, 53*(4), 712–717.

Epstein, R., & Kanwisher, N. (1998). A cortical representation of the local visual environment. *Nature, 392*(6676), 598–601. doi:10.1038/33402

Escobar, M. L., & Derrick, B. (2007). Long-term potentiation and depression as putative mechanisms for memory formation. In F. Bermúdez-Rattoni, F. Bermúdez-Rattoni, F. Bermúdez-Rattoni, F. Bermúdez-Rattoni, F. Bermúdez-Rattoni, & F. Bermúdez-Rattoni (Eds.), *Neural plasticity and memory: From genes to brain imaging.* CRC Press/Taylor & Francis.

Friston, K. (2010). The free-energy principle: a unified brain theory? *Nature Reviews Neuroscience, 11*(2), 127–138. doi:10.1038/nrn2787

Friston, K., Kilner, J., & Harrison, L. (2006). A free energy principle for the brain. *Journal of Physiology, Paris, 100*(1–3), 70–87. doi:10.1016/j.jphysparis.2006.10.001

Friston, K. J., Daunizeau, J., & Kiebel, S. J. (2009). Reinforcement learning or active inference? *Plos One, 4*(7), e6421. doi:10.1371/journal.pone.0006421

Fujii, M., Maesawa, S., Ishiai, S., Iwami, K., Futamura, M., & Saito, K. (2016). Neural basis of language: An overview of an evolving model. *Neurologia Medico-Chirurgica, 56*(7), 379–386. doi:10.2176/nmc.ra.2016-0014

Goh, J. O., & Park, D. C. (2009). Culture sculpts the perceptual brain. *Progress in Brain Research, 178*, 95–111. doi:10.1016/S0079-6123(09)17807-X

Goh, J. O., Tan, J. C., & Park, D. C. (2009). Culture modulates eye-movements to visual novelty. *Plos One, 4*(12), e8238. doi:10.1371/journal.pone.0008238

Goh, J. O. S., Chee, M., Tan, J. C., Venkatraman, V., Leshikar, E., Hebrank, A., Leshikar, E., Jenkins, L., Sutton, B. P., Gutchess, A. H., & Park, D. (2006, April 8–11). *Aging and culture modulate fMR-adaptation in the ventral visual area.* Annual Cognitive Neuroscience Society Meeting, San Francisco, CA, F39.

Goh, J. O. S., Chee, M. W., Tan, J. C., Venkatraman, V., Hebrank, A., Leshikar, E. D., Jenkins, L., Sutton, B. P., Gutchess, A. H., & Park, D. C. (2007). Age and culture modulate object processing and object-scene binding in the ventral visual area. *Cognitive, Affective & Behavioral Neuroscience, 7*(1), 44–52.

Goh, J. O. S., Hebrank, A. C., Sutton, B. P., Chee, M. W. L., Sim, S. K. Y., & Park, D. C. (2013). Culture-related differences in default network activity during visuo-spatial judgments. *Social Cognitive and Affective Neuroscience*, *8*(2), 134–142. doi:10.1093/scan/nsr077

Goh, J. O. S., & Huang, C.-M. (2012). Images of the cognitive brain across age and culture. In P. Bright (Ed.), *Neuroimaging—Cognitive and clinical neuroscience*. InTech.

Goh, J. O. S., Hung, H. Y., & Su, Y. S. (2018). A conceptual consideration of the free energy principle in cognitive maps: How cognitive maps reduce surprise. In K. Federmeier (Ed.), *Psychology of learning, and motivation, 69*, (pp. 205–240). Academic Press.

Goh, J. O. S., Leshikar, E. D., Sutton, B. P., Tan, J. C., Sim, S. K. Y., Hebrank, A. C., & Park, D. C. (2010). Culture differences in neural processing of faces and houses in the ventral visual cortex. *Social Cognitive and Affective Neuroscience*, *5*(2–3), 227–235. doi:10.1093/scan/nsq060

Goh, J. O. S., Li, C.-Y., Tu, Y.-Z., & Dallaire-Théroux, C. (2020). Visual cognition and culture. In O. Pedraza (Ed.), *Clinical cultural neuroscience: An integrative approach to cross-cultural neurospsychology*. Oxford University Press.

Goh, J. O. S., Siong, S. C., Park, D., Gutchess, A., Hebrank, A., & Chee, M. W. L. (2004). Cortical areas involved in object, background, and object-background processing revealed with functional magnetic resonance adaptation. *Journal of Neuroscience*, *24*(45), 10223–10228. doi:10.1523/JNEUROSCI.3373-04.2004

Goh, J. O. S., Su, Y. S., Tang, Y. J., McCarrey, A. C., Tereschenko, A., Elkins, W., & Resnick, S. M. (2016). Frontal, striatal, and medial temporal sensitivity to value distinguishes risk-taking from risk-aversive older adults during decision-making. *Journal of Neuroscience, 36*(49), 12498–12509. doi:10.1523/JNEUROSCI.1386-16.2016.

Graybiel, A. M. (2008). Habits, rituals, and the evaluative brain. *Annual Review of Neuroscience, 31*, 359–387. doi:10.1146/annurev.neuro.29.051605.112851

Greicius, M. D., Krasnow, B., Reiss, A. L., & Menon, V. (2003). Functional connectivity in the resting brain: A network analysis of the default mode hypothesis. *Proceedings of the National Academy of Sciences USA*, *100*(1), 253–258. doi:10.1073/pnas.0135058100

Grill-Spector, K., Henson, R., & Martin, A. (2006). Repetition and the brain: Neural models of stimulus-specific effects. *Trends in Cognitive Sciences, 10*(1), 14–23. doi:10.1016/j.tics.2005.11.006

Grill-Spector, K., Kourtzi, Z., & Kanwisher, N. (2001). The lateral occipital complex and its role in object recognition. *Vision Research, 41*(10–11), 1409–1422. doi:10.1016/S0042-6989(01)00073-6

Grill-Spector, K., Kushnir, T., Hendler, T., Edelman, S., Itzchak, Y., & Malach, R. (1998). A sequence of object-processing stages revealed by fMRI in the human occipital lobe. *Human Brain Mapping, 6*(4), 316–328. doi:10.1002/(SICI)1097-0193(1998)6:4<316::AID-HBM9>3.0.CO;2-6

Gusnard, D. A., Akbudak, E., Shulman, G. L., & Raichle, M. E. (2001). Medial prefrontal cortex and self-referential mental activity: Relation to a default mode of brain function. *Proceedings of the National Academy of Sciences USA, 98*(7), 4259–4264. doi:10.1073/pnas.071043098

Hagoort, P. (2014). Nodes and networks in the neural architecture for language: Broca's region and beyond. *Current Opinion in Neurobiology, 28*, 136–141. doi:10.1016/j.conb.2014.07.013

Han, H., Glover, G. H., & Jeong, C. (2014). Cultural influences on the neural correlate of moral decision making processes. *Behavioural Brain Research, 259*, 215–228. doi:10.1016/j.bbr.2013.11.012

Harris, C. S. (1963). Adaptation to displaced vision: Visual, motor, or proprioceptive change? *Science, 140*(3568), 812–813.

Harris, C. S. (1965). Perceptual adaptation to inverted, reversed, and displaced vision. *Psychological Review, 72*(6), 419–444.

Hebb, D. O. (1949). *The organization of behavior*. Wiley Press.

Hedden, T., Ketay, S., Aron, A., Markus, H. R., & Gabrieli, J. D. E. (2008). Cultural influences on neural substrates of attentional control. *Psychological Science, 19*(1), 12–17. doi:10.1111/j.1467-9280.2008.02038.x

Held, R., & Bossom, J. (1961). Neonatal deprivation and adult rearrangement: Complementary techniques for analyzing plastic sensory-motor coordinations. *Journal of Comparative and Physiological Psychology, 54*, 33–37.

Hirsch, H. V., & Spinelli, D. N. (1970). Visual experience modifies distribution of horizontally and vertically oriented receptive fields in cats. *Science, 168*(3933), 869–871.

Hitokoto, H., Glazer, J., & Kitayama, S. (2016). Cultural shaping of neural responses: Feedback-related potentials vary with self-construal and face priming. *Psychophysiology, 53*(1), 52–63. doi:10.1111/psyp.12554

Hofstede, G. (1980). Culture and organizations. *International Studies of Management & Organization, 10*(4), 15–41. doi:10.1080/00208825.1980.11656300

Hofstede, G. (2001). *Culture's consequences: Comparing values, behaviors, institutions, and organizations across nations.* Sage Publications.

Hofstede, G., & Bond, M. H. (1984). Hofstede's culture dimensions. *Journal of Cross-Cultural Psychology, 15*(4), 417–433. doi:10.1177/0022002184015004003

Hong, Y., Ip, G., Chiu, C., Morris, M. W., & Menon, T. (2001). Cultural identity and dynamic construction of the self: Collective duties and individual rights in Chinese and American cultures. *Social Cognition, 19*(3: Special issue), 251–268.

Hubel, D. H., & Wiesel, T. N. (1962). Receptive fields, binocular interaction and functional architecture in the cat's visual cortex. *Journal of Physiology, 160*, 106–154. doi:10.1113/jphysiol.1962.sp006837

Imbo, I., & LeFevre, J.-A. (2009). Cultural differences in complex addition: Efficient Chinese versus adaptive Belgians and Canadians. *Journal of Experimental Psychology. Learning, Memory, and Cognition, 35*(6), 1465–1476. doi:10.1037/a0017022

Izard, C. E. (1994). Innate and universal facial expressions: Evidence from developmental and cross-cultural research. *Psychological Bulletin, 115*(2), 288–299.

Izuma, K. (2013). The neural basis of social influence and attitude change. *Current Opinion in Neurobiology, 23*(3), 456–462. doi:10.1016/j.conb.2013.03.009

Jack, R. E., Blais, C., Scheepers, C., Schyns, P. G., & Caldara, R. (2009). Cultural confusions show that facial expressions are not universal. *Current Biology, 19*(18), 1543–1548. doi:10.1016/j.cub.2009.07.051

Jack, R. E., Sun, W., Delis, I., Garrod, O. G. B., & Schyns, P. G. (2016). Four not six: Revealing culturally common facial expressions of emotion. *Journal of Experimental Psychology. General, 145*(6), 708–730. doi:10.1037/xge0000162

Jenkins, L. J., Yang, Y.-J., Goh, J., Hong, Y.-Y., & Park, D. C. (2010). Cultural differences in the lateral occipital complex while viewing incongruent scenes. *Social Cognitive and Affective Neuroscience, 5*(2–3), 236–241. doi:10.1093/scan/nsp056

Kandel, E. R. (2001). The molecular biology of memory storage: A dialogue between genes and synapses. *Science, 294*(5544), 1030–1038. doi:10.1126/science.1067020

Kandel, E. R., Schwartz, J. H., Jessell, T. M., Siegelbaum, S. A., & Hudspeth, A. J. (Eds.). (2013). *Principles of neural science* (5th ed.). McGraw-Hill Companies.

Kanwisher, N., McDermott, J., & Chun, M. M. (1997). The fusiform face area: A module in human extrastriate cortex specialized for face perception. *Journal of Neuroscience, 17*(11), 4302–4311.

Kanwisher, N., & Yovel, G. (2006). The fusiform face area: A cortical region specialized for the perception of faces. *Philosophical Transactions of the Royal Society of London. Series B, Biological Sciences, 361*(1476), 2109–2128. doi:10.1098/rstb.2006.1934

Kitayama, S., Duffy, S., Kawamura, T., & Larsen, J. T. (2003). Perceiving an object and its context in different cultures: A cultural look at new look. *Psychological Science, 14*(3), 201–206. doi:10.1111/1467-9280.02432

Kitayama, S., King, A., Yoon, C., Tompson, S., Huff, S., & Liberzon, I. (2014). The dopamine D4 receptor gene (DRD4) moderates cultural difference in independent versus interdependent social orientation. *Psychological Science, 25*(6), 1169–1177. doi:10.1177/0956797614528338

Kitayama, S., & Park, J. (2010). Cultural neuroscience of the self: Understanding the social grounding of the brain. *Social Cognitive and Affective Neuroscience, 5*(2–3), 111–129. doi:10.1093/scan/nsq052

Klucharev, V., Hytönen, K., Rijpkema, M., Smidts, A., & Fernández, G. (2009). Reinforcement learning signal predicts social conformity. *Neuron, 61*(1), 140–151. doi:10.1016/j.neuron.2008.11.027

Knill, D. C., & Pouget, A. (2004). The Bayesian brain: The role of uncertainty in neural coding and computation. *Trends in Neurosciences, 27*(12), 712–719. doi:10.1016/j.tins.2004.10.007

Knudsen, E. I., & Knudsen, P. F. (1989). Visuomotor adaptation to displacing prisms by adult and baby barn owls. *Journal of Neuroscience, 9*(9), 3297–3305.

Kurihara, T., Kato, M., Sakamoto, S., Reverger, R., & Kitamura, T. (2000). Public attitudes towards the mentally ill: A cross-cultural study between Bali and Tokyo. *Psychiatry and Clinical Neurosciences, 54*(5), 547–552. https://doi.org/10.1046/j.1440- 1819.2000.00751.x

Laroche, S., Davis, S., & Jay, T. M. (2000). Plasticity at hippocampal to prefrontal cortex synapses: Dual roles in working memory and consolidation. *Hippocampus, 10*(4), 438–446. doi:10.1002/1098-1063(2000)10:4<438::AID-HIPO10>3.0.CO;2-3

LeCun, Y., Bengio, Y., & Hinton, G. (2015). Deep learning. *Nature, 521*(7553), 436–444. doi:10.1038/nature14539

Leventhal, A. G., & Hirsch, H. V. (1975). Cortical effect of early selective exposure to diagonal lines. *Science, 190*(4217), 902–904.

Lin, H. W., Tegmark, M., & Rolnick, D. (2017). Why does deep and cheap learning work so well? *Journal of Statistical Physics, 168*(6), 1223–1247. doi:10.1007/s10955-017-1836-5

Lochmann, T., & Deneve, S. (2011). Neural processing as causal inference. *Current Opinion in Neurobiology, 21*(5), 774–781. doi:10.1016/j.conb.2011.05.018

Ma, W. J., & Jazayeri, M. (2014). Neural coding of uncertainty and probability. *Annual Review of Neuroscience, 37*, 205–220. doi:10.1146/annurev-neuro-071013-014017

Malach, R., Reppas, J. B., Benson, R. R., Kwong, K. K., Jiang, H., Kennedy, W. A., Ledden, P. J., Brady, T. J., Rosen, B. R., & Tootell, R. B. (1995). Object-related activity revealed by functional magnetic resonance imaging in human occipital cortex. *Proceedings of the National Academy of Sciences USA, 92*(18), 8135–8139. doi:10.1073/pnas.92.18.8135

Masuda, T., Ellsworth, P. C., Mesquita, B., Leu, J., Tanida, S., & Van de Veerdonk, E. (2008). Placing the face in context: Cultural differences in the perception of facial emotion. *Journal of Personality and Social Psychology, 94*(3), 365–381. doi:10.1037/0022-3514.94.3.365

Masuda, T., & Nisbett, R. E. (2001). Attending holistically versus analytically: Comparing the context sensitivity of Japanese and Americans. *Journal of Personality and Social Psychology, 81*(5), 922–934.

Masuda, T., & Nisbett, R. E. (2006). Culture and change blindness. *Cognitive Science, 30*(2), 381–399. doi:10.1207/s15516709cog0000_63

Merabet, L., Thut, G., Murray, B., Andrews, J., Hsiao, S., & Pascual-Leone, A. (2004). Feeling by sight or seeing by touch? *Neuron, 42*(1), 173–179.

Miyamoto, Y., Nisbett, R. E., & Masuda, T. (2006). Culture and the physical environment. Holistic versus analytic perceptual affordances. *Psychological Science, 17*(2), 113–119. doi:10.1111/j.1467-9280.2006.01673.x

Miyazaki, K. W., Miyazaki, K., & Doya, K. (2012). Activation of dorsal raphe serotonin neurons is necessary for waiting for delayed rewards. *Journal of Neuroscience, 32*(31), 10451–10457. doi:10.1523/JNEUROSCI.0915-12.2012

Miyazaki, K. W., Miyazaki, K., Tanaka, K. F., Yamanaka, A., Takahashi, A., Tabuchi, S., & Doya, K. (2014). Optogenetic activation of dorsal raphe serotonin neurons enhances patience for future rewards. *Current Biology, 24*(17), 2033–2040. doi:10.1016/j.cub.2014.07.041

Mu, Y., Kitayama, S., Han, S., & Gelfand, M. J. (2015). How culture gets embrained: Cultural differences in event-related potentials of social norm violations. *Proceedings of the National Academy of Sciences USA, 112*(50), 15348–15353. doi:10.1073/pnas.1509839112

Nisbett, R E. (2003). *The geography of thought: How Asians and Westerners think differently—And why.* Free Press.

Nisbett, R. E., & Miyamoto, Y. (2005). The influence of culture: Holistic versus analytic perception. *Trends in Cognitive Sciences, 9*(10), 467–473. doi:10.1016/j.tics.2005.08.004

Nisbett, R. E., Peng, K., Choi, I., & Norenzayan, A. (2001). Culture and systems of thought: Holistic versus analytic cognition. *Psychological Review, 108*(2), 291–310. doi:10.1037/0033-295X.108.2.291

Nook, E. C., & Zaki, J. (2015). Social norms shift behavioral and neural responses to foods. *Journal of Cognitive Neuroscience, 27*(7), 1412–1426. doi:10.1162/jocn_a_00795

Oyserman, D., & Lee, S. W. S. (2008). Does culture influence what and how we think? Effects of priming individualism and collectivism. *Psychological Bulletin, 134*(2), 311–342. doi:10.1037/0033-2909.134.2.311

Park, D. C., & Huang, C.-M. (2010). Culture wires the brain: A cognitive neuroscience perspective. *Perspectives on Psychological Science, 5*(4), 391–400. doi:10.1177/1745691610374591

Park, J., & Kitayama, S. (2014). Interdependent selves show face-induced facilitation of error processing: Cultural neuroscience of self-threat. *Social Cognitive and Affective Neuroscience, 9*(2), 201–208. doi:10.1093/scan/nss125

Parr, T., & Friston, K. J. (2017). Uncertainty, epistemics and active inference. *Journal of the Royal Society, Interface, 14*(136), 1–10. doi:10.1098/rsif.2017.0376

Peters, A., Schweiger, U., Pellerin, L., Hubold, C., Oltmanns, K. M., Conrad, M., Schultex, B., Born, J., & Fehm, H. L. (2004). The selfish brain: Competition for energy resources. *Neuroscience and Biobehavioral Reviews, 28*(2), 143–180. doi:10.1016/j.neubiorev.2004.03.002

Plested, A. J. R. (2016). Structural mechanisms of activation and desensitization in neurotransmitter-gated ion channels. *Nature Structural & Molecular Biology, 23*(6), 494–502. doi:10.1038/nsmb.3214

Poirier, C., Collignon, O., Scheiber, C., Renier, L., Vanlierde, A., Tranduy, D., Veraart, C., & De Volder, A. G. (2006). Auditory motion perception activates visual motion areas in early blind subjects. *Neuroimage*, *31*(1), 279–285. doi:10.1016/j.neuroimage.2005.11.036

Preston, A. R., & Eichenbaum, H. (2013). Interplay of hippocampus and prefrontal cortex in memory. *Current Biology*, *23*(17), R764–R773. doi:10.1016/j.cub.2013.05.041

Price, C. J., & Devlin, J. T. (2003). The myth of the visual word form area. *Neuroimage*, *19*(3), 473–481. doi:10.1016/S1053-8119(03)00084-3

Purves, D., Augustine, G. J., Fitzpatrick, D., Hall, W. C., LaMantia, A.-S., McNamara, J. O., & Williams, S. M. (Eds.). (2004). *Neuroscience* (3rd ed.). Sinauer Associates.

Raichle, M. E., MacLeod, A. M., Snyder, A. Z., Powers, W. J., Gusnard, D. A., & Shulman, G. L. (2001). A default mode of brain function. *Proceedings of the National Academy of Sciences USA*, *98*(2), 676–682. doi:10.1073/pnas.98.2.676

Rodic, M., Zhou, X., Tikhomirova, T., Wei, W., Malykh, S., Ismatulina, V., Sabirova, E., Davidova, Y., Tosto, M. G., Lemelin, J. P., & Kovas, Y. (2015). Cross-cultural investigation into cognitive underpinnings of individual differences in early arithmetic. *Developmental Science*, *18*(1), 165–174. doi:10.1111/desc.12204

Rohan, M. J. (2000). A rose by any name? The values construct. *Personality and Social Psychology Review*, *4*(3), 255–277. doi:10.1207/S15327957PSPR0403_4

Ross, P. D., de Gelder, B., Crabbe, F., & Grosbras, M. H. (2014). Body-selective areas in the visual cortex are less active in children than in adults. *Frontiers in Human Neuroscience*, *8*, 941. doi:10.3389/fnhum.2014.00941

Rumelhart, D. E., Hinton, G. E., & Williams, R. J. (1986). *Learning internal representations by error propagation*. MIT Press.

Schmolesky, M. T., Wang, Y., Pu, M., & Leventhal, A. G. (2000). Degradation of stimulus selectivity of visual cortical cells in senescent rhesus monkeys. *Nature Neuroscience*, *3*(4), 384–390. doi:10.1038/73957

Schultz, W. (2016). Dopamine reward prediction error coding. *Dialogues in Clinical Neuroscience*, *18*(1), 23–32.

Schultz, W., & Dickinson, A. (2000). Neuronal coding of prediction errors. *Annual Review of Neuroscience*, *23*, 473–500. doi:10.1146/annurev.neuro.23.1.473

Schwartz, S. H. (1990). Individualism-collectivism: Critique and proposed refinements. *Journal of Cross-Cultural Psychology*, *21*(2), 139–157.

Schwartz, S. H. (1992). Universals in the content and structure of values: Theoretical advances and empirical tests in 20 countries. *Advances in Experimental Social Psychology*, *25*, 1–62.

Schwartz, S. H., & Bilsky, W. (1990). Toward a theory of the universal content and structure of values: Extensions and cross-cultural replications. *Journal of Personality and Social Psychology*, *58*(5), 878–891. doi:10.1037/0022-3514.58.5.878

Sekeres, M. J., Winocur, G., & Moscovitch, M. (2018). The hippocampus and related neocortical structures in memory transformation. *Neuroscience Letters*, *680*, 39–53. doi:10.1016/j.neulet.2018.05.006

Shams, L., & Beierholm, U. R. (2010). Causal inference in perception. *Trends in Cognitive Sciences*, *14*(9), 425–432. doi:10.1016/j.tics.2010.07.001

Spreng, R. N., Mar, R. A., & Kim, A. S. N. (2009). The common neural basis of autobiographical memory, prospection, navigation, theory of mind, and the default mode: A quantitative meta-analysis. *Journal of Cognitive Neuroscience*, *21*(3), 489–510. doi:10.1162/jocn.2008.21029

Squire, L. R. (2009). The legacy of patient H.M. for neuroscience. *Neuron*, *61*(1), 6–9. doi:10.1016/j.neuron.2008.12.023

Squire, L. R., Stark, C. E. L., & Clark, R. E. (2004). The medial temporal lobe. *Annual Review of Neuroscience*, *27*, 279–306. doi:10.1146/annurev.neuro.27.070203.144130

Steinberg, E. E., Keiflin, R., Boivin, J. R., Witten, I. B., Deisseroth, K., & Janak, P. H. (2013). A causal link between prediction errors, dopamine neurons and learning. *Nature Neuroscience*, *16*(7), 966–973. doi:10.1038/nn.3413

Sun, P., Gardner, J. L., Costagli, M., Ueno, K., Waggoner, R. A., Tanaka, K., & Cheng, K. (2013). Demonstration of tuning to stimulus orientation in the human visual cortex: A high-resolution fMRI study with a novel continuous and periodic stimulation paradigm. *Cerebral Cortex*, *23*(7), 1618–1629. doi:10.1093/cercor/bhs149

Talhelm, T., Zhang, X., Oishi, S., Shimin, C., Duan, D., Lan, X., & Kitayama, S. (2014). Large-scale psychological differences within China explained by rice versus wheat agriculture. *Science*, *344*(6184), 603–608. doi:10.1126/science.1246850

Tang, Y., Zhang, W., Chen, K., Feng, S., Ji, Y., Shen, J., Reiman, E. M., & Liu, Y. (2006). Arithmetic processing in the brain shaped by cultures. *Proceedings of the National Academy of Sciences USA, 103*(28), 10775–10780. doi:10.1073/pnas.0604416103

Tang, Y.-Y., & Liu, Y. (2009). Numbers in the cultural brain. *Progress in Brain Research, 178,* 151–157. doi:10.1016/S0079-6123(09)17810-X

Tenenbaum, J. B., Kemp, C., Griffiths, T. L., & Goodman, N. D. (2011). How to grow a mind: Statistics, structure, and abstraction. *Science, 331*(6022), 1279–1285. doi:10.1126/science.1192788

Tieman, S. B., & Hirsch, H. V. (1982). Exposure to lines of only one orientation modifies dendritic morphology of cells in the visual cortex of the cat. *Journal of Comparative Neurology, 211*(4), 353–362. doi:10.1002/cne.902110403

Tremblay, P., & Dick, A. S. (2016). Broca and Wernicke are dead, or moving past the classic model of language neurobiology. *Brain and Language, 162,* 60–71. doi:10.1016/j.bandl.2016.08.004

Triandis, H. C. (1995). *Individualism and collectivism.* Westview.

Triandis, H. C., Bontempo, R., Villareal, M. J., Asai, M., & Lucca, N. (1988). Individualism and collectivism: Cross-cultural perspectives on self-ingroup relationships. *Journal of Personality and Social Psychology, 54*(2), 323–338.

Tu, Y.-Z., Lin, D.-W., Suzuki, A., & Goh, J. O. S. (2018). East Asian young and older adult perceptions of emotional faces from an age- and sex-fair East Asian facial expression database. *Frontiers in Psychology, 9,* 2358. doi:10.3389/fpsyg.2018.02358

van der Schaaf, M. E., van Schouwenburg, M. R., Geurts, D. E. M., Schellekens, A. F. A., Buitelaar, J. K., Verkes, R. J., & Cools, R. (2014). Establishing the dopamine dependency of human striatal signals during reward and punishment reversal learning. *Cerebral Cortex, 24*(3), 633–642. doi:10.1093/cercor/bhs344

Vogel, A. C., Petersen, S. E., & Schlaggar, B. L. (2014). The VWFA: It's not just for words anymore. *Frontiers in Human Neuroscience, 8,* 88. doi:10.3389/fnhum.2014.00088

Waxman, S. G. (Ed.). (2013). *Clinical neuroanatomy* (27th ed.). McGraw-Hill Companies.

Wechsler, D. (1981). *Wechsler Adult Intelligence Scale—Revised.* Psychological Corporation.

Wiesel, T. N., & Hubel, D. H. (1965). Extent of recovery from the effects of visual deprivation in kittens. *Journal of Neurophysiology, 28*(6), 1060–1072. doi:10.1152/jn.1965.28.6.1060

Wiltgen, B. J., Brown, R. A. M., Talton, L. E., & Silva, A. J. (2004). New circuits for old memories: The role of the neocortex in consolidation. *Neuron, 44*(1), 101–108. doi:10.1016/j.neuron.2004.09.015

Xiang, T., Lohrenz, T., & Montague, P. R. (2013). Computational substrates of norms and their violations during social exchange. *Journal of Neuroscience, 33*(3), 1099–108a. doi:10.1523/JNEUROSCI.1642-12.2013

Zaki, J., Schirmer, J., & Mitchell, J. P. (2011). Social influence modulates the neural computation of value. *Psychological Science, 22*(7), 894–900. doi:10.1177/0956797611411057

Zhou, J., Jia, C., Feng, Q., Bao, J., & Luo, M. (2015). Prospective coding of dorsal raphe reward signals by the orbitofrontal cortex. *Journal of Neuroscience, 35*(6), 2717–2730. doi:10.1523/JNEUROSCI.4017-14.2015

Zhu, Y., Zhang, L., Fan, J., & Han, S. (2007). Neural basis of cultural influence on self-representation. *Neuroimage, 34*(3), 1310–1316. doi:10.1016/j.neuroimage.2006.08.047

Zinchenko, O., & Arsalidou, M. (2018). Brain responses to social norms: Meta-analyses of fMRI studies. *Human Brain Mapping, 39*(2), 955–970. doi:10.1002/hbm.23895

Culture and Technology

Joan Y. Chiao, Yoko Mano, and Norihiro Sadato

Abstract

This chapter provides an overview of the role of culture in technological innovation for global mental health. Culture influences basic mechanisms of psychological processes and neurobiological mechanisms of behavior. Technological innovation plays an important role in the discovery and delivery science of global mental health. Technological innovation that demonstrates cultural competence can strengthen the discovery of cures, preventions, and interventions of mental health disorders as well as the delivery of preventions and interventions for mental health promotion. Effective use of culture in technological innovation is a strategic development of mental health promotion for the achievement of health equity and health diplomacy. Implications for the role of culture in technology for closing the gap in population health disparities and addressing grand challenges in global mental health are discussed.

Key Words: cultural neuroscience, culture, technology, global mental health, health equity, health diplomacy

Introduction

Cultural neuroscience is an evidence-based resource for the development and implementation of prevention and early interventions in global mental health. Research in cultural neuroscience provides systematic investigation of the influence of culture on the organization and function of the nervous system. Theoretical foundations in cultural neuroscience expand the development of theoretical constructs and conceptual frameworks for formation of causal predictions of the mutual influence of culture and neurobiological circuitry. Methodological foundations in cultural neuroscience ensure tools for the observation and measurement of cultural influences on the nervous system across spatiotemporal scales. Empirical foundations in cultural neuroscience develop programs of research and standard paradigms for the systematic testing of theoretical frameworks.

The translation of research in cultural neuroscience into practice informs the development and implementation of prevention and early interventions in global mental health. The advancement of prevention and implementation of early interventions is a necessary component of the translation of research into practice. The development and implementation of effective strategies for the prevention of and implementation of early interventions for mental disorders rely on evidence-based resources in cultural neuroscience.

Cultural neuroscience as an evidence-based resource identifies the root causes and risk and protective factors of health and well-being. Understanding the cellular and molecular mechanisms of the brain enhances the potential for the design of effective preventions and interventions across cultural settings (Collins et al., 2011). The study of cultural influences on neurobiological mechanisms identifies regularity in the causal patterns of the brain that generate and maintain culture. Identification of the physical implementation of culture at the level of the nervous system demonstrates the set of physical or neural states that cause mental states of culture (Chiao, 2018). Reciprocally, mental states of culture instantiated as a causal pattern of neural states illustrates a fundamental role for culture as a protective factor in health and well-being.

Cultural Neuroscience

Culture affects psychological and neural mechanisms of social and emotional processes. Research in cultural neuroscience demonstrates cultural influences on neurobiological mechanisms of social and emotional behavior. Empirical studies in cultural neuroscience identify patterns of neural activity in brain regions related to culture (Chiao et al., 2017). Culture affects the neural response within brain regions of social behavior. Cultural variation is observed within the medial prefrontal cortex (MPFC) during social processes of the self (Chiao et al., 2009; Zhu et al., 2007). Priming culture modulates neural activation within the dorsal portion of the MPFC during self-processing (Harada et al., 2010). Temporarily heightening awareness of individualistic or collectivistic cultural norms in bicultural individuals increases dorsal MPFC response during self-evaluation. These findings show patterns of neural activity within the prefrontal cortex when people respond in a culturally congruent manner.

Culture influences neural mechanisms of intergroup empathy. People from interdependent cultures show greater empathic neural response for pain perceived in members of one's cultural group (Cheon et al., 2013). These findings suggest that cultural construal of interdependence is related to greater empathy for group members in neural and behavioral response. Interdependent cultures promote patterns of neural activity that support empathic responding. Racial identification modulates neural mechanisms of intergroup empathy. People who show greater racial identification demonstrate greater empathic neural response within cortical midline structures, including the MPFC, anterior cingulate cortex (ACC), and posterior cingulate cortex (PCC; Mathur et al., 2012). Racial identification increases neural activation within brain regions associated with empathic responding. Enhanced activation of empathic neural responding for group members reflects the recruitment of cultural resources to respond to the suffering of others. These findings illustrate the role of culture in shaping the neurobiological bases of social behavior.

Culture affects neural mechanisms of emotional behavior. Cultural variation in neural response to fear facial expressions is observed within the bilateral amygdala (Chiao et al., 2008). People show greater bilateral amygdala response to fear expressed by members of their cultural group. These findings illustrate the influence of culture on subcortical responses to threat-related emotional expressions. Ideal affect theory postulates that cultures vary in the valuation of ideal affect (Tsai, 2007). European Americans value high-arousal positive emotion, while East Asians prefer low-arousal positive emotion. Cultural differences in the ventral striatum to positive facial expressions are related to ideal affect (Park et al., 2016). Consistent with ideal affect theory, European Americans show greater neural activity within reward neural circuitry during perception of excited relative to calm facial expressions relative to East Asians. These findings support the notion that cultures differ in the valuation of positive affect.

Cultural variation in social and emotional processes arise through multilevel mechanisms. Empirical evidence shows the importance of culture in causal patterns of neural functioning. Culture plays a potent role in the identification of the root causes and risk and protective factors that affect health and well-being. The investigation of cultural processes in the human brain enhances understanding for the design of preventions and interventions in global mental health. The study of culture and human brain functioning is fundamental to discovery and delivery science in global mental health. Effective strategies for the advancement of health preventions and interventions across cultural settings are necessary for the achievement of health equity and health diplomacy.

Theoretical Foundations

Theoretical foundations in cultural neuroscience explain causal patterns in the functional organization of the nervous system that generate and maintain culture. Theoretical approaches in cultural neuroscience demonstrate causal pathways of culture and genetic systems that shape neural and mental architecture in response to environmental pressures. Dual inheritance theory posits that ecological and environmental factors contribute to the emergence of cultural systems. Cultural systems modify natural selection pressures of the environment to benefit the genetic adaptation of organisms. Cultural processes may modify environmental pressures that affect genetic inheritance through cultural biases of social interaction. Cultural systems act as regulatory mechanisms to modify environmental conditions of health and disease (Fincher et al., 2008; Chiao & Blizinsky, 2010) and ecological conditions of trade and warfare (Gelfand et al., 2011; Mrazek et al., 2013). Culture as a set of processes that guide social practices and epistemology affects reasoning and thought (Nisbett et al., 2001). Cultural processes affecting the rate and content of transmission of information for social learning modify genetic and behavioral expression for adaptation. The modification of ecological inheritance through processes of niche construction guides neural and mental architecture for the benefit of cultural and genetic inheritance.

Cumulative cultural evolution posits that cultural evolution is cumulative. Cultural changes build across generations in enhanced complexity through processes of social learning (Boyd & Richerson, 2005). The rate of cumulative cultural evolution is faster than that of biological evolution such that cultural change may accumulate faster than changes through environmental pressures. Cumulative cultural evolution reflects a difference between cultural evolution and slower processes of biological evolution.

As a byproduct of cumulative cultural evolution, technology supports cultural changes that accumulate through the rapid development and implementation of technologically driven applications and platforms. Technology represents a type of cumulative cultural evolution that illustrates the generation and maintenance of cultural inheritance through use of distinct tools. Digital culture as a type of technological innovation reflects modern tool use that builds in and responds to complexity. Digital culture is designed for the accumulation of cultural change through social learning and for the purpose of social feedback that builds cultural competence. Digital culture that transforms in the features and services of applications and underlying platforms enhances cultural resources for the benefit of future human potential.

Cultural processes contribute to the niche construction that guides cultural and ecological inheritance. Technology as a cultural process improves human capabilities for niche construction. Technology provides tools for the rapid transmission of information for social learning and feedback for cultural change (Laland et al., 2000). Technology enhances the cultural processes of model-based learning in social transmission. Model-based social learning enhances the transmission and persistence of cultural information across individuals and groups (Boyd & Richerson, 2005). Model-based social learning facilitates cultural transmission and the capability of feedback for cultural change.

Cultural processes of technological innovation improve the health and well-being of individuals, societies, and nations. Technological innovation designed to enhance health facilitates the sharing of information and access to health services across cultural settings (Minas, 2014). Technological innovation designed to promote well-being enables the social and economic development of communities. Programs in technological innovation seek to improve human choices and human capabilities that expand fundamental protections and freedoms.

Technological innovation for the sharing of information across individuals and groups promotes model-based learning and knowledge-based resources for cultural change. For patterns of environmental change or environmental shifts that occur rapidly across time, technological innovation may be particularly efficacious at providing individuals and groups with knowledge-based resources and adaptive feedback. Cultural processes that improve environmental regulation enhance constancy in the environment and transgenerational cultural transmission over time.

Technological innovation can enhance cultural biases in social learning for the benefit of health equity and social equality. Cultural evolutionary processes instantiated as cultural biases in social learning reflect patterns of cultural change (Mesoudi, 2009). Cultural biases based on popularity reflect a frequency-dependent cultural bias. Conformity reflects a cultural bias such that information is acquired because of its popularity or the level of frequency of content in the population. Model-based biases refer to the biases in social learning through cultural transmission based on the perception of cultural competence of the model. The perception of cultural competence in model-based biases is determinable by the prestige, success, or knowledge of the model. Cultural biases of content refer to the persistence in transmission of particular kinds of social information based on intrinsic properties. Cultural biases of content produce enhancement of memory and representational structure of information. Cultural group selection refers to cultural biases in social learning related to intergroup processes. The content of cultural transmission in cultural group selection is guided by the cultural bias to acquire information through the cooperation with groups guided by reason.

Culture demonstrates effective strategies for the design of technological innovation that promotes health equity. Programs and applications of technological innovation that promote health equity may benefit from the use of cultural strategies. Approaches to health communication that emphasize the acquisition of informational content that is popular, prestigious, memorable, or rational highlight the use of cultural strategies for the design of health preventions and interventions that are beneficial across cultural settings. Health messaging of preventative health behavior that enhances a perception of popularity or prestige illustrates the use of frequency- and model-based cultural strategies for health prevention and intervention. Health messaging that encourages a perception of preventative health behavior as rational and memorable shows the benefit of content-based cultural strategies for health communication.

Culture promotes a design of technological innovation that strengthens social equality. Programs that support knowledge-based resources for social equality enhance the sharing of informational content of cultural groups that is memorable and rational. Health messaging that promotes social inclusion and feelings of belonging among cultural groups strengthens social equality. The design of technological applications that build the perception of popularity or prestige of cultural groups illustrates the benefit of technological innovation for social equality. Health messaging that is consistent with larger societal preferences or goals promotes the popularity or prestige of cultural groups. Technological applications that build from informational content that is popular or prestigious across cultures enhance a culture of social equality. Technology that provides platforms for information content built on cultural identity strengthens its application for the maintenance of culture. Programs that include knowledge-based resources to enhance the participation of cultural groups in social and economic community development broaden opportunities for all.

The efficacy of technology for the achievement of social equality is demonstrated in the improvement in social and economic empowerment of community across cultures. The reduction of social and economic inequalities is achieved through the sharing of information and the achievement of empowerment. Technological innovation provides knowledge-based tools for the improvement in equal access to social practices and organizations across cultures. Broadening the participation of cultural groups in individual and collective action through the use of technology bolsters social equality.

The application of technology for social equality is beneficial across cultures. Technology as a resource for cultural change can be designed for the improvement of quality of life and the potential for human fulfillment. Technology as a modern human cultural adaptation is responsive to environmental and ecological pressures. Technology as a modern byproduct of cumulative cultural evolution demonstrates the importance of design capability for cultural niche construction. Cultural niche construction through technological innovation seeks to improve the ecological and cultural inheritance of the organism. Technological innovation enhances the capability and efficiency of cultural transmission for learning and adaptation. Technological innovation builds through recognition and implementation of the intention and goal states of the user design. Technological innovation enhances the capability for cultural regulation and cultural control of the environment.

Culture and Technological Innovation in Global Mental Health

Culture plays a foundational role in the development of technological innovation. Cultural processes guide the mental capacities and neurobiological mechanisms that facilitate the antecedents and consequences of technological innovation. Technological innovation reflects components of cultural dynamics whereby cultural processes enhance malleability as a behavioral adaptation. Technological innovation may be effective to provide knowledge-based resources for intercultural contact of individuals and groups. Intercultural knowledge-based resources may enhance capabilities for acculturation processes of plural societies.

Technology may be an effective tool to provide platforms that promote cultural processes of plural societies (Table 21.1). Technology supports trade and the exchange of information and ideas at a rapid pace. The cultural dimensions of plural societies depend on the mobility and voluntariness of contact of ethnocultural groups (Sam & Berry, 2006). Technological innovations designed for immigrants and refugees can improve their access

Table 21.1. Culture and Technological Innovation	
Level of Interaction	Technological Design
Individual	Improve intercultural knowledge, attitudes, and skills Train intercultural problem solving Enhance intercultural competence
Group	Cultural learning for intercultural relations Cultural learning for achievement Cultural learning for cooperation
National	Promote national cultural identity Form national cultural attitudes Build national culture

to cultural resources. For ethnocultural groups of plural societies, the cultural changes that arise due to intercultural contact affect acculturative processes of sociocultural and psychological adaptation.

Technology plays an important role in the advancement of tools for prevention and early intervention in global mental health. Technology as a health prevention and intervention may be designed to improve cultural knowledge, attitudes, and skills. Technology can provide knowledge-based resources for the sharing of information and ideas that may enhance intercultural contact and multilevel adaptation.

Technology demonstrates the capability for advancement of protections and empowerment. Technology may improve processes of acculturation for vulnerable populations, such as migrants and refugees. Training programs may be designed to assist individuals with the practicing of skills to produce behavioral shifts and to design coping strategies for sociocultural and psychological adaptation. Acculturation experiences that are perceived with ease and efficiency produce psychological adjustments and behavioral shifts. Other acculturation experiences that are perceived as high in conflict elicit cultural control through strategies that regulate social and emotional behavior.

Technology produces tools for the training of cognitive and behavioral skills that enhance cognitive performance and cognitive flexibility. Training programs that enhance cognitive skills lead to improvements in behavioral performance, such as improved accuracy and response time (Bavelier et al., 2011). Improvements of behavioral performance demonstrate cognitive flexibility. The improvement in cognitive flexibility from the use of training programs may reduce vulnerability and enhance resilience of mental health.

Behavioral performance that improves through training with technological tools demonstrates the efficacy of social learning. Cognitive training may be effective for building of behavioral skills that enhance cognitive flexibility for intercultural competence. Training programs that enhance cognitive flexibility with technological tools may illustrate the building of cognitive skills through social learning. Improvements in behavioral performance such as ease or accuracy in conformity to social norms reflect social learning for intercultural competence. Training programs may enhance the ease and efficiency of intercultural competence by strengthening intercultural knowledge, attitudes, and skills. Technological tools designed to support intercultural competence may train problem solving across cultural settings.

Technology may be beneficial for improvement in the cultural experience of control. Training programs that provide capabilities for sociocultural adaptation improve levels of cultural knowledge, positive cultural attitudes, and intercultural contact. Cultural applications designed to promote cultural experience seek to share cultural knowledge pertinent for effective and efficient intercultural contact. Cultural applications efficacious for providing multimedia messaging promote the maintenance of cultural heritage and cultural identity. Cultural applications that provide tracking of cultural behavior performance improve levels of cultural learning and acculturation experiences. Cultural applications for intercultural competence provide data collection and reporting of issues that benefit from intercultural knowledge or intercultural training.

Technological innovation facilitates cultural change. Technological platforms have the capability to support intercultural contact that enhances the quality of relations of social groups. Technological tools designed for cultural change are beneficial for the integration of attitudes toward the heritage and host culture that improve relations among ethnocultural groups. Training programs that enhance positive attitudes toward the heritage and host culture support intercultural competence and strengthen social relations of ethnocultural groups. Technological tools for building of behavioral skills to enhance the social and emotional preferences of individuals and groups promote strategies of integration of ethnocultural groups. Technological tools that build social and emotional flexibility facilitate learning that strengthens culture. Technological tools designed to eliminate racial discrimination support the reduction of societal exposure to risk factors and strengthen protective factors that contribute to social equality.

Digital culture as a form of technology improves the capability for social communication with other people. Social media, a type of digital culture, provides online tools for the sharing of social and emotional information through digital media across users. Social media improves communication for a range of social information across an identity-based social network. Behavioral paradigms may be designed for social and emotional training through digital media. Social media enhances behavioral training of social and emotion perception (e.g., visual images of people and groups), social attribution (e.g., causal reasoning of other people), and understanding of mental states (e.g., preferences, beliefs, intentions). Social media enhances the efficiency and quality of social communication through digital media to others. Behavioral performance on paradigms of social and emotional training may enhance social communication and social and emotional flexibility throughout life.

The culture of technology modulates neurobiological mechanisms of social behavior. Findings from neuroimaging studies of social media show the recruitment of social and emotional neural networks during a social preference "Like" task during visual perception. Behavioral performance on social media paradigms is related to greater neural activation within brain regions associated with reward and social processing, such as the ventral striatum and ventral medial prefrontal cortex (Sherman et al., 2018). These findings suggest that people find social media use rewarding and a reinforcement of positive social feedback. The use of social media may improve societal exposure to risk and protective factors in the social environment. Behavioral training of social and emotional knowledge may serve as an early prevention and intervention in the promotion of mental health.

Technology provides opportunities for the development and implementation of health prevention and interventions that build on social interaction with conversational agents and interfaces. The use of technology for health prevention and intervention shares considerations with those designed for naturalistic social interaction. People perceive agency and contingency through simple characteristics, such as animations (Blakemore et al., 2003; Mar et al., 2007; Frith & Frith, 2003). People show a preference for social interaction with agent-based technology that is similar to those of naturalistic social interaction (Cassell & Tartaro, 2008). Studies of human–computer interaction with embodied conversational agents show that people have a perception of communication with conversational agents as a social process (Cassell et al., 2000). People construct naturalistic conversational narratives to communicate with conversational agents. People show motivation and competence to train social skills with conversational agents. People respond to conversational agents of the same ethnicity as the user as a cultural ingroup member and perceive greater similarity in attitudes. People are more likely to show conformity with ingroup conversational agents. Findings from studies of human–computer interaction show that technology has the potential to train and improve social communication across cultures.

Technology shows capability for the development and implementation of health prevention and intervention of emotion processes across cultural settings. Emotion processes consist of antecedents and consequences of emotional experience, ranging from the generation to the regulation of emotion. People perceive and respond to emotional information in the environment that varies in valence, intensity, and arousal. Multilevel mechanisms respond preferentially to distinct dimensions of emotional processes. Cultural variations in emotion processes illustrate differential patterns of emotional experience.

Affective technology provides capability to the user to receive feedback about emotional information in the environment. Information about emotional states of the user may enable decision making that integrates affective biofeedback. Patterns of emotional processes that are unconscious may become recognizable through interaction with affective technology. With affective technology, people may produce informed signals of emotional communication with other people that complement those understood with emotional perception. Affective technology may provide knowledge-based resources for the design of system platforms and user-guided programs to train regulation of emotional communication with neurofeedback. Affective technology may provide user and system feedback for the design of emotional communication that is user guided and appropriate across cultural settings. Affective technology may be beneficial for the design of health prevention and intervention.

Affective wearable technology shows capability to measure and track emotional and physiological responding for the benefit of the user (Picard & Healey, 1997; Picard, 1997). Affective wearable technology may provide useful feedback for informed decision making of health. Affective wearable technology that interacts with the user provides a support platform for knowledge-based resources to guide user-guided programs. User-guided programs that provide information of cultural knowledge-based resources may be effective to generate user feedback appropriate across cultural settings. The use of affective wearable technology may be beneficial as an innovation for health prevention and intervention across cultures.

Culture and Technology for Health Equity

Technology provides tools and resources for the improvement of treatment and access to health care across nations. Technology builds capability for the sharing of information that improves the coordination and access to services. Digital health is set of scalable platforms designed to improve treatment and access to health care. Digital health encompasses mobile health (mHealth) initiatives for the use of mobile technology in medical and public health practice. mHealth includes the use of applications designed to support health communication, health monitoring, and access to health services between the health system and the public (World Health Organization [WHO], 2011). The wide-spread public use of mobile technology illustrates the practical benefits of technical tools for information sharing and personal use. mHealth programs aim to develop innovative and effective strategies for the public use of technology to improve health and well-being. mHealth programs enhance technical capability for the security and protection of public health, including preparation and recovery from natural disasters, and the restoration of access to health services in response to public health epidemics, among others.

mHealth programs design applications to address public health priorities in delivery science. The Global mHealth Initiative supports the advancement of technology for evidence-based health projects across nations. The Global mHealth Initiative is an invest-ment in the development of tools for health and community systems to boost health outcomes of vulnerable populations, including pregnant women, mothers, and children. Global mHealth programs coordinate the use of digital applications to provide service delivery including community-level health messaging and health information that sup-ports health programs across nations. Global mHealth programs are a component of the national health system developed within governmental strategy and policy. Global mHealth programs provide timely solutions to priority challenges in delivery science with government projects that support public–private partnerships. Filling the gaps in acces-sibility to health care requires the identification of priorities for policy and technical sup-port. Project implementation requires the design of digital platforms and applications and the training of community health workers and users to meet the goals of project models to improve the health of vulnerable populations.

Culture and Technology for Health Diplomacy

Government interest in mHealth includes the development and implementation of strategic initiatives of member-states to use technology to improve health and well-being across cultural settings. Policymakers benefit from the use of evidence-based resources to raise awareness regarding the benefits and barriers to the use of mHealth programs globally (WHO, 2011). Evaluation of mHealth programs of member-states at the coun-try level provides the greatest benefit for sharing best practices to inform standards and architecture of systems and applications. Evidence-based resources that provide infor-mation regarding the impact of mHealth for health outcomes and health systems may improve knowledge and understanding of mHealth programs and the priority application of mHealth practices for health systems. The evidence-based evaluation of the effective-ness and cost-effectiveness of mHealth programs may further inform international and national standards of implementation for member-states.

Strategic initiatives of mHealth policy include support for the systematic recognition of mHealth as an approach in health policy. Policymakers may promote the development and implementation of mHealth action plans, policy, and legislation. The policymaking

Box 21.1. Case Study of mHealth for Health Care in Ghana (WHO, 2011)

Health communication of providers provides essential information for the delivery of health care services across cultural settings. The mHealth program improves the technological capability of health communication for providers in rural cultural settings. Rural cultures may benefit from technical tools that enhance the efficiency and cultural competence of response in health care delivery.

The mHealth program MDNet promotes the transfer of knowledge across providers in Africa. The development of MDNet consists of an online communication tool for physicians as well as communication services for health care delivery through mobile technology. The mHealth program ensures the technical tools for the sharing of information of physicians to benefit the quality of health care delivery in Ghana. MDNet users access the technical tool to gain the professional advice of other providers and information regarding the availability of resources in rural and urban areas of Ghana. The mHealth program MDNet is effective at improving the connectivity of physicians across cultural settings.

The impact of the mHealth program to promote health care across cultural settings is considerable. The mHealth program has led to several improvements in delivery services for health care in the African region. The mHealth program demonstrates the feasibility of a scalable program designed to provide technical tools for the use of mobile technology to improve health communication of providers across cultural settings. The mHealth program illustrates the effectiveness of technology for improvements in health care delivery in rural and urban areas of the African region. The mHealth program is an efficacious model of the use of mobile technology in health care for the development and implementation of health policy in Africa.

process for the validation and support of mHealth programs in health policy includes public health campaigns, research and development, evaluation, and guidelines for use. The use of global standards in medical technology for health policy is important for cost-effectiveness and efficiency in the achievement of national health priorities and the Sustainable Goal Agenda.

Policy issues in mHealth focus on the areas of data security and citizen privacy that require proper protection. The development and implementation of security policies are important to protect health identity information, message transmission, and data storage of mHealth programs. Security policies are important to safeguard health information across the data cycle of health identity. Security policies can define technical standards as parameters of protections and capabilities that prevent data loss and strengthen privacy.

The development and implementation of health policy that supports mHealth programs consist of distinct barriers across global regions. For the African region, the lack

Box 21.2. Case Study of mHealth for Disease Control in Cambodia (WHO, 2011)

mHealth programs enhance technological capabilities to provide necessary protections for public health across cultures. Disease epidemics across cultures introduce a set of challenges to public health due to limitations in access to technology. Rural cultures may have limited technological capability, such as access to mobile technology and communication tools, for the protection of public health. Technical tools may be particularly effective for the efficient and accurate sharing of public health information in regions of limited capability. mHealth programs provide effective strategies for the development and implementation of technical tools that are necessary and beneficial for the protection of public health.

In 2003, the mHealth program in Cambodia, called Cam e-WARN, was designed to improve the control of disease spread and protection of public health with the use of mobile technology. Funding from the World Health Organization (WHO), Asia Development Bank, government, and other donors provided investment for equipment and training of personnel with the system. The mHealth program Cam e-WARN consists of health care workers who operate a surveillance system at different levels of the health structure. Local health care workers provide data related to disease to Cam e-WARN through mobile technology. District personnel communicate aggregate health information to the province and national levels. The Cam e-WARN system provides analyses regarding trends and incidences of disease by province. The Cam e-WARN system ensures early and accurate detection of disease spread by monitoring thresholds in trends and communicating an efficient response to afflicted regions.

The impact of the mHealth program for the benefit of public health in Cambodia is considerable. mHealth technology improves the technical capability to control the spread of disease and to protect the health of the Cambodian population. The Cam e-WARN system demonstrates the feasibility in design of applications to monitor disease outbreak in Cambodia. The Cam e-WARN system provides early detection of signs of disease or outbreak in the population using indicators. The Cam e-WARN system provides systematic data informatics on a set of diseases and syndromes affecting the Cambodian population, improving accuracy and recovery for public health.

The effectiveness of the Cam e-WARN system leads to several improvements in health delivery and health policy. The Cam e-WARN system was expanded in implementation to serve neighboring countries such as Laos, Indonesia, Papua New Guinea, and Vietnam. The Cam e-WARN system demonstrated the cost-effectiveness of investment in mHealth programs with public–private partnerships. The efficacy of the mHealth program has generated the interest of policymakers to support the system with a long-term funding strategy and integration into the health information system.

of infrastructure is a main barrier to the implementation of mHealth programs. The growth of mHealth in Africa may benefit from expanded infrastructure and network capacity for mobile technology (Box 21.1). For the European and Americas regions, the necessity of improved policy guidelines on security and privacy is the main barrier to the implementation of mHealth programs. The development of policy frameworks of eHealth may include considerations and technical solutions of mHealth. Policy frameworks that govern health information transfer and storage as well as health security and privacy are essential to enable eHealth and mHealth programs. For the South East Asian region, technical expertise is a main barrier such that mHealth programs in the region may benefit from greater availability of locally qualified personnel (Box 21.2). For most regions, the priority use of mHealth in health systems is an important barrier to mHealth programs. mHealth programs will benefit from expanded infrastructure to improve priority use in health systems. Relatedly, most regions require cost-effectiveness of mHealth initiatives to ensure efficient large-scale deployment. mHealth programs will benefit from cost-savings and cost–benefit studies across regions.

Global evaluation of mHealth programs characterizes the landscape of technological use for health delivery by region. Regional use of mHealth programs for health communication is considerable, while for disaster recovery it is relatively low in the African region. The use of mHealth programs for health communication suggests development of infrastructure and acceptance of technological use for delivery of health care across regions. The use of mHealth programs for delivery of disaster recovery in the African region may benefit from further investment in infrastructural support to respond efficiently and effectively to mobile communication related to natural disasters.

References

Bavelier, D., Green, C. S., Han, D. H., Renshaw, P. F., Merzenich, M. M., & Gentile, D. A. (2011). Brains on video games. *Nature Reviews Neuroscience, 12*, 763–768.

Blakemore, S. J., Boyer, P., Pachot-Clouard, M., Meltzoff, A., Segebarth, C., & Decety, J. (2003). The detection of contingency and animacy from simple animations in the human brain. *Cerebral Cortex, 13*(8), 837–844.

Boyd, R. & Richerson, P. J. (2005). *The origin and evolution of cultures.* Oxford University Press.

Cassell, J., & Tartaro, A. (2008). Intersubjectivity in human-agent interaction. *Interaction Studies 8*(3), 391–410.

Cassell, J., Sullivan, J., Prevost, S., & Churchill, E. F. (2000). *Embodied conversational agents.* MIT Press.

Cheon, B. K., Im, D-M., Harada, T., Kim, J.-S., Mathur, V. A., Scimeca, J. M., Parrish, T. B., Park, H., & Chiao, J. Y. (2013). Cultural modulation of the neural correlates of emotional pain perception: the role of other-focusedness. *Neuropsychologia, 51*(7), 1177–1186.

Chiao, J. Y. (2018). *Philosophy of cultural neuroscience.* New York: Routledge.

Chiao, J. Y. & Blizinsky K. D. (2010). Culture-gene coevolution of individualism-collectivism and the serotonin transporter gene. *Proceedings of the Biological Sciences, 277*(1681), 529–537.

Chiao, J. Y., Iidaka, T., Gordon, H. L., Nogawa, J., Bar, M., Aminoff, E., Sadato, N., & Ambady, N. (2008). Cultural specificity in amygdala response to fear faces. *Journal of Cognitive Neuroscience, 20*(12), 2167–2174,

Chiao, J. Y., Harada, T., Komeda, H., Li, Z., Mano, Y., Saito, D., Parrish, T. B., Sadato, N., & Iidaka, T. (2009). Neural basis of individualistic and collectivistic views of self. *Human Brain Mapping, 30*(9), 2813–2820.

Chiao, J. Y., Li, S. C., Turner, R., Lee-Tauler, S. Y., & Pringle, B. A. (2017). Cultural neuroscience and global mental health: Addressing grand challenges. *Culture and Brain, 5*(1), 4–13.

Collins, P. Y., Patel, V., Joestl, S. S., March, D., Insel, T. R., Daar, A. S., Scientific Advisory Board and the Executive Committee of the Grand Challenges on Global Mental Health, Anderson, W., Dhansay, M. A., Phillips, A., Shurin, S., Walport, M., Ewart, W., Savill, S. J., Bordin, I. A., Costello, E. J., Durkin, M., Fairburn, C., Glass, R. I., . . . Stein, D. J. (2011). Grand challenges in global mental health. *Nature, 475*(7354), 27–30.

Fincher, C. L., Thornill, R., Murray, D. R., & Schaller, M. (2008). Pathogen prevalence predicts human cross-cultural variability in individualism/collectivism. *Proceedings of the Biological Sciences, 275*(1640), 1279–1285.

Frith, U., & Frith, C. D. (2003). Development and neurophysiology of mentalizing. *Philosophical Transactions of the Royal Society London B: Biological Sciences, 358*(1431), 459–473.

Gelfand, M. J., Raver, J. L., Nishii, L., Leslie, L. M., Lun, J., Lim, B. C., Duan, L., Almaliach, A., Ang, S., Arnadottir, J., aycan, Z., Boehnke, K., Boski, P., Cabecinhas, R., Chan, D., Chhokar, J., D'Amato, A., Ferrer, M., Fischlmayr, I. C., Fischer, R., Fülöp, M., Georgas, J., Kashima, E. S., Kashima, Y., Kim, K., Lempereur, A., Marquez, P. Othman, R., Overlaet, B., Panagiotopoulou, P. Peltzer, K., Perez-Florizno, L. R., Ponomarenko, L., Realo, A., Schei, V., Schmitt, M., Smith, P. B., Soomro, N., Szabo, E., Taveesin, N., Toyama, M., Van de Vliert, E., Vohra, N., Ward, C., & Yamaguchi, S. (2011). Differences between tight and loose cultures: A 33-nation study. *Science, 332*(6033), 1100–1104.

Harada, T., Li, Z., & Chiao, J. Y. (2010). Differential dorsal and ventral medial prefrontal representations of the implicit self modulated by individualism and collectivism: An fMRI study. *Social Neuroscience, 5*(3), 257–271.

Laland, K. N., Odling-Smee, J., & Feldman, M. W. (2000). Niche construction, biological evolution, and cultural change. *Behavioral and Brain Sciences, 23*(1), 131–146.

Mar, R. A., Kelley, W. M., Heatherton, T. F., & Macrae, C. N. (2007). Detecting agency from the biological motion of veridical vs animated agents. *Social Cognitive and Affective Neuroscience, 2*(3), 199–205.

Mathur, V. A., Harada, T., & Chiao, J. Y. (2012). Racial identification modulates default network activity for same and other races. *Human Brain Mapping, 33*(8), 1883–1893.

Mesoudi, A. (2009). How cultural evolutionary theory can inform social psychology and vice versa. *Psychological Review, 116*(4), 929–952.

Minas, H. (2014). Human security, complexity and mental health system development. In Patel, V., Minas, H., Cohen, A., & Prince, M. J. (Eds.), *Global mental health: Principles and practice* (pp. 137–166). Oxford University Press.

Mrazek, A. J., Chiao, J. Y., Blizinsky, K. D., Lun, J., & Gelfand, M. J. (2013). The role of culture-gene coevolution in morality judgment: Examining the interplay between tightness-looseness and allelic variation of the serotonin transporter gene. *Culture and Brain, 1*(2–4), 100–117.

Nisbett, R. E., Peng, K., Choi, I., & Norenzayan, A. (2001). Culture and systems of thought: holistic versus analytic cognition. *Psychological Review, 108*(2), 291–310.

Park, B., Tsai, J. L., Chim, L. Blevins, E., & Knutson, B. (2016). Neural evidence for cultural differences in the valuation of positive facial expressions. *Social Cognitive and Affective Neuroscience, 11*(2), 243–252.

Picard, R. W. (1997). *Affective computing.* MIT Press.

Picard, R. W., & Healey, J. (1997, October). *Affective wearables.* Proceedings of the International Symposium on Wearable Computers, Cambridge, MA.

Sam, D. L. & Berry, J. W. (Eds.) (2006). *The Cambridge Handbook of Acculturation Psychology.* Cambridge University Press.

Sherman, L. E., Hernandez, L. M., Greenfield, P. M., & Dapretto, M. (2018). What the brain "Likes": Neural correlates of providing feedback on social media. *Social Cognitive and Affective Neuroscience, 13*(7), 699–707.

Tsai, J. L. (2007). Ideal affect: Cultural causes and behavioral consequences. *Perspectives in Psychological Science, 2*(3), 242–259.

World Health Organization (WHO). (2011). *mHealth: New horizons for health through mobile technologies. Global Observatory eHealth Series* (Vol. 3). World Health Organization Press.

Zhu, Y., Zhang, L., Fan, J., & Han, S. (2007). Neural basis of cultural influence on self-representation. *Neuroimage, 34*(3), 1310–1316.

Culture and Environment

Joan Y. Chiao, Yoko Mano, *and* Norihiro Sadato

Abstract

Cultural and environmental systems mutually influence the production and regulation of human behavior. Culture maintains and regulates the mental capacities important for the navigation of the social and physical environment. Geographic variation in environmental features are associated with cultural dimensions that serve as a protective factor. Identification of risk and protective factors in the environment across cultural settings is necessary for the development and implementation of prevention and intervention in global mental health. Implications of research on culture and the environment for population health disparities and global mental health are discussed.

Key Words: culture, social, environment, health equity, health disparities, global mental health

Introduction

One of the chief goals of sustainable development is to strengthen protections to environmental factors affecting global mental health. Environmental factors such as exposure to environmental hazards reflects risk factors to health. Improvements to environmental quality are a necessary component to the protection of environmental health. The identification of environmental problems may lead to the development of preventions and interventions for the benefit of human health. Global environmental health research identifies risk and protective factors in environmental health research. The translation of research in global environmental health for the implementation of preventions and interventions is important for the delivery of health equity. Building scientific capacity in global environmental health contributes to the enhancement of protections for global mental health.

Global concerns of climate change reflect one of the challenges in global mental health. Changes in environmental conditions impact health and well-being. Climate change contributes to the substantial morbidity and mortality due to natural disasters (Minas, 2014). Climate change may lead to increased prevalence of natural disasters and infectious diseases caused by changes to environmental conditions. Economic crises due to changes in food production may also result from changes in environmental conditions.

The capability of preparation for and recovery from environmental health conditions such as climate change is paramount to the strengthening of capacities for improved resilience and reduced vulnerabilities to environmental health hazards of nations. Understanding the capacities of individuals and societies to effectively prepare and respond to vulnerabilities brought about by climate change and related environmental conditions is important to addressing the public health impact of environmental health conditions (Swim et al., 2011; Weber & Stern, 2011).

Cultural change may result as a consequence of climate change given the possibility of the necessity for permanent or temporary migration to geographic regions with improved environmental quality. Complex environmental hazards such as climate change and natural disasters may result in a substantial flow of refugees seeking effective protection and recovery of health services. The cultural change due to increased cultural contact of refugees with a different culture requires the acquisition of acculturation capacities for sociocultural and psychological adaptation. The delivery of health equity relies on the capability to provide access to quality health care services across cultural settings.

The impact of environmental health conditions on global mental health is significant. Environmental hazards impact societal exposure to physical and social risk factors to well-being and mental health. The perceived experience of environmental conditions may also affect the physical and social risk factors that contribute to mental health. Preventions of and interventions for environmental hazards may include the development and implementation of cultural representations that improve the perceived experience of climate change. Understanding the risk and protective factors that enhance resilience and reduce vulnerabilities to environmental conditions is necessary for effective response and recovery in global mental health.

Theoretical Approaches

Theoretical approaches to the study of culture and the environment provide conceptual standards for the construction of scientific paradigms to postulate causal patterns or regularities in phenomena of the natural world. Dual inheritance theory posits that cultural and biological factors mutually influence behavioral adaptation. Natural selection holds that environmental conditions represent selective pressures that modify behavioral adaptation. Reciprocally, cultural niche construction postulates that organisms may change environmental conditions for their benefit (Boyd & Richerson, 2005). The ecological changes introduced by the organism through niche construction subsequently alter the environmental conditions of behavioral adaptation. Cumulative cultural evolution further articulates that cultural changes to environmental conditions may undergo rapid accumulation due to social learning. Cultural and genetic processes contribute to the maintenance and regulation of mental and neural architecture of behavioral adaptation. The conditions of the physical environment affect the regulation of cultural systems. The presence of environmental hazards, such as natural and man-made disasters, lead to changes in cultural systems. The increased prevalence of changes in environmental health conditions is related to cultural changes across geographic regions.

Environmental conditions such as climate change directly impact human health. Increases in severe weather conditions and natural disasters contribute to the hazardous environmental conditions that lead to greater prevalence of infectious diseases. Infectious diseases result from vulnerabilities or perceived vulnerabilities to hazards in physical health brought on by changes in environmental conditions. The capability to improve resilience and reduce perceptions of vulnerabilities is important for response and recovery from environmental health hazards.

Cultural systems provide the mental capital for effective protection to environmental health hazards. One protective factor of cultural systems is the reduction in societal exposure to the vulnerabilities of environmental health conditions. Cultural differences in societal practices, from food preparation to parenting, improve the resilience to and recovery from hazardous environmental health conditions (Fincher et al., 2008). Cultural differences in valuation of conformity or tolerance of uniqueness affect the vulnerability to adverse environmental health conditions. In geographic regions with higher historical pathogen prevalence, cultural systems of collectivism emphasize the value of tradition and conformity to reduce the societal exposure to risk factors to human health. In geographic regions with lower historical pathogen prevalence, cultural systems of individualism encourage tolerance of uniqueness to improve resilience to environmental health conditions. Cultural traditions and social norms serve as an effective protection for concerns of global environmental health.

Another protective factor of cultural systems is the reduction in societal exposure to the perception of vulnerabilities of environmental health hazards. Cultural systems of individualism and collectivism contribute to the reduction in the perceived vulnerabilities of environmental health hazards. Cultural variation in attitudes and behaviors of the social group reduce the societal exposure to risk factors to human health. In geographic regions with higher historical pathogen prevalence, cultural variation in the promotion of negative attitudes and behaviors may reduce the vulnerability to adverse environmental health conditions. In geographic regions with lower historical pathogen prevalence, cultural variation in the promotion of positive attitudes and behaviors may improve the resilience to environmental health conditions.

Cultural systems provide effective protection to environmental conditions affecting behavioral adaptation. In geographic regions with higher historical pathogen prevalence, cultural variation in attitudes and behaviors as a protective factor may become systematically refined through processes of social learning. Cultural acquisition of attitudes and behaviors through social learning that reduce the perception of vulnerability of the social group to environmental health hazards may serve as an effective health prevention or intervention. Cultural representations through media and popular culture regulate the perception of societal exposure to risk and protective factors of global environmental health. Cultural representations in the media and popular culture that promote the societal perception of protections, such as capabilities for preparation for, resilience to, and recovery from environmental health hazards, are effective preventions and interventions in global environmental health.

The impact of cultural systems on the perception and regulation of the environment is generated across time scales. Theoretical models of the mutual influence of culture and the environment posit reciprocal interactions of cultural and ecological inheritance across generations (Laland et al., 2000). Cultural inheritance modifies selective pressures of ecological inheritance through processes of niche construction. Ecological inheritance through selective processes modifies the gene pool of the population through cultural transmission across development. The parallel mechanisms of biological evolution and cultural change produce generational transmission as modified by ecological inheritance.

Ecological inheritance guides the generation and transmission of cultural systems. Culture provides a set of mental constructs and behavioral repertoire for behavioral adaptation in the social and physical environment (Sherman et al., 2009). Ecological pressures, including natural and man-made disasters, lead to population-level changes in the cultural and neurobiological systems of organisms across time (Gelfand et al., 2011; Mrazek et al., 2013). Ecological pressures may modify the social and physical environmental conditions of behavioral adaptation. Through processes of niche construction, organisms generate cultural change to modify the societal exposure to risk and protective factors of social and environmental conditions that produce changes at the level of the population. Cultural change consists of a set of processes for the development of effective preventions and interventions in global environmental health.

Cultural niche construction generates cultural change through mechanisms of social learning and biological evolution. Cultural transmission of social learning leads to the transfer and persistence of information across individuals in the social and physical environment. The modification of the social and physical environment for the transmission of cultural change modifies the gene pool of the population. The modification of the gene pool facilitates the reinforcement of changes in cultural systems and contributes to neurobiological changes of behavioral adaptation. Developmental epigenesis, as the dynamic process of genetic expression throughout the lifespan, modifies the neurodevelopmental pathway that maintains and regulates culture.

The mutual influence of culture and genes on the maintenance and regulation of mental and neural architecture demonstrates bidirectional pathways of development and generational inheritance. The identification of biomarkers underlying mental health and well-being requires theoretical constructs, from conceptual frameworks to pathway models, for characterization of the dynamic patterns of cultural and genetic variations in mind, brain, and behavior. The environment presents an important causal influence on cultural and genetic inheritance. Through interaction with environmental influences, patterns of cultural and epigenetic change modify the functionality of mental constructs and neuro-biological mechanisms of behavioral adaptation.

Theoretical approaches to the study of culture and the environment provide a set of concepts for understanding regularities and patterns in the structure of the natural world. Explanations of relations of culture and the environment posit multilevel mechanisms that detail the relations between parts of cultural and environmental systems and their distal and proximate causal influence on levels of sociocultural and behavioral adaptation. Explanations from theoretical models of culture and the environment are bidirectional, allowing for reliable predictions regarding expected and observed outcomes in environmental and cultural systems guided by laws of nature. Changes in patterns of cultural and environmental systems demonstrate the impact of relational causation on predicted and observed outcomes of the natural world.

Methodological Approaches

Methodological approaches to investigations of culture and the environment include a range of approaches from behavioral to genetic levels of analysis. Environmental influences on behavioral adaptation may lead to modifications in behavioral and genetic expression across cultural contexts. Cross-cultural research in psychology shows variation in the levels of behavioral expression of specific mental processes across cultural contexts (Matsumoto and Hwang, this volume, Chapter 3). Levels of psychological universalism may reflect differences in functionality, ease, or accessibility of use of particular mental processes due to sensitivity to cultural context. Culture guides the sensitivity to the social and physical environment observable in behavioral expression. Culture may interact with genes to alter the sensitivity of mental and neural processes to the social and physical environment in the production of behavioral adaptation.

Gene-by-culture interplay elaborates the notion that environmental influences modify the relation of genes to behavioral expression due to cultural context. Theories of gene-by-culture interplay examine the relation of specific genes to behavioral expression across cultural contexts (Sasaki et al., 2016). Studies of gene-by-culture interplay investigate the influence of culture on the genetic sensitivity of mental processes to the social and physical environment. Gene-by-culture interplay hypothesizes that the relation of genes to behavioral expression is relayed through mental constructs that are sensitized toward environmental influences such as the cultural context. Theories of gene-by-culture interplay postulate that genetic sensitivity in behavioral expression is modified toward the social and physical environment of a given cultural context. The mutual influence of culture and genes guides mental processes and the expression of behavior.

Culture and genes modify not only behavioral expression but also the functional organization of the brain. Culture and genes regulate the molecular and cellular mechanisms of the brain. Theories of cultural neurogenetics conceptualize the bidirectional influence of culture and genes, affecting the sensitivity of neural mechanisms to the cultural context.

Studies of cultural neurogenetics investigate the influence of culture on genetic regulation of neural bases of behavior. The modification of genetic sensitivity in functional neural activity to the social and physical environment toward the cultural context illustrates the mutual influence of culture and genes across levels of analyses. Culture plays an important role in guiding genetic expression of functional brain mechanisms underlying behavioral adaptation.

Theories of cultural genomics posit the notion that the relation of the human genome to behavioral phenotypes in the social and physical environment varies across ethnocultural groups at the level of population. Environmental influences affect the relation of the human genome and behavioral phenotypes across cultural contexts (Chen et al., 2016). Social and physical environment influences facilitate the behavioral expression of the human genome toward a given cultural context. Theories of cultural genomics hypothesize cultural variation in the functional relation of genomic processes and behavior due to influences of the social and physical environment.

Environmental influences on cultural systems lead to changes in mental and neural processes of behavioral adaptation. The influence of culture on the human genome and related behavioral expression is affected by the social and physical environment. Methodological approaches may systematically examine the mutual influence of culture and genes on psychological and neural processes of the social and physical environment across individuals and groups. Environmental factors serve to regulate changes in societal exposure to risk and protective factors maintained by cultural systems. The perception of environmental factors may similarly affect the maintenance and regulation of cultural systems.

Empirical Approaches

Empirical approaches to culture and the environment investigate the bidirectional influence of culture on global environmental health and the perception of the environment on representations of culture. Exposure to environmental hazards, including natural and man-made disasters, affects environmental quality. The regulation of societal exposure to risk and protective factors in global environmental health is important to improve environmental quality and the health benefits. The regulation of the perception of environmental hazards and its bidirectional influence on culture provides another important means for the development of preventions and interventions for global mental health.

Research in cultural neuroscience provides an evidence-based resource for understanding the impact of culture on the global environmental health of nations, societies, and individuals. Environmental factors affect cultural variation and related health outcomes across nations (Chiao & Blizinsky, 2010). Across nations, environmental conditions, such as pathogen prevalence, are related to the cultural conditions of individualism and collectivism. Cultural variation in individualism and collectivism relate to societal practices that provide an important defense to protect from pathogens. Collectivistic nations emphasize social norms that enhance the vigilance of members to social cues of group members and adherence to social conformity to a greater extent than individualistic nations (Oyserman et al., 2002). Greater vigilance to the social cues of cultural group members and social conformity ensure the social coordination of individual and collective action for the effective response to and recovery from risks and threats in environmental conditions. Cultural variation in individualism and collectivism provides an important protection from the environmental threat of pathogens.

Ecological conditions affect the cultural variation in the adherence to societal norms. The presence of distal and historical ecological conditions, including population density, resource scarcity, and natural disasters, among others, influences societal practices that strengthen the adherence to social norms across nations (Gelfand et al., 2011; Mrazek et al., 2013). Cultural variation in tightness and looseness enhance capacities for the regulation and prevention of the perception of threats in the environment. Ecological conditions affect cultural variation in broad and narrow socialization such as the range of characteristics that make up appropriate behavior. Tighter nations seek to strengthen the capabilities for the social regulation of nations and the capacities of self-regulation of individuals. Cultural variation due to ecological conditions affects the strength of capability and resilience for social organization and social coordination of collective action. Tighter nations regulate the protection of societal influences for religious and political participation. Cultural variation in mental and neural processes contributes to the effective response for behavioral adaptation. Tighter nations aim for greater adherence to situational constraints and the need for structure. Cultural variation in tightness and looseness serves as an effective protection from environmental conditions of ecological threats.

Cultural systems affect the perception and regulation of the social environment. Culture modifies the societal exposure to risk and protective factors in the social environment. Culture strengthens the functional activity of neural mechanisms important for social perception. People show greater response within brain regions located within the fusiform gyrus and parahippocampal gyrus during face perception for same relative to other races (Eberhardt, 2005; Golby et al., 2001). Neural activity for different race faces located within social brain regions, such as the amygdala and prefrontal cortex (PFC), is attenuated during the regulation of social processing (Lieberman et al., 2005; Richeson et al., 2003). Neural representations of different race faces show differential activation, suggesting variation in the ease and frequency of functional processing within neural circuits of social perception. Greater neural response to faces of members of the same race suggests enhanced processing of perceptual cues in the social environment that maintain culture. The cultural acquisition of neural processing for self and others enhances regularity of the perception of resilience and reduction of vulnerabilities in the social environment.

Culture influences the perception and regulation of the physical environment. Culture affects the analytic and holistic perception of the physical environment and its underlying neurobiological bases. Cultural and genetic variations regulate the locus of attention in the physical environment. Analytic perception of the physical environment refers to the locus of attention to the focal object, while holistic perception relies on the locus of attention to the focal object and the surrounding environment (Nisbett et al., 2001; Miyamoto et al., 2006). Cultural variation in the locus of attention is related to genetic variation of the serotonin receptor polymorphism (5-HTR1A) that reinforces the conscious preference for analytic or holistic perception (Kim et al., 2010). Cultural variation affects neural mechanisms of scene perception in aging (Gutchess et al., 2006; Goh et al., 2007; Jenkins et al., 2010; Park & Gutchess, 2002). East Asians demonstrate a pattern of greater selectivity in neural response within the lingual landmark area (LLA) relative to Westerners, consistent with cultural variation in perceptual processing style (Goh et al., 2010). Cultural variation in the neural mechanisms of scene perception illustrates the parallel influence of top-down and bottom-up perceptual processing of the physical environment.

Cultural experience affects the neurobiological bases of social learning. The mirror neuron system, including the inferior frontal gyrus, ventral premotor cortex, and rostral inferior parietal lobe, makes up the core neural circuitry of imitation (Iacoboni, 2005). Social learning of communicative gestures activates brain regions within the mirror neuron system when people observe and imitate motor action. Culture affects the neural mechanisms of social learning during the observation of gestures performed by different models. Neural activity within brain regions of the mirror neuron system, including frontal, parietal, and occipital areas, shows greater response during the imitation of models of different races (Losin et al., 2012, 2014; see Gianola and Losin, this volume, Chapter 17). Differential neural activation within the mirror neuron system exhibits functional variation of social learning. Cultural acquisition enhances neural processing of socially learned associations. The cultural acquisition of neural mechanisms for social learning demonstrates the capacity for flexibility of the imitative neuron system for effective response to environmental conditions.

Cultural processes modify the societal exposure to risk and protective factors that affect the perception of the physical and social environment. Cultural processes that strengthen the perception of protection in the physical and social environment improve resilience and reduce vulnerabilities to environmental conditions. Culture affects the perception of threat and protection in the physical and social environment. Culture influences the neural responses to the perception of natural disasters (Cheon et al., 2013). Cultural interdependence enhances the empathic neural response within the anterior cingulate cortex (ACC) and insula to social situations of emotional pain and distress due to exposure to natural disasters. Cultural interdependence strengthens the capacities of individuals and capability for collective action in effective response and recovery from hazardous environmental conditions.

Cultural and genetic variations strengthen sensitivity to the social environment. Cultural norms affect the behavioral expression related to the oxytocin receptor polymorphism (OXTR) rs53576 (Kim et al., 2010). Americans with the G/G or G/A genotype of the oxytocin receptor polymorphism who experience social distress show greater genetic sensitivity to the social environment and emotional support seeking relative to Koreans, who do not. These findings suggest cultural differences in the behavioral expression of genetic sensitivity to the social environment. Cultural variation in norms and practices also affects genetic sensitivity of the serotonin transporter polymorphism (5-HTTLPR) to the social environment. Japanese with the s/s genotype of the serotonin transporter polymorphism show greater genetic sensitivity to changes in emotional facial expressions in the social environment relative to Americans (Ishii et al., 2014). Cultural variation in genetic sensitivity to social and emotional cues affects the capacity to detect threat and protection in the social environment. Cultural variation in genetic sensitivity to social norms illustrates the importance of cultural norms on behavioral expression. Cultural and genetic variations in sensitivity to the social environment demonstrate multilevel mechanisms of behavioral adaptation.

Implications

The bidirectional influence of environmental and cultural systems demonstrates sources of malleability in risk and protective factors of the social and physical environment. The quality of environmental conditions is affected by the perception of threat and protection across cultural contexts. Cultural processes serve to strengthen the perception of protection and resilience for individual and collective action. Environmental conditions that are hazardous may lead to cultural changes that modify or reduce the societal exposure to risk and promote the effectiveness of protective factors. Reciprocally, cultural changes may modify the quality of environmental conditions for the benefit of health. Cultural systems impact the perception and regulation of environmental conditions to ensure the capability for effective response and recovery from environmental hazards. Cultural systems are an effective mechanism of protection from threat in the social and physical environment.

Population Health Disparities

Environmental conditions affect the quality of life and mental health across nations and individuals. The presence of environmental and ecological threats contributes to changes in the access to health care and services that benefit health. The geographic and cultural variations in societal exposure to risk and protective factors of environmental conditions contribute to population disparities in mental health. The development of preventions and interventions that reduce the societal exposure to risk factors and improve the quality of environmental health conditions ensures health equity across cultural contexts. Culture processes serve as a prevention and intervention that strengthen protection of capabilities and capacities for sociocultural and behavioral adaptation.

Global Mental Health

Environmental conditions demonstrate the direct and indirect effects on mortality and comorbidity of mental disorders. Environmental factors related to changes in environmental conditions, including climate change and natural disasters, may lead to population-level changes in cultural contact. Global concerns of changes in environmental conditions affect exposure to significant health and protective risk factors posed by exposure to environmental hazards. Environmental hazards affecting the perception of resilience and vulnerabilities of individuals may result in the necessity for an effective response and recovery from the adverse consequences of extreme environmental conditions.

Cultural systems serve as an important and necessary protection against threats in the social and physical environment. Culture acts as an effective protection to a range of threats, providing preparation for response, recovery, and demonstration of resilience in the social and physical environment. Culture modifies the societal exposure to risk and protective factors through strengthening of capabilities and capacities for sociocultural and behavioral adaptation. Culture ensures the ability to coordinate collective and individual action for health equity. Culture protects the plurality of social communities for social and financial investments that benefit all. Culture is an essential component of human security and human development, enhancing the quality of life and potential for human fulfillment.

Conclusion

The public health impact of environmental hazards is considerable and contributes to the global burden of disease. Environmental systems are composed of distal factors that are part of a complex causal pathway of cultural systems. The degradation of environmental conditions and its devastating consequences on social and economic conditions affect causal pathways in global mental health. Cultural systems provide effective preventions and interventions for the building of resilience and the reduction of vulnerabilities to environmental conditions in global mental health.

Building capacity in research on cultural neuroscience that investigates the complex causal influences of culture and the environment contributes to the development and implementation of effective protections in global mental health across cultural contexts. The translation of global environmental health research to understanding the design and preparation of health protection and promotion is necessary for priority setting and advocacy in global mental health. Understanding how the generation and maintenance of cultural systems improve environmental quality is necessary for the design and implementation of protections in global mental health that ensure the achievement of health equity for all.

References

Boyd, R., & Richerson, P. J. (2005). *The origin and evolution of cultures*. Oxford University Press.
Chen, C., Moyzis, R. K., Lei, X., Chen, C., & Dong, Q. (2016). The encultured genome: Molecular evidence for recent divergent evolution in human neurotransmitter genes. In J. Y. Chiao, S. C. Li, R. Seligman, & R. Turner (Eds.), *The Oxford handbook of cultural neuroscience* (pp. 315–338). Oxford University Press.

Cheon, B. K., Im, D. M., Harada, T., Kim, J. S., Mathur, V. A., Scimeca, J. M., Parrish, T. B., Park, H., & Chiao, J. Y. (2013). Cultural modulation of the neural correlates of emotional pain perception: The role of other-focusedness. *Neuropsychologia, 51*(7), 1177–1186.

Chiao, J. Y., & Blizinsky, K. D. (2010). Culture-gene coevolution of individualism-collectivism and the serotonin transporter gene. *Proceedings of the Royal Society B: Biological Sciences, 277*(1681), 529–537.

Eberhardt, J. L. (2005). Imaging race. *American Psychologist, 60*(2), 181–190.

Fincher, C. L., Thornhill, R., Murray, D. R., & Schaller, M. (2008). Pathogen prevalence predicts human cross-cultural variability in individualism/collectivism. *Proceedings of the Royal Society B, 275*, 1279–1285.

Gelfand, M. J., Raver, J. L., Nishii, L., Leslie, L. M., Lun, J., Lim B. C., Duan, L., Almaliach, A., Ang, S., Arnadottir, J., Aycan, Z., Boeknke, K., Boski, P., Cabecinhas, R., Chan, D., Chhokar, J., D'Amato, A., Ferrer, M., Fischlmayr, I. C., . . . Yamaguchi, S. (2011). Differences between tight and loose cultures: A 33-nation study. *Science, 332*(6033), 1100–1104.

Goh, J. O., Chee, M. W., Tan, J. C., Venkatraman, V., Hebrank, A., Leshikar, E. D., Jenkins, L., Sutton, B. P., Gutchess, A. H., & Park, D. C. (2007). Age and culture modulate object processing and object-scene binding in the ventral visual area. *Cognitive Affective Behavioral Neuroscience, 7*(1), 44–52.

Goh, J. O., Leshikar, E. D., Sutton, B. P., Tan, J. C., Sim, S. K., Hebrank, A. C., & Park, D. C. (2010). Culture differences in neural processing of faces and houses in the ventral visual cortex. *Social Cognitive and Affective Neuroscience, 5*(2–3), 227–235.

Golby, A. J., Gabrieli, J. D, Chiao, J. Y., & Eberhardt, J. L. (2001). Differential responses in the fusiform region to same-race and other-race faces. *Nature Neuroscience, 4*(8), 845–850.

Gutchess, A. H., Welsh, R. C., Boduroglu, A., & Park, D. C. (2006). Cultural differences in neural function associated with object processing. *Cognitive Affective Behavioral Neuroscience, 6*(2), 102–109.

Iacoboni, M. (2005). Neural mechanisms of imitation. *Current Opinion of Neurobiology, 15*(6), 632–637.

Ishii, K., Kim, H. S., Sasaki, J. Y., Shinada, M., & Kusumi, I. (2014). Culture modulates sensitivity to the disappearance of facial expression associated with serotonin transporter polymorphism (5-HTTLPR). *Culture and Brain, 2*, 72–88.

Jenkins, L. J., Yang, Y. J., Goh, J., Hong, Y. Y., & Park, D. C. (2010). Cultural differences in the lateral occipital complex while viewing incongruent scenes. *Social Cognitive Affective Neuroscience, 5*(2–3), 236–241.

Kim, H. S., Sherman, D. K., Sasaki, J. Y., Xu, J., Chu, T. Q., Ryu, C., Suh, E. M., Graham, K., & Taylor, S. E. (2010). Culture, distress and oxytocin receptor polymorphism (OXTR) interact to influence emotional support seeking. *Proceedings of the National Academy of Sciences, 107*(36), 15717–15721.

Kim, H. S, Sherman, D. K., Taylor, S. E., Sasaki, J. Y., Chu, T. Q., Ryu, C., Suh, E. M., & Xu, J. (2010). Culture, serotonin receptor polymorphism and locus of attention. *Social Cognitive and Affective Neuroscience, 5*(2–3), 212–218.

Laland, K. N., Odling-Smee, J., & Feldman, M. W. (2000). Niche construction, biological evolution, and cultural change. *Behavioral and Brain Sciences, 23*, 131–175.

Lieberman, M. D., Hariri, A., Jarcho, J. M., Eisenberger, N. I., & Bookheimer, S. Y. (2005). An fMRI investigation of race-related amygdala activity in African-American and Caucasian-American individuals. *Nature Neuroscience, 8*(6), 720–722.

Losin, E. A., Cross, K. A., Iacoboni, M., & Dapretto, M. (2014). Neural processing of race during imitation: Self-similarity versus social status. *Human Brain Mapping, 35*(4), 1723–1739.

Losin, E. A., Iacoboni, M., Martin, A., & Dapretto, M. (2012). Own-gender imitation activates the brain's reward circuitry. *Social Cognitive and Affective Neuroscience, 7*(7), 804–810.

Minas, H. (2014). Human security, complexity, and mental health system development. In V. Patel, H. Minas, A. Cohen, & M. J. Prince (Eds.), *Global mental health: Principles and practice* (pp. 137–166). Oxford University Press.

Miyamoto, Y., Nisbett, R. E., & Masuda, T. (2006). Culture and the physical environment: Holistic versus analytic perceptual affordances. *Psychological Science, 17*(2), 113–119.

Mrazek, A. J., Chiao, J. Y., Blizinsky, K. D., Lun, J., & Gelfand, M. J. (2013). The role of culture-gene coevolution in morality judgment: Examining the interplay between tightness-looseness and allelic variation of the serotonin transporter gene. *Culture and Brain, 1*, 100–117.

Nisbett, R. E., Peng, K., Choi, I., & Norenzayan, A. (2001). Culture and systems of thought: holistic versus analytic cognition. *Psychological Review, 108*(2), 291–310.

Oyserman, D., Coon, H. M., Kemmelmeier, M. (2002). Rethinking individualism and collectivism: evaluation of theoretical assumptions and meta-analyses. *Psychological Bulletin, 128*(1), 3–72.

Park, D. C., & Gutchess, A. H. (2002). Aging, cognition, and culture: A neuroscientific perspective. *Neuroscience and Biobehavioral Review, 26*(7), 859–867.

Richeson, J. A., Baird, A. A., Gordon, H. L., Heatherton, T. F., Wyland, C. L., Trawalter, S., & Shelton, J. N. (2003). An fMRI investigation of the impact of interracial contact on executive function. *Nature Neuroscience, 6*(12), 1323–1328.

Sasaki, J. Y., Le Clair, J., West, A. L., & Kim, H. S. (2016). The gene-culture interaction framework and implications for health. In J. Y. Chiao, S. C., Li, R. Seligman, & R. Turner (Eds.), *The Oxford handbook of cultural neuroscience* (pp. 279–297). Oxford University Press.

Sherman, D. K., Kim, H. S., & Taylor, S. E. (2009). Culture and social support: Neural bases and biological impact. In J. Y. Chiao (Ed.), *Cultural neuroscience: Cultural influences on brain function* (pp. 227–237). Elsevier.

Swim, J. K., Stern, P. C., Doherty, T. J., Clayton, S., Reser, J. P., Weber, E. U., Gifford, R., & Howard, G. S. (2011). Psychology's contributions to understanding and addressing global climate change. *American Psychologist, 66*(4), 241–250.

Weber, E. U., & Stern, P. C. (2011). Public understanding of climate change in the United States. *American Psychologist, 66*(4), 315–328.

Globalization: Human Development in a New Cultural Context

Lene Arnett Jensen

Abstract

Globalization—the flow across cultures of goods, people, and ideas at unprecedented speed, scope, and quantity—has profound implications for psychological development. In today's world, children seldom reach adulthood knowing of only one culture. Increasingly, they have interactions with people from diverse cultures, either firsthand or indirectly through various media. Exposure and openness to globalization are particularly pronounced among adolescents and emerging adults, and globalization impacts their development in a wide variety of areas, including moral values, relationships with parents, gender roles, health and body image, language development, and identity. Future research needs to pay more attention to younger children, local circumstances, and diverse responses to globalization.

Key Words: adolescence, culture, emerging adults, family relations, globalization, gender, health, human development, identity, moral values

Introduction

Globalization—the flow across cultures of goods, people, and ideas at unprecedented speed, scope, and quantity—has profound implications for psychological development. In today's world, children, adolescents, and emerging adults seldom, if ever, reach adulthood knowing of only one culture (Jensen, 2016). Rather, they increasingly have interactions with people from diverse cultures, either firsthand or indirectly through various media. Until fairly recently, this was not the case. It was common to have minimal exposure to other cultures.

Globalization impacts development in a variety of areas, including moral values, relationships with parents, gender roles, health and body image, language development, and identity. In this chapter, each of these areas of development will be addressed. The chapter will also point to future research directions. First, however, a description will be provided of the increasing scope and complexity of globalization, as well as an explanation for the present focus on adolescents and emerging adults.

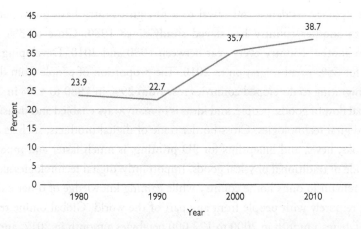

Figure 23.1. Percent of global gross domestic product (GDP) from international trade. Source: Based on data from McKinsey Global Institute (2014).

Globalization: A New Cultural Context

The flow of goods, people, and ideas across cultures is not new, but the global scope and complexity of this flow is unprecedented. In the 1990s, the entry into the global economy of Asia and Eastern European countries and the growth of transnational TV networks were important catalysts of globalization (Chalaby, 2016; McKinsey Global Institute, 2014). Since then, globalization has been accelerating.

A variety of indicators show this acceleration. One is the rapid growth in international trade. In every decade since 1990, as Figure 23.1 shows, there has been a substantial increase in the percent of the worldwide gross domestic product (GDP) that derives from the flow of goods, services, and finance across national borders. For example, the combined value of this flow went from 23% of GDP (US$5 trillion) in 1990 to 36% of GDP (US$26 trillion) in 2012.

The complexity of international trade has also changed. In 1990, 54% of all crossnational trade of goods was between economically developed countries. That number fell to 28% in 2012. Increasingly, economically developing countries are involved in international trade (McKinsey Global Institute, 2014). Developing countries trade with developed countries as well as with other developing countries. Trade between developing countries (known as South–South trade) grew from a mere 6% in 1990 to 24% in 2012.

Apart from the increase in international trade, there has also been a rapid growth since about 2000 in the flow of people across borders on a short-term basis (McKinsey Global Institute, 2014). Students enrolling in a foreign university grew by almost 5% every year between 2002 and 2010. During this same time period, short-term travel also increased by about 3.5% every year. In 2010, developing countries and developed countries accounted for 42% and 58%, respectively, of such short-term travel.

While temporary residence and travel to a foreign country have grown since 2000, migration to another country has stayed steady since 1980. Close to 3% of people migrated to another country every year between 1980 and 2010. Developing countries accounted for 65% of all migration in 2010. The proportion of people from developing countries migrating to developed countries rose from 29% in 1980 to 42% in 2010.

The global flow of goods, people, and ideas is in many ways enabled and transformed by the rise in digital technologies. Cross-border trade of digital products, such as entertainment, e-books, news, and blueprints for 3D printing, is much faster and much cheaper than the trade of traditional physical goods. Importantly, digital technologies also make it possible to remain in one's home country while gaining knowledge of other cultures and interacting remotely with people from any part of the world. Global online traffic grew from 84 petabytes a month in 2000 to 122,000 petabytes a month in 2017, and it is projected to rise to about 280,000 petabytes by 2021 (Statista, 2019).

While use of digital technologies is growing at amazing rates, a digital divide remains between developing countries and developed countries. Access to digital technologies is considerably lower in developing countries. Within developing countries, rural areas also lag notably behind urban areas in access to digital technologies (Onitsuka et al., 2018).

In sum, globalization is accelerating. It now reaches essentially every developed and developing country in the world. At the same time, however, it is important to recognize that experiences with globalization vary by location and entail differences in power between countries and groups. For example, the movement of migrants is more often from developing to developed countries than the other way around. Ideas and values pertaining to consumerism, however, flow largely from developed to developing countries. Also, globalization is more evident in urban than in rural areas, especially in developing countries.

A Focus on Adolescence and Emerging Adulthood

Psychological research on globalization mostly got underway in the late 1990s and early 2000s (e.g., Hermans & Kempen, 1998). It remains relatively sparse, especially in light of the ubiquitous nature of globalization. In developmental psychology, the primary focus of globalization research has been on adolescents (approximately the ages of 10 to 18) and emerging adults (approximately the ages of 19 to 29).

The psychological impact of globalization may be particularly salient in adolescence and emerging adulthood. Media such as television, movies, music, and the internet contribute to the rapid and extensive spread of ideas across cultures, and adolescents and emerging adults have more of an interest in popular and media culture compared to children or adults (Dasen, 2000; Onitsuka et al., 2018; Schlegel, 2001). For example, market researchers aim to sell to "global teens" because urban adolescents worldwide follow similar consumption patterns and have similar preferences for global brands of music, videos, clothing, and so on (Friedman, 2000).

Furthermore, adolescence and emerging adulthood constitute a time of life with a pronounced openness to diverse cultural beliefs and behaviors. Research has noted that, in many ways, adolescents and emerging adults have not yet settled on particular beliefs and behaviors (Arnett, 2015; Côté, 2006). Research with immigrants to the United States has also shown that adolescents change their behaviors, beliefs, values, and identifications more than adults do (Nguyen & Williams, 1989; Phinney et al., 2000). This phenomenon, also known as dissonant acculturation (Portes, 1997), may apply not only to immigrants but also more generally to adolescents and emerging adults who are exposed to globalization.

On the negative side, research with immigrants suggests that risks for psychological and social problems increase as a person moves from childhood into adolescence (Berry, 1997; Unger, 2011). With globalization, as with immigration, adolescence and emerging adulthood may be vulnerable developmental periods.

Finally, by 2008—for the first time in human history—more people were living in urban areas than in rural ones, and this migration has been led mainly by emerging adults (Hugo, 2005; Population Reference Bureau, 2008). In urban areas, youth encounter the diversity of ideas, products, and peoples promoted by the global economy. The projection is that, by 2050, close to 70% of the world's population will live in cities (United Nations, 2018).

Moral Values

Globalization promotes values pertaining to individual autonomy. For example, field experiments in Ethiopia have examined how the introduction of laptops and Western media influences adolescents' values (Hansen & Postmes, 2013; Hansen et al., 2012). In 2008, the Ethiopian government in collaboration with aid agencies decided to introduce laptops to 6,000 adolescents in schools in different parts of the country. Ethiopia is among the least economically developed countries in the world. In 2008, when the laptop program was started, 0.7% of the population owned a PC and 0.4% had access to the internet. (The comparable figures for the United States at that time were 81% and 74%; World Bank, 2009.) With respect to values, Ethiopian culture emphasizes collectivism and respect for elders. Adolescents, then, typically do not own much—let alone anything as valuable as a laptop. They also are not accustomed to making independent decisions.

Why might the introduction of a laptop into an Ethiopian adolescent's life matter? First, according to Hansen and colleagues, the use of a laptop introduces new information. Second, the use of a laptop requires new knowledge and action that would be foreign to parents and other elders. Third, possessing something as valuable as a laptop represents a radical change from the economic status quo and also a potential upheaval of the social hierarchy. Such a possession clearly distinguishes an adolescent from others.

In one study by Hansen and colleagues (2012), 169 adolescents in grades 7 and 8 were divided into three groups. In one group adolescents had fully functioning laptops; in another group the laptops had stopped functioning (as a result, for example, of broken parts); and the remaining group had no laptops. After 1 year, the three groups remained similar on interdependence and collectivism. However, the group with the functioning laptops scored significantly higher on independence as well as on individualistic values emphasizing autonomous decision making, achievement, and leadership. The findings indicate that it is not the mere ownership of a laptop that matters, but rather that the use of a laptop changes moral values.

A study of moral reasoning similarly found that globalization is related to autonomy-oriented values and thinking. The study also showed that this is more so for adolescents than adults. Interviews about moral issues were conducted with dyads of adolescents (aged 13 to 18) and parents (aged 35 to 65) who resided in rural and urban communities in Thailand (McKenzie, 2018). Although the two communities were located within 25 miles of one another, they constituted different cultural contexts. In the rural community, inhabitants had minimal exposure to globalization. For example, there were no tourists or restaurants selling foreign foods. Many rural homes did not have internet access, and some homes did not have cell phone reception. The urban community, in contrast, was undergoing rapid globalization. For example, advertisement billboards, typically in both English and Thai, featured such offerings as Western wedding attire, skin-whitening creams, and McDonald's. The urban households also had ready access to media, including televisions and laptops. Urban Thai adolescents and parents reported devoting many hours of their day to the use of a laptop or computer.

The moral reasoning of the rural and urban adolescents and parents were analyzed in terms of the Ethics of Autonomy, Community, and Divinity (Jensen, 2018). Briefly, the Ethic of Autonomy involves a focus on persons as individuals. Moral reasons within this ethic include the interests, well-being, and rights of individuals (self or other). The Ethic of Community focuses on persons as members of social groups, with attendant reasons such as duty to others, and concern with the customs and welfare of groups. The Ethic of Divinity focuses on persons as spiritual or religious entities, and attendant reasons encompass sacred lessons and laws as well as spiritual purity.

Findings showed that rural adolescents and adults were similar in their use of the three ethics, and they especially reasoned in terms of community consideration (McKenzie, 2018). Compared to the rural dyads, the urban ones reasoned less in terms of the Ethic of Community and more in terms of the Ethic of Autonomy. Globalization appears to have forged a gap between the urban and rural Thai communities in moral reasoning. There was also a gap within the urban dyads. Whereas urban parents used autonomy and community reasoning roughly equally, urban adolescents' moral reasoning was dominated by the Ethic of Autonomy. Thus, although urban adolescents and their parents both lived in a globalizing cultural community, their level of exposure to and developmental openness to experiences of globalization differed, as reflected in their moral reasoning.

A study of emerging adults also documented a change in values due to exposure to globalization. This study followed rural emerging adults in Chiapas, Mexico, who moved to an urban environment to attend university (Manago, 2012). With exposure to globalization through education and urbanization, the students gradually added new values to the traditional ones of respect for elders and obligation to family. Those new values centered on independence, individual exploration, self-fulfillment, and gender equality.

In sum, globalization does not erase the moral values of traditional cultures, although for some people their adherence to some traditional values may attenuate. Certainly, however, globalization introduces a new and notable emphasis on individual autonomy, especially among adolescents and emerging adults.

Relationships With Parents

With globalization, adolescents and emerging adults sometimes come to differ from their parents on views of children's autonomy and parental authority. In traditional cultures where adolescents spend the majority of their time with parents and are integrated into adult groups, adolescents and parents typically share common views of obedience, responsibility, self-reliance, and so forth. With globalization, however, differences of opinion emerge.

Research comparing immigrant adolescents and parents in the United States has shown that adolescents wish to make autonomous decisions about such matters as friends, dating, and leisure activities at an earlier age than what their parents regard as appropriate (Juang et al., 1999). Similarly, studies with immigrant groups in Canada have shown that parents sanction parental authority more than their adolescents, whereas adolescents desire more autonomy than their parents are willing to grant (Kwak & Berry, 2001).

It is not only in immigrant families that experiences with globalization forge a gap between adolescents and parents. As described earlier, Thai adolescents residing in a rapidly globalizing urban city placed more value on autonomy than their parents (McKenzie, 2018). Ethnographic research in Kathmandu, the capital of Nepal, has found that Nepalese adults use the terms "teen" and "teenager" in English, even when speaking Nepali, to refer to young people who are oriented toward Western tastes, especially Western media (Liechty, 1995, 2010). Not all Nepalese young people are "teenagers," even if they are in their teen years—the term is not an age category, but a social category that refers to young people who are pursuing a Western identity and style. Some adults use teenager with less favorable connotations to refer to young people who are disobedient, antisocial, and potentially violent. Their use of the term in this way reflects their view that Western media can have corrupting effects on many of their young people. In Japan, researchers have noted that emerging adults in their 20s who continue to rely on parental support while engaging in various forms of self-exploration and postponing marriage are termed "parasite singles" by their parents and older generations—a term that is hardly flattering (Naito & Gielen, 2002).

Taken together, these findings suggest that a division opens up between parents and their adolescents and emerging adults as they cease to share one traditional culture and instead are exposed to globalization. This division pertains to views and behaviors that revolve around autonomy and authority.

The extent to which this difference between parents and their children has negative repercussions on their relationship seems to be an open question. Some scholars have proposed that parents resent the division that globalization creates between themselves and their children (Friedman, 2000). However, with regard to the aforementioned study on Japanese "parasite singles," the researchers reported that, while parents clearly had some misgivings about their emerging adult children, some parents simultaneously expressed admiration for their children's self-assertiveness. Moreover, research has found that only 10% to 20% of Japanese adolescents report that their parents understand them, but at the same time 80% to 90% describe their family life as "fun" or "pleasant" and say that they communicate with their parents on a "fairly regular" basis (Stevenson & Zusho, 2002).

Among immigrant families, there has been a lot of research on the extent of conflict between adolescents and their parents, but findings are inconsistent (Jensen & Dost-Gozkan, 2015). Some studies report more conflict among immigrants than nonimmigrants; some find no differences; and some report less conflict among immigrants. Furthermore, very little of this research has attempted to demonstrate that division between adolescents and parents in views of authority and autonomy is predictive of higher levels of conflict.

In sum, extant research indicates that, with globalization, divisions can arise between parents and their adolescents and emerging adults in views of parents' authority and children's autonomy. The consequences of such divisions, however, require further research. Some findings suggest that resentment and conflict between parents and youth ensue. But findings also intimate that sometimes both parents and youth recognize the necessity or even desirability of their differences of opinion in a globalizing world. Finally, even as parents and their children come to differ in some areas due to globalization, they may continue to share views on interdependence, respect, and familial harmony (Jensen & Dost-Gozkan, 2015).

Gender Roles

Globalization contributes to changes in gender roles, including toward greater gender equality. Traditionally in many cultures around the world, girls and women have been subordinate to boys and men, and they have faced discrimination and inequality in many areas of life. Although inequality is still prevalent, today there is a global trend toward greater gender equality.

Evidence for the impact of globalization on gender roles comes from a variety of sources. Anthropologists and cultural psychologists have documented how global media promotes new views of gender in traditional cultures (Condon, 1988, 1995; Manago, 2012). One vivid and detailed illustration comes from ethnographic work in Morocco conducted over several decades (Davis & Davis, 1989, 1995, 2007, 2012). In the past, Moroccan culture, like many traditional cultures, had strictly defined gender roles (Arnett & Jensen, 2019). Marriages were arranged by parents primarily on the basis of economic considerations. Female—but not male—virginity at marriage was considered essential, and adolescent girls were forbidden to spend time in the company of adolescent boys. These gender differences continue to be part of Moroccan culture today, particularly in rural areas (Davis & Davis, 2007, 2012).

For both adolescent girls and boys, however, exposure to media is changing the way they view gender roles. The TV programs, songs, and movies they are exposed to are produced not only in Morocco and other Islamic countries but also in France (Morocco was once a French colony) and the United States. From these various sources, Moroccan adolescents are seeing portrayals of gender roles quite different from what they see among their parents, grandparents, and other adults around them. In the media that the adolescents use, romance and passion are central to female–male relationships. Love is the central basis for entering marriage, and the idea of accepting a marriage arranged by parents is either ignored or portrayed as something to be resisted. Young women are usually portrayed not in traditional roles but in professional occupations and as being in control of their lives and unashamed of their sexuality.

Young people in Morocco—and other places—are using these conceptions of gender to construct gender roles quite different from the traditional conceptions in their culture. Media are "used by adolescents in a period of rapid social change to reimagine many aspects of their lives, including a desire for more autonomy, for more variety in heterosexual interactions, and for more choice of a job" (Davis & Davis, 1995, p. 578).

Perhaps the trend toward greater gender equality is most evident in the area of education. Until recent decades, countries all over the world had customs and policies that favored boys' education over girls', for example, by discouraging or forbidding girls from obtaining education beyond primary school and by barring young women from entry to most colleges and universities.

In the majority of countries in the world today, however, girls and young women are equal to boys and young men in educational enrollment. The United Nations (UN) calculates the Gender Parity Index (GPI) to assess the extent to which educational attainment is equal for boys and girls. The GPI is calculated as a ratio of the value for females to that of males. A GPI value of 1.00 indicates parity between the sexes. Values below 1.00 indicate disparity in favor of boys, whereas values above 1.00 indicate disparity in favor of girls.

Table 23.1 shows the GPI for school enrollment rates in 1990 and 2016 for primary and secondary school in different regions of the world (World Bank, 2018). In 1990, there was a gender disparity in favor of boys for both primary and secondary education across large parts of the world. However, this gap between girls and boys has been closing.

Table 23.1. Gender Parity Index (GPI) for Primary and Secondary Education in 1990 and 2016

Geographic Region	Primary 1990	Primary 2016	Secondary 1990	Secondary 2016
World	0.88	1.01	0.85	0.99
Arab states	0.82	0.94	0.79	0.93
Central Europe and Baltics	0.99	1.00	0.99	0.99
East Asia and Pacific	0.93	0.99	0.90	1.00
European Union	1.00	1.00	1.00	1.00
Latin America and Caribbean	0.99	0.98	1.02	1.02
North America	0.99	1.00	1.00	1.01
South Asia	0.73	1.10	0.68	1.05
Sub-Saharan Africa	0.83	0.95	0.81	0.92

Source: Based on data from the World Bank (2018).

By 2016, girls had essentially reached parity with boys in all parts of the world, except the Arab states and Sub-Saharan Africa.

For enrollment in tertiary education, the picture is more complex. The numbers in Table 23.2, which shows the GPI for tertiary education in 1990 and 2017, indicate that there are two main regions of the world where females lag behind males in enrollment: South Asia and Sub-Saharan Africa (World Bank, 2018). For all other regions and on a worldwide scale, females now surpass males among students who reach the tertiary level of education.

There are two ways in which greater gender equality in education may be in part a consequence of globalization. First, in the global economy education is increasingly rewarded. The global economy is based mainly on information, technology, and services, and as this

Table 23.2. Gender Parity Index (GPI) for Tertiary Education in 1990 and 2017

Geographic Region	Tertiary 1990	Tertiary 2017
World	0.90	1.12
Arab states	0.60	1.09
Central Europe and Baltics	1.20	1.41
East Asia and Pacific	0.65	1.16
European Union	0.97	1.23
Latin America and Caribbean	0.95	1.32
North America	1.27	1.35
South Asia	0.48	0.96
Sub-Saharan Africa	0.45	0.73

Source: Based on data from the World Bank (2018).

economy spreads around the world it promotes social and cultural change. Families that may previously have viewed it as in their economic interest to keep girls at home working in the fields instead of sending them to school may now find it more advantageous to educate them so that they can take advantage of opportunities to participate in the global economy.

The second way in which globalization promotes gender equality in education (and other areas) is through international pressure on countries with customs and policies promoting discrimination. As described earlier, the United Nations publishes the GPI. The United Nations also calculates a yearly Gender Inequality Index (GII) for about 160 countries that combines statistics on educational attainment, women's economic and political participation, and female-specific health issues (such as maternal mortality). Indices such as the GPI and the GII are used by the United Nations and other organizations to lobby countries to improve their policies relating to girls and women. The explicit purpose of these kinds of indices is to make countries aware of international pressure to relieve gender discrimination and to promote greater equality.

In sum, girls and women continue to be subordinate to boys and men on a variety of measures across a wide swath of the globe. Globalization, however, appears to promote more egalitarian gender roles. Media and international aid organizations, for example, indirectly and directly promote equal educational aspirations and attainment for girls and boys.

Health and Body Image

As globalization makes foods available far from their original locales, changes to health and body image follow. While cuisines from every corner of the globe increasingly permeate the American and European food markets, the flow of foods also moves in the other direction. A rapid increase in the availability of Western—mainly American—fast foods and drinks is occurring in the developing world.

The global changes to diet have health effects. One such effect is the worldwide obesity epidemic, which the World Health Organization (2018) attributes primarily to economic growth and the globalization of food markets. Between 1975 and 2016, the proportion of 5- to 19-year-olds who were overweight rose from 4% to 18%, and the proportion who were obese rose from less than 1% to 7%. This dramatic rise has occurred similarly among boys and girls.

Rising obesity rates are pronounced among children and adolescents, who may be most likely to be attracted to unhealthy Western food. For example, research with early adolescents in Jamaica has shown that those who consume the most American media are also the most likely to be overweight and obese (Ferguson & Bornstein, 2015; Ferguson et al., 2018). The researchers argue that globalization prompts "remote acculturation." In other words, youth acquire behaviors based on indirect and intermittent exposure to foreign cultures. In this case, Jamaican adolescents acquire a taste for American fast foods based on exposure to American media featuring those foods, for example, in advertisements and product placements in films.

The promotion of unhealthy foods and drinks also occurs through other processes of globalization than media exposure and remote acculturation. Recent findings have documented that large fast food and beverage companies seek to influence research and public policy in developing countries to protect and increase their market share. For example, they seek to diminish attention to the role of unhealthy foods and drinks in obesity and instead advocate for research and policies focused on other factors such as exercise.

In China, for example, national efforts to address its rising rates of overweight and obesity largely center on exercise, without mentioning the prominent contribution of nutrition. One example is the Happy 10 Minutes program that encourages schoolchildren to exercise for 10 minutes a day (Greenhalgh, 2019a, 2019b). How did this focus on exercise come about? The program and others like it are supported by the International Life Sciences Institute in China (ILSI-China). ILSI-China is a branch of ILSI, a worldwide nonprofit organization founded by Coca-Cola and headquartered in Washington, DC. ILSI is funded by many of the largest food and drink corporations such as Coca-Cola, Nestlé, McDonald's, and PepsiCo. Created to promote ILSI's interests, ILSI-China emerged as the country's leading sponsor of research activities and policies on obesity beginning in the late 1990s. In fact, ILSI-China became so central to the nation's activities on obesity that it is housed inside the government's Center for Disease Control and Prevention in Beijing.

Recent quantitative and qualitative analyses of ILSI-China's newsletters and interviews with Chinese obesity specialists show that Chinese obesity science and policy shifted toward a predominant focus on exercise between 1999 and 2015 (Greenhalgh, 2019a, 2019b). Obesity activities sponsored by ILSI-China that focused exclusively on exercise rose significantly from 0% in 1999–2003 to 37% in 2004–2009 to 60% in 2010–2015. Over the course of this same time period, activities focused on nutrition fell from 42% in 1999–2003 to 23% in 2010–2015. Activities addressing both exercise and nutrition were consistently uncommon. This shift that has taken place in China's obesity research and policies aligns with Coca-Cola's message that exercise, not diet, is important to combat obesity. The author of the analyses concludes that "In putting its massive resources behind only one side of the science, and with no parties sufficiently resourced to champion more balanced solutions that included regulation of the food industry, the [Coca-Cola] company, working through ILSI, re-directed China's chronic disease science, potentially compromising the public's health" (Greenhalgh, 2019a, p. 1).

With sweetened beverage consumption on the decline in Europe and the United States, Coca-Cola as well as other large food and beverage corporations regard developing countries as key to maintaining and increasing their profits. ILSI not only has a branch in China but also has 16 other branches, most of them in developing countries such as India, Brazil, and Mexico (Jacobs, 2019).

With globalization comes not only a risk of becoming overweight but also an ideal of slimness. Studies have concluded that adolescent girls in developing countries have been influenced by Western media to develop a negative body image. Assessing themselves by the Western standard represented by models in advertisements and by actors on TV and in films, they conclude that their local norms of physical attractiveness are obsolete and seek to emulate the Western image they admire. For example, an interview study with adolescent girls in the Caribbean islands of Trinidad and Barbados found that 68% were concerned with their eating habits and extremely fearful of becoming fat (Bhugra et al., 2003). Based on their analyses, the authors concluded that the girls' anxieties about food and their weight were motivated by their aspiration to emulate Western ideals of slimness.

Related, research on the island nation of Fiji has documented the influence of global media on girls' body image. Traditionally the Fiji ideal body type for women was rounded and curvy. However, television was first introduced in 1995, mostly with programming from the United States and other Western countries, and subsequently the incidence of eating disorders rose substantially (Becker et al., 2007). Interviews with adolescent girls on Fiji showed that they admired the Western television characters and wanted to look like them, and that this goal in turn led to higher incidence of negative body image, preoccupation with weight, and purging behavior to control weight (Becker, 2004).

Eating disorders occur primarily in cultures that emphasize physical slimness. Until recently, this was mostly an ideal in Western countries, especially for White middle- to upper-middle-class females. By now, however, eating disorders occur worldwide (Pike & Dunne, 2015). A recent review of research, for example, documented the rise of eating disorders across Asian countries, including China, India, Japan, Malaysia, Pakistan, South Korea, Taiwan, and Thailand. The authors' analysis indicates that "Westernization" is a cause, and also that Western influence interacts in varied ways with urbanization and industrialization depending on the country. Their conclusion highlights the need for research to parse globalization processes between different cultures, a point discussed in the future directions section later.

In sum, globalization is contributing to changes in people's health across the world. Obesity is rising so rapidly that the World Health Organization has labeled it an "epidemic" (World Health Organization, 2019). Simultaneously, a slim physical ideal has become globally popular, and consequently eating disorders now afflict female youth across the world.

Language Development

In a globalizing world where the United States is the most influential economic power, English is increasingly an international language. As more and more people come into contact with each other, the need to communicate in a common language grows. The widespread presence and growth of English goes hand in hand with the diffusion of popular culture and technology and the expansion of international trade. Two children from

Japan and France teaming up in an online game are likely to communicate in English. At the Intel International Science and Engineering Fair (INSEF), the world's largest international science fair for high school students, with participation from more than 70 countries, all presentations are in English (Student Science, 2019). When emerging adults migrate to a different country in search of better job opportunities, they often use English to bridge the divide between their native language and the language of their country of destination.

Currently, English is the first language of about 400 million people and is spoken fluently by 500 million to 1 billion people worldwide (English Language, 2019). By the year 2050, the projection is that at least half of the world's population will be proficient English speakers. In part, this projection is based on the fact that children learn English in school in more and more countries. School systems increasingly seek to teach children English to enhance their ability to participate in the global economy. In China, for example, all children now begin learning English in primary school (Chang, 2008). In the European Union, more than 90% of students learn English in school (Rubenstein, 2017). In addition, students worldwide are increasingly seeking admission to universities in countries that teach in English.

Research has also shown that globalization is leading adolescents from around the world to incorporate English into their slang. One study of a group of Japanese adolescent girls found that they often created a Japanese–English hybrid language, for example, saying "*ikemen getto suru*" (I wanna get a cool dude; Miller, 2004). A study of Bulgarian 10th-grade adolescents also found frequent familiarity with and use of American English slang (Charkova, 2007). Common slang terms involved swear words, terms for sexual activities and body parts, derogatory terms for men and women, and positive terms for men and women. The adolescents reported that they primarily learned the terms and expressions from movies, television, and song lyrics. They also reported gaining prestige among their peers from knowing English slang. As one Bulgarian 10th-grade boy explained: "I want to learn English slang because when I tell my friends a new word or a phrase that they do not know, they look at me with respect and consider me an expert on a topic related to music, songs, movies, and so on" (Charkova, 2007, p. 401). Like the Japanese adolescent girls, the Bulgarian adolescents also often created a hybrid language interweaving Bulgarian and English (as in "*Toi e istinski asshole*").

Language is a vehicle of communication, but it also influences beliefs and ways of thinking. For example, it seems plausible that the export of English slang is about more than new words, but also about new thoughts regarding gender, body image, and sexuality, for example.

Research indicates that language even affects something as basic as spatial cognition. Spatial cognition may be differentiated between two broad types. An egocentric frame of reference is where the location of an object is determined in relation to the location of the self (e.g., "The cat is to the left of the house" from the perspective of the self). An allocentric frame of reference is where the object is located either in relation to another object (e.g., "The cat is by the front door of the house") or based on cardinal direction type systems (e.g., "The cat is on the west side of the house"). Some languages such as the Namibian language of ≠Akhoe Hai‖om primarily use an allocentric frame of reference, whereas other languages such as English and Dutch provide an egocentric frame of reference. Research has found that children between the ages of 3 and 5 commonly utilize allocentric spatial cognition. Older children and adults, however, vary according to their language. For example, 8-year-olds and adults who speak ≠Akhoe Hai‖om use allocentric reasoning, whereas Dutch 8-year-olds and adults use egocentric spatial reasoning (Haun et al., 2006).

In sum, more and more children, adolescents, and emerging adults across the world speak, read, and write English. They learn English in school and at work, through media, and in interactions with peers. As children, adolescents, and emerging adults learn English, they are also increasingly learning to see the world, others, and themselves in ways that are embedded in the English language.

Identity

Since the middle of the 20th century, when Erik Erikson (1950, 1968) first proposed the idea, developmental psychologists have examined identity formation. Erikson's focus was on how adolescents make choices about ideology, love, and work to arrive at an independent and unique sense of self *within* the culture in which they live. In a globalizing world, however, a new developmental identity task has arisen. It is the psychological task of forming a "cultural identity" (Jensen, 2003, in press; Jensen et al., 2011).

Whereas the Eriksonian identity formation task centers on deciding how one is distinct as an individual from the members of one's cultural community, forming a cultural identity involves deciding on the cultural communities to which one will belong. Forming a cultural identity becomes mainly a conscious process and decision when one has exposure to more than one culture. In today's world, most children are familiar with more than one culture. Even if they do not travel to or have the experience of living in more than one culture, the worldwide diffusion of media means that children are familiar with their local culture as well as being aware of the events, practices, styles, and information that are part of the global media culture.

It seems likely that the task of forming a cultural identity, just like the task of forming an individual identity, is most likely to arise in the course of adolescence and to continue into emerging adulthood. In societies that afford young people a stage of emerging adulthood, it is now generally accepted among scholars that this is the time when many of the most important steps in identity development take place (McLean & Syed, 2016; Schwartz et al., 2015).

There are multiple developmental pathways for forming a cultural identity. One model that has been used to understand how globalization promotes diverse cultural identities is the acculturation model, which was originally formulated to account for the experiences of immigrants. This acculturation model aimed to address the question of "What happens to individuals, who have developed in one cultural context, when they attempt to live in a new cultural context?" (Berry, 1997, p. 6). With respect to globalization, the question has been rephrased as "What happens in the identity development of adolescents and emerging adults when they are presented with multiple cultural contexts, including their local culture and other cultures they may come into contact with via globalization?" (Jensen et al., 2011, pp. 290–291).

The acculturation model comprises four possible pathways. *Integration* involves the original cultural identity being combined with elements of the new culture. *Assimilation* is where persons do not wish to maintain their original cultural identity; instead, they reject it and embrace their new culture as the basis of an entirely new cultural identity. The reverse, *separation* is where persons place value on holding onto their original culture and avoid contact with people in the new culture to which they have immigrated. *Marginalization* occurs when persons have little interest in maintaining their original culture but also reject or are rejected by the new culture.

While reviews of the literature have shown that all four pathways apply to adolescents' and emerging adults' experiences with globalization (Jensen & Arnett, 2012), integration and marginalization have received the most attention. An example of integration can be seen in India. India has a growing, vigorous high-tech economic sector, led largely by young people. However, even the better-educated young people who have become full-fledged members of the global economy still tend to prefer to have an arranged marriage, in accordance with Indian tradition (Verma & Saraswathi, 2002). They also generally expect to care for their parents in old age, again in accordance with Indian tradition. Thus, they have one identity for participating in the global economy and succeeding in the fast-paced world of high technology, and another identity, rooted in Indian tradition, that they maintain with respect to their families and their personal lives. These two identities are integrated in the daily lives of this segment of the Indian population.

In the process, new hybrid cultural practices also arise, such as "semiarranged" marriages, where parents no longer have sole or primary authority over the choice of a young person's spouse, but instead it is a mutual decision. Furthermore, the decision is no longer mainly based on socioeconomic considerations, as in traditional arranged marriages, but also involves romantic attraction. In short, integration preserves both local and global aspects of culture in one's identity. Moreover, integration may result in hybridization, where local and global cultures are merged to produce something new altogether (Hermans, 2015).

Marginalization may take place among people whose local culture is being rapidly altered by globalization. They may see their local culture changing beyond recognition, so that they no longer feel connected to it, but at the same time they may feel that the global culture has no place for them. There is some evidence that marginalization is related to problems such as substance abuse, prostitution, and suicide. In a study drawing on multiple data sources from the period between 1980 and 1991, researchers reported increases in suicide, drug abuse, and female and male prostitution in Ivory Coast youth aged 16 to 20 (Delafosse et al., 1993). The researchers attributed the increase in problems to the alienation that young people experienced from both the values of their traditional cultures and the values of the West.

Increases in recent decades, sometimes steep, in rates of suicide and suicide attempts have also been reported by a considerable number of researchers working in Pacific societies, parts of Sri Lanka, and Native American cultures (Booth, 1999; Hezel, 1987; Johnson & Tomren, 1999; Kearney & Miller, 1985; MacPherson & MacPherson, 1987; Novins et al., 1999; Reser, 1990; Robinson, 1990; Rubinstein, 1983). At a general level, researchers have attributed the increases in suicide to youth feeling alienated from both local and global values.

It should be added, however, that researchers working in different locations vary in their more specific explanations as to the ways that globalization and marginalization relate to suicide. The different specific emphases that researchers have highlighted include changing family roles, the irreconcilability of increased economic expectations and decreased opportunities, and the loss of traditional pathways of adolescent socialization.

Furthermore, a recent review of research found that an index measure of globalization (created by the authors) was associated both with increased suicide rates in Asia and Eastern Europe and with decreased suicide rates in Scandinavia (Milner et al., 2012). Thus, it is not globalization in and of itself that is related to suicide, but more likely the severe marginalization that some youth in some cultures experience from both local and global cultures.

Among some individuals, marginalization may also increase the risk of their showing hostility and aggression toward others. In the early 1990s, for example, researchers attributed increases in armed aggression by youth in the Ivory Coast to experiences of internal conflict between local and global values (Delafosse et al., 1993). On a broader level, some scholars have argued that "problems of identity" occur in some parts of Africa, South Asia, and the Middle East, where frustration with locally corrupt or unresponsive governments, coupled with alienation from global cultural values, leads to "rage" and sometimes violence, either locally or directed toward the West (Lieber & Weisberg, 2002). Thus, there is an empirical and theoretical basis for concern that globalization, marginalization, and serious internalizing and externalizing problems are connected. However, the specific nature of the connections and how they might manifest in different locales requires further research.

In sum, the developmental task of forming a cultural identity has become widespread with the advent of globalization. There is more than one pathway toward a cultural identity. Also, different kinds of cultural identities may be adaptive depending on local circumstances, and some identities, such as integration, may lead to entirely new hybrid cultural forms. Marginalization, however, seems fraught with risks to both individuals and communities.

Future Research

Research on the developmental implications of globalization is recent and somewhat sporadic. More research is needed altogether (Jensen, 2011). Nonetheless, there is a particularly notable dearth of research with younger children. Whereas adolescents and emerging adults may be in the eye of the globalization storm, many young children also cross borders and have extensive exposure to media. The developmental implications for this age group are essentially unknown.

Future research would also benefit from addressing globalization from different perspectives. For example, as noted, parents and their adolescents and emerging adults may not view and respond to globalization in the same ways. Research that takes multiple perspectives into account would be enlightening.

A related point is that globalization research needs to delve into local cultural contexts. The nature and extent of globalization varies widely from one group to another, or from one part of the world to another. Whereas some generalizations about globalization may sometimes be warranted, research that applies to local circumstances is also needed. Globalization is a multifaceted phenomenon and how it manifests in local contexts varies, depending, among other things, on the degree of urbanization and industrialization.

Conclusion

The last few decades likely represent only the beginnings of globalization. For example, China and India each have more than a billion people, of whom only a minority have fully entered the global economy and culture. The future, then, is likely to hold quite dramatic changes for even larger groups of children, adolescents, and emerging adults on a worldwide scale.

Future research on globalization not only will aid in our understanding of the phenomenon and its profound psychological implications but also holds the potential to help children develop new skills—the kinds of skills necessary for a world in which they increasingly interact with people from diverse cultures.

References

Arnett, J. J. (2015). *Emerging adulthood: The winding road from the late teens through the twenties* (2nd ed.). Oxford University Press.

Arnett, J. J., & Jensen, L. A. (2019). *Human development: A cultural approach* (3rd ed.). Pearson.

Becker, A. E. (2004). Television, disordered eating, and young women in Fiji: Negotiating body image and identity during rapid social change. *Culture, Medicine & Psychiatry, 28*, 533–559.

Becker, A. E., Fay, K., Gilman, S. E., & Striegel-Moore, R. (2007). Facets of acculturation and their diverse relations to body shape concern in Fiji. *International Journal of Eating Disorders, 40*, 42–50.

Berry, J. W. (1997). Immigration, acculturation, and adaptation. *International Journal of Applied Psychology, 46*, 5–34.

Bhugra, D., Mastrogianni, A., Maharajh, H., & Harvey, S. (2003). Prevalence of bulimic behaviors and eating attitudes in schoolgirls from Trinidad and Barbados. *Transcultural Psychiatry, 40*, 408–428.

Booth, H. (1999). Gender, power and social change: Youth suicide among Fiji Indians and Western Samoans. *Journal of the Polynesian Society, 108*, 39–68.

Chalaby, J. K. (2016). Television and globalization: The TV content global value chain. *Journal of Communication, 66*, 35–59.

Chang, L. (2008). *Factory girls: From village to city in a changing China.* Spiegel & Grau.

Charkova, K. D. (2007). A language without borders: English slang and Bulgarian learners of English. *Language Learning, 57*(3), 369–416.

Condon, R. G. (1988). *Inuit youth: Growth and change in the Canadian Arctic.* Rutgers University Press.

Condon, R. G. (1995). The rise of the leisure class: Adolescence and recreational acculturation in the Canadian Arctic. *Ethos, 23*, 47–68.

Côté, J. (2006). Emerging adulthood as an institutionalized moratorium: Risks and benefits to identity formation. In J. J. Arnett & J. L. Tanner (Eds.), *Emerging adults in America: Coming of age in the 21st century* (pp. 85–116). American Psychological Association Press.

Dasen, P. (2000). Rapid social change and the turmoil of adolescence: A cross-cultural perspective. *International Journal of Group Tensions, 29*, 17–49.

Davis, S., & Davis, D. (2012). Morocco. In J. J. Arnett (Ed.), *Adolescent psychology around the world* (pp. 47–60). Taylor & Francis.

Davis, S. S., & Davis, D. A. (1989). *Adolescence in a Moroccan town.* Rutgers.

Davis, S. S., & Davis, D. A. (1995). "The mosque and the satellite": Media and adolescence in a Moroccan town. *Journal of Youth & Adolescence, 24*, 577–594.

Davis, S. S., & Davis, D. A. (2007). Morocco. In J. J. Arnett, R. Ahmed, B. Nsamenang, T. S. Saraswathi, & R. Silbereisen (Eds.), *International encyclopedia of adolescence* (pp. 645–655). Routledge.

Delafosse, R. J. C., Fouraste, R. F., & Gbobouo, R. (1993). Entre hier et demain: Protocol d'étude des difficultés d'identité dans une population de jeunes ivoriens [Between yesterday and tomorrow: A study of identity difficulties in a population of young people in Cote d'Ivoire]. In F. Tanon & G. Vermes (Eds.), *L'individus et ses cultures* [Individuals and their culture] (pp. 156–164). L'Harmattan.

English Language. (2019). *English language statistics.* http://www.englishlanguageguide.com/facts/stats/

Erikson, E. H. (1950). *Childhood and society.* Norton.

Erikson, E. H. (1968). *Identity: Youth and crisis.* Norton.

Ferguson, G. M., & Bornstein, M. H. (2015). Remote acculturation of early adolescents in Jamaica towards European American culture: A replication and extension. *International Journal of Intercultural Relations, 45*, 24–35.

Ferguson, G. M., Muzaffar, H., Iturbide, M. I., Chu, H., & Meeks Gardner, J. (2018). Feel American, watch American, eat American? Remote acculturation, TV, and nutrition among adolescent–mother dyads in Jamaica. *Child Development, 89*, 1360–1377.

Friedman, T. L. (2000). *The Lexus and the olive tree: Understanding globalization.* Anchor.

Greenhalgh, S. (2019a). Soda industry influence on obesity science and policy in China. *Journal of Public Health Policy, 40*(1), 5–16.

Greenhalgh, S. (2019b). Making China safe for Coke: How Coca-Cola shaped obesity science and policy in China. *BMJ, 364*, 1–8.

Hansen, N., & Postmes, T. (2013). Broadening the scope of societal change research: Psychological, cultural, and political impacts of development aid. *Journal of Social and Political Psychology, 1*, 273–292.

Hansen, N., Postmes, T., van der Vinne, N., & van Thiel, W. (2012). Information and communication technology and cultural change: How ICT changes self-construal and values. *Social Psychology, 43*, 222–231.

Haun, D. B. M., Rapold, C. J., Call, J., Janzen, G., & Levinson, S. C. (2006). Cognitive cladistics and cultural override in Hominid spatial cognition. *Proceedings of the National Academy of the Sciences of the United States of America, 103*, 17568–17573.

Hermans, H. J. M. (2015). Human development in today's globalizing world: Implications for self and identity. In L. A. Jensen (Ed.), *Oxford handbook of human development and culture: An interdisciplinary perspective* (pp. 28–42). Oxford University Press.

Hermans, H. J. M., & Kempen, H. J. G. (1998). Moving cultures: The perilous problems of cultural dichotomies in a globalizing society. *American Psychologist, 53*, 1111–1120.

Hezel, F. X. (1987). Truk suicide epidemic and social change. *Human Organ, 46*, 283–291.

Hugo, G. (2005). A demographic view of changing youth in Asia. In F. Gale & S. Fahey (Eds.), *Youth in transition: The challenge of generational change in Asia* (pp. 59–88). Association of Asian Social Science Research Councils.

Jacobs, A. (2019, January 10). With obesity rising in China, Coke helps set nutrition policy. *New York Times*, A1, A9.

Jensen, L. A. (2003). Coming of age in a multicultural world: Globalization and adolescent cultural identity formation. *Applied Developmental Science, 7,* 188–195.

Jensen, L. A. (Ed.). (2011). *Bridging cultural and developmental approaches to psychology: New syntheses in theory, research and policy.* Oxford University Press.

Jensen, L. A. (Ed.). (2016). *The Oxford handbook of human development and culture: An interdisciplinary perspective.* Oxford University Press.

Jensen, L. A. (2018). The cultural-developmental approach to moral psychology: Autonomy, community, and divinity across cultures and ages. In M. J. Gelfand, C.-Y. Chiu, & Y.-Y. Hong (Eds.), *Handbook of advances in culture and psychology* (Vol. 7, pp. 107–143). Oxford University Press.

Jensen, L. A. (in press). Globalization. In S. Hupp & J. Jewell (Eds.), *The encyclopedia of child and adolescent development.* Wiley.

Jensen, L. A., & Arnett, J. J. (2012). Going global: New pathways for adolescents and emerging adults in a changing world. *Journal of Social Issues, 68,* 472–491.

Jensen, L. A., Arnett, J. J., & McKenzie, J. (2011). Globalization and cultural identity developments in adolescence and emerging adulthood. In S. J. Schwartz, K. Luyckx, & V. L. Vignoles (Eds.), *Handbook of identity theory and research* (pp. 285–301). Springer Publishing Company.

Jensen, L. A., & Dost-Gozkan, A. (2015). Adolescent-parent relations in Asian Indian and Salvadoran immigrant families: A cultural-developmental analysis of authority, autonomy, conflict and cohesion. *Journal of Research on Adolescence, 25,* 340–351.

Johnson, T., & Tomren, H. (1999). Helplessness, hopelessness, and despair: Identifying the precursors to Indian youth suicide. *American Indian Culture Research Journal, 23,* 287–301.

Juang, P. L., Lerner, J. V., McKinney, J. P., & von Eye, A. (1999). The goodness of fit in autonomy timetable expectations between Asian-American late adolescents and their parents. *International Journal of Behavioral Development, 23*(4), 1023–1048.

Kearney, R. N., & Miller, B. D. (1985). The spiral of suicide and social change in Sri Lanka. *Journal of Asian Studies, 45,* 81–101.

Kwak, K., & Berry, J. W. (2001). Generational differences in acculturation among Asian families in Canada: A comparison of Vietnamese, Korean, and East-Indian groups. *International Journal of Psychology, 36,* 152–162.

Lieber, R. J., & Weisberg, R. E. (2002). Globalization, culture, and identities in crisis. *International Journal of Politics, Culture, and Society, 16,* 273–296.

Liechty, M. (1995). Media, markets, and modernization: Youth identities and the experience of modernity in Kathmandu, Nepal. In V. Amit-Talai & H. Wulff (Eds.), *Youth cultures: A cross-cultural perspective* (pp. 166–201). Routledge.

Liechty, M. (2010). *Out here in Kathmandu: Modernity on the global periphery.* Martin Chautari Press.

MacPherson, C., & MacPherson, L. (1987). Towards an explanation of recent trends in suicide in Western Samoa. *Man, 22,* 305–330.

Manago, A. M. (2012). The new emerging adult in Chiapas, Mexico: Perceptions of traditional values and value change among first-generation Maya university students. *Journal of Adolescent Research, 27,* 663–713.

McKenzie, J. (2018). Globalization and moral personhood: Dyadic perspectives of the moral self in rural and urban Thai communities. *Journal of Adolescent Research, 33*(2), 209–246.

McKinsey Global Institute. (2014). *Global flows in a digital age: How trade, finance, people, and data connect the world economy.* https://www.mckinsey.com/~/media/mckinsey/featured%20insights/Globalization/Global%20flows%20in%20a%20digital%20age/MGI%20Global%20flows%20in%20a%20digial%20age%20Executive%20summary.ashx

McLean, K. C., & Syed, M. (2016). Personal, master, and alternative narratives: An integrative framework for understanding identity development in context. *Human Development, 58*(6), 318–349.

Miller, L. (2004). Those naughty teenage girls: Japanese kogals, slang, and media assessments. *Journal of Linguistic Anthropology, 14*(2), 225–247.

Milner, A., McClure, R., & De Leo, D. (2012). Globalization and suicide: An ecological study across five regions of the world. *Archives of Suicide Research, 16,* 238–249.

Naito, T., & Gielen, U. P. (2002). The changing Japanese family: A psychological portrait. In J. L. Roopnarine & U. P. Gielen (Eds.), *Families in global perspective*. Allyn & Bacon.

Nguyen, N. A., & Williams, H. L. (1989). Transition from East to West: Vietnamese adolescents and their parents. *Journal of the American Academy of Child and Adolescent Psychiatry, 28*, 505–15.

Novins, D. K., Beals, J., Roberts, R. E., & Manson, S. M. (1999). Factors associated with suicide ideation among American Indian adolescents: Does culture matter? *Suicide and Life-Threatening Behavior, 29*, 332–346.

Onitsuka, K., Hidayat, A. R. T., & Huang, W. (2018). Challenges for the next level of digital divide in rural Indonesian communities. *Electronic Journal of Information Systems in Developing Countries, 84*, e12021.

Phinney, J., Ong, A., & Madden, T. (2000). Cultural values and intergenerational value discrepancies in immigrant and non-immigrant families. *Child Development, 71*, 528–539.

Pike, K. M., & Dunne, P. E. (2015). The rise of eating disorders in Asia: A review. *Journal of Eating Disorders, 33*, 1–14.

Population Reference Bureau. (2008). *World population data sheet.*

Portes, A. (1997). Immigration theory for a new century: Some problems and opportunities. *International Migration Review, 31*, 799–825.

Reser, J. (1990). The cultural context of aboriginal suicide: Myths, meanings, and critical analysis. *Oceania, 61*, 177–184.

Robinson, G. (1990). Separation, retaliation and suicide: Mourning and the conflicts of young Tiwi men. *Oceania, 60*, 161–178.

Rubenstein, J. M. (2017). *The cultural landscape: An introduction to human geography* (12th ed.). Pearson.

Rubinstein, D. H. (1983). Epidemic suicide among Micronesian adolescents. *Social Science and Medicine, 17*, 657–665.

Schlegel, A. (2001). The global spread of adolescent culture. In L. J. Crockett & R. K. Silbereisen (Eds.), *Negotiating adolescence in times of social change*. Cambridge University Press.

Schwartz, S. J., Zamboanga, B. L., Luyckx, K., Meca, A., & Ritchie, R. (2015). Identity development in emerging adulthood. In J. J. Arnett (Ed.), *Oxford handbook of emerging adulthood* (pp. 401–420). Oxford University Press.

Statista. (2019). *Global IP traffic from 2016 to 2021*. https://www.statista.com/statistics/499431/global-ip-data-traffic-forecast/

Stevenson, H. W., & Zusho, A. (2002). Adolescents in China and Japan: Adapting to a changing environment. In R. Larson & T. S. Saraswathi (Eds.), *The world's youth: Adolescence in eight regions of the globe*. Cambridge University Press.

Student Science. (2019). *About Intel ISEF*. https://student.societyforscience.org/intel-isef

Unger, J. B. (2011). Cultural identity and public health. In S. J. Schwartz, K. Luyckx, & V. L. Vignoles (Eds.), *Handbook of identity theory and research* (pp. 811–825). Springer.

United Nations. (2018). *Department of Economic and Social Affairs: News*. https://www.un.org/development/desa/en/news/population/2018-revision-of-world-urbanization-prospects.html

Verma, S., & Saraswathi, T. S. (2002). Adolescents in India: Street urchins or Silicon Valley millionaires? In R. Larson & T. S. Saraswathi (Eds.), *The world's youth: Adolescence in eight regions of the globe* (pp. 105–140). Cambridge University Press.

World Bank. (2009). *Information and communications for development 2009: Extending research and increasing impact*. http://www.worldbank.org

World Bank. (2018). *Data: UNESCO Institute for Statistics*. https://data.worldbank.org/indicator/SE.ENR.PRIM.FM.ZS?year_high_desc=false

World Health Organization. (2018). *Obesity and overweight*. https://www.who.int/news-room/fact-sheets/detail/obesity-and-overweight

World Health Organization. (2019). *Controlling the global obesity epidemic*. https://www.who.int/nutrition/topics/obesity/en/

Treatment and Access to Care for Global Mental Health

PART IV

Religion and Risk of Suicide: A Cross-National Study of Cultural Differences

Tetsuya Iidaka

Abstract

Preventing death from suicide remains a major issue in global mental health even though the suicide rate worldwide has been gradually decreasing over the last 15 years. The trend is decreasing, but the change is small; therefore, more effective sex- and culture-specific treatments for suicide prevention are needed. This chapter focuses on religion, which is a major factor in culture and belief and plays an important role in people's lives and deaths, and reports the relationship between suicide and self-declared religion worldwide. The chapter discusses an analysis that used a cross-national approach in which suicide rates and religious composition were correlated across countries based on a large census dataset from 2015. There was a strong preventive effect of religion on suicide; however, the effect was weaker in religions originating from Eastern cultures than Western and Middle Eastern cultures. A weak preventive effect on suicide was observed mainly in women living in Eastern cultures. The chapter also briefly describes the rise and fall of the suicide rate in Japan, which paralleled the downturn and upturn of the economic condition of the nation. Some psychological characteristics of Japanese workers based on its culture are discussed.

Key Words: suicide rate, sex ratio, income, religion, economic crisis

Introduction

According to the World Health Organization (WHO), there were more than 788,000 suicide deaths worldwide in 2015, indicating an annual age-standardized suicide rate of 10.7 per 100,000 people (http://www.who.int/gho/mental_health/). The global rate has gradually decreased over several years (an approximately 8% decrease from 2000 to 2015 in both sexes); however, death from suicidal behavior is still a major cause of global mortality. In addition, there is a large difference in suicide rate trends across regions and by sex, such that the rate is decreasing most significantly in the male population in Europe. However, there has also been a large decrease in suicide in the female population in Southeast Asia. Several reasons, such as secure economic, political, and governmental conditions, may explain these differences. Another issue that should be addressed is the high male-to-female ratio of suicide—that is, men commit suicide three times more frequently than women. The high sex ratio may be affected by changes in the social roles of each sex, which are based on cultural tradition and belief, and by the economic condition of the country, both of which may correlate with suicidality in sex-specific ways.

It is difficult to precisely identify a cause of suicide because the reason is often unperceivable and multifactorial; however, both promotive and preventive factors should be considered when analyzing a person's commitment to suicide. Among these factors, which include personality, culture, genetics, family and social support, economy, religion, mental health, and others, religion appears to have a particularly strong preventive effect on suicide (Gearing & Lizardi, 2009; Goldsmith et al., 2002; Kleiman & Liu, 2014; Koenig, 2012; Norko et al., 2017; Shah & Chandia, 2010; Stack & Laubepin, 2019; VanderWeele et al., 2016; Wu et al., 2015). Religion constitutes a major part of cultural traditions and beliefs and plays an important role in people's lives and deaths in each region and country; therefore, we analyzed religious composition and suicide rates to reveal cultural differences in suicidality across countries. The main part of the study took a cross-national approach in which the data related to religious composition and suicide rates in a particular year were correlated across countries, and then a longitudinal approach was applied across four time points from 2000 to 2015 at 5-year intervals. A study using a cross-national design may commit the ecological fallacy because the unit of analysis is a nation or region of interest and not the people who actually commit suicide; however, this approach has been used and validated in many studies to investigate the involvement of socioeconomic factors in suicide (Shah & Chandia, 2010; Stack, 2000; Stack & Laubepin, 2019).

After World War II, Japan achieved economic restoration and growth through the 1970s and 1980s and encountered a major recession in the 1990s; the changes produced a rise and fall of socioeconomic conditions that paralleled the suicide rate. At its maximum, the number of committed suicides exceeded 34,000 per year (27.0 per 100,000 population) in 2003; the rate was more than double the global rate in 2008 and was the highest among the developed countries of the world (Varnik, 2012). This increased suicide rate lasted more than 10 years. Fortunately, due to several effective treatments by the Japanese government and private concerns, the rate gradually returned to normal in 2015, but it is still higher than the global mean. Here we present a brief overview of the changes in the suicide rate in Japan from the Meiji era, when the emperor regained rule over the nation, until now. We correlate the suicide rate with the unemployment rate and the annual changes in gross domestic product (GDP) and discuss the results in relation to specific characteristics of Japanese culture.

The present study consists of three sections: (a) a global trend of suicide in association with gender and income, (b) effects of religious composition on suicide, and (c) changes of suicide rate and economic status in Japan. In the first section, the data regarding suicide rates from the WHO were analyzed to reveal a global trend in the suicide rate, its difference between the sexes, and its correlation with income. In the second section, which is the major part of the study, we describe the relationship between religious composition and the suicide rate across countries using a simple correlation analysis and principal component analysis (PCA). The third section describes the historical changes in Japan from 1901 to 2015 to show rises and falls of the suicide rate in relation to warfare, economic restoration, growth, and recession. Finally, the characteristics of suicidality based on Japanese culture are discussed.

Overview of Data and Analyses

In the first section of the study, the datasets for the suicide rate and other demographic characteristics in 183 countries downloaded from the WHO website (http://www.who.int/en/) were used for analysis. The data consisted of year (2000, 2005, 2010, and 2015), region (Africa, Americas, Southeast Asia, Europe, Eastern Mediterranean, and Western Pacific), country (183 nations), sex (both sexes, male, and female), suicide rate (age-standardized, per 100,000 population), World Bank income group (low, lower middle, upper middle, and high, in 2012), and population (total, percentage of population under 15 and over 60 years old). The data were analyzed to visualize the changes in suicide rate in each country, which were classified into three groups according to increasing, decreasing, and stable trends (Figure 24.1) from 2000 to 2015. Sex ratio was computed by dividing male by female rates in each country and averaging across the regions (Figure 24.2). Changes of suicide rate across the regions from 2000 to 2015 are shown in Figure 24.3. Because our specific interest is the relationship between suicide rate and economic status in each country, we conducted a one-way analysis of variance (ANOVA) of suicide rates in 2015 using the World Bank income group as a factor (Figure 24.4). Finally, correlation analysis (Pearson's correlation coefficient) was conducted between the suicide rate in 2015 and the proportion of population under 15 and over 60 years old (Figure 24.5). The

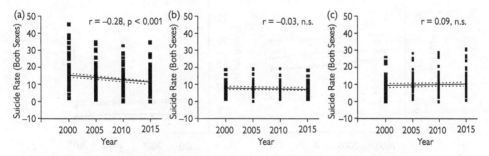

Figure 24.1. Longitudinal changes in the suicide rate for both sexes (vertical axis) in 183 countries worldwide from 2000 to 2015 (horizontal axis) are plotted. The dot indicates the rate for each country. (a) In 98 countries (54%), there was a decrease (above 1%) in the suicide rate from 2000 to 2015. (b) In 40 countries (22%), the suicide rate showed no change from 2000 to 2015. (c) In 45 countries (25%), the suicide rate slightly increased from 2000 to 2015. The regression line (filled), 95% confidence line (broken), correlation coefficient, and *p* value are noted in the figure.

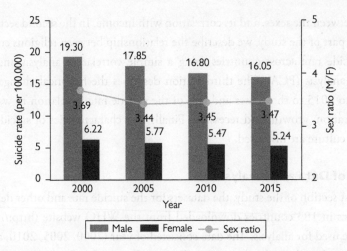

Figure 24.2. Longitudinal changes in the suicide rate worldwide (left axis, per 100,000 population) from 2000 to 2015. The grey bars indicate the male population and the black bars the female population. The change of sex ratio (light grey, right axis) is also shown.

statistical threshold was set at $p < 0.05$ with Bonferroni's correction for multiple comparisons when necessary.

In the second section, a research report regarding the size and geographic distribution of eight major religious groups, including the religiously unaffiliated, in each country was used for analysis. The report, which was published by the Pew Research Center in 2012, tabulated the religious composition of each country as the percentage of Christian, Muslim, Unaffiliated, Hindu, Buddhist, Folk religion, Other religion, and Jewish people

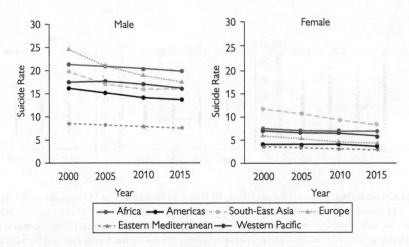

Figure 24.3. Longitudinal changes of the suicide rate (per 100,000 population) for male (left) and female (right) populations in each region from 2000 to 2015. Six regions are displayed.

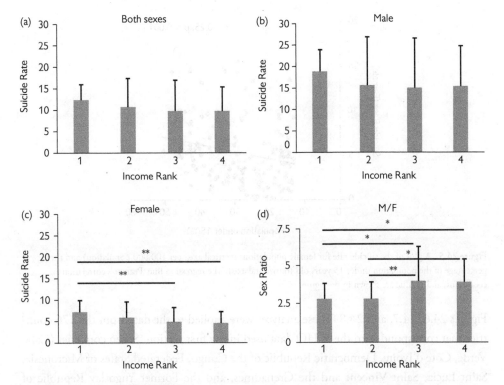

Figure 24.4. The relationship between income group rank and the suicide rate. The mean (column) and standard deviation (bar) of suicide rate (per 100,000 population) for a) both sexes, b) male, and c) female. d) The relationship between income group rank and sex ratio (M/F). Four income group ranks were according to the World Bank: 1: low-income group, 2: lower-middle-income group, 3: upper-middle-income group, and 4: upper income group. Double and single asterisks indicate significance at $p < 0.01$ and $p < 0.05$ after Bonferroni's correction for multiple comparisons, respectively.

in the population.[1] The report by the Pew Research Institute was used only to extract the percentage of each religious group in each country, and the following data analysis is original with the author. The percentage of each religious group was correlated with the suicide rate (both sexes, male, and female) and the sex ratio in 2015 worldwide using Pearson's correlation coefficients (Table 24.1). Because the religious homogeneity of a region or country is a predictor of the suicide rate (Wu et al., 2015), we took the highest percentage among the religious groups except for unaffiliated as an index of the religious homogeneity of each, which was then correlated with the suicide rate and the sex ratio. The statistical threshold was set at $p < 0.05$, and Bonferroni's correction for multiple comparisons was applied when necessary (e.g., across eight religious groups). The plots of the rate/ratio and the percentage of religious groups and homogeneity indices are shown in

---

[1] Examples of folk religions include African traditional religions, Chinese folk religions, Native American religions, and Australian Aboriginal religions. Other religions include the Baha'i faith, Jainism, Shintoism, Sikhism, Taoism, Tenrikyo, Wicca, Zoroastrianism, and many others. The religiously unaffiliated include atheists, agnostics, and people who do not identify with any particular religion (Pew Research Center, 2012).

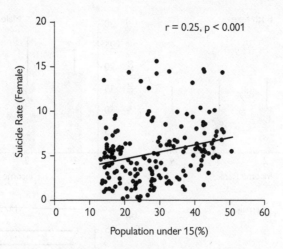

Figure 24.5. A plot of the suicide rate for female populations (vertical axis, per 100,000 population) and the percentage of the population under 15 years old (horizontal axis). The regression line, Pearson's correlation coefficient, and p value are shown in the figure.

Figures 24.6, 24.7, and 24.8. These analyses were applied to the data from the 176 countries that corresponded to the WHO data used in the first section. Seven countries (Cabo Verde, Côte d'Ivoire, Democratic Republic of the Congo, Federated States of Micronesia, Saint Lucia, Saint Vincent and the Grenadines, and the Former Yugoslav Republic of Macedonia) were excluded from the analysis because religious data were not available.

The religious group data were subjected to PCA to reduce their dimensionality and make a predictive model of religion in each country. Among the components produced by the PCA, two components (PC1 and PC2) had an eigenvalue greater than 1.5 and were used for further analysis. The principal component loadings for PC1 and PC2 are shown in Figure 24.9. The Pearson's correlation coefficient was computed between the principal

Table 24.1. Correlation Coefficients Between suicide Rate, Sex Ratio, and Religious Composition

	Suicide Rate Both Sexes	Suicide Rate Male	Suicide Rate Female	Sex Ratio Male/ Female
Christian	0.06	0.15*	–0.12	0.41**
Muslim	–0.25**	–0.30**	–0.13	–0.30**
Unaffiliated	0.23**	0.22**	0.20*	0.07
Buddhist	0.19*	0.15*	0.24**	–0.16*
Hindu	0.09	0.03	0.19*	–0.12
Folk religion	0.06	0.03	0.17*	–0.16*
Jewish	–0.06	–0.06	–0.07	0.02
Other religion	0.06	0.01	0.22**	–0.13

* $p < 0.05$ (uncorrected); ** $p < 0.05$ (Bonferroni's correction).

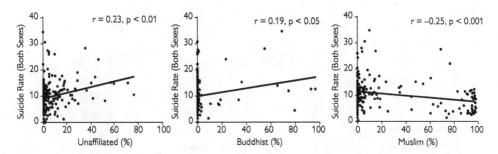

Figure 24.6. Plots of the suicide rate for both sexes (vertical axis, per 100,000 population) and the percentage of religion (horizontal axis) across countries. The results for Unaffiliated (left), Buddhist (middle), and Muslim (right) are shown. The regression line, Pearson's correlation coefficient, and p value are shown in the figure.

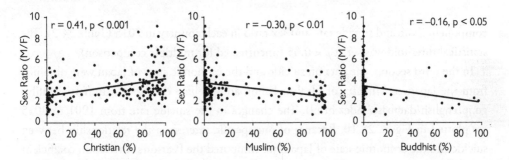

Figure 24.7. Plots of the sex ratio (vertical axis) and the percentage of religion (horizontal axis) across countries. The results for Christian (left), Muslim (middle), and Buddhist (right) are shown. The regression line, Pearson's correlation coefficient, and p value are shown in the figure.

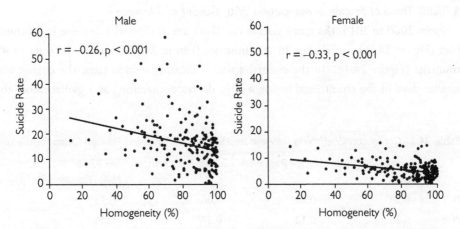

Figure 24.8. Plots of the suicide rate (vertical axis, per 100,000 population) and the religious homogeneity index (horizontal axis) across countries are shown for male (left) and female (right) groups. The regression line, Pearson's correlation coefficient, and p value are shown in the figure.

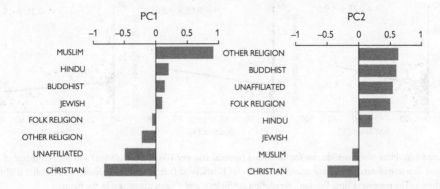

Figure 24.9. The results of principal component loadings are shown for PC1 (left) and PC2 (right). PC1 has strong positive loading for Muslim and strong negative loading for Christian and Unaffiliated, and PC2 has strong negative loading for Christian, weak negative loading for Muslim, and neutral or positive loading for other groups.

component score and suicide rate and sex ratio in each country in 2015 (Table 24.2). The statistical threshold was set at $p < 0.05$ (uncorrected for multiple comparison).

In the third section, the data on suicide and the economic state of Japan were obtained from the Japanese Ministry of Health, Labor, and Welfare database (http://www.mhlw.go.jp/english/database/index.html). The changes in the suicide rate from 1901 to 2015 are plotted in Figure 24.10. Because of our specific interest in the relationship between suicide and the economic state of Japan, we computed the Pearson's correlation coefficient between the unemployment rate (from 1975 to 2015), annual increment of GDP (from 1981 to 2015), suicide rate, and sex ratio. (The statistical threshold was set at $p < 0.05$; plots are shown in Figure 24.11.)

Results

A Global Trend of Suicide in Association With Gender and Income

From 2000 to 2015, the mean suicide rate (both sexes) showed a decrease in 98 countries (Figure 24.1a), no change in 40 countries (Figure 24.1b), and an increase in 45 countries (Figure 24.1c). In the countries with increasing suicide rates, the change was smaller than in the countries showing a large decrease; therefore, as a global trend, the

Table 24.2. Correlation Coefficients Between suicide Rate, Sex Ratio, and Principal Component Scores

	Suicide Rate Both Sexes	Suicide Rate Male	Suicide Rate Female	Sex Ratio Male/Female
PC1	–0.20*	–0.26**	–0.06	–0.35**
PC2	0.20*	0.12	0.37**	–0.26**

* $p < 0.01$ (uncorrected); ** $p < 0.001$.

PC1 has positive loading for Muslim and negative loading for Christian and Unaffiliated. PC2 has negative loading for Christian and positive loading for Other religion, Buddhist, Unaffiliated, and Folk religion.

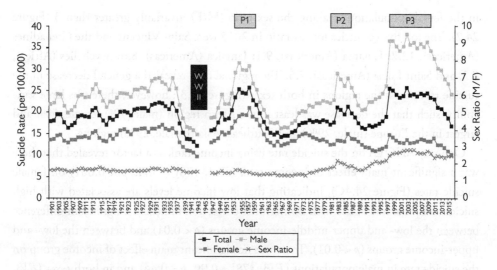

Figure 24.10. Changes of the suicide rate (total, male, and female, left vertical axis) and the sex ratio (right vertical axis) are plotted by year (horizontal axis) from 1901 to 2016. The beginning of the modern era of Japan was 1868, and the emperor ruled the nation until the end of World War II (from 1941 to 1945). No data were reported for the period from 1944 to 1946 during wartime. Even before World War II, the suicide rate in Japan was not as low as in the years after the war. There was a large decrease in the suicide rate before the war and an increase after the war, which produced the first peak (P1) from 1955 to 1958. The second peak (P2) was observed from 1983 to 1986, while the third and largest increase was observed from 1998 to 2010 (P3).

suicide rate in both sexes decreased over 15 years. The top five countries for suicide rates (per 100,000 population) in 2015 for both sexes were Sri Lanka (Southeast Asia), 34.6; Guyana (Americas), 30.6; Mongolia (Western Pacific), 28.1; Kazakhstan (Europe), 27.5; and Côte d'Ivoire (Africa), 27.2. The suicide rate was greater in the male population than

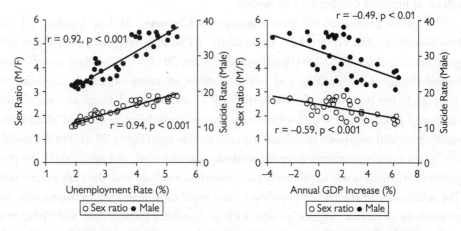

Figure 24.11. Left: The unemployment rate (%, horizontal axis), sex ratio (open circle, left vertical axis), and suicide rate in the male population (closed circle, right vertical axis) are plotted. Right: The annual gross domestic product increase (%, horizontal axis), sex ratio (open circle, left vertical axis), and suicide rate in males (closed circle, right vertical axis) are plotted. In both figures, the regression line, Pearson's correlation coefficient, and p value are shown.

in the female population, making the sex ratio (M/F) invariably greater than 3 (Figure 24.2). The top five countries for sex ratio in 2015 were Saint Vincent and the Grenadines (Americas), 12.2; Panama (Americas), 9.1; Jamaica (Americas), 8.6; Seychelles (Africa), 8.2; and Saint Lucia (Americas), 7.5. The regional data revealed a general decrease in the suicide rate across the regions in both sexes (Figure 24.3); however, there was large variability, such that the decrease was least in the Africa region (male, 7%; female, 5%) and largest in the Europe (male, 29%) and Southeast Asia (female, 29%) regions.

One-way ANOVA on the suicide rate using income rank as a factor revealed that there was a significant main effect of income rank (F [3, 178] = 5.72, $p < 0.001$) on female suicide rates (Figure 24.4C), indicating that low income levels are associated with high suicide risk. Post hoc t-tests with Bonferroni's correction indicated a significant difference between the low- and upper-middle-income groups ($p < 0.01$) and between the low- and upper-income groups ($p < 0.01$). There was no significant main effect of income group on the suicide rate in male populations (F [3, 178] = 0.90, $p = 0.44$) and in both sexes (F [3, 178] = 1.59, $p = 0.19$). One-way ANOVA on the sex ratio using income rank as a factor revealed that there was a significant main effect of income rank (F [3, 177] = 6.49, $p < 0.001$) on the ratio (Figure 24.4D). Post hoc t-tests with Bonferroni's correction indicated a significant difference between the low-income and the upper-middle- ($p < 0.05$) and upper-income ($p < 0.05$) groups and between the lower-middle-income and the upper-middle- ($p < 0.01$) and upper-income groups ($p < 0.05$), indicating that high income is associated with a high male-to-female ratio. Finally, there was a significant positive correlation between the female suicide rate and the percentage of the population under 15 years old ($r = 0.25$, $p < 0.001$, Figure 24.5), while the percentage of population over 60 years old did not significantly correlate with the female suicide rate ($r = -0.10$, $p = 0.17$).

Effects of Religious Composition on Suicide

The global proportion of each religion was Christian, 31.5%; Muslim, 23.2%; Unaffiliated, 16.3%; Hindu, 15.0%; Buddhist, 7.1%; Folk religion, 5.9%; Other religion, 0.8%; and Jewish, 0.2% (Pew Research Center, 2012). The correlation coefficients between religious composition and suicide rates or sex ratios worldwide are shown in Table 24.1. For both sexes, the proportions of Unaffiliated and Buddhist were significantly and positively correlated with suicide rate, whereas the proportion of Muslim was significantly and negatively correlated with the suicide rate (Figure 24.6). For the suicide rate in the male populations, a similar tendency was observed, and additionally the proportion of Christians was significantly and positively correlated with the male suicide rate. The suicide rate in the female populations had significant positive correlations with the proportions of several religious groups, such as Buddhist, Hindu, Folk and Other religions, and Unaffiliated. The sex ratio was strongly and positively correlated with the proportion of Christian, strongly and negatively correlated with the proportion of Muslim, and weakly and negatively correlated with the proportion of Buddhist and Folk religion

(Figure 24.7). The homogeneity index was significantly and negatively correlated with the suicide rate for both sexes ($r = -0.31$, $p < 0.001$), male ($r = -0.26$, $p < 0.001$, Figure 24.8, left), and female ($r = -0.33$, $p < 0.001$, Figure 24.8, right), but was not correlated with the sex ratio ($r = 0.07$, $p = 0.33$).

The results of PCA revealed that the eigenvalues (contribution ratios) of PC1 and PC2 were 1.91 (23.9%) and 1.58 (19.8%), respectively. PC1 had a strong positive loading for Muslim and strong negative loading for Christian and Unaffiliated, while the PC2 had strong negative loading for Christian and neutral or negative loading for other groups (Figure 24.9). The variation of the loading factor indicates that PC1 is characterized by the contrast between Christian/Unaffiliated and Muslim and PC2 by the contrast between Christian and Other groups. The correlation analysis between the suicide rate and the principal component scores across countries revealed that PC1 had a significant negative correlation with the rate in both sexes and male populations, whereas PC2 had a significant positive correlation with the rate in both sexes and female populations (Table 24.2). These results yielded strong negative correlations between the principal component score and the sex ratio across countries for both PC1 and PC2.

Changes of Suicide Rate and Economic Status in Japan

In 1868, Japan completed the historical transformation of its political system from the Tokugawa shogunate to the Meiji era, in which the emperor ruled the nation directly. Reliable annual data of mortality and cause of death have been recorded from 1901 to today (Figure 24.10). Before World War II (from 1941 to 1945), the suicide rate in Japan from the last quarter of the Meiji era to the early Showa era was relatively high compared with the lowest period since the war, around 1967. This high suicide rate is expected to be related to the political, economic, and cultural transformation from a feudal system to the modern system achieved during this period. In the beginning, and during the critical period when Japan shifted to the wartime regime from 1936 to 1943, the suicide rate decreased to a great extent, a phenomenon reported by Durkheim in the 19th century. He wrote that vital and emotional feeling is extraordinarily elevated during wartime and collective unity among people is strengthened, both of which decrease suicidality (Durkheim, 1897).

The decrease in the suicide rate turned to a sharp rise after defeat in the war and reached its first peak in 1955 (P1 in Figure 24.10), when economic growth was beginning in Japan. This rise in the suicide rate could have been due to the psychological aftermath and terrible consequences of the war, and to the rapid changes of the social system from an imperial government to democracy. The rise in the suicide rate continued for several years and then showed a rapid fall until 1967, when the rate was the lowest ever (14.2 for both sexes) apart from the wartime period. Japan's gross national product (GNP) in 1968 had risen to the second largest in the world, following the United States. The historical implication here is that the rise and fall of the suicide rate is significantly associated with modernization, the crisis caused by the war, and the remarkable rehabilitation of postwar Japan.

Economic growth in Japan continued throughout the 1970s; however, interestingly, the suicide rate gradually increased from 1967 to 1979 and showed a sharp rise in 1983, which lasted until 1986 (P2 in Figure 24.10). The year 1979 was memorable for the world economy because an economist at Harvard University published a book titled *Japan as Number One: Lessons for America* (Vogel, 1979). This book described how the island nation had achieved highly efficient industrial productivity after defeat in the war by analyzing not only the economy but also the culture, educational system, and security of the nation. On the other hand, the fact that a high suicide rate under economic growth and industrial prosperity was observed in Japan in the 1980s would be in accordance with a statement by Durkheim that the suicide rate increases when the balance of a nation collapses, not only under hard times but also under good times, with reference to the cases of Italy and Prussia (Durkheim, 1897). In addition, the sex ratio exceeded 2.0 for the first time in Japan in 1983 (2.15) and reached a maximum (2.81) in 2003.

The economic condition from 1986 to 1991 is known as the period of the bubble economy in Japan, during which time the suicide rate decreased from 21.2 to 16.1 (both sexes). An economic crisis after 1992 was considered a major cause of the increasing suicide rate from 1992, which showed a further rise in 1998 and continued to be high thereafter, producing the third and largest peak in the modern era of Japan (P3 in Figure 24.10). The highest rate was 25.5 (both sexes) in 2003, which was 1st, ironically, in the Group of Seven (France, United States, United Kingdom, Germany, Italy, Canada, and Japan), 8th in the Organization for Economic and Co-operation and Development, and 23rd in the world (WHO data in 2005). Responding to nationwide concern regarding the high suicide rate, the Japanese Diet and Government enacted legislation on suicide prevention in 2005; however, it was not until 2015 that the rate returned to a level comparable to that before the peak. Although the suicide prevention act was effective to some extent, the decrease in the rate was most likely associated with the economic recovery in Japan.

The relationship between the economic recovery and decreasing suicidality is seen in more detail in the correlation analysis between the unemployment rate and the suicide rate from 1975 to 2015 (Figure 24.11, left). A significant and positive correlation between these values was found only for the male population (male, $r = 0.92$, $p < 0.001$, female, $r = 0.07$, n.s.). The sex ratio (M/F) also showed a significant and positive correlation with the unemployment rate ($r = 0.94$, $p < 0.01$). Similarly, the annual increase in GDP had a significant and negative correlation with the suicide rate (Figure 24.11, right) in the male population ($r = -0.49$, $p < 0.01$) and the sex ratio ($r = -0.59$, $p < 0.001$) but not with the suicide rate in the female population ($r = 0.05$, n.s.). These results indicate that economic depression and loss of jobs, which usually occur at the same time, were major causes of the increasing number of suicides, particularly in the male population.

Discussion

A Global Trend of Suicide in Association With Gender and Income

In approximately half of the countries worldwide (54%), between 2000 and 2015, the suicide rate decreased by more than 1%; in one-fourth of the countries (25%) the rate increased; and in the remaining countries the rate was stable. The decreasing trend in 98 countries from 2000 to 2015 was statistically significant (Figure 24.1a), while the increasing trend in 45 countries was not (Figure 24.1c), suggesting a global trend of decreasing suicide rate in these 15 years. However, this decreasing trend is not large or universal; therefore, suicide prevention programs are still needed in many countries. The sex ratio was universally greater than 1.0 except in Bangladesh, China, and Grenada, indicating that more men completed suicide than women in almost every country. The sex ratio gradually decreased from 2000 to 2015; however, this trend is not predominant for the last decade. A regional variation in suicide rate was observed, indicating that the decreasing trend was large among men in Europe and among women in Southeast Asia (Figure 24.3).

The economic state of the country significantly affected the suicide rate for women and the sex ratio. The female suicide rate was low and the sex ratio was high in the high-income group compared with other income rank groups (Figure 24.4). Although the analyses using regional data suggested that the suicide rate was the highest in low-income areas in several countries (Sweden, Canada, Australia, and London; Goldsmith et al., 2002), there was no report of the gender differences in this correlation shown in the present study. In particular, a significant positive correlation between the female suicide rate and the population under 15 years old was observed, a finding probably due to the significant negative correlation between income rank and population under 15 years old ($r = -0.82$, $p < 0.001$). These results suggest that the high frequency of childbearing and burden of fostering in low-income countries may be associated with the high suicide rate in the female population.

Effects of Religious Composition on the Suicide Rate

A significant and positive correlation was observed between the suicide rate and the proportion of religiously unaffiliated groups worldwide in both sexes, findings that inversely mirror a protective effect of religion on suicidality regardless of sex. The proportion of Muslims showed a significant negative correlation with the suicide rate in both sexes and the male population, suggesting high religiosity among Muslims in which suicide is forbidden, as discussed later in this section. In contrast, the proportion of Buddhists showed a moderate but significant positive correlation with the suicide rate in both sexes and the male population and, in particular, a strong positive correlation with the suicide rate in the female population, indicating a finding opposed to the protective role of religion in suicidality.

A novel finding of the present study is that the proportion of Christians showed a significant positive relationship with male suicide rate and a nonsignificant negative relationship with female suicide rate, increasing the sex ratio of suicide rate significantly, showing a positive correlation with the proportion of Christians across countries. This indicates that the larger the population of Christians in a country is, the more men commit suicide compared to women. Such a relationship between the sex ratio and the proportion of a religious group was not observed in other groups, including the religiously unaffiliated; therefore, the result appears to be specific to Christians. In addition, the religious homogeneity index was strongly and negatively correlated with the suicide rate for all gender groups, suggesting that predominance of a particular religion in a country would be protective of suicidality.

Extracting principal components from the worldwide religious composition data was a novel approach that showed that two components were significantly related with the suicide rates. The loading factor of PC1 indicated that Christian in combination with Unaffiliated was contrasted to Muslim, and those countries with a high proportion of Muslims had lower suicide rates in the male population and a lower sex ratio than countries with a high proportion of Christians/Unaffiliated. The loading factor of PC2 indicated that this component is specifically related to the proportion of Christians as contrasted with other religious groups, ignoring the proportions of Muslims and Jewish people. Surprisingly, the countries with high PC2 scores had high suicide rates in the female population, making the correlation of PC2 and the sex ratio significantly negative. The results suggest that women commit suicide more frequently in countries with higher proportions of Other religion, Buddhist, Unaffiliated, Folk religion, and Hindu compared with the countries with high proportions of Christians.

A recent meta-analysis indicated that religion plays a protective role against suicide; however, this effect varies according to the cultural and religious context (Wu et al., 2015). This study, based on case-control and retrospective cohort studies conducted in the United States, China, Indonesia, and Hungary, revealed that the protective effect was significant in Western cultures but not in Eastern cultures. In addition, the protective role of religion in suicide was significant in the older population and in religiously homogenous groups but not in the younger population or less homogenous groups. These results suggest that mechanisms of religion such as peer support, coping strategy, altruism, and charity, which may reduce the risk of suicidality, are not universal, but are likely to be regionally and culturally specific. The effect of religious homogeneity on suicide may suggest that a strong sense of unity derived from shared belief and thought in the community is beneficial to mitigate suicidality.

Although the research is limited, Islamic countries showed lower rates of suicide (Stack, 2000) than did other countries, probably due to higher religiosity among Muslims, whose religion strictly forbids suicide (Gearing & Lizardi, 2009). A cross-national study investigating the relationship between suicide and Islam showed a significant negative correlation between the suicide rate in the general population and the percentage of Muslims in men and women, when controlling for socioeconomic status and income (Shah & Chandia,

2010). This study used WHO and United Nations data involving suicide rates and the percentage of people in the population adhering to Islam in 27 countries in 2000. Thus, the results of the present study accord with those by Shah and Chandia and extend the negative relationship between suicide and Islam further using a more recent global dataset.

A descriptive review indicates that, although religiosity has been shown to be associated with a reduced risk of suicidality, its protective role for suicide varies across religions (Gearing & Lizardi, 2009). The view of suicide as a sin dominates current Christian attitudes across the various denominations; however, relatively higher suicide rates were observed among Protestants than Catholics. Judaism also has strict prohibitions against suicide, and the suicide rates among Jewish individuals in the United States and Israel have been low. In contrast to the three monotheistic religions noted earlier, Hindu scriptures are relatively ambivalent on the issue of intentional death, although Hindu teachers condemn suicide as the destruction of a sacred life. Finally, Buddhist practice is focused on the relief from human suffering and pain, which fill all stages of life. Buddhists believe that if one takes one's life through suicide, the results are rebirth into a lower level of life and future pain, but not relief from suffering (Lizardi & Gearing, 2010). Although suicide may be seen as a form of suffering, Buddhist countries often reported higher suicide rates than other countries (Norko et al., 2017); the findings accord with the results of the present study.

Two points that should be discussed in the present study are that (a) a higher proportion of Christians is associated with a larger male-to-female ratio of suicide rate (Table 24.1), and (b) a greater proportion of religious groups excluding Christian, Muslim, and Jewish was associated with a larger suicide rate in the female population; the results were derived from both correlation analyses (Table 24.1) and PCA (Table 24.2). The first point, that the larger the Christian proportion, the greater the sex ratio is, would be partly due to a strong negative correlation between the proportions of Christian and Muslim; the latter is associated with a lower sex ratio. Another explanation for this is that the countries with both a high sex ratio and a high proportion of Christians were found in Eastern Europe (Romania, Poland, and Lithuania) and former members of the Soviet Union (Armenia, Moldova, and Georgia). Therefore, several problems such as ethnic and ideological conflicts that elevate the suicide rate in the male population may exist in these countries. The second point, that the greater proportion of Buddhist, Hindu, and Folk/Other religions was associated with a higher suicide rate in the female population, is more difficult to explain. It appears that the gender gap in social roles still exists because these countries are in the Western Pacific and Southeast Asia regions.

The present study used a cross-national design, and the unit of analysis was nations of the world showing large variances in total population, developmental state, and secularization. In a recent cross-sectional study of 162 European regions in which the developmental state is high and the population is secular, religiousness was significantly and negatively correlated with the suicide rate, as observed in the present study (Stack &

Laubepin, 2019). Several other studies using an individual-level analysis also showed that religiosity has a protective role in suicidality. Frequent attendance at religious services was a protective factor against suicide in a long-term, longitudinal prospective study (Kleiman & Liu, 2014). A large prospective long-term cohort study of U.S. women showed that frequent religious service attendance was associated with lower suicide risk (VanderWeele et al., 2016). Although most prospective studies have been conducted in the countries in which Christianity is predominant, the present study using a cross-national design and worldwide data corresponds with those studies using analyses of finer units or individual-level analysis.

Changes of Suicide Rate and Economic Status in Japan

We described historical changes in the suicide rate and sex ratio along with changes in the social system and economic conditions in Japan from 1901 to 2015, including a sharp drop during wartime. As noted in the second section, the cross-sectional study of the relationship between income rank and suicide rate showed that poverty itself does not necessarily increase suicidality in the total or male populations (Figure 24.4A and B). On the other hand, it is known that sudden changes of economic state, particularly a downturn, may have a predominantly upward effect on the suicide rate (Goldsmith et al., 2002), as observed in the postwar period of Japan. Unrecognized in recent analyses, a previously mentioned issue in the relationship between socioeconomic condition and suicidality is that even an upturn period of national changes in the social situation can elevate the number of suicides committed (Durkheim, 1897). The reasons people commit suicide during such good times are not clear, and further analysis is needed to clarify this issue.

Although a strong association between unemployment and suicide has been predicted from the literature (Arya et al., 2018; Chuang & Huang, 1996; Fountoulakis et al., 2014; Goldsmith et al., 2002; Helbich et al., 2017; Preti & Miotto, 1999), there were a few exceptions regarding the relationship. For example, in Canadian youth, the unemployment rate did not show a positive relationship with the suicide rate in 1971, and even demonstrated a negative relationship with the rate in 1981 (Trovato, 1992). In addition, in a study of the relationship of suicide rate with economic variables in Europe from 2000 to 2011, the correlation coefficients varied greatly across countries, from -0.77 (Hungary) to 0.89 (Italy) in men (Fountoulakis et al., 2014). Thus, the varying nature of such a relationship appears to be culture and region specific. The GDP (or GNP) and the growth rate have been strongly linked to the suicide rate, as reported by several authors; however, there is also considerable variation across countries, and it is unclear whether the variations are related with severity of recession, social support, religion, the health and welfare system, or other factors (Chuang & Huang, 1996; Fountoulakis et al., 2014).

Finally, we briefly describe some important aspects of the Japanese value system regarding suicide. It is well known that samurai warriors in the feudal era committed honorable suicide by ritual disembowelment; however, the contemporary Japanese do not accept this custom or react in this way in response to harshness. On the other hand, the general attitude of Japanese toward suicide is somewhat different from that of Americans, such that Japanese are more likely to think that suicide is not always abnormal behavior and might be permissible in certain situations (Takahashi, 1997). Japanese college students had a higher degree of accepting suicide as a natural way to end one's life than did U.S. students (Saito et al., 2013). There is little effect of religion on such attitudes toward suicide, because one-third of Japanese are Buddhist (36%) and more than half are unaffiliated with any religious group (57%; Pew Research Center, 2012). Both Buddhist and Unaffiliated groups are associated with increasing suicide rates across countries, as shown in the second section (Table 24.1). Although Shintoism is a Japanese faith that has been part of religious life in Japan for many centuries and Shinto rituals are widely practiced, only a minority of the Japanese population (less than 3%; Nishi, 2009) identifies with Shintoism (Pew Research Center, 2012). Shintoism and medical issues have usually been discussed in relation to brain death and organ transplantation (McConnell, 1999), but rarely to suicidality.

In addition to these basic characteristics of the Japanese, changes in the social situation since the 1990s may impose a tremendous burden on Japanese workers, particularly on men. Because many Japanese workers tended to dedicate their whole lives to their company, losing a job directly leads to a loss of income and one's social network. Difficulty in finding another job and continued unemployment cause a feeling of shame, and Japanese men have difficulty in expressing such feelings and asking for help (Russell et al., 2017). Durkheim (1897) describes well the role of shame in a particular class of suicides. Furthermore, Japanese workers often identify themselves with their profession, and such an attitude may lead to suicide to take responsibility for failure in the workplace (Takahashi, 1997). Given that the cause of suicide is always multifactorial, we assume that a combination of such characteristics of Japanese workers and changes in social situations could be closely linked to the elevated suicidal risk in Japan.

Limitations

The present study has several limitations. First, the method of the present study is descriptive, and a further controlled study is needed to fully reveal the relationship between religion and suicide. Second, most of the present results are correlational; therefore, causal relationships between religion and suicide have not yet been determined. Third, information on the prevalence of depression and other psychiatric disorders in each country that appear to have a strong influence on suicide is not available in the present study. Fourth, the timeframes used in the present study are limited, and data obtained from a longer time scale should be used in future studies. Finally, figures for the suicide rates as well as the religious compositions of some countries may not be as reliable as those for developed countries; therefore, the results in the present study should be treated with caution.

Conclusions

The present study revealed that although the global suicide rate has decreased over the last 15 years or so, the degree of change was small and further progress in suicide prevention programs is needed. The decreasing trend of suicide rates varies across regions and sexes; thus, prevention strategies should be tailored in culture- and sex-specific ways. In a cross-national approach, the income of the country does not necessarily relate to the suicide rate in men; however, as seen in the case of Japan, time-course changes in economic conditions were strongly correlated with the suicide rate in men. Religion was one of the strongest preventive factors for suicide, as found in the present study; however, there was a huge variation in the effect, such that the religions originating from Eastern cultures were less preventive than those originating from Western and Middle Eastern cultures. The changes in the suicide rate in Japan after World War II were strongly linked with economic upturns and downturns. In particular, specific characteristics of middle-aged Japanese workers, such as commitment to a job and long working time, in combination with financial depression, were major factors of the elevated suicide rate.

References

Arya, V., Page, A., River, J., Armstrong, G., & Mayer, P. (2018). Trends and socio-economic determinants of suicide in India: 2001–2013. *Social Psychiatry and Psychiatric Epidemiology, 53*, 269–278.

Chuang, H. L., & Huang, W. C. (1996). A reexamination of "sociological and economic theories of suicide: A comparison of the U.S.A. and Taiwan." *Social Science and Medicine, 43*, 421–423.

Durkheim, E. (1897). *Le Suicide: étude de sociologie*. Alcan.

Fountoulakis, K. N., Kawohl, W., Theodorakis, P. N., Kerkhof, A. J., Navickas, A., Hoschl, C., Lecic-Tosevski, D., Sorel, E., Rancans, E., Palova, E., Juckel, G., Isacsson, G., Jagodic, H. K., Botezat-Antonescu, I., Warnke, I., Rybakowski, J., Azorin, J. M., Cookson, J., Waddington, J., . . . Lopez-Ibor, J. (2014). Relationship of suicide rates to economic variables in Europe: 2000–2011. *British Journal of Psychiatry, 205*, 486–496.

Gearing, R. E., & Lizardi, D. (2009). Religion and suicide. *Journal of Religion and Health, 48*, 332–341.

Goldsmith, S. K., Pellmar, T. C., Kleinman, A. M., Bunney, W. E., (Eds.) Committee on Pathophysiology and Prevention of Adolescent and Adult Suicide Board on Neuroscience and Behavioral Health (2002). Society and culture. In *Reducing suicide: A national imperative* (pp. 193–227). The National Academies Press, Washington, D.C.

Helbich, M., Plener, P. L., Hartung, S., & Bluml, V. (2017). Spatiotemporal suicide risk in Germany: A longitudinal study 2007–11. *Scientific Reports, 7*, 7673.

Kleiman, E. M., & Liu, R. T. (2014). Prospective prediction of suicide in a nationally representative sample: Religious service attendance as a protective factor. *British Journal of Psychiatry, 204*, 262–266.

Koenig, H. G. (2012). Religion, spirituality, and health: The research and clinical implications. *ISRN Psychiatry, 2012*, 278730.

Lizardi, D., & Gearing, R. E. (2010). Religion and suicide: Buddhism, Native American and African religions, atheism, and agnosticism. *Journal of Religion and Health, 49*, 377–384.

McConnell, J. R., 3rd. (1999). The ambiguity about death in Japan: An ethical implication for organ procurement. *Journal of Medical Ethics, 25*, 322–324.

Nishi, K. (2009, May). *The NHK monthly report on broadcast research* (pp. 66–81). NHK Broadcasting Culture Research Institute.

Norko, M. A., Freeman, D., Phillips, J., Hunter, W., Lewis, R., & Viswanathan, R. (2017). Can religion protect against suicide? *Journal of Nervous and Mental Disorders, 205*, 9–14.

Pew Research Center. (2012). *The global religious landscape. A report on the size and distribution of the world's major religious groups as of 2010.*

Preti, A., & Miotto, P. (1999). Suicide and unemployment in Italy, 1982–1994. *Journal of Epidemiology and Community Health, 53*, 694–701.

Russell, R., Metraux, D., & Tohen, M. (2017). Cultural influences on suicide in Japan. *Psychiatry and Clinical Neuroscience, 71*, 2–5.

Saito, M., Klibert, J., & Langhinrichsen-Rohling, J. (2013). Suicide proneness in American and Japanese college students: Associations with suicide acceptability and emotional expressivity. *Death Studies, 37*, 848–865.

Shah, A., & Chandia, M. (2010). The relationship between suicide and Islam: A cross-national study. *Journal of Injury and Violence Research, 2*, 93–97.

Stack, S. (2000). Suicide: A 15-year review of the sociological literature. Part II: Modernization and social integration perspectives. *Suicide and Life-Threatening Behavior, 30*, 163–176.

Stack, S., & Laubepin, F. (2019). Religiousness as a predictor of suicide: An analysis of 162 European regions. *Suicide and Life-Threatening Behavior, 49*, 371–381. doi:10.1111/sltb.12435

Takahashi, Y. (1997). Culture and suicide: From a Japanese psychiatrist's perspective. *Suicide and Life-Threatening Behavior, 27*, 137–145.

Trovato, F. (1992). A Durkheimian analysis of youth suicide: Canada, 1971 and 1981. *Suicide and Life-Threatening Behavior, 22*, 413–427.

VanderWeele, T. J., Li, S., Tsai, A. C., & Kawachi, I. (2016). Association between religious service attendance and lower suicide rates among US women. *JAMA Psychiatry, 73*, 845–851.

Varnik, P. (2012). Suicide in the world. *International Journal of Environmental Research and Public Health, 9*, 760–771.

Vogel, E. F. (1979). *Japan as number one: Lessons for America.* Harvard University Press.

Wu, A., Wang, J. Y., & Jia, C. X. (2015). Religion and completed suicide: A meta-analysis. *PLoS One, 10*, e0131715.

Cross-Cultural Mental Health Promotion and Prevention for Global Mental Health

Yi-Yuan Tang *and* Rongxiang Tang

Abstract

Global mental health has increasingly adopted a medicalized approach to addressing challenges and problems. However, medicalizing global mental health produces a narrow view of the problems and solutions because it mainly emphasizes biomedical factors in the globalization of mental health and is disputed cross-culturally. The focus of this chapter is to summarize the cultural differences associated with mental health such as attention, beliefs and attitudes, and feelings and experiences of symptoms and mental disorders, and conclude with suggestive future directions of research pertaining to cultural influences on global mental health. The chapter proposes an integrative health model to promote global mental health and prevent mental disorders cross-culturally.

Key Words: cultural differences, mental health, medicalization, promotion and prevention, attention, beliefs and attitudes, integrative health model

Introduction

If you have two choices (e.g., taking a pill vs. physical exercise) to treat one symptom or disorder, what would be your decision? Most will certainly choose to take a pill for a quick solution with less effort even though any medication has side effects to a certain extent. Given the dominance of medicalizing global mental health (Clark, 2014), even healthy individuals without mental disorders often take pills to handle daily stress and discomfort. For instance, the stimulant Adderall, widely used to treat attention deficit hyperactivity disorder, is often used to sustain attention, improve cognitive performance, and relieve emotional discomfort, especially in healthy adults such as students. Nowadays, this phenomenon is observed globally across both Western and Eastern cultures, which raises a serious concern on how to effectively promote global mental health and prevent mental disorders in addition to the dominant medicalization approach (Chase et al., 2018). This chapter will mainly focus on cultural factors associated with mental health such as *cognitive, affective, and social processes* (i.e., attention and attentional bias, beliefs and attitudes, and feelings and experiences of symptoms of mental disorders, with an emphasis on cultural differences in these processes). We use Americans versus Chinese to represent Western and Eastern cultures, consistent with the large body of literature (Nisbett, 2004; Tang & Liu, 2009; Tang et al., 2006). We will also discuss the potential of developing culture-specific prevention and intervention programs for promoting mental health. Finally, we will provide suggestions of new research directions to promote global mental health and prevent mental disorders through an integrative health model in different cultures.

Cultural Differences in Cognitive and Affective Processes

Studies have shown that people from Western cultures (e.g., Americans) are inclined to attend to focal objects and perform better on tasks emphasizing independent (absolute) dimensions, whereas East Asians (e.g., Chinese) are more likely to attend to context and perform better on tasks emphasizing interdependent (relative) dimensions (Chiao et al., 2016; Nisbett, 2004; Nisbett & Masuda, 2003). In other words, Westerners and Easterners pay attention to, perceive, and receive information very differently even if they are placed in the same context and environment, suggesting fundamental differences in perception, attention, and subsequent cognitive processing such as decision making between two cultures (Markus & Conner, 2014; Nisbett, 2004). One influential explanation for these findings is that aside from potential differences in biology (e.g., genes) across cultures, social factors can also play an important role in directing attention and decision making. For example, East Asians live in a complex social system, which often involves large families with extended relatives living together; thus, attention to context is important to effective functioning in daily life. Moreover, the external environments of the East are also far more complex and compacted, containing more people and objects such as skyscrapers and public infrastructure than those of the West, which may further influences perception, cognition, and emotion (Chiao et al., 2016; Nisbett, 2004; Nisbett & Masuda, 2003).

Most importantly, convergent lines of evidence have shown that the brain can be changed by culture. For example, culture can influence neural substrates of attentional control, inhibitory control, and diverse cognitive tasks (Han & Ma, 2014, 2015; Hedden et al., 2008; Nisbett & Masuda, 2003; Pornpattananangkul et al., 2016; Tang et al., 2006). Moreover, these holistic versus analytic or interdependent versus independent processes in cognition and behavior between Eastern and Western cultures also correspond to the different neural networks. For example, increasing evidence suggests that cultural influences on brain activity are associated with multiple cognitive and affective processes (Han & Ma, 2015). A quantitative meta-analysis of functional magnetic resonance imaging studies on cultural differences indicated that East Asian cultures are associated with increased brain activity in the regions related to inference of others' minds and emotion regulation, whereas Western cultures are associated with enhanced brain activity in areas related to self-relevance encoding and emotional responses during social cognitive/affective processes (Han & Ma, 2014). Given that our social cognitive and affective processes are associated with how we believe and perceive mental health and how we feel, interpret, and experience symptoms and cope with disorders, these research findings provide evidence that cultures may shape our beliefs and attitudes about mental health, influence our feelings and experiences of symptoms and mental disorders, and even shape our treatment preferences (Jimenez et al., 2012, 2013; Kramer et al., 2002).

In the same vein, research has shown that behavior change is also related to cultural differences in responses to behavioral interventions or treatments (Jimenez et al., 2012, 2013; Kramer et al., 2002). Because fundamental differences in perception, attention, and subsequent cognitive processing such as decision making exist between Western and Eastern cultures (e.g. American and Chinese) (Markus & Conner, 2014; Nisbett, 2004), these data suggest that more work is necessary to understand how interventions or treatments should be tailored with respect to different cultures for effective improvement in outcomes (e.g., development of individualized culture-specific interventions or treatments).

Cultural Differences in the Experience of Symptoms and Mental Disorders

Our experience is associated with attention and interoception. Attentional bias refers to the tendency of our perception to be affected by our recurring thoughts and may explain our failure to consider alternatives. For example, smokers often have attentional bias for smoking-related cues; sleep-related attentional bias plays an important role in the development and maintenance of insomnia (Bar-Haim et al., 2007; Harris et al., 2015). Attentional bias also involves the exacerbation and maintenance of chronic pain (Rusu et al., 2018) and is associated with symptoms and disorders such as anxiety, depression, and posttraumatic stress disorder (PTSD; Browning et al., 2010). In a cross-cultural study of attentional bias in chronic fatigue syndrome, compared to controls, Dutch and U.K. chronic fatigue patients showed a significant attentional bias for illness-related words and were significantly more likely to interpret ambiguous information in a somatic way (Hughes et al., 2018). A review article examines cross-cultural differences in interoception and the role of culturally bound epistemologies and contemplative practices. Specifically, the review summarizes that people from Western and non-Western cultures (a) exhibit differential levels of interoceptive accuracy and somatic awareness(b), as well as different culturally bound psychopathologies, including somatization, body dysmorphia, pain sensitivity, eating disorders, and mood disorders (Di Lernia et al., 2016; Ma-Kellams, 2014). One explanation is that culture may influence attentional allocation and subsequent cognitive, affective, and social processes, and people in different cultures pay different attention to the same "thing" in the same context, which may lead to different interpretations of mental health and experiences of symptoms and mental disorders (Boduroglu et al.,

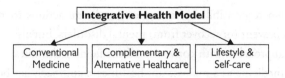

Figure 25.1. Integrative health model.

2009). Taken together, these results suggest that culture as a set of beliefs, attitudes, and values can shape experiences of disorders, including symptom experience, expression, and treatment seeking (Chase et al., 2018). It should be noted that the elements of "self" (i.e., a set of beliefs, attitudes, values, and emotions) in different cultures are central to understanding conceptions of mental health and psychological well-being and subsequent stigma (Kohrt & Harper, 2008; Liddell & Jobson, 2016). Is there a cross-cultural health model in global mental health and prevention of mental disorders?

An Integrative Health Model

Although cultural differences in attention, emotions, beliefs, feelings, and experiences of symptoms and disorders have been shown, there is an increasing trend in global mental health of using integrative health approaches. Here, we propose an integrative health model (IHM) to address the concerns in global mental health and prevention of mental disorders (see Figure 25.1). The IHM has three components: (a) Conventional medicine, which is taught in accredited medical schools and widely adopted by mainstream health care that focuses on disease treatment. Under this framework, people often believe symptom relief is equal to health and well-being and patients have the mindset that physicians should fix their problems and symptoms. Therefore, many patients keep a passive attitude, mindset, and action in response to treatment. (b) Complementary and alternative health care (CAH), which consists of nonmainstream traditional health practices but focuses more on prevention. These methods can translate into practices such as meditation, yoga, Tai Chi, herbs, and acupuncture. Although the United States mainly emphasizes biomedical factors in mental health and has adopted the medicalization model for mental health, about 38% of U.S. adults and 12% of children are using some forms of CAH approaches that mainly focus on the self-regulation of body, mind, and behavior for health and well-being. The latest data from the National Health Interview Survey, published by the National Center for Complementary and Integrative Health of the National Institutes of Health and the National Center for Health Statistics, show that many more Americans meditated or practiced yoga in 2017 than in 2012 (Black et al., 2018; Clarke et al., 2018). CAH approaches such as mindfulness meditation are popular in both research and application (Tang & Posner, 2009; Tang et al., 2015). (c) Lifestyle and self-care, which mainly includes behavioral and nutritional approaches to promote health and wellness, and more focuses on prevention and healthy lifestyle. Both CAH and self-care approaches emphasize our own responsibilities, awareness, and care actions to respond to health-related issues and prevent (or recover from) mental disorders, but also encourage the combination of such approaches with conventional medicine techniques.

Conventional medicine as a mainstream health care approach has been widely applied in disease treatment; however, medical spending has increased significantly (e.g., prescription drug spending is the fastest growing one). In the 1950s, about 2% to 3% of U.S. gross domestic product (GDP) was for health care/medical spending, but in the 2000s it increased to almost 20% of GDP (Wilson, 2017). Unfortunately, we have not received the highest quality of health care as we expect. People joke about "sick care" versus "health care" under this system. Therefore, a new health care model is urgently needed. Fortunately, the IHM has been accepted by leading institutions such as Harvard, Stanford, and Columbia University and has become a promising model for promoting global mental health and prevention of mental disorders in both Western and Eastern cultures (Chase et al., 2018), but the implementation may be different cross-culturally. This raises an important question on how to develop the individualized and culturally adapted interventions or treatments to promote global mental health.

Cross-Cultural Mental Health Promotion

Clearly, the IHM's global implementation will be heavily affected by the beliefs, attitudes, emotions, and thinking processes in different cultures. Based on the IHM, we propose two strategies to promote mental health cross-culturally: (a) Understanding our experiences associated with symptoms and disorders in different cultures. Given that culture influences our experiences, it affects the way we describe our symptoms. For instance, Asian patients tend to report somatic symptoms first and then later describe emotional afflictions, indicating that people selectively present symptoms in a "culturally appropriate" way that won't reflect badly on them (U.S. Department of Health and Human Services [DHHS], 2001). In Western culture, we are socially asked how we feel and name our emotional states from a very early age. Yet this is not the case everywhere, such as in some Eastern and African cultures. In reality, whether we describe emotional or physical symptoms relies on our cultural beliefs and norms. Without considering these cultural differences, physicians may misunderstand and interpret the symptoms and diagnose incorrectly. Likewise, patients are not aware of the cultural influences and only express the "culturally appropriate" symptoms that may mislead the diagnosis (Chase et al., 2018; Jimenez et al., 2013; Kohrt et al., 2008; Kramer et al., 2002). (b) Selecting interventions or treatments following cultural differences. Given the cultural effects on beliefs, attitudes, and values, people will decide how they cope with mental disorders and seek treatments from psychiatrists, psychologists, physicians, or traditional healers. For example, some Asian patients prefer avoidance of upsetting thoughts with regard to personal problems rather than explicit expression of the distress. Compared to White Americans, African Americans are more likely to handle personal problems and distress on their own or turn to their spirituality for support. Moreover, cultural factors often determine how much support we have from our families and communities in seeking help; people in the Eastern "collectivism" culture versus the Western "individualism" culture behave very differently (DHHS, 2001; Hunt et al., 2013; Jimenez et al., 2013). Therefore, some symptoms and mental disorders may be more prevalent in certain cultures, but it should be noted that this is largely determined by whether that particular symptom or disorder is rooted more in genetic or social factors. For example, the prevalence of schizophrenia is consistent throughout the world cross-culturally, but pain, anxiety, depression, PTSD, and suicide rates are more attributed to cultural factors (Chiao et al, 2017; DHHS, 2001). If we plan to develop culture-specific prevention for mood disorders (using meditation as an example), we should consider the cultural differences in Easterners versus Westerners (e.g., global vs. local or holistic vs. analytic information processing). Should we tailor the meditation program for Chinese or Americans using more a global or holistic strategy (e.g., open-monitoring meditation that focuses on any stimuli or thoughts that arise at the present moment) that may promote intervention effects? Or should we take an opposite approach of using a more local or analytic strategy (i.e., focus-based meditation) to adjust and balance the cultural influences? These research gaps warrant further investigation.

Conclusions and Future Directions

In this chapter, we focused on cultural factors associated with mental health and summarized how cultures (e.g., Western and Eastern) may influence and shape our brain and behavior differently and thus affect our beliefs, attitudes, and experiences of symptoms and mental disorders. The potential implications of cultural differences in the development of culturally adapted interventions or treatments for mental health promotion were also discussed. We proposed the IHM to address the global medicalization issue, promote global mental health, and prevent mental disorders cross-culturally. It is important to note that culture is a multifaceted concept encompassing a variety of factors that interact with one another and has far-reaching impacts on not only mental health but also other critical aspects of our daily lives. Given that research on cultural differences in mental health is still fairly limited, there is still a lot to be learned regarding which cultural factors play the greatest role in differentially affecting diagnosis and treatment of mental disorders across different cultures. Therefore, future research needs to delineate the exact mechanisms and factors underlying the contribution of cultures in shaping the interpretations and experiences of symptoms and disorders.

Another important domain concerns the genetic contribution to cultural differences and its relation to mental health. The culture–gene coevolutionary theory suggests that cultural values have evolved, are adaptive and may influence the social and physical environments under which genetic selection operates. For example, a study across 29 nations suggested the culture–gene coevolution between allelic frequency of the serotonin transporter gene (5-HTTLPR) and the cultural values of individualism–collectivism, and cultural values buffer genetically susceptible populations from increased prevalence of affective disorders such as depression. In other words, people from Eastern "collectivist" cultures are more likely to have gene variations that buffers them from depression than people from Western cultures (Chiao & Blizinsky, 2010; Chiao et al., 2016; Mrazek et al., 2013). The gene × environment interaction is not a new concept in psychology and neuroscience, but not much has been done with regard to how genetic variations between different cultures may exert an influence over the behavioral expression of symptoms and mental disorders or how distinct cultural experiences as part of our environment may reciprocally interact with genes to affect mental health. To integrate dynamic interactions between culture, behavior, brain, and gene, some proposed a culture–behavior–brain (CBB) loop model of human development that states that culture shapes the brain by contextualizing behavior, and the brain fits and modifies culture via behavioral influences. Genes provide a fundamental basis for, and interact with, the CBB loop at both individual and population levels (Han & Ma, 2015).

Finally, another important topic is personalizing health promotion cross-culturally to increase participants' interest and engagement in maintaining mental health. We propose that personalizing health promotion should follow individuals' cultural beliefs, values, interests, and preferences to develop different types of interventions aimed at personalizing mental health, but so far effective integrative health programs in different cultures remain underdeveloped (Tang, 2017). In sum, we are in a stage of research that requires both exploratory and large-scale studies to fill in these research gaps. Without them, we will inadvertently constrain ourselves with the basic yet incomplete knowledge about the relationship between culture and mental health.

Acknowledgment

This work was supported by the Office of Naval Research and Presidential Endowment.

References

Bar-Haim, Y., Lamy, D., Pergamin, L., Bakermans-Kranenburg, M. J., & van IJzendoorn, M. H. (2007). Threat-related attentional bias in anxious and nonanxious individuals: A meta-analytic study. *Psychological Bulletin, 133*(1), 1–24.

Black, L. I., Barnes, P. M., Clarke, T. C., Stussman, B. J., & Nahin, R. L. (2018). *Use of yoga, meditation, and chiropractors among U.S. children aged 4–17 years.* NCHS Data Brief, 324. National Center for Health Statistics.

Boduroglu, A., Shah, P., & Nisbett, R. E. (2009). Cultural differences in allocation of attention in visual information processing. *Journal of Cross-Cultural Psychology, 40*, 349–360.

Browning, M., Holmes, E. A., & Harmer, C. J. (2010). The modification of attentional bias to emotional information: A review of the techniques, mechanisms, and relevance to emotional disorders. *Cognitive, Affective, & Behavioral Neuroscience, 10*(1), 8–20.

Chase, L. E., Sapkota, R. P., Crafa, D., & Kirmayer, L. J. (2018). Culture and mental health in Nepal: An interdisciplinary scoping review. *Global Mental Health (Cambridge), 5*, e36.

Chiao, J. Y., & Blizinsky, K. D. (2010). Culture-gene coevolution of individualism-collectivism and the serotonin transporter gene (5-HTTLPR). *Proceedings of the Royal Society B: Biological Sciences, 277*(1681), 529–537.

Chiao, J. Y., Li, S.-C., Seligman, R., & Turner, R. (Eds.). (2016). *Oxford handbook of cultural neuroscience.* Oxford University Press.

Chiao, J. Y., Li, S.-C., Turner, R., Lee-Tauler, S. Y., & Pringle, B. A. (2017). Cultural neuroscience and global mental health: Addressing grand challenges. *Culture and Brain, 5*(1), 4–13.

Clark, J. (2014). Medicalization of global health 2: The medicalization of global mental health. *Glob Health Action, 7*, 24000.

Clarke, T. C., Barnes, P. M., Black, L. I., Stussman, B. J., & Nahin, R. L. (2018). *Use of yoga, meditation, and chiropractors among U.S. adults aged 18 and over.* NCHS Data Brief, 325. National Center for Health Statistics.

Di Lernia, D., Serino, S., & Riva, G. (2016). Pain in the body. Altered interoception in chronic pain conditions: A systematic review. *Neuroscience & Biobehavioral Reviews, 71*, 328–341.

Han, S., & Ma, Y. (2014). Cultural differences in human brain activity: A quantitative meta-analysis. *Neuroimage, 99*, 293–300.

Han, S., & Ma, Y. (2015). A culture-behavior-brain loop model of human development. *Trends in Cognitive Sciences, 19*(11), 666–676.

Harris, K., Spiegelhalder, K., Espie, C. A., MacMahon, K. M., Woods, H. C., & Kyle, S. D. (2015). Sleep-related attentional bias in insomnia: A state-of-the-science review. *Clinical Psychology Review, 42*, 16–27.

Hedden, T., Ketay, S., Aron, A., Markus, H. R., & Gabrieli, J. D. E. (2008). Cultural influences on neural substrates of attentional control. *Psychological Science, 19*, 12–17.

Hughes, A. M., Hirsch, C. R., Nikolaus, S., Chalder, T., Knoop, H., & Moss-Morris, R. (2018). Cross-cultural study of information processing biases in chronic fatigue syndrome: Comparison of Dutch and UK chronic fatigue patients. *International Journal of Behavioral Medicine, 25*(1), 49–54.

Hunt, J., Sullivan, G., Chavira, D. A., Stein, M. B., Craske, M. G., Golinelli, D., Roy-Byrne, P. P., & Sherbourne, C. D. (2013). Race and beliefs about mental health treatment among anxious primary care patients. *The Journal of Nervous and Mental Disease, 201*(3), 188–195.

Jimenez, D. E., Bartels, S. J., Cardenas, V., & Alegría, M. (2013). Stigmatizing attitudes toward mental illness among racial/ethnic older adults in primary care. *International Journal of Geriatric Psychiatry, 28*(10), 1061–1068.

Jimenez, D. E., Bartels, S. J., Cardenas, V., Dhaliwal, S. S., & Alegría, M. (2012). Cultural beliefs and mental health treatment preferences of ethnically diverse older adult consumers in primary care. *The American Journal of Geriatric Psychiatry, 20*(6), 533–542.

Kohrt, B. A., & Harper, I. (2008). Navigating diagnoses: Understanding mind-body relations, mental health, and stigma in Nepal. *Culture, Medicine and Psychiatry, 32*, 462–491.

Kramer, E. J., Kwong, K., Lee, E., & Chung, H. (2002). Cultural factors influencing the mental health of Asian Americans. *Western Journal of Medicine, 176*(4), 227–231.

Liddell, B. J., & Jobson, L. (2016). The impact of cultural differences in self-representation on the neural substrates of posttraumatic stress disorder. *European Journal of Psychotraumatology, 7*, 30464.

Ma-Kellams, C. (2014). Cross-cultural differences in somatic awareness and interoceptive accuracy: A review of the literature and directions for future research. *Frontiers in Psychology, 5*, 1379.

Markus, H. R., & Conner, A. C. (2014). *Clash! How to thrive in a multicultural world.* Penguin (Hudson Street Press).

Mrazek, A. J., Chiao, J. Y., Blizinsky, K. D., Lun, J., & Gelfand, M. J. (2013). The role of culture–gene coevolution in morality judgment: Examining the interplay between tightness–looseness and allelic variation of the serotonin transporter gene. *Culture and Brain, 1*(2–4), 100–117.

Nisbett, R. E. (2004). *The geography of thought: How Asians and Westerners think differently and why.* Free Press.

Nisbett, R. E., & Masuda, T. (2003). Culture and point of view. *Proceedings of the National Academy of Sciences, 100*(19), 11163–11170.

Pornpattananangkul, N., Hariri, A. R., Harada, T., Mano, Y., Komeda, H., Parrish, T. B., Sadato, N., Iidaka, T., & Chiao, J. Y. (2016). Cultural influences on neural basis of inhibitory control. *Neuroimage, 139*, 114–126.

Rusu, A. C., Gajsar, H., Schlüter, M. C., & Bremer, Y. I. (2018). Cognitive biases towards pain: Implications for a neurocognitive processing perspective in chronic pain and its interaction with depression. *The Clinical Journal of Pain,35*(3), 252–260.

Tang, Y. Y., & Posner, M. I. (2009). Attention training and attention state training. *Trends in cognitive sciences, 13*(5), 222–227.

Tang, Y., Zhang, W., Chen, K., Feng, S., Ji, Y., Shen, Ji, Y., Shen, J., Reiman, E. M., & Liu, Y. (2006). Arithmetic processing in the brain shaped by cultures. *Proceedings of the National Academy of Sciences, 103*(28), 10775–10780.

Tang, Y. Y. (2017). Rethinking future directions of the mindfulness field. *The neuroscience of mindfulness meditation: How the body and mind work together to change our behavior?* (pp. 83–91). Springer Nature.

Tang, Y. Y., Holzel, B., & Posner, M. I. (2015). The neuroscience of mindfulness meditation. *Nature Reviews Neuroscience, 16*(4), 213–225.

Tang, Y. Y., & Liu, Y. (2009). Numbers in the cultural brain. *Progress in Brain Research, 178,* 151–157.

U.S. Department of Health and Human Services (DHHS). (2001). *Mental health: Culture, race, and ethnicity— A supplement to mental health: A report of the Surgeon General.* U.S. Department of Health and Human Services, Substance Abuse and Mental Health Services Administration, Center for Mental Health Services.

Wilson, K. (2017). Health care costs 101: Spending rose with more coverage and care. https://www.chcf.org/publication/health-care-costs-101-spending-rose-with-more-coverage-and-care/

PART V

Awareness of Global Burden of Mental Health Disorders

Population Disparities in Mental Health

Joan Y. Chiao *and* Katherine D. Blizinsky

Abstract

Population disparities in mental health refer to the wide variation in the prevalence of mental, neurological, and substance use (MNS) disorders that result from unequal or unfair conditions across racial and ethnic groups. Mental health disparities of ethnic and racial groups suggest challenges and opportunities for research, policy, and action for cures, preventions, and interventions in global mental health. Due to mental health disparities across racial and ethnic groups, it is important to understand how cultural factors affect root causes and mechanisms of MNS disorders. Research in cultural neuroscience aims to investigate the etiology of MNS disorders across racial and ethnic groups. Advances in cultural neuroscience address a key priority for closing the gap in population health disparities. The amelioration of racial and ethnic disparities in mental health reflects the achievement of the goal for improvement of health equity in global mental health.

Key Words: population health disparities, health equity, cultural neuroscience, MNS disorders, global mental health

Introduction

Global mental health aims to improve health and health equity for all individuals, societies, and nations. Health disparities across racial and ethnic groups within and across nations reflect differences of health equity. The prevalence of mental, neurological, and substance use (MNS) disorders varies across nations (Collins et al., 2011; Patel et al., 2014) and within nations across racial and ethnic groups (Kessler & Ustün, 2008), and contributes to premature mortality and morbidity. Mental health is vital to the well-being of individuals and the growth of societies and nations. Mental health is an achievement of human development and human security for all people.

The 2012 World Health Organization World Mental Health Report highlighted the notion that health equity requires global research across nations (Collins et al., 2014). Research in cultural neuroscience examines the etiology of mental health and behavior across cultures. Evidence-based understanding of the cultural and biological factors that contribute to mental health is a necessary component of research in global mental health (Chiao et al., 2017). Research in cultural neuroscience and global mental health builds the culture of science that strengthens the capability for the discovery and delivery of health equity.

The goal of this chapter is to examine population disparities in mental health across racial and ethnic groups. First, the principles of global mental health illustrate the considerations in improvements to health equity. Second, a historical perspective articulates the rationale for the use of race and ethnicity in medicine and health policy. Third, a review of health disparities among racial and ethnic groups provides an evidence-based approach to understanding population-level differences in health equity. Fourth, theoretical approaches to health disparities among racial and ethnic groups postulate the causes and consequences of differences in health equity. Fifth, health issues of racial and ethnic groups provide a comprehensive analysis of the impact of historical, political, and social conditions of racial and ethnic groups on health equity. Finally, the need to address racial and ethnic disparities in mental health with the development and implementation of mental health research, policy, and programs across nations is discussed.

Global Mental Health

The Commission on Human Security reports that human security encompasses the protection of fundamental freedoms and protection from threats. Differences in mental health equity reflect concerns of human security and threat (Minas, 2014). Human security is obtained with protection from threats that reduce freedoms and capabilities, and empowerment that strengthens resilience, reduces vulnerabilities, and builds capability. Effective protection in human security includes the capability to facilitate the preparation of and recovery from natural and man-made threats. Threats reduce the quality of life and policy choices that are optimal for government and nongovernmental entities. Threats reduce the capability of individuals and groups to control events and circumstances around them.

Across nations, differences in capabilities for human security affect levels of human development. Human development illustrates the capability to protect from threats. Nations with the highest levels of human development[1] are the least likely to experience violent conflict. Political, economic, and social factors, such as the absence of competition for land, resources, and influence, are factors that reduce the likelihood for violent conflict. Natural disasters and climate change may cause loss of life and social and economic devastation. Recovery from conflict and disasters is procured with humanitarian responses of reconstruction and development.

---

[1] Human development refers to a composite index of the life expectancy, education, and income of nations.

Social and financial investment in regions of nations afflicted by conflict or disaster increases capabilities for effective governance and innovation in social systems that provide health, education, and other services. The economic growth of nations is an important protection from the threat of poverty and economic crises. Financial security from income and employment protects the well-being of populations. Permanent and temporary migration of people living outside their nation of origin may contribute to the capabilities of nations for social and economic growth.

Empowerment enhances human freedoms and fulfillment of potential with capabilities for human rights, good governance, education, and health care. Human rights ensure capabilities in equal access to education, work, and health care across nations. Good governance builds capabilities that protect from threats and fulfill freedoms. Education and health care are components of social systems that encourage human fulfillment and protect the dignity and well-being of all.

Research is an integral component of the development of nations. Research guides international and national health policy and health system strategies with evidence-based plans of action. The translation of international and national policies into social and cultural practices of the community demonstrates effective implementation of mental health programs. Community and economic development programs that perform within the social and cultural context achieve health equity. The achievement of health equity within and across nations represents the achievement of global objectives and partnership for equality and advancement in human development.

Historical Perspectives in Race, Ethnicity, and Health

The use of race and ethnicity in national health policy and health programs reflects the demographic characteristics of plural societies. Demographic changes in the population due to migration suggest the potential for changes in health status based on racial composition. International comparisons of health status reflect patterns of global health based on race and ethnicity defined by ancestral geographic origin.

The notions of race and ethnicity refer to categories of groups of people based on ancestral geographic origin and shared cultural traits such as identification with and commitment to the social practices and norms of the cultural group. The development of the conceptualization of race and ethnicity reflects the categorization of groups of people based on the rationale of biological and social construction (Smedley & Smedley, 2005). Race as a biological concept reflects the notion that people belong to a social group or a population based on geographic origin and biological inheritance. Early historical attempts to develop a classification system for the concepts of race and ethnicity suggest that while notions of race and ethnicity as based at least in part on biological inheritance are shared, the societal considerations in the use of race and ethnicity yield distinctions in favor of the social construction of race and ethnicity as social categories.

The historical distinction of classification systems for the notions of race and ethnicity across nations for demographic purposes illustrates the cultural and political aspects of the conceptualization. The designation of a race of people with the same biological inheritance may be different depending on their nationality. Shared cultural and ethnic heritage may similarly lead to different racial or ethnic classification based on nationality. The development and implementation of the notions of race and ethnicity across nations are guided by public policy and health programs.

The historical origin of the conceptualization of race and ethnicity as based in part on biological inheritance has led to the use of the notions of race and ethnicity in medicine and health policy. One of the rationales for the usage of race and ethnicity in medicine and health policy is that social categories may provide practical considerations for the prediction of risk factors and preventions that affect health and health behavior (LaVeist, 2005). The patterns in health behavior that characterize the social group may yield benefits in the identification of risk factors and preventions in health. Racial and ethnic disparities in health status reflect differences due to injustice or unfairness.

Health Disparities Among Racial and Ethnic Groups

Racial and ethnic disparities in health refer to differences in prevalence of health risk factors and disease. Racial and ethnic variation in mortality rates reflect the health status of racial and ethnic groups. The National Center for Health Statistics (NCHS) in the United States reports that the health status of all racial and ethnic groups has shown steady improvement in the 20th century (NCHS, 2003). Overall, mortality rates have demonstrated a steady decline across all racial and ethnic groups in the United States during this historical period. Lower rates of mortality across racial and ethnic groups reflect and strengthen effective protection in human security.

Racial and ethnic differences in health status may result from variation in morbidity or prevalence of health risk factors that contribute to mortality. Differences in morbidity rates across racial and ethnic groups reflect disparities in perceived physical and mental health status. Perceived health status serves as a predictor for future health outcomes and an indicator of the general health of a population. The perceived health status of racial and ethnic groups shows a pattern similar to the health status as defined by age-adjusted mortality rates. White and Asian populations in the United States demonstrate lower rates of poor perceived health than that of Black, American Indian, and Hispanic populations. The planned use of health services is predicted to be lower for White and Asian populations based on perceived health status.

While the health status across all ethnic and racial groups has steadily improved, racial and ethnic disparities in health risk factors and disease have persisted. Racial and ethnic health disparities reflect differences in unmet needs and societal burden of disease due to unequal and unfair treatment in health and health care (Williams et al., 1997). Disparities in health status across racial and ethnic groups illustrate the need for development and implementation of preventions and interventions in health behavior that improve the perceived and actual health status of all.

Mental Health Disparities Among Racial and Ethnic Groups

Mental health is the state of complete physical, mental, and social well-being of individuals and nations. Mental health is important to the development of societies and countries, reflecting the fulfillment of the goals for reduction of human suffering and improvement in quality of life. Health disparities across racial and ethnic groups reflect differences of health equity that may be ameliorated with improvements to human security, including protection from threat and protection for empowerment.

Racial and ethnic disparities in mental health refer to differences in the prevalence of MNS disorders across racial and ethnic groups. In the United States, Asian Americans and African Americans show lower prevalence of common mental disorders than White Americans (LaVeist, 2005; IOM, 2002). In international comparisons, cross-national prevalence of mental health disorders across geographic regions is similar to those of national comparisons of racial and ethnic groups within the United States (Kessler & Ustun, 2008). Nations in the African and Asian regions, such as Nigeria, China, and Japan, show the lowest prevalence of MNS disorders in the North and South American regions.

Disparities in mental health may arise due to differences in risk and protective factors across racial and ethnic groups. Racial and ethnic minorities demonstrate mental health despite exposure to risk factors. Racial and ethnic minorities may be more exposed to risk factors, such as racial discrimination, due to social factors, such as negative cultural attitudes and behaviors. On the other hand, racial and ethnic minorities are more likely to rely on protective factors, such as spirituality and family, as resources for coping with stressors. Social resources ameliorate the societal burden due to exposure to risk factors and contribute to the achievement of mental health for ethnic and racial minorities. Historical and contemporary periods of social and economic inequality contribute to racial and ethnic disparities in mental health. Racial and ethnic discrimination are one of the social factors affecting differences in prevalence of mental health disorders as well as access to and use of mental health care services.

Disparities in Health Care Across Racial and Ethnic Groups

Differences in the access to, use of, or quality of health care services across racial and ethnic groups represent a barrier to health equity. The Institute of Medicine (IOM) reported differences in quality of care among minorities and nonminorities in the United States (IOM, 2002). Nonminorities are more likely to receive better quality of care than racial minorities. Differences in quality of care result from health care disparities and health care dissimilarities. Health care dissimilarities refer to differences in quality of care due to the cultural preferences of the patient. Health care disparities refer to differences in quality of care due to injustice of the health care system or the behavior of health care providers. Racial and ethnic disparities in health care reflect social and economic inequality based on historical contexts. Processes of racial discrimination, including stereotyping and prejudice, contribute to differences in the access to, use of, or quality of health care among racial and ethnic groups.

Racial and ethnic groups differ in access to and use of health care. White Americans and Asian Americans are more likely to have health insurance and access to health services than American Indians, African Americans, and Hispanic Americans. White Americans and African Americans are also more likely to be satisfied with their quality of health care services than Hispanic Americans and Asian Americans. White Americans and Asian Americans are less likely to plan to use health care services due to greater levels of perceived health status.

Cultural competence contributes to differences in quality of health care among racial and ethnic groups. Cultural competence refers to awareness of attitudes and behaviors that enable effective social communication in cultural settings. Across racial and ethnic groups, patients who are race concordant with their provider report the highest level of satisfaction (LaVeist & Nuru-Jeter, 2002). White Americans represent a greater proportion of total providers than minorities within the nation. White Americans are more likely to receive health care services from providers who are of the same race or ethnicity than minorities. Differences in racial and ethnic distribution of the provider affect levels of race concordance and quality of health care.

Cultural competence enhances the quality of health care among racial and ethnic groups. White Americans report greater trust and less perceived discrimination in health care than minorities. Physicians are more likely to report negative cultural attitudes about African American than White American patients. Cultural competence due to race concordance contributes to levels of trust, perceived discrimination, and positive attitudes about racial and ethnic groups in health care. Greater equity in the racial and ethnic distribution of health care providers may lead to overall improvements in quality of health care for all.

The Role of Socioeconomic Status in Racial and Ethnic Disparities in Mental Health

Socioeconomic status (SES) contributes to the capabilities for mental health within and across nations. The alleviation of poverty is a focus of policy programs for human development. High- and middle- to low-income countries demonstrate varying levels of resources for the development and implementation of social systems that promote mental health. Across nations, communities with lower levels of poverty show the least vulnerability to mental health disorders.

In recent years, poverty rates have been in steady decline across all racial and ethnic groups in the United States. Differences among racial and ethnic groups in SES based on income and poverty are observed. Asian Americans and White Americans report higher median incomes and lower poverty rates than African Americans and Hispanics (U.S. Bureau of Census, 2002). Differences in poverty rates across racial and ethnic groups may reflect geographic variation in cost of living. Geographic regions with predominantly Asians or White Americans may yield a higher cost of living than those with predominantly African Americans and Hispanics.

Racial and ethnic group differences in SES are not primary contributors to disparities in health status among racial and ethnic groups. On the one hand, lower levels of exposure to risk factors in high-SES communities may enhance the health status of racial and ethnic groups. On the other hand, greater perceived health status may lead to higher SES across racial and ethnic groups. Nevertheless, levels of exposure to risk factors due to economic factors are unrelated to the health status of racial and ethnic groups across nations. Differences in economic factors are not a predictor of cross-national prevalence of anxiety and mood disorders across nations (Chiao & Blizinsky, 2010). Moreover, within the United States, irrespective of level of income, White Americans are more likely to report lower levels of poor perceived health status than African Americans and Hispanics. Thus, while racial and ethnic group differences in SES are observed, disparities in health status across racial and ethnic groups are not due to SES per se.

Health Issues of Racial and Ethnic Groups
African and African American Health

African mental health policy reflects the plan and action for development of African national mental health. Mental health policy in Nigeria consists of mandates for improvements in the mental health care system of the African nation. Research on African mental health in Nigeria represents a health policy initiative to identify the unmet needs and societal burden of disease due to mental health disorders. Large-scale epidemiological surveys reflect a social and financial investment in resources for national mental health in the African region.

Nations in the African region show lower prevalence of common mental disorders than other regions in the world, ranging from 6.0% to 16.7%. Nigeria exhibits the lowest prevalence of mental disorders in a 12-month period. Most of the proportion of disorders are considered mild in severity (74.7%) with minimal limitations. Use of mental health services in Nigeria in a 12-month period (1.6%) is lower than other developed nations. Knowledge of and attitudes about mental health are relatively limited across Africa (Gureje et al., 2005).

Mental health policy of South Africa is characterized as the reconstruction and development of the nation postapartheid. The African National Congress (ANC) generated a broad health care policy framework of legislation in the National Health Act of 2003 and Mental Health Act of 2002 to establish delivery of health care services in South Africa. Substantial investments in discovery and delivery science of mental health were made to address the unmet needs and societal burden of disease in the South African nation. The South African Stress and Health (SASH) study of the World Health Organization World Mental Health (WMH) Survey Initiative represents the first large-scale epidemiological survey of mental health in South Africa (Kessler et al., 2006).

The prevalence of common mental disorders in South Africa of 16.7% is higher than Nigeria and other nations in the world. The proportions of mental disorders considered mild (42.8%), moderate (31.5%), and serious (25.7%) in severity were relatively evenly distributed. Greater national prevalence of mental disorders in South Africa than other nations in Sub-Saharan Africa may be due to the political, social, and economic conditions of the nation.

Racial and ethnic disparities in mental health in South Africa reflect the impact of apartheid policy on health across provincial regions. Provinces with the greatest implementation of apartheid policy such as Free State (24.3%) show the greatest prevalence of mental health disorders, while those with the least implementation such as Eastern Cape (12.0%) show the least prevalence of mental health disorders (Kessler et al., 2006). Use of health services differs across racial and ethnic groups in South Africa. Whites (1.7%) exhibit greater use of health care than Coloreds (0.8%) and Indians (1.0%) in a 12-month period. Knowledge and attitudes of mental health vary across racial and ethnic groups in South Africa (Pretorius, 1995). Beliefs and conceptualization of mental health differ among Blacks and Whites. The notion of a distinction between physical and mental health may be more common for Whites than Blacks. Cultural competence affects the use and quality of health care in South Africa. Across both racial groups, Blacks and Whites prefer race concordance with their health provider.

National policies in the United States that protect racial equity arose from the civil rights movement with the Civil Rights Act of 1964 and the Voting Rights Act of 1965. Policies reducing exposure to risk factors, such as racial discrimination, enhanced conditions that promote health equity. The post–civil rights period in the United States reflects development of resources for health and health care of racial and ethnic minorities.

African Americans represent approximately 13% of the U.S. population and are one of the largest racial and ethnic groups in the nation. African Americans show lower prevalence of mood disorders than White Americans in the United States. Nevertheless, health care disparities reflect considerations of social and economic inequality in health issues for African Americans. Access to and use of health care services for African Americans depend on the availability of resources and cultural competence of providers. Levels of poverty and SES reflect the greatest risk factors to health and health care of African Americans in the United States. Improvements in financial security may strengthen resilience and reduce vulnerabilities for African Americans. Cultural competence is also a main contributor to quality of care. African Americans experience greater quality of care with race concordance of the provider. Health care and social systems that address the needs of social and economic equality promote mental health and human development for African

Americans. The achievement of health care equity for African Americans encourages human fulfillment and dignity for all.

American Indian and Alaska Native Health

American Indian and Alaska Native health policy is the result of development in the United States during the civil rights era to provide health care to Native Americans. The Bureau of Indian Affairs (BIA) and the Indian Health Service (IHS) in 1955 were established to provide health care to the American Indian population. The IHS provides health care insurance and services to Native Americans through tribal health programs and private health care providers.

American Indians and Alaska Natives are the indigenous people of North and South America and make up approximately 1.5% of the U.S. population. One of the greatest health issues for American Indians and Alaska Natives is unintentional injuries due to unmet needs of development. The age-adjusted mortality rate for American Indians related to unintentional injuries is higher than for other racial and ethnic groups. A mental health issue for the American Indian and Alaska Native population is substance abuse. American Indians and Alaska Natives exhibit greater prevalence of substance use disorder than other racial and ethnic groups in the United States. Mental health disparities result from social and economic inequality in the American Indian and Alaska Native population.

The health status of American Indians and Alaska Natives may be improved with development. Levels of poverty and SES are the greatest risk factors to improved health status for American Indians and Alaska Natives. Lower levels of exposure to environmental risk factors are a main consideration for health status. Greater social and financial investment in American Indian and Alaska Native communities may enhance health status. Another barrier in health status for American Indians and Alaska Natives is availability and access to quality health care due to language and culture. Cultural competence is a main consideration to quality health care for American Indians and Alaska Natives. Similar to other racial and ethnic groups, cultural competence in social communication in health care for American Indians and Alaska Natives may be enhanced with race concordance of the provider.

The mental capital of American Indians and Alaska Natives as an indigenous population may be considered a resource of resilience in health. Traditionalism as a cultural dimension is considered a protective factor bolstering resilience in health. Traditionalism includes the nurturance of spirituality and healing practices. American Indians and Alaska Natives benefit from traditional healing practices and experience fewer risk factors to mental health with the traditional medicine of their culture (Coe et al., 2004; P. K. Han et al., 1994). Cultural maintenance of positive attitudes toward traditional culture and identity and relations among groups reflects the strengthening of mental capital.

Asian and Pacific Islander Health

Asians make up more than 56% of the world's population. Asian and Pacific Islanders are a diverse population of ethnic groups including ancestry from China, Korea, Japan, Taiwan, and other Southeast Asian nations, as well as Native Hawaiians and other Pacific Islanders. Prevalence of mental health disorders is among the lowest in the Asian region. Nations in the Asian region, such as China (7.1%) and Japan (7.4%), show lower prevalence of mental disorders than other regions in the world. Most of the proportion of disorders are considered mild (41% to 54%) to moderate (32% to 45%) in severity. Knowledge of and attitudes about mental health are considerable in traditional medicine. Research in mental health is a component for the development of national mental health policy in the Asian region.

Asians and Pacific Islanders make up 4.2% of the U.S. population. The Asian and Pacific Islander population is considered to have one of the best health statuses across racial and ethnic groups in the United States, with fewer health risks and effective protective factors. Asians and Pacific Islanders are considered to have better perceived health status among racial and ethnic groups in the United States. The higher levels of perceived health status result in less planned use of health care.

Language and culture affect quality of health care for the Asian population. Asians utilize both traditional Asian and Western medicine practices, sometimes preferring traditional Asian medicine (Ngo-Metzger et al., 2003). Another factor affecting access to and use of quality health care is cultural competence. Consistent with White Americans, Asian Americans are more likely to be race concordant with their health provider. Asian Americans report greater levels of satisfaction with the quality of health care than other racial and ethnic groups due to race concordance (LaVeist & Nuru-Jeter, 2002).

Mental and social capital strengthen the health profile of the Asian and Pacific Islander population. Cultural factors impact the mental health of the Asian and Pacific Islander population. The East Asian cultural dimension of collectivism emphasizes harmonious social relations with others (Oyserman et al., 2002). Greater cultural collectivism is associated with improved mental health outcomes across nations (Chiao & Blizinsky, 2010). Cultural beliefs may also influence the use of and access to quality health care, including preference for traditional medicine and race concordance with the health provider (Yang & Benson, 2016). Cultural maintenance of positive attitudes about the traditions of the heritage culture and meaningful social relations with others act as protective factors of health for the Asian and Pacific Islander population.

Hispanic and Latino Health

Central and South American mental health policy reflects the plan and action of development and implementation of national health policy. Nations in the Central and South American region show higher prevalence of mental disorders than other regions in the world, ranging from 13.4% to 21.0%. Mexico shows the lowest prevalence of mental disorders of 13.4% in a 12-month period of the nations in the Central and South American region. Colombia exhibits a higher prevalence of mental disorders of 21% in a 12-month period than other nations in the Central and South American region. Most of the proportion of disorders are considered mild (21% to 36%) to moderate (34% to 41%) in severity. Research in mental health is a component for the development and implementation of mental health policy in the Central and South American region.

Hispanics and Latinos make up approximately 14% of the U.S. population and are considered one of the largest minority groups in the United States. The Hispanic and Latino population is diverse, including ancestry from Central and South America. Hispanics and Latinos in the United States are considered to have a perceived health status comparable to the American Indian and Alaska Native population. Language and culture are thought to affect quality of and access to health care for the Hispanic and Latino population. Lack of health insurance is a barrier to quality health care. Another factor in quality health care is cultural competence. The Hispanic and Latino population represents 14% of the U.S. population, but only 2% of health providers in the United States (Carrillo et al., 2001). The need for Hispanic and Latino health care providers in the United States affects race concordance and satisfaction with quality of health care for the Hispanic and Latino population.

Levels of poverty and SES of the Hispanic and Latino population are among the greatest risk factors in health status. However, the mortality rate of the Hispanic and Latino population is better than that of the non-Hispanic and Latino population. Despite the risk factors of poverty and SES, Hispanics and Latinos show a better health profile than non-Hispanics and non-Latinos in the United States.

Acculturation is thought to have considerable impact on the health of the Hispanic and Latino population. Cultural dimensions of Hispanic and Latino culture, such as *familismo* (family) and *respeto* (respect for elders), strengthen mental and social capital, serving as protective factors of health. Cultural maintenance of positive attitudes for the heritage culture and social relations among others may improve the capability of the Hispanic and Latino population to maintain a better health profile.

Theories of Health Disparities Across Racial and Ethnic Groups

Theories in cultural neuroscience contribute to evidence-based research on the study of cultural and biological factors underlying health disparities across racial and ethnic groups. Theoretical models in cultural neuroscience postulate that cultural and biological factors interacting with social and environmental exposures cause differences in health status across racial and ethnic groups. Health behavior may cause changes in health status through increased exposure to risk factors that change the quality of the social and physical environment in cultural settings. Racial and ethnic variation in the exposure to risk factors in the social and physical environment within cultural settings lead to differences in health outcomes. Differences in exposure to social or environmental health risks among racial and ethnic groups across cultural contexts contribute to differences in prevalence of disease and mortality across racial and ethnic groups.

Levels of exposure to social or environmental health risks among racial and ethnic groups may vary due to differences in patterns of health behavior of individuals across racial and ethnic groups that affect the quality of the social and physical environment in cultural settings. Cultural stereotypes of different racial and ethnic groups may contribute to patterns of behaviors that change levels of exposure to risk factors in the social and physical environment. Positive stereotypes toward a particular racial or ethnic group may lead to lower levels of exposure to risk factors, while negative stereotypes may contribute to higher levels of exposure to risk factors in the social and physical environment.

Positive stereotypes of racial and ethnic groups may improve access to community infrastructure that support health behavior, while negative stereotypes may generate barriers in access to community resources that support health behavior. Positive stereotypes of racial and ethnic groups may strengthen social and financial investment in community infrastructure that supports health behavior. By motivating cultural expectation and social investment in health behavior, positive stereotypes may serve as a prevention and intervention strategy for improving the health status of racial and ethnic groups. Positive stereotypes of racial and ethnic groups may lead to lower prevalence of disease and mortality by improving the quality of the social and physical environment.

Behavioral or psychological factors of the individual cause racial and ethnic disparities in mental health. Mental and social capital affect the capability of the individual to maintain mental health. Racial and ethnic variation in mental and social capital affect differences in health outcomes. Differences in the mental and social capital of racial and ethnic groups reflect differences in the social resources for coping with stressors. Exposure to racial discrimination is associated with negative mental and physical health outcomes. Individual coping resources such as positive cultural attitudes may reduce or alleviate the negative impact of psychological and physiological stressors on health.

The mental and social capital of racial and ethnic groups may differ due to historical considerations. Due to a history of settlement, the mental and social capital of immigrants and ethnocultural groups consists of attitudes and behaviors defined by cultural maintenance and social relations. Positive cultural attitudes lead to behaviors that integrate members of racial and ethnic groups. Integration of members of racial and ethnic groups may result in cultural benefits due to meaningful social interaction with members of other racial and ethnic groups. Negative cultural attitudes produce behaviors that marginalize members of racial and ethnic groups. Marginalization of members of racial and ethnic groups may lead to cultural losses due to social exclusion and racial discrimination.

Cultural factors that interact with genetic or biological processes cause health disparities across racial and ethnic groups. Interactions of genetics with culture and the environment modify exposure to risk factors and cause changes in the consequence of health behavior.

Racial and ethnic variation in genetic or biological processes and their interaction with socioenvironmental factors in cultural settings lead to differences in health outcomes.

Cultural factors that interact with biological or genetic differences among racial or ethnic groups may contribute to varying levels of disease susceptibility. Differences in the allelic frequency for specific genes across racial and ethnic groups may cause variation in prevalence of mental health disorders (Chiao & Blizinsky, 2013). Neurobiological differences in specific brain regions across racial and ethnic groups may cause behavior that leads to variation in prevalence of mental health disorders. Interactions of genes with cultural and environmental factors may cause varying levels of disease (Sasaki et al., 2016). Exposure to risk factors in the social and physical environment in cultural settings may increase genetic susceptibility to disease. Exposure to negative cultural attitudes in the social and physical environment may increase genetic susceptibility to negative health behavior (Cheon et al., 2014). Biological or genetic differences among racial or ethnic groups may result from genetic predispositions for health outcomes that enhance adaptation (Chen et al., 2016).

Research on Racial and Ethnic Disparities in Health

Research in cultural neuroscience provides programs of study on the cultural and biological factors underlying health disparities across racial and ethnic groups. Empirical evaluation of theoretical models in cultural neuroscience involves advancement of empirical paradigms and methodological tools for discovery in cultural neuroscience (Chiao & Ambady, 2007; S. Han & Northoff, 2008; Kim & Sasaki, 2014; Kitayama & Uskul, 2011; Park & Gutchess, 2002). Programs of study in cultural neuroscience investigate exposure to factors of risk and resilience in the social and physical environment that contribute to behavior across cultural contexts. Cultural differences in exposure to social or environmental health risks across racial and ethnic groups contribute to differences in prevalence of disease (Chiao & Blizinsky, 2010; Fincher et al., 2008) and mortality (Gelfand et al., 2011; Mrazek et al., 2013) across racial and ethnic groups.

Cultural maintenance of social attitudes affects risk and resilience in the social and physical environment to behavior. Positive social attitudes of the heritage culture and identity serve as a protective buffer reducing the negative impact of psychological and physiological health stressors (Mathur et al., 2012; Telzer et al., 2010). The amelioration of negative attitudes of other racial and ethnic groups also acts as a protective factor promoting meaningful social interaction with members of other racial and ethnic groups (Cunningham et al., 2003; Lieberman et al., 2005; Masten et al., 2011; Richeson et al., 2003; Telzer et al., 2013). Cultural maintenance of positive social attitudes about the heritage culture and identity as well as meaningful social interaction with other racial and ethnic groups promotes strategies of integration and multiculturalism in plural societies (Berry, 1997).

Cultural factors that interact with genetic or neurobiological processes cause health disparities among racial and ethnic groups. Interactions of cultural and genetic factors with the environment modify risk factors and consequences of health behavior (Sasaki et al., 2016). Cultural factors interact with genetic processes that affect health outcomes across racial and ethnic groups (Kim et al., 2010; Kim & Sasaki, 2012). Cultural factors that interact with biological differences among racial and ethnic groups contribute to varying levels of disease susceptibility. Cultural influences on neurobiological differences in specific brain regions across racial and ethnic groups affect behavior underlying variation in mental health (Chiao et al., 2008; Mathur et al., 2012; Telzer et al., 2010). Interaction of cultural and genetic factors with neurobiological mechanisms modifies risk factors and consequences of health behavior (Luo et al., 2015). Cultural acquisition alters neurobiological mechanisms of social learning (Losin et al., 2014; Telzer et al., 2013). Culture acts as a protective buffer of neurobiological differences during aging across racial and ethnic groups (Goh et al., 2007; Gutchess et al., 2010).

Addressing Racial and Ethnic Disparities in Health

Research on racial and ethnic disparities in health contributes to the development and implementation of mental health policy of nations. Racial and ethnic disparities in mental health illustrate the impact of cultural and biological factors on the etiology of mental health. One of the primary research priorities is the identification of the etiology of mental health disorders across cultures. Research in cultural neuroscience contributes to the identification of biomarkers of mental health across cultures. Discovery in cultural neuroscience contributes to the development and implementation of evidence-based strategies for effective delivery science in global mental health. Evidence-based approaches contribute to the setting of research priorities in cultural neuroscience and global mental health and the development of mental health research and policy that address racial and ethnic disparities in health.

Building capacity for research in cultural neuroscience and global mental health requires human resources. Social and financial investment in effective national research programs involves providing the infrastructure for conducting research. Effective research environments include intellectual and human resources for building capacity in research. Sustained research funding requires the cooperation of individuals, institutions, and nations to engage in program planning of research that guides policy and practice. The mental health research workforce is a necessary component to establish and implement international and national programs for research, education, and clinical work in cultural neuroscience and global mental health. Initiatives of targeted capacity development build research capabilities, while those of integrated capacity development include a training component for the mental health research workforce in development or research programs that strengthen mental health (Collins et al., 2014; Thornicroft et al., 2012).

Partnerships and networks in cultural neuroscience and global mental health develop platforms and collaborations for international and national research and education. International partnerships of institutional programs support individual research and education in cultural neuroscience and global mental health. International networks facilitate research collaborations and networks that provide opportunities for individuals, groups, teams, or organizations in the mental health research workforce to build research capacity. Global research networks may enhance cooperation in research priority settings to ensure that global priorities are developed and implemented in national, regional, and local research networks. Research priority setting of global research networks may further ensure the coordination and cooperation of funders, policymakers, and research communities in the development and implementation of evidence-based research, policy, and practice in global mental health.

Research in cultural neuroscience and global mental health contributes to the development and implementation of mental health policy that addresses racial and ethnic disparities in health. The development of national mental health policy across nations refers to policy instruments generated based on guidelines regarding key elements of mental health policy developed by the World Health Organization (WHO), country-specific experience, and evidence-based rationale of the epidemiology of mental disorders in the nation. The WHO mental health Gap Action Program (mhGAP) establishes guidelines for the implementation of national mental health services. Mental health policy development that addresses racial and ethnic disparities in health may be enhanced with consideration of priorities in health policy and other social systems, such as education, that improve mental health. Health policy that enhances quality health care and educational level across racial and ethnic groups improves health equity. Health policy that is developed within the cultural context to recognize the values, principles, and objectives of the local community promotes health diplomacy. National mental health policy implementation ensures the ownership and practice of health policy with the local country stakeholders. The coordination of national policy content with the standards of international policy ensures effective policy implementation across cultural settings. Building capacity for mental health policy through educational programs and regional networks is important for the effective implementation of delivery services and interventions in global mental health.

The achievement of health equity relies on the effective coordination, development, and implementation of international and national health policy across nations. Health policy protects the human right to equal access to health care and development that empowers communities. Health diplomacy ensures humanitarian responses of development and recovery after conflict and disaster. The development and implementation of research, practice, and policy that addresses racial and ethnic health disparities strengthens the human security necessary for the protection of freedoms and fulfillment of human potential for all.

Acknowledgments

Research reported in this publication was supported by the National Institutes of Health under award number R13DA33065 and R21NS074017-01A1 0. The content is solely the responsibility of the authors and does not necessarily represent the official views of the National Institutes of Health.

References

Berry, J. W. (1997). Immigration, acculturation and adaptation. *Applied Psychology*, *46*(1), 5–68.

Carrillo, J. E., Trevino, F. M., Betancourt, J. R., & Coustasse, A. (2001). Latino access to health care: The role of insurance, managed care, and institutional barriers. In M. Aguirre-Molina, C. Molina, & R. E. Zambrana (Eds.), *Health issues in the Latino community* (pp. 55–76). Jossey-Bass.

Chen, C., Moyzis, R. K., Lei, X., Chen, C., & Dong, Q. (2016). The enculturated genome: Molecular evidence for recent divergent evolution in human neurotransmitter genes. In J. Y. Chiao, S.-C. Li, R. Seligman, & R. Turner (Eds.), *The Oxford handbook of cultural neuroscience* (pp. 315–338). Oxford University Press.

Cheon, B. K., Livingston, R. W., Hong, Y. Y., & Chioa, J. Y. (2014). Gene x environment interaction on intergroup bias: The role of 5-HTTLPR and perceived outgroup threat. *Social Cognitive and Affective Neuroscience*, *9*(9), 1268–1275.

Chiao, J. Y., & Ambady, N. (2007). Cultural neuroscience: Parsing universality and diversity across levels of analysis. In S. Kitayama & D. Cohen (Eds.), *Handbook of cultural psychology* (pp. 237–254). Guilford Press.

Chiao, J. Y., & Blizinsky, K. D. (2010). Culture-gene coevolution of individualism-collectivism and the serotonin transporter gene (5-HTTLPR). *Proceedings of the Royal Society (Series B): Biological Sciences*, *277*(1681), 529–537.

Chiao, J. Y., & Blizinsky, K. D. (2013). Population disparities in mental health: Insights from cultural neuroscience. *American Journal of Public Health*, *103*(11), S122–S132.

Chiao, J. Y., Iidaka, T., Gordon, H. L., Nogawa, J., Bar, M., Aminoff, E., Sadato, N., & Ambady, N. (2008). Cultural specificity in amygdala response to fear faces. *Journal of Cognitive Neuroscience*, *20*(12), 2167–2174.

Chiao, J. Y., Li, S.-C., Turner, R., Lee-Tauler, S. Y., & Pringle, B. A. (2017). Cultural neuroscience and global mental health. *Culture and Brain*, *5*(1), 4–13.

Collins, P. Y., Patel, V., Joestl, S. S., March, D., Insel, T. R., Daar, A. S., Scientific Advisory Board and the Executive Committee of the Grand Challenges on Global Mental Health, Anderson, W., Dhansay, M. A., Phillips, A., Shurin, S., Walport, M., Ewart, W., Savill, S. J., Bordin, I. A., Costello, E. J., Durkin, M., Fairburn, C., Glass, R. I., . . . Stein, D. J. (2011). Grand challenges in global mental health. *Nature*, *475*(7354), 27–30.

Collins, P. Y., Tomlinson, M., Kakuma, R., Awuba, J., & Minas, H. (2014). Research priorities, capacity, and networks in global mental health. In V. Patel, H. Minas, A. Cohen, & M. J. Prince (Eds.), *Global mental health: Practices and principles* (pp. 423–449). Oxford University Press.

Coe, K., Attakai, A., Papenfuss, M., Giuliano, A., Martin, L., & Nuvayestewa, L. (2004). Traditionalism and its relationship to disease risk and protective behaviors of women living on the Hopi reservation. *Health Care for Women International*, *25*(5), 391–410.

Cunningham, W. A., Johnson, M. K., Gatenby, J. C., Gore, J. C., & Banaji, M. R. (2003). Neural components of social evaluation. *Journal of Personality and Social Psychology*, *85*(4), 639–649.

Fincher, C. L., Thornhill, R., Murray, D. R., & Schaller, M. (2008). Pathogen prevalence predicts human cross-cultural variability in individualism/collectivism. *Proceedings of the Royal Society B: Biological Sciences*, *275*, 1279–1285.

Gelfand, M. J., Raver, J. L., Nishii, L., Leslie, L. M., Lun, J., Lim, B. C., Duan, L., Almaliach, A., Ang, S., Arnadottir, J., Aycan, Z., Boehnke, K., Boski, P., Cabecinhas, R., Chan, D., Chhokar, J., D'Amato, A., Ferrer, M., Fischlmayer, I. C., . . . Yamaguchi, S. (2011). Differences between tight and loose cultures: A 33-nation study. *Science*, *332*(6033), 1100–1104.

Goh, J. O., Chee, M. W., Tan, J. C., Venkatraman, V., Hebrank, A., Leshikar, E. D., Jenkins, L., Sutton, B. P., Gutchess, A. H., & Park, D. C. (2007). Age and culture modulate object processing and object-scene binding in the ventral visual area. *Cognitive Affective and Behavioral Neuroscience*, *7*(1), 44–52.

Gureje, O., Lasebikan, V. O., Ephraim-Oluwanuga, O., Olley, B. O., & Kola, L. (2005). Community study of knowledge of and attitude to mental illness in Nigeria. *British Journal of Psychiatry, 186,* 436–441.

Gutchess, A. H., Hedden, T., Ketay, S., Aron, A., & Gabrieli, J. D. (2010). Neural differences in the processing of semantic relationships across cultures. *Social Cognitive and Affective Neuroscience, 5*(2–3), 254–263.

Han, P. K., Hagel, J., Welty, T. K., Ross, R., Leonardson, G., & Keckler, A. (1994). Cultural factors associated with health-risk behavior among the Cheyenne River Sioux. *American Indian/Alaska Native Mental Health Research, 5*(3), 15–29.

Han, S., & Northoff, G. (2008). Culture-sensitive neural substrates of human cognition: A transcultural neuroimaging approach. *Nature Reviews Neuroscience, 9*(8), 646–654.

Institute of Medicine (IOM). (2002). *Unequal treatment: Confronting racial and ethnic disparities of health care.* National Academies Press.

Kessler, R. C., Haro, J. M., Heeringa, S. G., Pennell, B. E., & Ustun, T. B. (2006). The World Health Organization World Mental Health Survey Initiative. *Epidemiologia e Psichiatria Sociale, 15,* 161–166.

Kessler, R. C., & Ustun, T. U. (Eds.). (2008). *The WHO World Mental Health Surveys: Global perspectives of mental disorders.* Cambridge University Press.

Kim, H. S., & Sasaki, J. Y. (2012). Emotion regulation: The interplay of culture and genes. *Social and Personality Psychology Compass, 6,* 865–877.

Kim, H. S., & Sasaki, J. Y. (2014). Cultural neuroscience: Biology of the mind in cultural context. *Annual Review of Psychology, 65,* 487–514.

Kim, H. S., Sherman, D. K., Sasaki, J. Y., Xu, J., Chu, T. Q., Ryu, C., Suh, E. M., Graham, K., & Taylor, S. E. (2010). Culture, distress, and oxytocin receptor polymorphism (OXTR) interact to influence emotional support seeking. *Proceedings of the National Academy of Sciences, 107*(36), 15717–15721.

Kitayama, S., & Uskul, A. K. (2011). Culture, mind, and the brain: Current evidence and future directions. *Annual Review of Psychology, 62,* 419–449.

LaVeist, T. A. (2005). *Minority populations and health: An introduction to health disparities in the United States.* Wiley.

LaVeist, T. A., & Nuru-Jeter, A. (2002). Is doctor-patient race concordance associated with greater satisfaction with care? *Journal of Health and Social Behavior, 43*(3), 296–306.

Lieberman, M. D., Hariri, A., Jarcho, J. M., Eisenberger, N. I., & Bookheimer, S. Y. (2005). An fMRI investigation of race-related amygdala activity in African-American and Caucasian-American individuals. *Nature Neuroscience, 8*(6), 720–722.

Losin, E. A., Cross, K. A., Iacoboni, M., & Dapretto, M. (2014). Neural processing of race during imitation: Self-similarity versus social status. *Human Brain Mapping, 35*(4), 1723–1739.

Luo, S., Ma, Y., Liu, Y., Li, B., Wang, C., Shi, Z., Li, X., Zhang, W., Rao, Y., & Han, S. (2015). Interaction between oxytocin receptor polymorphism and interdependent culture values on human empathy. *Social Cognitive and Affective Neuroscience, 10*(9), 1273–1281.

Masten, C. L., Telzer, E. H., & Eisenberger, N. I. (2011). An fMRI investigation of attributing negative social treatment to racial discrimination. *Journal of Cognitive Neuroscience, 23*(5), 1042–1051.

Mathur, V. A. Harada, T., & Chiao, J. Y. (2012). Racial identification modulates default network activity for same and other races. *Human Brain Mapping, 33*(8), 1883–1893.

Minas, H. (2014). Human security, complexity, and the mental health system development. In V. Patel, H. Minas, A. Cohen, & M. J. Prince (Eds.), *Global mental health: Principles and practice* (pp. 137–166). Oxford University Press.

Mrazek, A. J., Chiao, J. Y., Blizinsky, K. D., Lun, J., & Gelfand, M. J. (2013). The role of culture-gene coevolution in morality judgment: Examining the interplay between tightness-looseness and allelic variation of the serotonin transporter gene. *Culture and Brain, 1*(2–4), 100–117.

National Center for Health Statistics (NCHS). (2003). *Health, United States, 2003.* Centers for Disease Control and Prevention, U.S. Department of Health and Human Services.

Ngo-Metzger, Q., Massagli, M. P., Clarridge, B. R., Manocchia, M., Davis, R. B., Iezzoni, L. I., et al. (2003). Linguistic and cultural barriers to care. *Journal of General Internal Medicine, 18*(1), 44–52.

Oyserman, D., Coon, H. M., & Kemmelmeier, M. (2002). Rethinking individualism and collectivism: Evaluation and theoretical assumptions and meta-analyses. *Psychological Bulletin, 128*(1), 3–72.

Park, D. C., & Gutchess, A. H. (2002). Aging, cognition, and culture: A neuroscientific perspective. *Neuroscience and Biobehavioral Review, 26*(7), 859–867.

Patel, V., Minas, H., Cohen, A., & Prince, M. J. (2014). *Global mental health: Principles and practice*. Oxford University Press.

Pretorius, H. W. (1995). Mental disorders and disability across cultures: A view from South Africa. *Lancet, 345*, 534.

Richeson, J. A., Baird, A. A, Gordon, H. L., Heatherton, T. F., Wyland, C. L., Trawalter, S., & Shelton, J. N. (2003). An fMRI investigation of the impact of interracial contact on executive function. *Nature Neuroscience, 6*(12), 1323–1328.

Sasaki, J. Y., LeClair, J., West, A. L., & Kim, H. S. (2016). Application of the gene-culture interaction framework in health contexts. In J. Y. Chiao, S.-C. Li, R. Seligman, & R. Turner (Eds.), *The Oxford handbook of cultural neuroscience* (pp. 279–298). Oxford University Press.

Smedley, A., & Smedley, B. D. (2005). Race as biology is fiction, racism as a social problem is real: Anthropological and historical perspectives on the social construction of race. *American Psychologist, 60*(1), 16–26.

Telzer, E. H., Humphreys, K. L., Shapiro, M., & Tottenham, N. (2013). Amygdala sensitivity to race is not present in childhood but emerges over adolescence. *Journal of Cognitive Neuroscience, 25*(2), 234–244.

Telzer, E. H., Masten, C. L., Berkman, E. T., Lieberman, M. D., & Fuligni, A. J. (2010). Gaining while giving: An fMRI study of the rewards of family assistance among white and Latino youth. *Social Neuroscience, 5*(5–6), 508–518.

Thornicroft, G., Cooper, S., Bortel, T. V., Kakuma, R., & Lund, C. (2012). Capacity building in global mental health research. *Harvard Review of Psychiatry, 20*, 13–24.

U.S. Bureau of Census. (2002). Population by race and Hispanic or Latino origin for the United States. http://www.census.gov/population/cen2000/phc-t1/tab01.pdf

Williams, D. R., Yu, Y., Jackson, J. S., & Anderson, N. B. (1997). Racial differences in physical and mental health: Socioeconomic status, stress and discrimination. *Journal of Health Psychology, 2*(3), 335–351.

Yang, L. H., & Benson, J. M. (2016). The role of culture in population mental health: Prevalence of mental disorder among Asian and Asian American populations. In J. Y. Chiao, S. C. Li, R. Seligman, & R. Turner (Eds.), *Oxford handbook of cultural neuroscience* (pp. 339–354). Oxford University Press.

Stigma and Health Disparities

Diane-Jo Bart-Plange *and* Sophie Trawalter

Abstract

Members of many socially stigmatized and historically exploited groups are more likely to be ill, to be injured, and to die prematurely relative to members of socially privileged and historically advantaged groups. This is true in the United States and elsewhere. These disparities are often large, pervasive, and persistent, and constitute a public health crisis. Although pervasive, such large and pervasive disparities along lines of stigma are not obligatory. In the present chapter, we examine how stigma operates at the individual, interpersonal, and structural level to produce broad patterns of mental and physical health disparities. We then suggest some initial steps at the individual, interpersonal, and structural levels to reduce health disparities along the lines of stigma.

Key Words: Stigma, prejudice, discrimination, health, disparities, inequality

Members of many socially stigmatized and historically exploited groups are more likely to be ill, to be injured, and to die prematurely relative to members of socially privileged and historically advantaged groups. This is true in the United States and elsewhere. Indeed, such health disparities exist in at least 126 countries, representing over 90% of the world's population (see Penner et al., 2010). These disparities are often large, pervasive, and persistent, and constitute a public health crisis. Although pervasive, such large and pervasive disparities along lines of stigma are not obligatory. Stigma is socially constructed. It is an attribute *deemed* deeply discrediting, one that reduces someone "from a whole and usual person to a tainted, discounted one" (Goffman, 1963, p. 265). Of note, it is contextual; stigma is an attribute deemed deeply discrediting *in some particular social contexts and not others* (Crocker et al., 1998). Stigma is also system justifying; *it creates and maintains social hierarchies*. Stigmatization requires social, political, and economic capital; power to decide what attributes are good or bad, right or wrong, normal or abnormal; power to place and label people into groups and construct stereotypes about those groups; and power to not only disapprove but also reject, exclude, and discriminate against people from those groups (Link & Phelan, 2001). In the context of the United States, stigma along the lines of race, class, gender, gender identity, sexual identity, and other dimensions is rooted in a long history of white supremacy, patriarchy, and heteronormativity, and in a long history of power-based exploitation, violence, and oppression.

Here, we focus on stigma related to race and ethnicity as well as social class, sexual identity, weight, and substance abuse. We focus on these stigmas because they span many "types" of stigmas, as described by Goffman and others. We consider ways in which stigma operates at the structural, interpersonal, and individual levels to produce broad patterns of mental and physical health disparities; in other words, we adopt a socioecological framework that acknowledges that individuals are nested in social networks and contexts, nested in society with a particular history and set of cultural norms. We focus on the United States because such a framework requires attention to a specific historical and cultural context, and also because the bulk of the research on stigma, particularly in psychology, has been done in the context of the United States. Finally, we honor the critical race tradition in other fields—sociology, law, and others—and discuss disparities both in terms of interpersonal and *systemic* disadvantage and in terms of *privilege*. Our aim, then, is to shed light on the ways in which stigma produces and maintains health inequity.

Structural Level

Laws, policies, and institutional and cultural norms create and maintain societal hierarchies and disparities (Hatzenbuehler & Link, 2014; Link & Phelan, 2001). In this section, we focus on the social construction of health, how structural stigma impacts stigmatized groups, and how these systems are under the control of the powerful. We draw from Feagin, Link, Phelan, Hatzenbuehler, and others, and complement their analysis with psychological research when appropriate.

Health and Systems of Control

The majority of public health researchers, medical school faculty members, physicians, and other health care professionals are White (Feagin & Bennefield, 2014; U.S. Census Bureau, 2018). Outside of the health care context, predominantly White lawmakers write and pass legislation controlling access to and standards of health care and funding allocations for research pertaining to health. In other words, health care is very much under White control.

Perhaps not surprisingly, then, public health crises that predominantly affect people of color are often met with ineffective and punitive responses, or no response at all (Pomeranz, 2008). Consider, for instance, the response to the crack cocaine epidemic that ravaged Black and poor communities in the 1980s and 1990s. The crack cocaine epidemic was considered a threat to public safety and was met with a "War on Drugs" and "tough on crime" laws. The "tough on crime" Anti-Drug Abuse Act of 1986 included mandatory minimum sentences for the distribution of crack cocaine that were significantly harsher than those for powder cocaine, a drug associated with White Americans. A few years later in 1988, Congress extended this legislation; they increased punitive measures for even first-time-possession offenders and precluded drug offenders from receiving public housing and federal benefits (Alexander, 2012). It was not until the passing of the Fair

Sentencing Act of 2010 that the penalties for crack cocaine (vs. powder cocaine) were reduced (U.S. Sentencing Commission, 2015), but the damage had been done. These laws increased the disproportionate incarceration of poor, Black and Latino people and those with mental illness (Alexander, 2012; Hansen & Netherland, 2016). Notably, the more recent opioid epidemic, which has been largely seen as a "White problem," has been considered a public health crisis requiring public health solutions. In fact, in 2018, Congress passed the Support for Patients and Communities Act, making addiction treatment and education more accessible and providing federal funding for addiction and pain research.

The War on Drugs is not an isolated incident. Other laws and policies have promoted White health and undermined the health of people of color. For instance, a 2011 Alabama law precluding undocumented immigrants from using public services left many Latina immigrants feeling marginalized. Not only that, the law left these women and clinic staff unsure about health care eligibility requirements and ultimately decreased Latina immigrant women's access to care for themselves and their foreign-born children (White et al., 2014). The passing of SB 1070, "Supporting Our Law Enforcement and Safe Neighborhoods Act," in Arizona in 2010 had similar effects. This law allowed law enforcement officials with "reasonable suspicions of unlawful presence" to determine any individuals' immigration status during any lawful stops, detentions, or arrests. After its passing, Mexican-born and Mexican American families were less likely to use preventative health care and seek out public assistance (Toomey et al., 2014). SB 1070 and other policies targeting Latinx immigrants have also been shown to have negative effects on mental health among Latinx populations; they can lead to anxiety and depression, stress, and more days of poor mental health (Salas et al., 2013; Hatzenbuehler et al., 2017).

Outside the context of race and ethnicity, laws and policies can create and maintain health disparities between sexual majority and sexual minority groups. For example, in one study, researchers interviewed lesbian, gay, and bisexual (LGB) people in 2001 and in 2005, after several states banned same-sex marriage in 2004. Results showed that anxiety and mood disorders and alcohol use disorders increased significantly among LGB adults living in states that banned same-sex marriage. These disorders did not increase among LGB adults living in states without marriage bans (Hatzenbuehler et al., 2010). Similarly, other work has shown that state laws that fail to protect LGB people (e.g., from hate crimes or employment discrimination) and community-level anti-gay prejudice are associated with health disparities ranging from stress and anxiety-related disorders to cardiovascular disease, suicide, and mortality (Hatzenbuehler, 2018; Hatzenbuehler et al., 2009).

In some cases, it is not the presence of harsh and punitive laws but the absence of laws that set the stage for disparities. Although discrimination against higher-weight individuals is well documented in domains such as employment and health care, there are no federal laws making such discrimination illegal (Pomeranz & Puhl, 2013; Puhl et al., 2015). Individuals seeking legal redress for weight discrimination often must do so under the Americans With Disabilities Act. In other words, they must claim that their size is an impairment, a physiological disorder or condition. This legal avenue has been largely unsuccessful for plaintiffs claiming weight discrimination and has further pathologized weight. It allows the stigmatization of higher-weight people to remain acceptable (Pomeranz, 2008). Some proposed legislation has even tried to legalize weight discrimination; for example, Mississippi House Bill 282, a bill aimed at reducing obesity in the state, would have made it illegal for some restaurants to serve obese customers (Pomeranz, 2008).

Taken together, these examples illustrate how institutions and the powerful individuals within them stigmatize groups and individuals and create disparities through laws and policies.

Social Construction of Health

Institutions and the powerful individuals within them also define who is deemed healthy or unhealthy and who is capable of obtaining health (Burr, 2015). Often, this has meant pathologizing the behaviors of stigmatized people, thereby reinforcing their stigmatized status. Indeed, across history, pathologies have been imagined and reimagined to uphold social, political, and economic hierarchies with adverse consequences for the health of stigmatized people. Consider the following examples:

In the 18th and 19th centuries, physicians, scientists, and enslavers pathologized enslaved people's resistance to captivity. Prominent physicians and scientists conjectured diseases such as *drapetomania*, *rascality*, and *dysaesthesia aethiopica*, diseases that allegedly caused enslaved people to try to escape, commit petty offenses, and become lazy and indifferent to punishment (Willoughby, 2018). These so-called diseases were used to legitimize slavery as the right and natural state of the world.

In 1952, the first edition of the American Psychological Association *Diagnostic and Statistical Manual of Mental Disorders* (DSM) described homosexuality as a mental disorder, specifically, a "sociopathic personality disturbance." It was reclassified as sexual deviancy in 1968 (Drescher, 2015) before being dropped from the DSM in 1987. The formal pathologizing of sexual minorities legitimized the public's stigmatizing beliefs and treatment of sexual minorities, and likely biased health care professionals.

In 1992, the World Health Organization (WHO) established labels of underweight, normal, overweight, and obese, based on the body mass index (BMI; i.e., body weight in kilograms divided by height squared in meters; Nuttall, 2015). Today, BMI is the most utilized metric of obesity, used by the WHO and U.S. Centers for Disease Control and Prevention (CDC). This is despite growing knowledge that BMI does not distinguish between lean body mass and fat, leading to incorrect classifications and diagnoses (Bener et al., 2013; Nuttall, 2015). Misclassifications and misdiagnoses have clear negative health implications for individuals with higher BMIs, such as higher health insurance premiums (Carels et al., 2015; Pollitz & Rae, 2016). Psychologically, the mere classification of individuals into weight categories, regardless of actual size, has implications for health.

A recent study, for instance, found that labeling 10 year-old girls as "fat" increased their likelihood of becoming obese at age 19 (Hunger & Tomiyama, 2014).

More recently, the Personal Responsibility and Work Opportunity Act of 1996 (among other policies) arguably pathologized the poor. This act introduced new restrictions for welfare recipients. It capped benefits at 5 years, which effectively restricted access to health care. As a result, many had to seek out and receive a medical or psychiatric diagnosis to qualify for Social Security Insurance to retain or regain access to health care (Angell, 2011). This, in effect, medicalized support for the poor and further contributed to stereotypes of the poor as "disabled," "crazy," and "unworthy" (Hansen et al., 2014).

Taken together, these examples demonstrate how various institutions and the powerful individuals within them shape narratives of health. These narratives paint stigmatized groups and individuals as deviant and diseased and paint nonstigmatized groups and individuals as normal and healthy. As such, these narratives create barriers for stigmatized people to achieve health and, ultimately, maintain health disparities.

Medical Training

These social constructions and narratives of health have implications for health care professionals and their training. As an example, historically, medical education reinforced false notions that Black bodies are biologically different. From the early to mid-19th century until the mid-20th century, polygenism—the belief that different racial groups are different species, descending from separate ancestors—was popular among physicians and scientists (Keel, 2013; Willoughby, 2018). Medical textbooks and reports by prominent physicians claimed that relative to Whites, Africans had smaller brains, denser bones, and darker blood, were more capable of withstanding heat, pain, and disease, and they recommended different medical treatment based on patient race (Morton, 1842; Mustakeem, 2016; Willoughby, 2018). Although polygenism has long been discredited by modern research, many people still treat race as a biologically meaningful category. A case in point: a 2016 study found that medical students and residents who believe in biological differences between Black and White people (e.g., that Black people have less sensitive nerve endings; that Black people have denser bones) also believed that Black patients feel less pain and require less pain medication (Hoffman et al., 2016). Importantly, perceptions that Black people feel less pain do not appear to be related to modern-day racist attitudes (Druckman et al., 2018; cf. Mathur et al., 2014). Instead, many of the biological beliefs measured in the 2016 study can be directly traced to centuries-old beliefs that were used to justify slavery.

Outside the context of race, research suggests that medical training fails to provide adequate education about weight and nutrition (Stanford et al., 2015; Jay et al., 2010). A recent survey found that most medical schools do not provide the recommended 25 hours of nutrition education (Adams et al., 2015). Not surprisingly then, large percentages of physicians feel either moderately qualified or unqualified to treat higher-weight patients

(Block et al., 2003; Kristeller & Hoerr, 1997). At the institutional level, this lack of education and understanding may exacerbate negative attitudes toward individuals labeled as overweight and obese among health care professionals (Hebl & Xu, 2001; J. A. Lee & Pausé, 2016).

Segregation and Health

Outside of the health care context, racist government legislation and practices (e.g., slavery, Black Codes, Jim Crow laws, banking and housing policies such as redlining and restrictive covenants) and "White flight" from urban areas have led to residential segregation (Hatzenbuehler, 2017; Mehra et al., 2017; Williams & Collins, 2001). Segregation, in turn, has limited socioeconomic mobility and opportunity for Black Americans (Massey & Denton, 1993; Quillian, 2012). As of 2010, 28% of African Americans lived below the poverty line (Massey & Wagner, 2018), and one-third of Black people in metropolitan areas lived in hypersegregated areas (Massey & Tannen, 2015).

Segregation restricts access to basic resources and consequently, health. For example, Bower and colleagues examined census data and found that low-income and urban Black neighborhoods have severely restricted access to food (Bower et al., 2013). Moreover, studies have found that poor and marginalized communities often lack health care and mental health services (Dai, 2010; Dinwiddie et al., 2013; cf. Gaskin et al., 2012). Qato and colleagues, for instance, investigated pharmacy access in the city of Chicago from 2000 to 2012; they found that segregated Black and Hispanic (vs. White) communities had fewer pharmacies (Qato et al., 2014). These studies exemplify how obstacles in obtaining basic necessities (in these cases, food and medicine) are maintained through segregation. These barriers then have downstream consequences for health.

In fact, the links between poverty and poor health are well known (Ferguson et al., 2007; Garmezy, 1991; Graif et al., 2014; Ludwig et al., 2011; Rodriguez, 2018). What is perhaps less well known is that segregation amplifies the negative health effects of poverty. For example, Kershaw and colleagues (2011) have found that racial disparities in hypertension cases are the largest in highly segregated, low-poverty areas. More generally, segregation is linked to late-stage breast and lung cancer diagnoses, preterm birth and low birth weight, and higher mortality rates for Black Americans (Landrine et al., 2017; Mehra et al., 2017). For instance, Clarke and colleagues (2007), have found that both Pennsylvania and Virginia hospitals are highly segregated, and that hospitals in Virginia with a higher proportion of Black patients had higher mortality rates for surgical procedures and other medical conditions (e.g., pneumonia).

Although much of the research on the impact of segregation on health has focused on non-Hispanic populations, more recent studies have begun to examine how segregation affects Hispanic populations. Some of this research suggests that Hispanic people in the United States experience segregation as a result of housing discrimination but also immigration patterns; many immigrants move to immigrant enclaves for a shared cultural experience, economic reasons, and social support (Iceland & Scopilliti, 2008; Kershaw et al., 2013; Massey & Denton, 1987; see also Portes & Manning, 2012). Perhaps because of this, research on the relationship between residential segregation and health outcomes for Hispanics has been mixed. Some researchers have found that Hispanics living in segregated (vs. less segregated) areas are more likely to die of breast cancer (Haas et al., 2008; Pruitt et al., 2015). Other research suggests a more complex relationship between segregation and health among multiple Hispanic populations (Lee & Ferraro, 2007). For example, a recent study found a U-shaped relationship between segregation and self-reported health such that self-reported health of Latinxs decreased when segregation increased in low-segregation areas but increased when segregation increased in high-segregation areas (Plascak et al., 2016). More research on the association between segregation and health outcomes is clearly needed; this research will need to disaggregate data for specific Hispanic and Latinx subgroups and consider the causes and extent of the segregation they experience.

Environmental Injustice

The impact of residential segregation is compounded by inequitable access to public transportation. Indeed, survey data from multiple U.S. cities have found that lack of transportation is often a barrier to receiving necessary medical care for low-income patients (Ahmed et al., 2001) and Black and Hispanic patients (Guidry et al., 1997). Residential segregation and lack of public transportation set the stage for environmental racism, whereby people of color in poor communities are forced to live and stay in toxic environments.

Extant work has documented glaring racial disparities in lead exposure, air pollution, and proximity to toxic waste (Bravo et al., 2016; R. L. Jones et al., 2009; Mohai & Saha, 2015; Pirkle et al., 1998; Sampson & Winter, 2016). For example, Sampson and Winter used blood test data from 1995 to 2013 in Chicago to examine lead levels. They found that residents in Black neighborhoods had the highest levels, followed by residents in Hispanic neighborhoods; residents in predominantly White neighborhoods had the lowest levels. This continued to be true even after the city's efforts to reduce high levels of lead exposure, when lead levels decreased substantially over a decade (Sampson & Winter, 2016). A 2016 study similarly found that residents in highly segregated neighborhoods are exposed to more air pollution (Bravo et al., 2016). It has also found that Black people are much more likely to live near hazardous waste facilities (Chakraborty et al., 2011; Hunter et al., 2003; Saha & Mohai, 2005). In fact, a longitudinal study found that the number of low-income people of color in an area predicts where hazardous waste sites are located, challenging the idea that people of color simply move to geographical areas where hazardous sites are already located (Mohai & Saha, 2015). This study then suggests that disparities are a consequence not only of past policies and decisions but also of contemporary policies and choices.

These residential disparities are concerning given their adverse health effects. Indeed, several studies have found a relationship between segregation, pollution, and poor health including higher rates of asthma and even cancers (T. Hill et al., 2011; M. R. Jones et al., 2014; Rice et al., 2014). Other studies have shown that lead exposure impairs the mental and physical development of children (e.g., Banks et al., 1997). In fact, as recently as 2000, lead poisoning has been recognized as "a public health problem of global dimension," contributing to health disparities in the United States and elsewhere (Tong et al., 2000). Finally, several studies have shown that proximity to hazardous waste is associated with poor health including higher risk of asthma, cancers, developmental and skeletal abnormalities, and adverse birth outcomes (Fazzo et al., 2017).

Structural Level Summary

Laws, policies, and the institutional and cultural norms they engender, create, and maintain societal hierarchies and disparities. Inside of the health care context, laws, policies, and norms can effectually restrict health care access and pathologize stigmatized group members. Those same laws, policies, and norms also provide, and in some cases expand, health care access for advantaged group members and reinforce cultural narratives that benefit these groups. Narratives of health can also be transmitted in medical education and affect patient health. Outside of the health care context, segregation and environmental injustice are just two examples of how structural stigma affects health, leaving geographically isolated and marginalized groups—particularly poor and Black people—at greater risk.

Interpersonal Level

These structural factors, in turn, have downstream consequences for interpersonal interactions, both inside and outside the health care setting. Inside the health care setting, unequal access to health care, the social construction of health, and the demographics of health care professionals all have implications for patient–physician interactions and health. More generally, inside and outside of the health care setting, cultural narratives about who is valued and who is not have implications for intergroup interactions and health. Here, we draw on recent reviews by Major and colleagues (2013) and Penner and colleagues (2018) to highlight ways that interpersonal interactions—particularly interactions in which prejudice and discrimination are possible, likely, or certain—undermine the health of stigmatized individuals and not-privileged individuals. Where appropriate, we supplement these with newer work and work outside of psychology.

Inside of Health Care: Interactions With Health Care Providers

Disparities in health are at least partly driven by disparities in health care and, by extension, health care professionals. According to the 2016 National Healthcare Quality and Disparities Report published by the Agency for Healthcare Research and Quality (2017),

Black and Hispanic patients received worse care on about 40% of health care measures collected; low-income patients received worse care on more than 50% compared with high-income patients. There is also evidence that sexual minorities, substance users, and higher-weight patients receive lower-quality care (e.g., Elliott et al., 2015; Hebl & Xu, 2001; Phelan et al., 2015; van Boekel et al., 2013).

Health care professionals are privileged by virtue of their high-status profession and often by virtue of their other identities. Recall, for example, that a majority of health care professionals are White. In addition, health care professionals often hold negative attitudes and biases toward stigmatized people, much like the rest of the population. Extant research suggests that health care professionals are biased against patients of color (e.g., Green et al., 2007; van Ryn, 2002), higher-weight patients (e.g., Phelan et al., 2015; Schwartz et al., 2003; Teachman & Brownell, 2001), patients who struggle with substance abuse (e.g., Brener et al., 2010; van Boekel et al., 2013), poor patients (e.g., Boylston & O'Rourke, 2013; Smith-Campbell, 2005), and lesbian and gay patients (Burke et al., 2015; Sabin et al., 2015). These biases, in the context of health care, often lead to perceptions that stigmatized patients are bad patients—noncompliant, ignorant, and/or apathetic—and can affect patient health in at least two ways (Penner et al., 2018).

First, health care professionals' bias might affect treatment. And indeed, some evidence suggests that health care professionals' bias affects patient treatment directly. To our knowledge, the bulk of the evidence comes from work examining the impact of explicit (conscious) and/or implicit (less conscious) bias and treatment of Black patients, although some studies have examined the impact of implicit and/or explicit bias on treatment of patients from other stigmatized groups, such as higher-weight patients (e.g., Hebl & Xu, 2001, Persky & Eccleston, 2011). In one study, for instance, medical students believed that a Black (vs. White) patient at risk of human immunodeficiency virus (HIV) would be more likely to engage in sexually risky activities. In turn, they were less likely to prescribe the Black patient prophylactic antiretroviral drugs (Calabrese et al., 2014). In another study, pediatricians who had more negative stereotypes of Black (vs. White) patients were less likely to agree with prescribing pain medication for Black patients (Sabin & Greenwald, 2012). In both cases, then, explicit racial bias predicted bias in treatment (see also van Ryn et al., 2006). Research has also shown that implicit bias can predict treatment. For example, in one study, medical residents higher in implicit bias were less likely to recommend thrombolysis for a Black (vs. White) patient suffering from an acute coronary syndrome (Green et al., 2007). In another study, pediatricians higher in implicit bias were less likely to prescribe a narcotic for pain following surgery (Sabin & Greenwald, 2012). It is worth noting that other studies have not found significant associations between bias and treatment (e.g., Blair et al., 2014; Oliver et al., 2014; Sabin & Greenwald, 2012). And indeed, a systematic review published by Hall and colleagues (2015) suggests that implicit bias and health care outcomes are sometimes but not always related. In other words, results are mixed, suggesting that there might be boundary conditions to when implicit bias impacts treatment.

Second, health care professionals' bias might affect the tone and tenor of interactions with patients and have negative consequences. Here, the literature is robust and across stigmas. Indeed, that same systematic review by Hall and colleagues (2015) found quite strong and consistent evidence that health care providers' implicit bias is related to patient–provider interactions and health outcomes. For example, studies have shown that non-Black physicians higher in implicit racial bias are more likely to dominate the conversation with a Black (vs. White) patient (Hagiwara et al., 2013) and speak faster and end the visit sooner (Cooper et al., 2012). More generally, non-Black physicians higher in explicit racial bias say that they involve their Black patients less in medical decision making and are generally less warm toward their Black patients (Penner et al., 2010; see also Blair et al., 2013). In the context of weight bias, Persky and Eccleston (2011) found that medical students make less eye contact with an obese than nonobese virtual patient. In the context of substance use, van Boekel and colleagues' (2013) systematic review revealed that physicians take a more task-oriented, less person-centered approach to treating patients with substance use problems, resulting in reduced empathy toward these patients and less patient empowerment. These kinds of behaviors do not go unrecognized. Stigmatized individuals report feeling devalued and disrespected by health care professionals (e.g., Blair et al., 2013; Penner et al., 2013; Rintamaki et al., 2007).

The negative tone and tenor of these interactions have implications for patient behavior. Health care professionals' negative behavior can confirm stigmatized patients' suspicions of medicine and health care professionals. It can increase anxiety and mistrust (Cooper et al., 2012; Dovidio et al., 2008; Penner et al., 2010, 2014), making patients less comfortable revealing private information, less likely to ask questions, more likely to discount information from health care professionals, and ultimately less likely to adhere to recommendations by health care professionals (Burgess et al., 2010; Casagrande et al., 2007; Hagiwara et al., 2013; Kinsler et al., 2007; Thrasher et al., 2008). It can even lead to avoidance of health care in the future (Aldrich & Hackley, 2010; Drury & Louis, 2002; Fortenberry et al., 2002; Thompson et al., 2004).

Notably, work in economics suggests these strained interactions might have measurable impacts on patient health. In a study examining the impact of matching patient race to physician race, A. Hill and colleagues (2018) estimate that having a same-race physician can reduce mortality rates substantially. This study highlights, then, both the disadvantage of patients of color and privilege of White patients in a society where a majority of physicians are White.

Outside of Health Care: Interactions With Nonstigmatized Others and Identity Threat, Cognitive Load, and Stress

Research has shown that intergroup interactions—especially interactions in which prejudice and discrimination are possible, probable, or certain—can be threatening, cognitively depleting, and stressful. Here, we consider how these features of intergroup contact relate to health-related responses among stigmatized individuals.

Social identity threat and health behaviors. Extant work has shown that intergroup contact can be psychologically threatening. It can elicit concerns about being or becoming the target of prejudice, stereotypes, and/or discrimination (Major & Schmader, 2018; Steele et al., 2002). These concerns can lead to stress and, ultimately, negative outcomes. In one study by Guendelman and colleagues (2011), for instance, Asian American participants interacted with a White research assistant who either asked participants if they spoke English or did not ask this question (making the interaction discriminatory vs. not). Students were then asked to write down their favorite food. Students who had been asked if they spoke English were significantly more likely to list (less healthy) American food than (healthier) Asian food in order to reassert their American identity. In another study, Asian American participants again interacted with a White research assistant. Upon their arrival to the lab, the White assistant informed the participants that "actually, you have to be an American to be in this study" or did not say this. Next, participants were asked to order food from a food delivery website. Students who had been informed that the study was for Americans were more likely to choose (less healthy) American food than (healthier) Asian food in order to reassert their American identity. The authors of this work concluded that identity threat among Asian Americans can lead to less healthy eating (see also Inzlicht & Kang, 2010, for evidence that identity threat among women can also lead to unhealthy eating).

In the case of weight-based stigma, weight-based identity threat can lead to decreased self-efficacy and in turn, decreased healthy eating and exercising and decreased success with weight loss (Gudzune et al., 2014; Major et al., 2014; Pearl et al., 2015; Puhl et al., 2013; Wott & Carels, 2010). For example, in one study, self-perceived overweight women who were reminded of stigma felt less able to exert self-control and ate more calories compared with self-perceived overweight women who were not reminded of stigma (Major et al., 2014). In the case of substance use and smoking specifically, nonsmokers with lung cancer experience the worst outcomes if they fear others assume they are responsible for their disease, for fear of identity threat (Criswell et al., 2016). Across many stigmatized identities, being aware that one might be evaluated negatively because of a stigmatized identity and managing that stigmatized identity can have negative health-related consequences.

Cognitive load and healthy behaviors. Studies have also shown that intergroup contact—particularly interactions in which prejudice and discrimination are possible, likely, or certain—can exert a cognitive load (Johnson et al, 2011; Major et al., 2012;

Murphy et al., 2013; Richeson et al., 2005; Salvatore & Shelton, 2007; cf. Johnson et al., 2010). It can disrupt working memory capacity and undermine cognitive performance. In one study, for instance, Black participants exposed to prejudice—particularly subtle prejudice—were more cognitively depleted than were Black participants not exposed to prejudice; they performed more poorly on a Stroop task, a cognitive task used to measure response inhibition (Salvatore & Shelton, 2007).

Cognitive depletion, in turn, has been linked with a number of suboptimal behaviors and choices. In the context of health, it could be that depletion makes healthy choices more difficult. For example, a 30-day diary study of college students found that students felt more cognitively depleted on days they reported being mistreated and disrespected, an experience central to the experience of stigma. They also were more likely to binge drink on those days (DeHart et al., 2014). Likewise, studies by Major and colleagues suggest that stigma is depleting for higher-weight women and can lead to unhealthy behavior. In one study (Major et al., 2012), for example, higher-weight women gave a videotaped or audiotaped speech about dating and then completed a Stroop task. Results revealed that women in the videotaped condition, who presumably expected to be the target of stigma by virtue of being seen and not just heard, performed more poorly on the Stroop task. In a related study (Major et al., 2014), self-perceived overweight women who anticipated stigma (they read an article about discrimination against higher-weight individuals) ate more junk food compared with women who did not anticipate stigma. These data suggest that cognitive load associated with intergroup contact—and more specifically, stigma—can undermine response inhibition and, specifically, health behavior.

Stress and health. More generally, studies have shown that intergroup contact—particularly interactions in which prejudice and discrimination are possible, likely, or certain—can be quite stressful (e.g., Clark et al., 1999; Meyer, 1995; Meyer et al., 2008; Tomiyama, 2014). Studies have shown, for instance, that interracial interactions can trigger physiological stress responses, particularly among people of color concerned about being the target of prejudice and discrimination (Page-Gould et al., 2008). Likewise, interactions with peers who hold anti-fat attitudes can trigger physiological stress responses among higher-weight women (Hunger et al., 2018).

Over time, these stress responses can lead to disparities. Correlational research has shown that interpersonal discrimination—or at least self-reported interpersonal discrimination—is associated with unhealthy behaviors such as smoking, substance abuse, disordered eating, and risky sexual behavior, behaviors that can provide comfort and reduce stress in the short term but that have negative consequences for health in the longer term (e.g., Bariola et al., 2016; Brondolo et al., 2015; Puhl & Brownell, 2006; Sanders-Phillips et al., 2014; Terrell et al., 2006; Whitebeck et al., 2001; see Richman et al., 2018, for a review across stigmas). More generally, studies have shown that stigma and the stress associated with stigma are associated with poorer mental health and physical health (e.g., Amato & Zuo, 1992; Bogart et al., 2011; Frost et al., 2015; Mays et al., 2007; Schafer & Ferraro,

2011; Sutin et al., 2015; Whitbeck et al., 2002; Williams & Mohammed, 2009; again, see Richman et al., 2018, for a review across stigmas).

Here, two caveats are in order. First, the bulk of the evidence regarding the longer-term effects of stigma-related stress on health is correlational; experiences with stigma are most often measured, not manipulated. This means that the direction of causality is unclear. It could be that stigma-related stress leads to poor health outcomes. Alternatively, it could be that poor health leads to stigma and stigma-related stress, or that a third variable leads to both stigma-related stress and poor health. The experimental work—in which exposure to stigma is manipulated—converges nicely with the correlational research on stigma and health, however. It has shown that stigma induces stress (e.g., Hunger et al., 2018; Page-Gould et al., 2008). And research has shown that, over time, stress can "wear and tear" the body (McEwen, 1998). In fact, at least one analysis suggests that stress reactivity to in-lab stressors predicts later cardiovascular disease risk (Chida & Steptoe, 2010). There is thus good reason to think that momentary stress responses to stigma are related to longer-term, health-related physiological function and health outside of the lab.

A second caveat is that the bulk of the evidence regarding the health effects of stigma-related stress relies on self-reported stigma, not observed experiences of stigma. This may create some doubt as to whether it is merely the perception or anticipation of prejudice and discrimination that impacts health (even in the absence of actual prejudice and discrimination) or whether it is the "actual" experience of prejudice and discrimination that impacts health. Here, let us make three points. First, there is no doubt that prejudice and discrimination are real; large public opinion polls and careful audit studies have made this clear (e.g., Bertrand & Mullainathan, 2004; Neal, 2017). Second, as just noted, experiments in which prejudice and discrimination are manipulated and not measured show that "actual" experiences with prejudice and discrimination lead to increased stress and cognitive load (e.g., Hunger et al., 2018; Salvatore & Shelton, 2007). And third, research suggests that self-reported measures are valid and reliable (Krieger et al., 2005). If anything, some researchers believe self-reported measures *underestimate* the extent to which individuals experience prejudice and discrimination, and thus underestimate the impact of prejudice and discrimination on health (Krieger, 2012; Richman et al., 2018). Our assessment, then, is that the case that interpersonal stigma leads to stress and affects health is compelling, although we acknowledge that perceiving and/or anticipating prejudice and discrimination (even in the absence of actual prejudice and discrimination) might further undermine the health of stigmatized individuals (see Major & Schmader, 2018, for a recent discussion).

Outside of Health Care: Interactions With Stigmatized Others and Social Norms

Finally, extant work has shown that people are quite sensitive to the health behavior and health status of those around them. People are more likely to be obese and to smoke if they know others who are obese and who smoke (Christakis & Fowler, 2007, 2008).

People living in concentrated poverty are more likely to struggle and live in communities in which others struggle with substance use, obesity, and disease (Hannon & Cuddy, 2006; Ludwig et al., 2011; Piontak & Schulman, 2016; R. J. Sampson, 2012; Tamburlini & Cattaneo, 2007). Seeing close others struggle with health can make unhealthy behaviors and poor health itself not salient, even normative (e.g., Oyserman et al., 2014; Smith & Christakis, 2008). This is especially troubling given that health behavior and health status "cluster" socially and geographically due to segregation.

Interpersonal Level Summary

Taken together, these lines of work show that those who are stigmatized must contend with identity threat, cognitive load, and stress, which can make healthy choices more difficult. Independent of choices people make, intergroup interactions, particularly those characterized by prejudice and discrimination, are stressful. And over time, that stress can be damaging; it can "wear and tear" the body. These deleterious effects are compounded by the fact that health care providers are often biased against stigmatized individuals, sometimes resulting in substandard care and often resulting in more negative interactions between patients and health care providers. The latter can further undermine trust and compliance with health care professionals' recommendations. In other words, interpersonal interactions promote disparities along lines of stigma, disparities borne out of structural factors that are then amplified by interpersonal interactions.

These lines of work also reveal that those who are not stigmatized benefit from a very different reality. They receive better and friendlier care from health care professionals. They enjoy better rapport with their health care providers. More generally, their daily interactions are less likely to trigger identity threat, and although they surely have stressful and depleting interactions, these interactions are fewer. That is at least in part because nonstigmatized people have more control over their interactions with others. They can choose to interact mostly with other nonstigmatized people (e.g., Mallet et al., 2016. As such, their daily interactions are less likely to create a chronic state of stress that "wears and tears" on their bodies.

Individual Level

The structural and interpersonal dynamics of stigma also have implications for individual behavior. As already noted earlier, structural and interpersonal barriers can make it difficult to engage in healthy behavior; for example, cognitive depletion and stress can promote drinking, smoking, and other coping behaviors that provide comfort in the short term but undermine health in the longer term. In explaining health differences between stigmatized and privileged groups and individuals, some theories and studies have focused on individual behavior and the proximal, intrapsychic processes that guide such behavior. Here, we provide examples of this work as it relates to race and ethnicity, social class, weight, sexual identity, and substance use.

Identity and Unhealthy Habits

Stigmatized group members are more likely to engage in unhealthy behavior. Critically, data suggest that stigmatized group members are more likely to engage in such behavior if and when they are more highly identified with their group or if and when their group membership is more salient. The identity-based motivation theory provides one lens through which to understand these effects (Oyserman et al., 2014; see also Hackel et al., 2018). According to the theory, "people prefer to act and make sense of the world in ways that fit the identities that are on their mind." And indeed, studies have shown that low-income students and ethnic minority students perceive "eating healthy," "getting enough sleep," and "exercising" as things higher-income White people do and *not* things members of their own groups do. That is because stigmatized individuals often lack choice and control over their environment and the health choices they can make; this can lead stigmatized individuals to reason that making an effort to be healthier is pointless and "not for people like me" (Oyserman et al., 2014; Rivera, 2014). Moreover, studies have shown that priming stigmatized identity—making one's stigmatized identity salient—can undermine health behavior (Oyserman et al., 2014). In one study, for example, participants answered demographic questions (i.e., their race/ethnicity, social class status) either before or after rating the extent to which they agree with fatalistic statements such as "some people are healthy, others die young, that is just the way it is." Results revealed that students who answered the demographic questions first—for whom identity was made salient—were more fatalistic. In another study, participants answered demographic questions before or after answering questions about health, for example, questions about the benefits of exercise and the number of daily servings of each food group. Results revealed that students who answered demographic questions first—for whom identity was made salient—answered fewer questions correctly; they had less "access" to health-related information. Together, these studies suggest that identity salience, particularly if tied to unhealthy norms, could lead to less-healthy behavior. If true, this is especially concerning given that stigmatized identity often looms large and that stigmatized group members are often highly identified with their group (at least more identified than are nonstigmatized group members whose group membership and privilege are often invisible to them).

A literature on the internalization of stigma, also called self-stigma, suggests another way in which identity can become the source of unhealthy behavior (Rivera & Paredez, 2014; Vartanian & Novak, 2011). It suggests that endorsing stereotypes and negative attitudes toward one's own group undermines mental health and physical health. For example, in one study, Latinx participants who reported possessing more stereotypical characteristics—being lazy, poor, stupid, freeloading—were also more likely to be categorized as overweight and obese based on their BMIs (Rivera & Paredez, 2014). Moreover, this relationship was mediated by self-esteem. Rivera and Paredez (2014) argued that the internalization of stigma likely lowered participants' self-esteem, and that lowered self-esteem in turn impaired participants' ability to maintain a healthy weight. Similarly, work has shown that the internalizing of weight stigma is associated with negative outcomes including disordered eating, lower levels of exercise, and worse mental and physical health more generally (Latner et al., 2014; Pearl et al., 2015; Vartanian & Novak, 2011; Vartanian & Porter, 2016). Beyond internalized weight stigma, studies have found that the internalization of gender identity—and race-based stigma predicts poorer mental health (Fredriksen-Goldsen, 2016; Kuyper & Vanwesenbeeck, 2011; Meyer, 1995; Mouzon & McLean, 2017; Williams & Mohammed, 2009).

These two areas of research—on identity and internalization—suggest that stigmatized identity is associated with unhealthy behavior and that stigmatized identity salience can become the trigger—can become the "cause" of—unhealthy behavior. This work exemplifies how intrapsychic processes can undermine health behaviors and exacerbate health disparities.

Cognitive Depletion and Proximal Goals

Another literature suggests that stigmatized individuals often cope with stress, injury, and illness in unhealthy ways, perhaps due to self-control failure. This is perhaps most common in research trying to make sense of the psychology of substance use. In a widely cited article, for instance, Baumeister and Heatherton (1996) write, "Many patterns of self-regulation break down when people are under stress, presumably because the stress depletes their self-regulatory capacities. People become more emotional and irritable, they are more likely to increase smoking, break diets or overeat, abuse alcohol or other drugs, and so forth when under stress", p. 3. This analysis is consistent with some work in public health. Jackson and colleagues (2010) have found that stress can lead to unhealthy behaviors that can have protective mental health effects but that, in the long run, can contribute to existing health inequities between groups. Work by Pascoe and Richman (2011) showed that both participants who recalled incidents of discrimination more frequently and women facing gender discrimination in the form of non-merit based negative feedback were more likely to choose the unhealthier snack option, a candy bar, compared to the "healthier" granola bar. Discrimination is stressful and depletes cognitive resources, which in turn can contribute to unhealthy behavior (Cohen & Babey, 2012). Similarly, stressors associated with poverty such as uncertainty or instability in employment, food, and housing also increase cognitive burden, and this combined with less ability to purchase healthier food contributes to lower quality dietary choices (Laraia et al., 2017). This work suggests that stigmatized individuals might be prioritizing short-term gains over longer-term costs (see Shah et al., 2012). Focus on distal vs proximal goals is a privilege that many stigmatized individuals do not have, particularly in the face of immediate barriers, threats, and uncertainty. In this way, traditional notions of "self-control"—choosing long-term gains over short-term outcomes- do not always make sense. Individuals with socioeconomic stigma may focus on needs or outcomes that are short-term as a rational adaptation to an unstable environment, which can in turn have consequences for health

(Sheehy-Skeffington & Rea, 2017). Taken together, this work suggests that, in the face of stress, illness, or injury, stigmatized group members sometimes engage in "maladaptive" coping, perhaps because of self-control depletion or reasoned focus on proximal goals.

Underuse of Health Care Services and Distrust

Finally, research suggests that stigmatized group members often distrust the health care system and health care professionals; not surprisingly, then, they are less likely to seek out and use health care services (Ashton et al., 2003; Dovidio et al., 2008; Fingerhut & Abdou, 2017; Gornick et al., 1996; Gornick, 2000; Ostertag et al., 2006; Phelan et al., 2015; Schectman et al., 2008; Thompson et al., 2004; Trivedi & Ayanian, 2006). This distrust also affects stigmatized patients' behavior when they do seek out and use health care services. Work by Penner and colleagues (2016), for example, has shown that Black cancer patients who are less trusting of the health care system are less willing to cooperate with their physicians.

Individual Level Summary

Research on the individual level of analysis has shown that stigmatized individuals sometimes behave in unhealthy ways. And although these behaviors are often described as unhealthy *choices,* hinting at individual responsibility, it is clear from work on structural and interpersonal stigma why and how such behaviors might result. The effects of identity and internalized stigma can be tied to social norms and, in turn, segregation and narratives of health. The effects of self-control (or lack thereof) can be tied to cognitively depleting interactions, stigma-related stress, and a lack of access to resources. The effects of distrust can be tied to negative interactions with health care professionals and a history of harmful policies and systems of control. In other words, research on the individual level of analysis is perhaps best understood as revealing the downstream, intrapsychic consequences of interpersonal and structural stigma. Although not the focus, research focusing on the individual level of analysis also suggests that nonstigmatized individuals often behave in healthy ways. And again, although these behaviors can be described as choices, it is clear from the work on structural and interpersonal stigma how nonstigmatized individuals benefit from a different reality, one that makes healthy behavior easier and more attainable.

Cultural Neuroscience and Psychophysiology: Pathways From Systems to Individuals

Cultural neuroscience and psychophysiology have played an important role in establishing the pathways from structures and interactions to individuals. This research has shown that stigma impacts health-related systems; it heightens physiological responses—blood pressure, heart rate, cortisol reactivity, and immune response—that, over time, "wear and tear" the body. We think, however, that another and often underappreciated contribution is laying bare the ways is which stigma is biologized, the way in which stigma is made real and tangible, reified. Here, we draw on a recent review on neural and cardiovascular pathways by Derks and Scheepers (2018). We focus on research that has examined how stigmatized individuals respond to stigma (we do not include research on how nonstigmatized individuals respond to stigma-like conditions such as rejection).

Laboratory experiments have shown that intergroup contact and the prospect of stigma can activate health-related and, specifically, stress-related systems. It has shown that experiences with stigma, real or anticipated, are associated with neural activity linked to negative emotion processing and central to self-regulation and cardiovascular reactivity. For example, research has shown that identity threat is associated with heightened brain activation in areas of the anterior cingulate cortex (ACC) and dorsolateral prefrontal cortex (dlPFC), brain regions associated with negative emotion processing and regulation (Forbes & Leitner, 2014; Krendl et al., 2008). It is also associated with increased blood pressure (Blascovich et al., 2001; Eliezer et al., 2010; Major, et al., 2012) and inflammation (John-Henderson et al., 2014). Of note, some research suggests that subtle rather than blatant stigma can be more stressful (Merritt et al., 2006; cf. K. P. Jones et al., 2016; Salomon et al., 2015), perhaps because subtle bias is less easy to identity and resolve, and more cognitively taxing (Salvatore & Shelton, 2007).

In addition, studies have revealed correlations between stigma and stigma-related experiences outside of the laboratory and psychophysiology inside the laboratory. For instance, research has shown that students from a low socioeconomic status show increased physiological responses to social threats; specifically, they show increased amygdala reactivity to angry faces (Gianaros et al., 2008). And studies have shown that Latinx students who are chronically concerned about stigma exhibit heightened physiological responses—specifically, cortisol reactivity—during interracial contact with a White student during an in-lab encounter; those unconcerned about stigma do not exhibit this pattern of reactivity (Page-Gould et al., 2008; see also Clark, 2006). Taken together, these studies and studies like these suggest that stigma has measurable effects on physiology, both centrally (in the brain) and peripherally (in cardiovascular systems). Moreover, these patterns of physiological responses suggest that stigma increases vigilance for negative information while, at the same time, reducing one's ability to reduce stress. These findings are important given other work showing that stress reactivity, over time, can "wear and tear" the body (e.g., McEwen & Gianaros, 2010) and that stress reactivity in lab settings predicts later risk for cardiovascular disease (Chida & Steptoe, 2010).

Outside of the laboratory, research has shown that stigma is related to negative cardiovascular health and dysregulated diurnal cortisol rhythms over time. For example, in one study, high school students who reported more interpersonal discrimination on the basis of race, gender, weight, or age also exhibited dysregulated diurnal cortisol rhythms; specifically, they had flatter cortisol slopes across the day (Huynh et al., 2016). In another study, Mexican American teens had higher cortisol levels overall the more ethnic discrimination they reported (Zeiders et al., 2012). This is important because dysregulated cortisol rhythms have been linked to heart disease and diabetes (Chida & Steptoe, 2010) and poor mental health (Adam et al., 2010; Gunnar & Vazquez, 2001). In addition, other work has shown that prejudice and discrimination at work can be stressful and that work stress is associated with both heightened blood pressure and increased risk of hypertension (Din-Dzietham et al., 2004). This is important because hypertension is a major risk factor for cardiovascular disease. Finally, more recent work suggests that discrimination—or at least self-reported discrimination—might have epigenetic effects (Brody et al., 2016).

Taken together, these works lay bare the outcomes of stigma, in concrete, biological terms. They provide compelling evidence that stigma impacts individual health and wellness. At the same time, such evidence must be regarded with caution. As Jonathan Kahn (2017) warns, a focus on the biological manifestations of stigma can obscure interpersonal and structural stigma. It can make stigma seem natural, a "timeliness attribute of the human brain" devoid of historical context. It might give rise to technological and, in this case, biological solutions to stigma rather than societal, structural ones. Indeed, Kahn points to research showing that a drug used to reduce high blood pressure can also reduce implicit racial bias, and worries that, as a society, we might attempt to fix the ills of stigma and oppression through drug therapies rather than social change. In addition, because this work links stigma and stigmatized identities to biology, it can also reinforce notions that stigmatized individuals are biologically—fundamentally and essentially—different from nonstigmatized others. Previous work has theorized and shown that essentializing and biologizing race can be dangerous; it can increase prejudice, stereotyping, and discrimination (e.g., Allport et al., 1954; Haslam et al., 2006; Hoffman et al., 2016; Prentice & Miller, 2007).

Final Words

Extant work makes clear that stigma operates at the structural, interpersonal, and individual levels to create and maintain health disparities. More research is needed to better understand the impact of stigma—to understand the links between structural, interpersonal, and individual stigma and to understand how multiple stigmatized identities, in combinations, produce different patterns of inequity. More research is also needed to better understand the impact of stigma outside of the U.S. context; the bulk of the research and most of the research cited in the present chapter have been conducted in the United States. These calls for research have been made elsewhere and we refer interested readers to these important calls (e.g., Keusch et al., 2006; Major et al., 2018; Ngui et al., 2010). With respect to global health, Ngui and colleagues have made clear how the relative dearth of research on stigma and health across nations is problematic; they note, "Data limitations put mental health needs on the backburner for most policy makers and make it difficult for governments and international agencies to devote more resources to address mental disorders. Strategies, such as adding reliable mental health measures to ongoing population surveys (e.g. The Demographic Health Survey) can significantly improve availability of data for advocacy, programme planning and policy formation in many countries", p. 7. Here, we focus on potential solutions suggested by the existing research on the individual, interpersonal, and structural dynamics of stigma, focusing on the U.S. context. The extant work makes clear that reducing and eliminating disparities will require interventions at each level and, notably, will require interventions at the structural level.

At the individual level, research suggests that (a) framing healthy behaviors as identity congruent, (b) bolstering self-control, and/or (c) increasing trust of the health care system could help reduce disparities. These solutions at the individual level will require change at the interpersonal level, however. Here, the research suggests that interventions ought to (a) challenge unhealthy norms within stigmatized communities, perhaps by creating health-promoting identity-consistent messages; (b) improve interpersonal interactions, inside and outside of health care, by reducing bias, perhaps through intergroup contact (e.g., Pettigrew & Tropp, 2006); and (c) improve interpersonal interactions, inside and outside of health care, by decreasing the impact of bias on behavior, perhaps by promoting egalitarian social norms (e.g., Blanchard et al., 1994).

The structural section of this chapter puts interpersonal and individual level stigma into context, making clear that institutional and cultural changes are also necessary. Here, we propose actions necessary to reduce and eliminate structural stigma, drawing on the research and calls to action of others (e.g., Alexander, 2012; Asaria et al., 2016; Feagin & Bennefield, 2014; Zewde, 2018). Their works suggest that systems of control must change. Concretely, this means (a) broadening participation and representation of decision makers, (b) eliminating laws and policies that harm stigmatized groups, and (c) replacing them with laws and policies that protect vulnerable groups. What might those laws and policies look like? Others have suggested "baby bonds," universal health care, and universal basic income as potential policy solutions (Asaria et al., 2016; Forget, 2011; Veugelers & Yip, 2003; Zewde, 2018). More generally, policies should improve access to health and health care, and policies related to the labor market, education, and family welfare should aim not only to improve the common good but also to reduce social disparities (Wilkinson & Marmot, 2003).

In addition, reducing social disparities in health will require (d) changing medical education and (e) challenging social constructions of health. It will require broadening the representation and participation of underrepresented students, perhaps through "bridge" programs that help underrepresented students transition from college to medical school (Campbell et al., 2018). It will also require additional specialized training (e.g., more nutrition education to address weight bias and improve health care for higher-weight people) and additional cultural competency training (e.g., offering language and labels that do not reinforce stigmatizing attitudes such as "higher weight" instead of overweight; Meadows & Daníelsdóttir, 2016). Importantly, such training will need to focus students on social and historical determinants of health and make clear that race and other dimensions of stigma do not represent fixed biological categories (e.g., Metzl & Hansen, 2014). This is no trivial undertaking; research suggests that, at present, race is often discussed in biological terms in medical school curricula (Tsai et al., 2016).

Outside of the health care context, (f) segregation and environmental injustice must be eliminated. Clearly, this represents a gargantuan undertaking, but others have suggested first steps. These include aggressive enforcement of the Fair Housing Act by governmental agencies, re-establishing the President's Fair Housing Council, increasing funding for the Fair Housing Initiatives program and returning its control to knowledgeable and experienced fair housing organizations, and expanding access to credit for communities of color (Abedin et al., 2017). Eliminating segregation requires not only ending ongoing housing discrimination but also rectifying the damage caused by segregation. Many researchers, activists, and scholars have proposed reparations for slavery, Jim Crow, and continued racial discrimination (Coates, 2014; Feagin, 2004; Westley, 1998). Congressman John Conyers has repeatedly presented legislation to create a national congressional commission to create and carry out modes of reparation since 1989. Such a commission could be modeled after South Africa's Truth and Reconciliation Commission, which recommended community programs in education, health, and housing in addition to payments to victims and survivors of apartheid. This will not be easy. Reparations are widely unpopular among White Americans. For this reason, some scholars have proposed focusing on group programs such as job training programs and collective policies such as educational and housing policies aimed at reducing disparities rather than cash payments (e.g., Feagin, 2004).

To promote environmental justice, scholars, advocates, and policymakers have proposed laws prohibiting political suppression of Environmental Protection Agency research from the public (Shulman, 2004); increasing funding for environmental justice research; monitoring environmental toxins, toxic waste, and air pollution (National Environmental Justice Advisory Council, 2003); and using monitoring data in policy decisions. School settings offer a concrete example of what this might look like in practice. Currently, most states do not have laws that require an environmental assessment to build a school, and most states do not have laws that stop schools from being built near sources of toxic waste (N. Sampson, 2012). Such laws, however, could be implemented and enforced using monitoring data.

Ultimately, change at all of these levels—individual, interpersonal, and structural—will be necessary to reduce social disparities in health, in the United States, and around the globe (Link & Hatzenbuehler, 2016; Wilkinson & Marmot, 2003).

References

Abedin, S., Cloud, C., Goldberg, D., Rice, L., & Williams, M. (2017). *The case for fair housing: 2017 Fair housing trends report.* National Fair Housing Alliance.

Adam, E. K., Doane, L. D., Zinbarg, R. E., Mineka, S., Craske, M. G., & Griffith, J. W. (2010). Prospective prediction of major depressive disorder from cortisol awakening responses in adolescence. *Psychoneuroendocrinology, 35*, 921–931.

Adams, K. M., Butsch, W. S., & Kohlmeier, M. (2015). The state of nutrition education at US medical schools. *Journal of Biomedical Education, 2015*, 1–7.

Agency for Healthcare Research and Quality. (2017, July). *2016 National healthcare quality and disparities report.* AHRQ Pub. No. 17-0001.

Ahmed, S. M., Lemkau, J. P., Nealeigh, N., & Mann, B. (2001). Barriers to healthcare access in a non-elderly urban poor American population. *Health and Social Care in the Community, 9*, 445–453. doi:10.1046/j.1365-2524.2001.00318.x

Aldrich, T., & Hackley, B. (2010). The impact of obesity on gynecologic cancer screening: An integrative literature review. *Journal of Midwifery and Women's Health, 55*, 344–356.

Alexander, M. (2012). *The new Jim Crow: Mass incarceration in the age of colorblindness.* New Press.

Allport, G. W., Clark, K., & Pettigrew, T. (1954). *The nature of prejudice.* Addison-Wesley.

Amato, P. R., & Zuo, J. (1992). Rural poverty, urban poverty, and psychological well-being. *Sociological Quarterly, 33*, 229–240.

Angell, M. (2011). Illusions of psychiatry. *New York Review of Books.* July 14 http:// www.nybooks.com/articles/archives/2011/jul/14/illusions-of-psychiatry/? Page=1 Accessed 3.10.19.

Asaria, M., Ali, S., Doran, T., Ferguson, B., Fleetcroft, R., Goddard, M., Goldblatt, P., Laudicella, M., Raine, R., & Cookson, R. (2016). How a universal health system reduces inequalities: Lessons from England. *Journal of Epidemiology and Community Health, 70*, 637–643.

Ashton, C. M., Haidet, P., Paterniti, D. A., Collins, T. C., Gordon, H. S., O'Malley, K., Petersen, L. A., Sharf, B. F., Suarez-Almazor, M. E., Wray, N. P., & Street Jr., R. L. (2003). Racial and ethnic disparities in the use of health services: Bias, preferences, or poor communication? *Journal of General Internal Medicine, 18*, 146–152.

Banks, E. C., Ferretti, L. E., & Shucard, D. W. (1997). Effects of low level lead exposure on cognitive function in children: A review of behavioral, neuropsychological and biological evidence. *Neurotoxicology, 18*, 237–281.

Bariola, E., Lyons, A., & Leonard, W. (2016). Gender-specific health implications of minority stress among lesbians and gay men. *Australian and New Zealand Journal of Public Health, 40*, 506–512.

Baumeister, R. F., & Heatherton, T. F. (1996). Self-regulation failure: An overview. *Psychological Inquiry, 7*, 1–15.

Bener, A., Yousafzai, M. T., Darwish, S., Al-Hamaq, A. O., Nasralla, E. A., & Abdul-Ghani, M. (2013). Obesity index that better predict metabolic syndrome: Body mass index, waist circumference, waist hip ratio, or waist height ratio. *Journal of Obesity, 2013*, 1–9.

Bertrand, M., & Mullainathan, S. (2004). Are Emily and Greg more employable than Lakisha and Jamal? A field experiment on labor market discrimination. *American Economic Review, 94*, 991–1013.

Blair, I. V., Steiner, J. F., Fairclough, D. L., Hanratty, R., Price, D. W., Hirsh, H. K., . . . Havranek, E. P. (2013). Clinicians' implicit ethnic/racial bias and perceptions of care among Black and Latino patients. *Annals of Family Medicine, 11*, 43–52.

Blair, I. V., Steiner, J. F., Hanratty, R., Price, D. W., Fairclough, D. L., Daugherty, S. L., Bronsert, M., Magid, D. J., & Havranek, E. P. (2014). An investigation of associations between clinicians' ethnic or racial bias and hypertension treatment, medication adherence and blood pressure control. *Journal of General Internal Medicine, 29*, 987–995.

Blanchard, F. A., Crandall, C. S., Brigham, J. C., & Vaughn, L. A. (1994). Condemning and condoning racism: A social context approach to interracial settings. *Journal of Applied Psychology, 79*, 993–997.

Blascovich, J., Spencer, S. J., Quinn, D., & Steele, C. (2001). African Americans and high blood pressure: The role of stereotype threat. *Psychological Science, 12*, 225–229.

Block, J. P., Desalvo, K. B., & Fisher, W. P. (2003). Are physicians equipped to address the obesity epidemic? Knowledge and attitudes of internal medicine residents. *Preventive Medicine, 36*, 669–675.

Bogart, L. M., Wagner, G. J., Galvan, F. H., Landrine, H., Klein, D. J., & Sticklor, L. A. (2011). Perceived discrimination and mental health symptoms among Black men with HIV. *Cultural Diversity and Ethnic Minority Psychology, 17*, 295–302.

Bower, K. M., Thorpe, R. J., Rohde, C., & Gaskin, D. J. (2013). The intersection of neighborhood racial segregation, poverty, and urbanicity and its impact on food store availability in the United States. *Preventive Medicine, 58*, 33–39.

Boylston, M. T., & O'Rourke, R. (2013). Second-degree bachelor of science in nursing students' preconceived attitudes toward the homeless and poor: A pilot study. *Journal of Professional Nursing, 29*, 309–317.

Bravo, M. A., Anthopolos, R., Bell, M. L., & Miranda, M. L. (2016). Racial isolation and exposure to airborne particulate matter and ozone in understudied US populations: Environmental justice applications of downscaled numerical model output. *Environment International, 92–93*, 247–255.

Brener, L., Von Hippel, W., Von Hippel, C., Resnick, I., & Treloar, C. (2010). Perceptions of discriminatory treatment by staff as predictors of drug treatment completion: Utility of a mixed methods approach. *Drug and Alcohol Review, 29*, 491–497.

Brody, G. H., Miller, G. E., Yu, T., Beach, S. R., & Chen, E. (2016). Supportive family environments ameliorate the link between racial discrimination and epigenetic aging: A replication across two longitudinal cohorts. *Psychological Science, 27*, 530–541.

Brondolo, E., Monge, A., Agosta, J., Tobin, J. N., Cassells, A., Stanton, C., & Schwartz, J. (2015). Perceived ethnic discrimination and cigarette smoking: Examining the moderating effects of race/ethnicity and gender in a sample of Black and Latino urban adults. *Journal of Behavioral Medicine, 38*, 689–700.

Burgess, D. J., Warren, J., Phelan, S., Dovidio, J., & Van Ryn, M. (2010). Stereotype threat and health disparities: What medical educators and future physicians need to know. *Journal of General Internal Medicine, 25*, 169–177.

Burke, S. E., Dovidio, J. F., Przedworski, J. M., Hardeman, R. R., Perry, S. P., Phelan, S. M., Sean, M., Nelson, D. B., Burgess, D. J., Yeazel, M. W., & Van Ryn, M. (2015). Do contact and empathy mitigate bias against gay and lesbian people among heterosexual medical students? A report from Medical Student CHANGES. *Academic Medicine, 90*, 645–651.

Burr, V. (2015). *Social constructionism*. Routledge.

Calabrese, S. K., Earnshaw, V. A., Underhill, K., Hansen, N. B., & Dovidio, J. F. (2014). The impact of patient race on clinical decisions related to prescribing HIV pre-exposure prophylaxis (PrEP): Assumptions about sexual risk compensation and implications for access. *AIDS and Behavior, 18*, 226–240.

Campbell, K. M., Brownstein, N. C., Livingston, H., & Rodríguez, J. E. (2018). Improving underrepresented minority in medicine representation in medical school. *Southern Medical Journal, 111*, 203–208.

Carels, R. A., Rossi, J., Borushok, J., Taylor, M. B., Kiefner-Burmeister, A., Cross, N., Hinman, N., & Burmeister, J. M. (2015). Changes in weight bias and perceived employability following weight loss and gain. *Obesity Surgery, 25*, 568–570.

Casagrande, S. S., Gary, T. L., LaVeist, T. A., Gaskin, D. J., & Cooper, L. A. (2007). Perceived discrimination and adherence to medical care in a racially integrated community. *Journal of General Internal Medicine, 22*, 389–395.

Chakraborty, J., Maantay, J. A., & Brender, J. D. (2011). Disproportionate proximity to environmental health hazards: Methods, models, and measurement. *American Journal of Public Health, 101*(Suppl 1), S27–S36.

Chida, Y., & Steptoe, A. (2010). Greater cardiovascular responses to laboratory mental stress are associated with poor subsequent cardiovascular risk status: A meta-analysis of prospective evidence. *Hypertension, 55*, 1026–1032.

Christakis, N. A., & Fowler, J. H. (2007). The spread of obesity in a large social network over 32 years. *New England Journal of Medicine, 357*, 370–379.

Christakis, N. A., & Fowler, J. H. (2008). The collective dynamics of smoking in a large social network. *New England Journal of Medicine, 358*, 2249–2258.

Clark, R. (2006). Perceived racism and vascular reactivity in black college women: Moderating effects of seeking social support. *Health Psychology, 25*, 20–25.

Clark, R., Anderson, N. B., Clark, V. R., & Williams, D. R. (1999). Racism as a stressor for African Americans: A biopsychosocial model. *American Psychologist, 54*, 805–816.

Clarke, S. P., Davis, B. L., & Nailon, R. E. (2007). Racial Segregation and Differential Outcomes in Hospital Care. *Western Journal of Nursing Research, 29*, 739–757.

Coates, T. N. (2014, June). The case for reparations. *The Atlantic*, 54–71.

Cohen, D. A., & Babey, S. H. (2012). Contextual influences on eating behaviours: heuristic processing and dietary choices. *Obesity reviews: An official journal of the International Association for the Study of Obesity, 13*(9), 766–779.

Cooper, L. A., Roter, D. L., Carson, K. A., Beach, M. C., Sabin, J. A., Greenwald, A. G., & Inui, T. S. (2012). The associations of clinicians' implicit attitudes about race with medical visit communication and patient ratings of interpersonal care. *American Journal of Public Health, 102,* 979–987.

Criswell, K. R., Owen, J. E., Thornton, A. A., & Stanton, A. L. (2016). Personal responsibility, regret, and medical stigma among individuals living with lung cancer. *Journal of Behavioral Medicine, 39,* 241–253.

Crocker, J., Major, B., & Steele, C. (1998). Social stigma: The psychology of marked relationships. *Handbook of Social Psychology, 2,* 504–553.

Dai, D. (2010). Black residential segregation, disparities in spatial access to health care facilities, and late-stage breast cancer diagnosis in metropolitan Detroit. *Health & Place, 16,* 1038–1052.

DeHart, T., Longua Peterson, J., Richeson, J. A., & Hamilton, H. R. (2014). A diary study of daily perceived mistreatment and alcohol consumption in college students. *Basic and Applied Social Psychology, 36,* 443–451.

Derks, B., & Scheepers, D. (2018). Neural and cardiovascular pathways from stigma to suboptimal health. In Major, B., Dovidio, J. F., & Link, B. G. (Eds.), *The Oxford handbook of stigma, discrimination, and health* (pp. 85–104). Oxford University Press.

Din-Dzietham, R., Nembhard, W. N., Collins, R., & Davis, S. K. (2004). Perceived stress following race-based discrimination at work is associated with hypertension in African-Americans. The metro Atlanta heart disease study, 1999–2001. *Social Science & Medicine, 58,* 449–461.

Dinwiddie, G. Y., Gaskin, D. J., Chan, K. S., Norrington, J., & McCleary, R. (2013). Residential segregation, geographic proximity and type of services used: Evidence for racial/ethnic disparities in mental health. *Social Science & Medicine, 80,* 67–75.

Dovidio, J. F., Penner, L. A., Albrecht, T. L., Norton, W. E., Gaertner, S. L., & Shelton, J. N. (2008). Disparities and distrust: The implications of psychological processes for understanding racial disparities in health and health care. *Social Science and Medicine, 67,* 478–486.

Drescher, J. (2015). Out of DSM: Depathologizing homosexuality. *Behavioral Sciences, 5,* 565–575.

Druckman, J. N., Trawalter, S., Montes, I., Fredendall, A., Kanter, N., & Rubenstein, A. P. (2018). Racial bias in sport medical staff's perceptions of others' pain. *Journal of Social Psychology, 158,* 721–729.

Drury, C. A. A., & Louis, M. (2002). Exploring the association between body weight, stigma of obesity, and health care avoidance. *Journal of the American Academy of Nurse Practitioners, 14,* 554–561.

Eliezer, D., Major, B., & Mendes, W. B. (2010). The costs of caring: Gender identification increases threat following exposure to sexism. *Journal of Experimental Social Psychology, 46,* 159–165.

Elliott, M. N., Kanouse, D. E., Burkhart, Q., Abel, G. A., Lyratzopoulos, G., Beckett, M. K., Schuster, M. A., & Roland, M. (2015). Sexual minorities in England have poorer health and worse health care experiences: A national survey. *Journal of General Internal Medicine, 30,* 9–16.

Fazzo, L., Minichilli, F., Santoro, M., Ceccarini, A., Della Seta, M., Bianchi, F., Comba, P., & Martuzzi, M. (2017). Hazardous waste and health impact: A systematic review of the scientific literature. *Environmental Health, 16,* 107. doi:10.1186/s12940-017-0311-8

Feagin, J. (2004). Documenting the costs of slavery, segregation, and contemporary racism: Why reparations are in order for African Americans. *Harvard Black Letter Law Journal, 20,* 49–81.

Feagin, J., & Bennefield, Z. (2014). Systemic racism and U.S. healthcare. *Social Science Medicine, 103,* 7–14.

Ferguson, H., Bovaird, S., & Mueller, M. (2007). The impact of poverty on educational outcomes for children. *Paediatrics & Child Health, 12,* 701–706.

Fingerhut, A. W., & Abdou, C. M. (2017). The role of healthcare stereotype threat and social identity threat in LGB health disparities. *Journal of Social Issues, 73,* 493–507.

Forbes, C. E., & Leitner, J. B. (2014). Stereotype threat engenders neural attentional bias toward negative feedback to undermine performance. *Biological Psychology, 102,* 98–107.

Forget, E. L. (2011). The town with no poverty: The health effects of a Canadian guaranteed annual income field experiment. *Canadian Public Policy, 37,* 283–305.

Fortenberry, J. D., McFarlane, M., Bleakley, A., Bull, S., Fishbein, M., Grimley, D. M., Malotte, K. C., & Stoner, B. P. (2002). Relationships of stigma and shame to gonorrhea and HIV screening. *American Journal of Public Health, 92,* 378–381.

Fredriksen-Goldsen, K. I., Shiu, C., Bryan, A. E., Goldsen, J., & Kim, H. J. (2016). Health equity and aging of bisexual older adults: Pathways of risk and resilience. *Journals of Gerontology Series B: Psychological Sciences and Social Sciences, 72,* 468–478.

Frost, D. M., Lehavot, K., & Meyer, I. H. (2015). Minority stress and physical health among sexual minority individuals. *Journal of Behavioral Medicine, 38*, 1–8.

Garmezy, N., (1991). Resiliency and vulnerability to adverse developmental outcomes associated with poverty. *American Behavioral Scientist, 34*, 416–430.

Gaskin, D. J., Dinwiddie, G. Y., Chan, K. S., & McCleary, R. R. (2012). Residential segregation and the availability of primary care physicians. *Health Services Research, 47*, 2353–2376.

Gianaros, P. J., Horenstein, J. A., Hariri, A. R., Sheu, L. K., Manuck, S. B., Matthews, K. A., & Cohen, S. (2008). Potential neural embedding of parental social standing. *Social Cognitive and Affective Neuroscience, 3*, 91–96.

Goffman, E. (1963). *Stigma: Notes on a spoiled identity.* Jenkins, JH & Carpenter.

Gornick, M. E., Eggers, P. W., Reilly, T. W., Mentnech, R. M., Fitterman, L. K., Kucken, L. E., & Vladeck, B. C. (1996). Effects of race and income on mortality and use of services among Medicare beneficiaries. *New England Journal of Medicine, 335*, 791–799.

Gornick M. E. (2000). Disparities in Medicare services: potential causes, plausible explanations, and recommendations. *Health care financing review, 21*(4), 23–43.

Graif, C., Gladfelter, A. S., & Matthews, S. A. (2014). Urban poverty and neighborhood effects on crime: Incorporating spatial and network perspectives. *Sociology Compass, 8*, 1140–1155.

Green, A. R., Carney, D. R., Pallin, D. J., Ngo, L. H., Raymond, K. L., Iezzoni, L. I., & Banaji, M. R. (2007). Implicit bias among physicians and its prediction of thrombolysis decisions for black and white patients. *Journal of General Internal Medicine, 22*, 1231–1238.

Gudzune, K. A., Bennett, W. L., Cooper, L. A., & Bleich, S. N. (2014). Perceived judgment about weight can negatively influence weight loss: A cross-sectional study of overweight and obese patients. *Preventive Medicine, 62*, 103–107.

Guendelman, M. D., Cheryan, S., & Monin, B. (2011). Fitting in but getting fat: Identity threat and dietary choices among US immigrant groups. *Psychological Science, 22*, 959–967.

Guidry, J. J., Aday, L. A., Zhang, D., & Winn, R. J. (1997). Transportation as a barrier to cancer treatment. *Cancer Practice, 5*, 361–366.

Gunnar, M. R., & Vazquez, D. M. (2001). Low cortisol and a flattening of expected daytime rhythm: Potential indices of risk in human development. *Development and Psychopathology, 13*, 515–538.

Haas, J. S., Earle, C. C., Orav, J. E., Brawarsky, P., Keohane, M., Neville, B. A., & Williams, D. R. (2008). Racial segregation and disparities in breast cancer care and mortality. *Cancer, 113*, 2166–2172.

Hackel, L. M., Coppin, G., Wohl, M. J., & Van Bavel, J. J. (2018). From groups to grits: Social identity shapes evaluations of food pleasantness. *Journal of Experimental Social Psychology, 74*, 270–280.

Hagiwara, N., Penner, L. A., Gonzalez, R., Eggly, S., Dovidio, J. F., Gaertner, S. L., West, T., & Albrecht, T. L. (2013). Racial attitudes, physician-patient talk time ratio, and adherence in racially discordant medical interactions. *Social Science and Medicine, 87*, 123–131.

Hall, W. J., Chapman, M. V., Lee, K. M., Merino, Y. M., Thomas, T. W., Payne, B. K., Eng, E., Day, S. H., & Coyne-Beasley, T. (2015). Implicit racial/ethnic bias among health care professionals and its influence on health care outcomes: A systematic review. *American Journal of Public Health, 105*, e60–e76.

Hansen, H., Bourgois, P., & Drucker, E. (2014). Pathologizing poverty: New forms of diagnosis, disability, and structural stigma under welfare reform. *Social Science & Medicine, 103*, 76.

Hansen, H., & Netherland, J. (2016). Is the prescription opioid epidemic a white problem? *American Journal of Public Health, 106*, 2127–2129.

Haslam, N., Bastian, B., Bain, P., & Kashima, Y. (2006). Psychological essentialism, implicit theories, and intergroup relations. *Group Processes and Intergroup Relations, 9*, 63–76.

Hatzenbuehler, M. L. (2018). *Structural stigma and health.* In Major B., Dovidio, J. F. & Link, B. G. (Eds.), *The Oxford handbook of stigma, discrimination, and health* (pp. 105–121). Oxford University Press.

Hatzenbuehler, M. L., Keyes, K. M., & Hasin, D. S. (2009). State-level policies and psychiatric morbidity in lesbian, gay, and bisexual populations. *American Journal of Public Health, 99*(12), 2275–2281.

Hatzenbuehler, M. L., & Link, B. G. (2014). Introduction to the special issue on structural stigma and health. *Social Science and Medicine, 103*, 1–6.

Hatzenbuehler, M. L., McLaughlin, K. A., Keyes, K. M., & Hasin, D. S. (2010). The impact of institutional discrimination on psychiatric disorders in lesbian, gay, and bisexual populations: A prospective study. *American Journal of Public Health, 100*, 452–459.

Hatzenbuehler, M. L., Prins, S. J., Flake, M., Philbin, M., Frazer, M. S., Hagen, D., & Hirsch, J. (2017). Immigration policies and mental health morbidity among Latinos: A state-level analysis. *Social Science and Medicine, 174*, 169–178.

Hebl, M. R., & Xu, J. (2001). Weighing the care: Physicians' reactions to the size of a patient. *International Journal of Obesity, 25*, 1246–1252.

Hill, A., Jones, D., & Woodworth, L. (2018). A doctor like me: Physician-patient race-match and patient outcomes. Available at SSRN: https://ssrn.com/abstract=3211276 or http://dx.doi.org/10.2139/ssrn.3211276

Hill, T., Graham, L., & Divgi, V. (2011). Racial disparities in pediatric asthma: A review of the literature. *Current Allergy and Asthma Reports, 11*, 85–90.

Hoffman, K. M., Trawalter, S., Axt, J. R., & Oliver, M. N. (2016). Racial bias in pain assessment and treatment recommendations, and false beliefs about biological differences between blacks and whites. *Proceedings of the National Academy of Sciences, 113*, 4296–4301.

Hunger, J. M., Blodorn, A., Miller, C. T., & Major, B. (2018). The psychological and physiological effects of interacting with an anti-fat peer. *Body Image, 27*, 148–155.

Hunger, J. M., & Tomiyama, A. J. (2014) Weight labeling and obesity: A longitudinal study of girls aged 10 to 19 years. *JAMA Pediatrics, 168*, 579–580.

Hunter, L. M., White, M. J., Little, J. S., & Sutton, J. (2003). Environmental hazards, migration, and race. *Population & Environment, 25*, 23–39.

Huynh, V. W., Guan, S. S. A., Almeida, D. M., McCreath, H., & Fuligni, A. J. (2016). Everyday discrimination and diurnal cortisol during adolescence. *Hormones and Behavior, 80*, 76–81.

Iceland, J., & Scopilliti, M. (2008). Immigrant residential segregation in U.S. metropolitan areas, 1990–2000. *Demography, 45*, 79–94.

Inzlicht, M., & Kang, S. K. (2010). Stereotype threat spillover: How coping with threats to social identity affects aggression, eating, decision making, and attention. *Journal of Personality and Social Psychology, 99*, 467–481.

Jackson, J. S., Knight, K. M., & Rafferty, J. A. (2010). Race and unhealthy behaviors: Chronic stress, the HPA axis, and physical and mental health disparities over the life course. *American Journal of Public Health, 100*, 933–939.

Jay, M., Schlair, S., Caldwell, R., Kalet, A., Sherman, S., & Gillespie, C. (2010). From the patient's perspective: The impact of training on resident physician's obesity counseling. *Journal of General Internal Medicine, 25*, 415–422.

John-Henderson, N. A., Rheinschmidt, M. L., Mendoza-Denton, R., & Francis, D. D. (2014). Performance and inflammation outcomes are predicted by different facets of SES under stereotype threat. *Social Psychological and Personality Science, 5*, 301–309.

Johnson, S. E., Mitchell, M. A., Bean, M. G., Richeson, J. A., & Shelton, J. N. (2010). Gender moderates the self-regulatory consequences of suppressing emotional reactions to sexism. *Group Processes & Intergroup Relations, 13*, 215–226.

Johnson, S. E., Richeson, J. A., & Finkel, E. J. (2011). Middle class and marginal? Socioeconomic status, stigma, and self-regulation at an elite university. *Journal of Personality and Social Psychology, 100*, 838.

Jones, K. P., Peddie, C. I., Gilrane, V. L., King, E. B., & Gray, A. L. (2016). Not so subtle: A meta-analytic investigation of the correlates of subtle and overt discrimination. *Journal of Management, 42*, 1588–1613.

Jones, M. R., Diez-Roux, A. V., Hajat, A., Kershaw, K. N., O'Neill, M. S., Guallar, E., Post, W. S., Kaufman, J. D., & Navas-Acien, A. (2014). Race/ethnicity, residential segregation, and exposure to ambient air pollution: the Multi-Ethnic Study of Atherosclerosis (MESA). *American Journal of Public Health, 104*(11), 2130–2137.

Jones, R. L., Homa, D. M., Meyer, P. A., Brody, D. J., Caldwell, K. L., Pirkle, J. L., & Brown, M. J. (2009). Trends in blood lead levels and blood lead testing among U.S. children aged 1 to 5 years, 1988–2004. *Pediatrics, 123*, e376–e385.

Kahn, J. (2017). *Race on the brain: What implicit bias gets wrong about the struggle for racial justice.* Columbia University Press.

Keel, T. D. (2013). Religion, polygenism and the early science of human origins. *History of the Human Sciences, 26*, 3–32.

Kershaw, K. N., Albrecht, S. S., & Carnethon, M. R. (2013). Racial and ethnic residential segregation, the neighborhood socioeconomic environment, and obesity among Blacks and Mexican Americans. *American Journal of Epidemiology, 177*, 299–309.

Kershaw, K. N., Diez Roux, A. V., Burgard, S. A., Lisabeth, L. D., Mujahid, M. S., & Schulz, A. J. (2011). Metropolitan-level racial residential segregation and black-white disparities in hypertension. *American Journal of Epidemiology, 174*, 537–545.

Keusch, G. T., Wilentz, J., & Kleinman, A. (2006). Stigma and global health: Developing a research agenda. *The Lancet, 367*, 525–527.

Kinsler, J. J., Wong, M. D., Sayles, J. N., Davis, C., & Cunningham, W. E. (2007). The effect of perceived stigma from a health care provider on access to care among a low-income HIV-positive population. *AIDS Patient Care and STDs, 21*, 584–592.

Krendl, A. C., Richeson, J. A., Kelley, W. M., & Heatherton, T. F. (2008). The negative consequences of threat: A functional magnetic resonance imaging investigation of the neural mechanisms underlying women's underperformance in math. *Psychological Science, 19*, 168–175.

Krieger, N. (2012). Methods for the scientific study of discrimination and health: An ecosocial approach. *American Journal of Public Health, 102*, 936–944.

Krieger, N., Smith, K., Naishadham, D., Hartman, C., & Barbeau, E. M. (2005). Experiences of discrimination: Validity and reliability of a self-report measure for population health research on racism and health. *Social Science & Medicine, 61*, 1576–1596.

Kristeller, J., & Hoerr, R. (1997). Physician attitudes toward managing obesity: Differences among six specialty groups. *Prevention Medicine, 26*, 542–549.

Kuyper, L., & Vanwesenbeeck, I. (2011). Examining sexual health differences between lesbian, gay, bisexual, and heterosexual adults: The role of sociodemographics, sexual behavior characteristics, and minority stress. *Journal of Sex Research, 48*, 263–274.

Landrine, H., Corral, I., Joseph, G. L., Lee, J., Efird, J., Hall, M., & Bess, J. (2017). Residential segregation and racial cancer disparities: A systematic review. *Journal of Racial Ethnic Health Disparities, 4*, 1195–1205. doi:10.1007/s40615-016-0326-9

Laraia, B. A., Leak, T. A., Tester, J. M., Leung, C. W. (2017). Biobehavioral Factors That Shape Nutrition in Low-Income Populations: A Narrative Review. *American Journal of Preventive Medicine. 52*(2), S118–S126.

Latner, J. D., Barile, J. P., Durso, L. E., & O'Brien, K. S. (2014). Weight and health-related quality of life: The moderating role of weight discrimination and internalized weight bias. *Eating Behaviors, 15*, 586–590.

Lee, J. A., & Pausé, C. J. (2016). Stigma in practice: Barriers to health for fat women. *Frontiers in Psychology, 7*, 2063.

Lee, M.-A., & Ferraro, K. F. (2007). Neighborhood residential segregation and physical health among Hispanic Americans: Good, bad, or benign? *Journal of Health and Social Behavior, 48*, 131–148.

Link, B., & Hatzenbuehler, M. L. (2016). Stigma as an unrecognized determinant of population health: Research and policy implications. *Journal of Health Politics, Policy and Law, 41*, 653–673.

Link, B. G., & Phelan, J. C. (2001). Conceptualizing stigma. *Annual Review of Sociology, 27*, 363–385.

Ludwig, J., Sanbonmatsu, L., Gennetian, L., Adam, E., Duncan, G. J., Katz, L. F., Kessler, R. C., Kling, J. R., Lindau, S. T., Whitaker, R. C., & McDade, T. W. (2011). Neighborhoods, obesity, and diabetes—A randomized social experiment. *New England Journal of Medicine, 365*, 1509–1519.

Major, B., Dovidio, J. F., & Link, B. G. (2018). *The Oxford handbook of stigma, discrimination, and health.* Oxford University Press.

Major, B., Eliezer, D., & Rieck, H. (2012). The psychological weight of weight stigma. *Social Psychological and Personality Science, 3*, 651–658.

Major, B., Hunger, J. M., Bunyan, D. P., & Miller, C. T. (2014). The ironic effects of weight stigma. *Journal of Experimental Social Psychology, 51*, 74–80.

Major, B., Mendes, W. B., & Dovidio, J. F. (2013). Intergroup relations and health disparities: A social psychological perspective. *Health Psychology, 32*, 514.

Major, B., & Scmader, T. (2018). Stigma, social identity threat, and health. In Major, B., Dovidio, J. F., & Link, B. G. (Eds.), *The Oxford handbook of stigma, discrimination, and health* (pp. 85–104). Oxford University Press.

Massey, D. S., & Denton, N. A. (1993). *American apartheid: Segregation and the making of the underclass.* Harvard University Press.

Massey, D. S., & Tannen, J. (2015). A research note on trends in Black hypersegregation. *Demography, 52*, 1025–1034.

Massey, D. S., & Wagner, B. (2018). Segregation, stigma, and stratification: A biosocial model. In Major, B., Dovidio, J. F., & Link, B. G. (Eds.), *The Oxford handbook of stigma, discrimination, and health* (pp. 147–162). Oxford University Press.

Mathur, V. A., Richeson, J. A., Paice, J. A., Muzyka, M., & Chiao, J. Y. (2014). Racial bias in pain perception and response: Experimental examination of automatic and deliberate processes. *Journal of Pain, 15*, 476–484.

Mays, V. M., Cochran, S. D., & Barnes, N. W. (2007). Race, race-based discrimination, and health outcomes among African Americans. *Annual Review of Psychology, 58*, 201–225.

McEwen, B. S. (1998). Protective and damaging effects of stress mediators. *New England Journal of Medicine, 338*, 171–179.

McEwen, B. S., & Gianaros, P. J. (2010). Central role of the brain in stress and adaptation: Links to socioeconomic status, health, and disease. *Annals of the New York Academy of Sciences, 1186*, 190–222.

Meadows, A., & Daníelsdóttir, S. (2016). What's in a word? On weight stigma and terminology. *Frontiers in Psychology, 7*, 1527. doi:10.3389/fpsyg.2016.01527

Mehra, R., Boyd, L., & Ickovics, J. (2017). Racial residential segregation and adverse birth outcomes: A systematic review and meta-analysis. *Social Science & Medicine, 191*, 237–250.

Merritt, M. M., Bennett Jr., G. G., Williams, R. B., Edwards, C. L., & Sollers III, J. J. (2006). Perceived racism and cardiovascular reactivity and recovery to personally relevant stress. *Health Psychology, 25*, 364.

Metzl, J. M., & Hansen, H. (2014). Structural competency: Theorizing a new medical engagement with stigma and inequality. *Social Science & Medicine, 103*, 126–133.

Meyer, I. H. (1995). Minority stress and mental health in gay men. *Journal of Health and Social Behavior, 36*, 38–56.

Meyer, I. H., Schwartz, S., & Frost, D. M. (2008). Social patterning of stress and coping: Does disadvantaged social statuses confer more stress and fewer coping resources? *Social Science & Medicine, 67*, 368–379.

Mohai, P., & Saha, R. (2015). Which came first, people or pollution? Assessing the disparate siting and post-siting demographic change hypotheses of environmental injustice. *Environmental Research Letters, 2015*, 1–17.

Morton, S. G. (1842, November 1). Brief remarks on the diversities of the human species, and on some kindred subjects: Being an introductory lecture delivered before the class of Pennsylvania Medical College, in Philadelphia.

Mouzon, D. M., & McLean, J. S. (2017). Internalized racism and mental health among African-Americans, US-born Caribbean Blacks, and foreign-born Caribbean Blacks. *Ethnicity & Health, 22*, 36–48.

Murphy, M. C., Richeson, J. A., Shelton, J. N., Rheinschmidt, M. L., & Bergsieker, H. B. (2013). Cognitive costs of contemporary prejudice. *Group Processes & Intergroup Relations, 16*, 560–571.

Mustakeem, S. M. (2016). *Slavery at sea: Terror, sex, and sickness in the Middle Passage.* University of Illinois Press.

National Environmental Justice Advisory Council. (2003). *Advancing environmental justice through pollution prevention* (pp. 1–155).

Neal, S. (2017). *Views of racism as a major problem increase sharply, especially among Democrats.* Pew Research Center. http://www.pewresearch.org/fact-tank/2017/08/29/views-of-racism-as-a-major-problem-increase-sharply-especially-among-democrats/

Ngui, E. M., Khasakhala, L., Ndetei, D., & Roberts, L. W. (2010). Mental disorders, health inequalities and ethics: A global perspective. *International Review of Psychiatry, 22*, 235–244.

Nuttall, F. Q. (2015). Body mass index: Obesity, BMI, and health: A critical review. *Nutrition Today, 50*, 117–128.

Oliver, M. N., Wells, K. M., Joy-Gaba, J. A., Hawkins, C. B., & Nosek, B. A. (2014). Do physicians' implicit views of African Americans affect clinical decision making? *Journal of the American Board of Family Medicine, 27*, 177–188.

Ostertag, S., Wright, B. R., Broadhead, R. S., & Altice, F. L. (2006). Trust and other characteristics associated with health care utilization by injection drug users. *Journal of Drug Issues, 36*, 953–974.

Oyserman, D., Smith, G. C., & Elmore, K. (2014). Identity-based motivation: Implications for health and health disparities. *Journal of Social Issues, 70*, 206–225.

Page-Gould, E., Mendoza-Denton, R., & Tropp, L. R. (2008). With a little help from my cross-group friend: Reducing anxiety in intergroup contexts through cross-group friendship. *Journal of Personality and Social Psychology, 95*, 1080–1094.

Pascoe, E. A. & Richman, L. S. (2011) Effect of discrimination on food decisions. *Self and Identity, 10*(3), 396–406.

Pearl, R. L., Puhl, R. M., & Dovidio, J. F. (2015). Differential effects of weight bias experiences and internalization on exercise among women with overweight and obesity. *Journal of Health Psychology, 20*, 1626–1632.

Penner, L. A., Albrecht, T. L., Orom, H., Coleman, D. K., & Underwood III, W. (2010). Health and health care disparities. In J. F. Dovidio, M. Hewstone, & P. Glick, (Eds.), *The Sage handbook of prejudice, stereotyping and discrimination* (pp. 472–490). SAGE Publications Ltd.

Penner, L. A., Dovidio, J. F., Hagiwara, N., Foster, T., Albrecht, T. L., Chapman, R. A., & Eggly, S. (2016). An analysis of race-related attitudes and beliefs in black cancer patients: Implications for health care disparities. *Journal of Health Care for the Poor and Underserved, 27*, 1503–1520.

Penner, L. A., Gaertner, S., Dovidio, J. F., Hagiwara, N., Porcerelli, J., Markova, T., & Albrecht, T. L. (2013). A social psychological approach to improving the outcomes of racially discordant medical interactions. *Journal of General Internal Medicine, 28*, 1143–1149.

Penner, L. A., Phelan, S. M., Earnshaw, V., Albrecht, T. L., & Dovidio, J. F. (2018). Patient stigma, medical interactions, and health care disparities. In B. Major, J. F. Dovidio, & B. G. Link (Eds.), *The Oxford handbook of stigma, discrimination, and health* (pp. 183–218). Oxford University Press.

Persky, S., & Eccleston, C. P. (2011). Medical student bias and care recommendations for an obese versus non-obese virtual patient. *International Journal of Obesity, 35*, 728–735.

Pettigrew, T. F., & Tropp, L. R. (2006). A meta-analytic test of intergroup contact theory. *Journal of Personality and Social Psychology, 90*, 751–783.

Phelan, S. M., Burgess, D. J., Yeazel, M. W., Hellerstedt, W. L., Griffin, J. M., & van Ryn, M. (2015). Impact of weight bias and stigma on quality of care and outcomes for patients with obesity. *Obesity Reviews, 16*, 319–326.

Pirkle, J. L., Kaufmann, R. B., Brody, D. J., Hickman, T., Gunter, E. W., & Paschal, D. C. (1998). Exposure of the U.S. population to lead, 1991–1994. *Environmental Health Perspectives, 106*, 745–750.

Plascak, J. J., Molina, Y., Wu-Georges, S., Idris, A., & Thompson, B. (2016). Latino residential segregation and self-rated health among Latinos: Washington State Behavioral Risk Factor Surveillance System, 2012–2014. *Social Science & Medicine, 159*, 38–47.

Pollitz, K., & Rae, M. R. (2016). *Workplace wellness programs characteristics and requirements.* Henry J. Kaiser Family Foundation Issue Brief.

Pomeranz, J. L. (2008). A historical analysis of public health, the law, and stigmatized social groups: The need for both obesity and weight bias legislation. *Obesity, 16*, 93–102.

Pomeranz, J. L., & Puhl, R. M. (2013). New developments in the law for obesity discrimination protection. *Obesity, 21*(3), 469–471.

Portes, A., & Manning, R. D. (2012). The immigrant enclave: Theory and empirical examples. In *The urban sociology reader* (pp. 216–227). Routledge.

Prentice, D. A., & Miller, D. T. (2007). Psychological essentialism of human categories. *Current Directions in Psychological Science, 16*, 202–206.

Pruitt, S. L., Lee, S. J., Tiro, J. A., Xuan, L., Ruiz, J. M., & Inrig, S. (2015). Residential racial segregation and mortality among black, white, and Hispanic urban breast cancer patients in Texas, 1995 to 2009. *Cancer, 121*, 1845–1855.

Puhl, R., Peterson, J. L., & Luedicke, J. (2013). Fighting obesity or obese persons? Public perceptions of obesity-related health messages. *International Journal of Obesity, 37*, 774.

Puhl, R. M., & Brownell, K. D. (2006). Confronting and coping with weight stigma: An investigation of overweight and obese adults. *Obesity, 14*, 1802–1815.

Puhl, R. M., Latner, J. D., O'Brien, K. S., Luedicke, J., Danielsdottir, S., & Salas, X. R. (2015). Potential policies and laws to prohibit weight discrimination: Public views from 4 countries. *Milbank Quarterly, 93*, 691–731.

Qato, D. M., Daviglus, M. L., Wilder, J., Lee, T., Qato, D., & Lambert, B. (2014). Pharmacy deserts' are prevalent in Chicago's predominantly minority communities, raising medication access concerns. *Health Affairs, 33*, 1958–1965.

Quillian, L. (2012). Segregation and poverty concentration: The role of three segregations. *American Sociological Review, 77*(3), 354–379.

Rice, L. J., Jiang, C., Wilson, S. M., Burwell-Naney, K., Samantapudi, A., & Zhang, H., (2014). Use of segregation indices, Townsend index, and air toxics data to assess lifetime cancer risk disparities in metropolitan

Charleston, South Carolina, USA. *International Journal Environmental Research and Public Health, 11,* 5510–5526.

Richeson, J. A., Trawalter, S., & Shelton, J. N. (2005). African Americans' implicit racial attitudes and the depletion of executive function after interracial interactions. *Social Cognition, 23,* 336–352.

Richman, L. S., Pascoe, E., & Lattanner, M. (2018). Interpersonal discrimination and physical health. In B. Major, J. F. Dovidio, & B. G. Link (Eds.), *The Oxford handbook of stigma, discrimination, and health* (pp. 203–218). Oxford University Press.

Rintamaki, L. S., Scott, A. M., Kosenko, K. A., & Jensen, R. E. (2007). Male patient perceptions of HIV stigma in health care contexts. *AIDS Patient Care and STDs, 21,* 956–969.

Rivera, L. M. (2014). Ethnic-racial stigma and health disparities: From psychological theory and evidence to public policy solutions. *Journal of Social Issues, 70,* 198–205.

Rivera, L. M., & Paredez, S. M. (2014). Stereotypes can "get under the skin": Testing a self-stereotyping and psychological resource model of overweight and obesity. *Journal of Social Issues, 70,* 226–240.

Rodriguez, J. (2018). Health disparities, politics, and the maintenance of the status quo: A new theory of inequality. *Social Science and Medicine, 200,* 36–43.

Sabin, J. A., & Greenwald, A. G. (2012). The influence of implicit bias on treatment recommendations for 4 common pediatric conditions: Pain, urinary tract infection, attention deficit hyperactivity disorder, and asthma. *American Journal of Public Health, 102,* 988–995.

Sabin, J. A., Riskind, R. G., & Nosek, B. A. (2015). Health care providers' implicit and explicit attitudes toward lesbian women and gay men. *American Journal of Public Health, 105*(9), 1831–1841.

Saha, R., & Mohai, P. (2005). Historical context and hazardous waste facility siting: Understanding temporal patterns in Michigan. *Social Problems, 42,* 618–642.

Salas, L. M., Ayón, C., & Gurrola, M. (2013). Estamos traumados: The effect of anti-immigrant sentiment and policies on the mental health of Mexican immigrant families. *Journal of Community Psychology, 41,* 1005–1020. https://doi.org/10.1002/jcop.21589

Salomon, K., Burgess, K. D., & Bosson, J. K. (2015). Flash fire and slow burn: Women's cardiovascular reactivity and recovery following hostile and benevolent sexism. *Journal of Experimental Psychology: General, 144,* 469.

Salvatore, J., & Shelton, J. N. (2007). Cognitive costs of exposure to racial prejudice. *Psychological Science, 18,* 810–815.

Sampson, R. J., & Winter, A. (2016). The racial ecology of lead poisoning: Toxic inequality in Chicago neighborhoods, 1995-2013. *DuBois Review: Social Science Research on Race, 13*(2), 261–283.

Sampson, N. (2012). Environmental justice at school: Understanding research, policy, and practice to improve our children's health. *Journal of School Health, 82*(5), 246–252.

Sampson, R. J. (2012). *Great American city: Chicago and the enduring neighborhood effect.* University of Chicago Press.

Sanders-Phillips, K., Kliewer, W., Tirmazi, T., Nebbitt, V., Carter, T., & Key, H. (2014). Perceived racial discrimination, drug use, and psychological distress in African American youth: A pathway to child health disparities. *Journal of Social Issues, 70,* 279–297.

Schafer, M. H., & Ferraro, K. F. (2011). The stigma of obesity: Does perceived weight discrimination affect identity and physical health? *Social Psychology Quarterly, 74,* 76–97.

Schectman, J. M., Schorling, J. B., & Voss, J. D. (2008). Appointment adherence and disparities in outcomes among patients with diabetes. *Journal of General Internal Medicine, 23,* 1685.

Schwartz, M. B., Chambliss, H. O. N., Brownell, K. D., Blair, S. N., & Billington, C. (2003). Weight bias among health professionals specializing in obesity. *Obesity Research, 11,* 1033–1039.

Shah, A. K., Mullainathan, S., & Shafir, E. (2012). Some consequences of having too little. *Science, 338,* 682–685.

Sheehy-Skeffington, J. & Rea, J. (2017). *How Poverty Affects People's Decision-Making Processes.* Joseph Rowntree Foundation. https://www.jrf.org.uk/.

Shulman, S. (2004). *Scientific integrity in policymaking: An investigation into the Bush administration's misuse of science* (pp. 1–41). Union of Concerned Scientists.

Smith, K. P., & Christakis, N. A. (2008). Social networks and health. *Annual Review of Sociology, 34,* 405–429.

Smith-Campbell, B. (2005). Health professional students' cultural competence and attitudes toward the poor: The influence of a clinical practicum supported by the National Health Service Corps. *Journal of Allied Health, 34,* 56–62.

Stanford, F. C., Johnson, E. D., Claridy, M. D., Earle, R. L., & Kaplan, L. M. (2015). The role of obesity training in medical school and residency on bariatric surgery knowledge in primary care physicians. *International Journal of Family Medicine, 2015*, 841249.

Steele, C. M., Spencer, S. J., & Aronson, J. (2002). Contending with group image: The psychology of stereotype and social identity threat. In M. P. Zanna (Ed.), *Advances in experimental social psychology* (Vol. 34, pp. 379–440). Academic Press.

Sutin, A. R., Stephan, Y., & Terracciano, A. (2015). Weight discrimination and risk of mortality. *Psychological Science, 26*, 1803–1811.

Tamburlini, G., & Cattaneo, A. (2007). The spread of obesity in a social network. *New England Journal of Medicine, 357*, 1866.

Teachman, B. A., & Brownell, K. D. (2001). Implicit anti-fat bias among health professionals: Is anyone immune? *International Journal of Obesity, 25*, 1525.

Terrell, F., Miller, A. R., Foster, K., & Watkins Jr., C. E. (2006). Racial discrimination-induced anger and alcohol use among black adolescents. *Adolescence, 41*, 485–493.

Thompson, H. S., Valdimarsdottir, H. B., Winkel, G., Jandorf, L., & Redd, W. (2004). The Group-Based Medical Mistrust Scale: Psychometric properties and association with breast cancer screening. *Preventive Medicine, 38*, 209–218.

Thrasher, A. D., Earp, J. A. L., Golin, C. E., & Zimmer, C. R. (2008). Discrimination, distrust, and racial/ethnic disparities in antiretroviral therapy adherence among a national sample of HIV-infected patients. *JAIDS: Journal of Acquired Immune Deficiency Syndromes, 49*, 84–93.

Tomiyama, A. J. (2014). Weight stigma is stressful. A review of evidence for the Cyclic Obesity/Weight-Based Stigma model. *Appetite, 82*, 8–15.

Tong, S., Schirnding, Y. E. V., & Prapamontol, T. (2000). Environmental lead exposure: A public health problem of global dimensions. *Bulletin of the World Health Organization, 78*, 1068–1077.

Toomey, R. B., Umaña-Taylor, A. J., Williams, D. R., Harvey-Mendoza, E., Jahromi, L. B., & Updegraff, K. A. (2014). Impact of Arizona's SB 1070 immigration law on utilization of health care and public assistance among Mexican-origin adolescent mothers and their mother figures. *American Journal of Public Health, 104*, 28–34.

Trivedi, A. N., & Ayanian, J. Z. (2006). Perceived discrimination and use of preventive health services. *Journal of General Internal Medicine, 21*, 553–558.

Tsai, J., Ucik, L., Baldwin, N., Hasslinger, C., & George, P. (2016). Race matters? Examining and rethinking race portrayal in preclinical medical education. *Academic Medicine, 91*(7), 916–920.

U.S. Census Bureau. (2018, October 11). American Community Survey (ACS). https://www.census.gov/programs-surveys/acs/data/pums.html

U.S. Sentencing Commission. (2015, August 3). *U.S. Sentencing Commission Reports on Impact of Fair Sentencing Act of 2010* [Press release]. https://www.ussc.gov/sites/default/files/pdf/news/press-releases-and-news-advisories/press-releases/20150803_Press_Release.pdf

Van Boekel, L. C., Brouwers, E. P., Van Weeghel, J., & Garretsen, H. F. (2013). Stigma among health professionals towards patients with substance use disorders and its consequences for healthcare delivery: Systematic review. *Drug and Alcohol Dependence, 131*, 23–35.

Van Ryn, M. (2002). Research on the provider contribution to race/ethnicity disparities in medical care. *Medical Care, 40*, I140–I151.

Van Ryn, M., Burgess, D., Malat, J., & Griffin, J. (2006). Physicians' perceptions of patients' social and behavioral characteristics and race disparities in treatment recommendations for men with coronary artery disease. *American Journal of Public Health, 96*, 351–357.

Vartanian, L. R., & Novak, S. A. (2011). Internalized societal attitudes moderate the impact of weight stigma on avoidance of exercise. *Obesity, 19*, 757–762.

Vartanian, L. R., & Porter, A. M. (2016). Weight stigma and eating behavior: A review of the literature. *Appetite, 102*, 3–14.

Veugelers, P. J., & Yip, A. M. (2003). Socioeconomic disparities in health care use: Does universal coverage reduce inequalities in health? *Journal of Epidemiology and Community Health, 57*, 424–428.

Westley, R. (1998). Many billions gone: Is it time to reconsider the case for Black reparations. *Boston College Third World Law Journal, 19*, 429.

Whitbeck, L. B., Hoyt, D. R., McMorris, B. J., Chen, X., & Stubben, J. D. (2001). Perceived discrimination and early substance abuse among American Indian children. *Journal of Health and Social Behavior, 42,* 405–424.

Whitbeck, L. B., McMorris, B. J., Hoyt, D. R., Stubben, J. D., & LaFromboise, T. (2002). Perceived discrimination, traditional practices, and depressive symptoms among American Indians in the upper Midwest. *Journal of Health and Social Behavior, 43,* 400–418.

White, K., Yeager, V. A., Menachemi, N., & Scarinci, I. C. (2014). Impact of Alabama's immigration law on access to health care among Latina immigrants and children: Implications for national reform. *American Journal of Public Health, 104,* 397–405.

Wilkinson, R. G., & Marmot, M. (Eds.). (2003). *Social determinants of health: The solid facts.* World Health Organization.

Williams, D. R., & Collins, C. (2001). Racial residential segregation: A fundamental cause of racial disparities in health. *Public Health Reports (Washington, DC: 1974), 116,* 404–416.

Williams, D. R., & Mohammed, S. (2009). Discrimination and racial disparities in health: Evidence and needed research. *Journal of Behavioral Medicine, 32,* 20–47.

Willoughby, C. D. E. (2018). Running away from drapetomania: Samuel A. Cartwright, medicine, and race in the antebellum South. *Journal of Southern History, 84,* 579–614.

Wott, C. B., & Carels, R. A. (2010). Overt weight stigma, psychological distress and weight loss treatment outcomes. *Journal of Health Psychology, 15,* 608–614.

Zeiders, K. H., Doane, L. D., & Roosa, M. W. (2012). Perceived discrimination and diurnal cortisol: Examining relations among Mexican American adolescents. *Hormones and Behavior, 61,* 541–548.

Zewde, N., (2018). *Universal baby bonds reduce black-white wealth inequality, progressively raise net worth of all young adults.* Center for Poverty and Social Policy.

A Cultural Neuroscience Perspective on Socioeconomic Disparities in Global Mental Health

Gabriella M. Alvarez *and* Keely A. Muscatell

Abstract

This chapter reviews the neural and physiological mechanisms that may underlie socioeconomic disparities in global mental health through a cultural neuroscience lens. First, it discusses the cultural and psychological processes (namely, interdependence and "cultural mismatch") that may be experienced by individuals with lower socioeconomic status (SES) and could contribute to alterations in physiological and neural responses to stress and consequently put individuals at greater risk for the development of depression and anxiety. Next, it discusses the physiological systems, both peripheral (e.g., hypothalamic-pituitary-adrenal axis, autonomic nervous system, inflammation) and central (e.g., brain structure and function), that are implicated in responding to stress and confer risk for negative mental health outcomes, and how these systems are modulated by SES. The chapter concludes with a discussion of the resilience factors that might promote better outcomes among lower-SES individuals and the ethical and scientific considerations involved in this field of study.

Key Words: socioeconomic disparities, cultural neuroscience, stress, neurobiology, physiology

In 2008, the World Health Organization Commission on Social Determinants of Health published a striking statement in their final report: "Social injustice is killing on a grand scale" (Marmot et al., 2012). Indeed, socioeconomic disparities in physical and mental health outcomes exist across the globe, from India (Vellakkal et al., 2013) to Brazil (Andrade et al., 2012), from Europe (Ladin, 2008) to Pakistan (Maselko et al., 2018), and in the United States (Kessler, 1994) and nearly every country in between (see Chapter 26 on "Population Disparities in Mental Health" for more discussion). Results from multinational epidemiological studies have consistently demonstrated that individuals with lower levels of education, household income, and occupational prestige are more likely to suffer from mental, neurological, and substance abuse disorders compared to those with higher education, income, and occupational prestige (Andrade et al., 2012; Kessler, 1994; Ladin, 2008; Vellakkal et al., 2013). But how do socioeconomic factors, which seem to exist outside of the brain and body, come to affect neurobiology in ways that could lead to the development of psychological disorders?

In the present chapter, we present a cultural neuroscience perspective on the mechanisms by which socioeconomic factors may influence global mental health. More specifically, we present evidence suggesting that different socioeconomic groups may have distinct cultural values and experiences, which in turn can shape psychological, physiological, and neural functioning. Over time, these patterns of neurobiological activation could lead to increased risk for mental health problems (see Figure 28.1 for an illustration of the conceptual model guiding the chapter). Thus, the goal is to review past findings that have examined the associations between socioeconomic status (SES), physiological activation, and brain structure and function, and to view these results through a cultural neuroscience lens, thus shedding new light on how and why SES-based disparities in mental health outcomes may exist across the globe. Within the broader topic of global mental health, we focus on major depressive disorder (MDD) and anxiety disorders, as combined they constitute almost 50% of the total burden of psychiatric disease (Vos et al., 2012). Given the prevalence of these disorders and the high comorbidity between the two, this chapter will focus on reviewing the neurobiological underpinnings of depression and anxiety and their links to SES.

Before diving into the cultural, physiological, and neural mechanisms that may link SES and mental health, it is important to acknowledge that there are multiple, interacting pathways that undoubtedly contribute to mental health disparities. Though we focus here on a cultural neuroscience approach that emphasizes cultural, psychological, physiological, and neural factors, it is undeniable that lack of access to resources (e.g., quality health care, food, opportunities for exercise and outdoor space, etc.) is another important mechanism that links SES and mental health. In support of the role that material resources may play, one recent epidemiological study found that increased food insecurity was associated with poorer mental health and greater psychosocial stress across 149 countries (Jones, 2017), documenting that material deprivation undoubtedly contributes to SES disparities

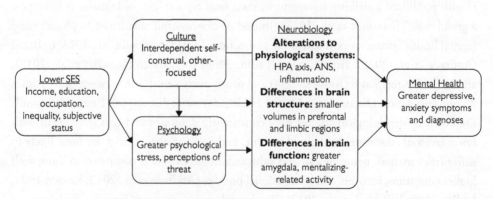

Figure 28.1. Conceptual model outlined in the chapter.

in mental health. However, it is also important to recognize that other pathways, including those more involved in the psychological experiences of being lower in SES, play a role. For example, although poverty alleviation programs effectively decrease depression in certain contexts (Burmaster et al., 2015), there are also findings showing that income inequality at a societal level independently affects mental health (Chiavegatto Filho et al., 2013). In other words, it is not just how much (education, income) one has but also how much one has *relative to others* that seems to matter for mental health, which emphasizes the role of psychological processes in mental health disparities.

Noteworthy here is that although SES disparities in mental health exist across racial/ethnic groups, even when controlling for SES, ethnicity and race exert a unique influence on mental health outcomes. Although beyond the scope of this chapter (see Chapter 27 on "Stigma and Health Disparities" for more discussion), the intersectionality between SES and ethnicity/race is a meaningful consideration, as differential mechanisms likely produce risk for psychopathology across ethnic/racial groups (e.g., discrimination, acculturative stress, historical trauma) and in some cases may also serve as protective factors against low-SES environments (e.g., familial values, length of residence, ethnic identity) in the United States and across countries (Alegría et al., 2008; Gone & Trimble, 2012; Walters & Simoni, 2002; Williams, 1999). This chapter will focus on SES as a distilled factor that cuts across groups and will explore the underlying cultural and psychological experiences, and their associated physiological and neural alterations, that may put lower-SES individuals at greater risk for developing psychopathology.

Cultural and Psychological Contributions to Socioeconomic Status Disparities in Mental Health

Cultural Perspective on Socioeconomic Status

Cultural psychologists and cultural neuroscientists have long appreciated that there can be substantial variability in the cultural values held by particular groups or even particular individuals within a country (S. Han et al., 2013). More recently within the United States, social psychologists who are interested in the effects of SES on thoughts, feelings, and behaviors have begun to view different social class groups within the United States as having different cultural orientations (Grossmann & Varnum, 2011; Kraus et al., 2011; Stephens, Markus, & Fryberg, 2012). For example, individuals from higher-SES groups in the United States are thought to have a more *independent* self-construal, conceptualized as a view of the self in relation to others that stresses the importance of the self as autonomous, an appreciation of one's uniqueness from others, and the need to assert the self (Markus & Kitayama, 1991). Meanwhile, individuals from lower-SES groups tend to have a more *interdependent* self-construal, conceptualized as stressing the importance of attending to and fitting in with other people and maintaining interpersonal harmony, sometimes even at the expense of the self (Markus & Kitayama, 1991). In other words, within the same country, and within what some might consider the same "culture" (i.e., the United States), there may be stark differences in cultural values that are patterned by SES.

Indeed, consistent with predictions from a theoretical view of "social class as culture" mentioned earlier, a growing number of empirical findings have demonstrated that higher-SES individuals behave in more "independent" ways, while lower-SES individuals behave in more "interdependent" ways. For example, in one of the earliest findings in this domain, Snibbe and Markus (2005) examined SES-based differences in choice and agency, demonstrating that individuals from higher-SES backgrounds (i.e., with higher levels of education) preferred cultural products that emphasized uniqueness and individuality, while those from lower-SES backgrounds preferred cultural products that emphasized interpersonal integrity and adjusting the self to fit the situation. Since this initial work, a number of other related findings have emerged, including those showing that lower-SES individuals (compared to higher-SES individuals) are more engaged in social interactions (Kraus & Keltner, 2009), are better at reading others' emotional states (Kraus et al., 2010), are more compassionate toward the suffering of others (Stellar et al., 2012), and rely more on social connection and community (rather than material wealth) in the face of chaos (Piff et al., 2012). Together, this growing theoretical and empirical literature suggests that different SES groups may have distinct cultural values, particularly those related to the way one should view the self in relation to others. These cultural values have implications for cognition, emotion, and behavior, and may also relate to mental health.

Initial cross-country work suggests that these SES differences in behavior may not be confined to the United States, but rather may also exist in other countries. Along these lines, in a study of individuals from both the United States and Russia, lower SES was associated with lower dispositional bias, greater interdependent self-views, and greater holistic cognition, compared to higher SES (Grossmann & Varnum, 2011). This effect held among individuals regardless of whether they were from the United States (typically conceptualized as an independent culture) or from Russia (typically conceptualized as an interdependent culture). These findings demonstrate that social class may confer similar cultural values across countries, although much more cross-national work is needed to replicate these findings in other countries across the globe.

In light of this emerging work highlighting SES differences in cultural values and self-construal, it is important to consider the role that cultural orientation may play in potentially contributing to mental health among individuals from different SES backgrounds. Although no known research has directly explored how SES and culture interact to influence mental health, hints can be drawn from other literatures linking interdependent self-construal (and its corresponding cognitions, emotions, and behaviors) to mental health. For example, work on culture and social support seeking suggests that Asians and Asian Americans, both groups that score high on interdependence, are hesitant to ask for support from close others during times of stress (compared to European Americans) and are less likely to utilize mental health services, due in part to concerns about disrupting interpersonal harmony and potential negative relational consequences of such support-seeking behaviors (Kim et al., 2008). Given the importance of social support for mental health, it is possible that the hesitancy to seek support may be associated with greater experiences of depression and anxiety. Thus, one hypothesis is that, due to a similar interdependent cultural orientation as some Asian and Asian Americans, individuals from lower-SES backgrounds may be less likely to seek emotional support during times of stress, which could lead to poor mental health outcomes. A separate but related line of work suggests that greater empathy and perspective taking, two common correlates of interdependence and characteristic of lower-SES individuals (Kraus et al., 2010), can have physiological costs, including increases in levels of inflammation in the body, which may put individuals at risk for the development of anxiety and depressive symptoms (see section on inflammation later in this chapter for more details; Manczak, Basu, & Chen, 2016; Manczak, DeLongis, & Chen, 2016). Finally, a number of clinical conditions are characterized by disruptions in perspective taking and theory of mind (e.g., social anxiety, generalized anxiety; see Hezel & McNally, 2014; Tibi-Elhanany & Shamay-Tsoory, 2011; Zainal & Newman, 2018), suggesting that greater attention to others and emphasis on relational harmony might come with psychological and physiological costs that could put individuals at risk for mental health problems.

While there are cultural tendencies and behavioral patterns among individuals *within* similar contexts (i.e., low-SES culture), the interaction *between* cultural groups (i.e., lower vs. higher SES) within the larger U.S. context might generate value-based conflicts that themselves could be stressful, ultimately contributing to risk for psychiatric conditions. This constant awareness of one's relative position and juggling of competing values and schemas might be particularly difficult for someone whose cultural practices (i.e., not discussing one's own accomplishments because it could disrupt group cohesion) differ more widely from "mainstream" ideas and values (i.e., working at a company in which one needs to point out their accomplishments to be promoted). Considering this "values mismatch," cultural consonance is a theory borrowed from cultural anthropology that provides a useful lens for understanding the cultural and psychological underpinnings of SES-based mental health disparities. Cultural consonance is a measure of the "degree to which individuals approximate, in their own beliefs and behaviors, the prototypes for belief and behavior encoded in shared cultural models" (Dressler, 2007, p. 2058). This theory attempts to fill gaps in cultural research by explicitly linking societal-level beliefs and practices to behavior at the individual level to improve our understanding of the psychological and health consequences of low SES. As Dressler and colleagues (2017) state, "Without connecting culture to the individual in some theoretically and methodologically satisfying way, how culture influences mental health remains something of a mystery" (Dressler et al., 2017, p. 43). Cultural consonance attempts to capture how one internalizes and behaves in a way that mirrors the model for what makes an individual and their life "culturally successful" (also known as social status). The idea is that lower-SES experiences do not mirror broader society's "model" of success, resulting in less cultural consonance for the individual, possibly leading to more stress. Along these lines, Dressler and colleagues argue that less cultural consonance might be stressful because perceptions of lower status can exacerbate negative social sanctions in banal interactions, blunt an individual's receipt of reassuring positive feedback, and amplify feelings of failure due to not living up to the widely shared expectations (Dressler et al., 2017). Over time, an accumulation of such experiences may lead to negative mental health outcomes. A test of this hypothesized link between cultural consonance and mental health outcomes in a Brazilian sample found that change in cultural consonance was associated with depressive symptoms 2 years later, such that increases in cultural consonance over time led to decreases in symptoms (Dressler et al., 2007). Further, in domains in which cultural consensus was the greatest (e.g., family life), greater cultural consonance scores related to those domains were associated with decreased psychiatric symptoms. These findings propose that the extent to which an individual's life approximates society's model of success relates to psychological distress and may be a mechanism explaining why low-SES individuals might be at greater risk for psychopathology.

Similar to cultural consonance, a growing literature in the educational domain suggests other ways in which a mismatch between the cultural values instilled in a person growing up in a lower-SES community can come into conflict with the cultural values present in the U.S. higher education system. This conflict can in turn perpetuate disparities and produce negative mental health outcomes for those from lower-SES backgrounds striving for upward mobility (Stephens et al., 2019). From this perspective, individuals from lower-SES backgrounds may arrive to college with a relatively interdependent self-construal, which might not be compatible with the independent culture of higher education, in which the need for students to pave their own paths, challenge norms and rules, and express their personal preferences is emphasized (Stephens, Fryberg, et al., 2012). As a result of this cultural mismatch, lower-SES students might perform worse in school and show higher levels of stress, both of which have negative mental health consequences. Thus, considering the cultural values instilled by different SES groups may shed light on disparities in educational outcomes as well as mental health. Interventions that focus on creating a more interdependent environment in higher education contexts could improve both education and psychological outcomes for individuals from lower-SES backgrounds (Dittmann & Stephens, 2017).

Psychological Theories of Socioeconomic Status, Stress, and Mental Health

While the cultural perspectives on social class reviewed previously are relatively new to the study of SES-based mental health disparities, other important theories examine relationships between SES, psychological processes, and mental (and physical) health. Although an extensive review of each of these theories is beyond the scope of the current chapter, it is worth noting that, at their core, many of these perspectives emphasize psychological stress experiences and coping responses as critical contributors to SES disparities. For example, the seminal work of Sir Michael Marmot argues that relative deprivation, or an individual's concern about their position in a social hierarchy, is undergirded by several psychological characteristics that increase stress. Specifically, Marmot argues that relative deprivation decreases perceptions of self-esteem and induces "status anxiety," consisting of an acute awareness of status differences, pain in losing status, and preoccupation with others having too much, and that ultimately, this stress can affect health (Marmot, 2004). More recently, Brosschot and colleagues' generalized unsafety theory of stress argues that a lower-SES individual's physiological response to stress is not hyperactive because of an accumulation of stress exposure in their life, but rather that it is the continual absence of perceived safety that generates a prolonged stress response that is ultimately harmful for well-being (Brosschot et al., 2017, 2018). Finally, Gallo's reserve capacity theory argues that low SES is characterized by stressful environments that reduce an individual's reserved capacity to manage subsequent stress, thus leaving an individual more vulnerable to continued distress (Gallo & Matthews, 2003). Though distinct in some ways, these various "stress and coping" theories overlap in their idea that low SES affects one's experience of stress, control, and resources, which can increase negative emotions and threat perceptions.

Because this chapter outlines a neuroscience perspective and neurobiology encompasses both peripheral and central nervous system mechanisms, this next section of the chapter will review a diversity of systems involved in the stress response as they relate to SES and psychiatric diseases. Specifically, we will focus on six different systems that appear to be involved in responding to and affected by psychological stress, including the hypothalamic-pituitary-adrenal (HPA) axis, the autonomic nervous system (ANS), the inflammatory response, multisystem dysregulation, and brain structure and function. Within each section, we will first provide a brief overview of the system and its function, following which we will review evidence linking alterations in the system with mental health outcomes. We close each section by reviewing the literature linking SES to the functioning of each neurobiological system, in an effort to provide context for how activation of that system may link with SES disparities in mental health outcomes.

Physiological Mechanisms Linking Socioeconomic Status and Mental Health

Socioeconomic Status and Activation of the Hypothalamic-Pituitary-Adrenal Axis

Arguably the most commonly studied physiological system in the context of mental health disparities, particularly in children and younger adults, is the HPA axis. The HPA axis is a neuroendocrine system that relies on hormone-secreting glands to help regulate the body's response to perceived challenges, threats, and other situational demands (Sapolsky, 2004). Briefly, the axis functions such that when, for example, a threat is perceived, the hypothalamus secretes corticotropin-releasing hormone (CRH) to communicate with the pituitary gland. The pituitary gland then signals to the adrenal glands, above the kidney, via adrenocorticotropic hormone (ACTH). The product of this response cascade is cortisol, which is the most commonly studied marker of HPA axis function. In the brain, cortisol regulates neuron survival, neurogenesis, and hippocampal size (Herbert et al., 2006; Pariante & Lightman, 2008). Cortisol can be collected from humans in saliva, blood, urine, and even hair samples, making it relatively noninvasive to obtain and therefore widely used in the literature.

HPA axis dysfunction is thought to occur due to a rapid, repeated rise in cortisol in response to accumulating stressors, coupled with weak HPA feedback regulation of this response, resulting in persistent hypersecretion of the cortisol hormone. Certainly, this pattern of HPA functioning appears to have negative consequences for physiological and neural processes important for mental health (Herbert et al., 2006). Given that cortisol is an endpoint of HPA axis function, it has been extensively studied in the context of psychiatric disease.

Along these lines, alterations in HPA functioning have been found in both depression and anxiety. In a 2001 review paper, Varghese and Brown reported that aberrant HPA axis activity is common in depressed patients, such that these patients exhibit elevated CRH and cortisol, as well as smaller hippocampal volume. Greater cortisol and CRH were also linked to increased depression relapse and suicide risk. Prior research demonstrates that cortisol has a diurnal rhythm, peaking in the morning upon awakening, and that the magnitude of this response predicted the new onset of MDD and recurrence of depressive episodes (Adam et al., 2010), as well as anxiety more than 6 years later (Adam et al., 2014). Further, this study found that depressed patients exhibited greater levels of cortisol at baseline compared to those without depression. Elevated levels of cortisol have also been reported for patients with anxiety disorders. For example, several studies report greater levels of basal cortisol in patients with posttraumatic stress disorder (PTSD), obsessive-compulsive disorder (OCD), panic disorder (PD), social anxiety, and generalized anxiety disorder (GAD), although some studies find lower levels of basal cortisol among individuals with anxiety disorders, which is discussed in more detail later (Faravelli et al., 2012). Finally, recent theory and empirical research converge to suggest that early life stress can cause alterations in HPA functioning, and as such, dysregulation of the HPA axis due to early life stress may serve as a risk factor for the development of depression and anxiety (Heim & Binder, 2012; Juruena, 2014; Pariante & Lightman, 2008). Thus, findings indicate that early environmental factors such as stress exposure may enact changes in HPA axis function that have important implications for the development of psychopathology.

Although several studies report hyperactivation of the HPA axis in both depression and anxiety, other research has found that hypoactivation of the HPA axis has also been linked to risk and maintenance of psychopathology. For example, one study found that older adults with an anxiety diagnosis had lower cortisol levels in the morning than those without the disorder (Hek et al., 2013). These authors concluded that their results support a competing theory that chronic stress results in *downregulation* of HPA axis activity, which may have important implications for the development of anxiety. A recent meta-analysis reported that depression was associated with varied responses that include blunted cortisol responses following a laboratory stressor (Belvederi Murri et al., 2014). Thus, depression and anxiety may also be associated with hypoactivation of the HPA axis.

Taken together, these findings lead to inconclusive evidence regarding the pattern of cortisol activation that is most predictive of mental health or what factors drive heterogeneity within the cortisol activation pattern. Factors that may contribute to this variability in the results could first encompass methodological differences across studies. For example, some work shows that different findings may emerge depending on whether the cortisol sample was derived from saliva or blood, the type of quantification of the cortisol response (e.g., mean concentration vs. change scores), and even that associations may vary depending on the time of day that the samples were collected. For example, depression may be most associated with elevated cortisol levels in samples collected in the afternoon and among older adults (Belvederi Murri et al., 2014; Burke, Davis, et al., 2005). Thus, although it is currently unclear whether hypo- versus hyperactivation of the HPA axis is most closely linked to depression and anxiety, there does exist a consistent finding that *dysregulation* (be it hypo- or hyperactivity) in this system is implicated in the development of psychopathology. Further, given the variability in findings, it is also pertinent to examine demographic and psychosocial characteristics of individuals that may put one at risk for dysregulation of HPA axis function.

Indeed, other factors related to variability in cortisol findings include cultural and SES differences. For example, in one study, researchers examined cortisol reactivity to a laboratory stressor in Mexican women all living in low-income contexts (Burke, Fernald, et al., 2005). Specifically, researchers explored whether there was an interaction between depressive symptoms and cortisol reactivity to a stressor, finding that women who reported greater levels of depression exhibited blunted cortisol responses compared to women who reported no symptoms or mild symptoms. Other research in this area has examined how depression in low-SES mothers affects their children's HPA responses. Studies have found that children from low-SES families exhibit hypoactivation of the HPA axis such that they demonstrate blunted cortisol levels (Fernald et al., 2008; Sheridan et al., 2013) as well as hyperactivation (Lupien et al., 2000), relative to children from higher-SES families. More recently, some work has moved beyond simply documenting associations between SES, HPA dysregulation, and negative symptoms to examine the psychosocial processes that might account for chronic activations in the HPA axis by measuring cortisol in hair samples. Measuring hair cortisol not only captures chronic stress build-up but also circumvents discrepancies that may be due to daily fluctuations in salivary cortisol measurement. Utilizing this novel marker of HPA axis activity, researchers measured hair cortisol levels in parents and children from diverse SES backgrounds and found that lower SES was associated with elevated hair cortisol levels in families (Ursache et al., 2017). Further, the link between SES and parent anxiety symptoms was marginally associated with hair cortisol amount. Thus, these exciting recent findings suggest that the HPA axis may play a critical role in linking SES to depressive and anxiety symptoms, thus contributing to our understanding of the mechanisms that underlie SES disparities in global mental health. However, many questions remain regarding the specificity and directionality of findings, which will need to be addressed in future research.

Socioeconomic Status and Activation of the Autonomic Nervous System

Another physiological system that is responsive to stress and may play a role in contributing to SES-based mental health disparities is the ANS. The ANS enervates and helps regulate most visceral organs in the body, including the cardiovascular, respiratory, and gastrointestinal systems, and is increasingly viewed as a central component of affective states (Barrett, 2017; Critchley & Garfinkel, 2017; MacCormack & Lindquist, 2017). Several emotion theorists debate the nature of ANS activity for constructing or responding to different emotional responses (Kreibig, 2010); nonetheless, the consensus is that the ANS is fundamentally linked to affective responses to environmental demands, including stress. The ANS is most often characterized by an interaction of the sympathetic nervous system (SNS) and parasympathetic nervous system (PNS; Berntson et al., 1993). The "acceleratory" SNS stimulates the infamous "fight or flight" response to a threat, or energy utilization. Conversely, the "deceleratory" PNS encourages the body to "rest and digest," or conserve energy. One way to measure ANS activity is by collecting data regarding the electrical activity of the heart during its cardiac cycle, and the mechanical movement of blood to derive indicators of heart rate and blood pressure. Both are influenced by the SNS and PNS. More sophisticated psychophysiological measures such as the pre-ejection period (PEP), as well as concentrations of norepinephrine and epinephrine, can be gathered as indicators of SNS activation (Cohen et al., 2006), while cardiac vagal tone, or heart rate variability, is an indicator of PNS activity. Given that the ANS is relevant for affective states, stress responses, and possibly emotion regulation, it is not surprising that this system is also highly relevant in psychopathology.

ANS dysregulation is documented across several psychiatric diseases. Specific to the SNS, blunted PEP reactivity is associated with greater depressed mood and anhedonia (Brinkmann & Franzen, 2013; Brinkmann et al., 2009; Franzen & Brinkmann, 2015). Another study tested the relationship between symptoms of depression and anxiety during a 24-hour urinary catecholamine excretion in a sample of 91 women (Hughes et al., 2004). Analyses indicated that greater depression and anxiety symptoms were associated with increased norepinephrine excretion over time such that women with higher depression were excreting norepinephrine at a 25% higher rate than women with lower depression scores. A treatment study explored the link between MDD and cardiac risk by measuring changes in SNS activity over the course of 12 weeks and then administered selective serotonin reuptake inhibitors (SSRIs) to examine whether treatment moderated

SNS activity (Barton et al., 2007). A subset of patients with high SNS activity were identified and SSRI treatment in this group significantly reduced the excessive SNS activation. These results suggest that aberrant SNS activity is implicated in depression and anxiety.

Turning to the PNS, lower cardiac vagal tone, a measure of the variation in time between each heartbeat, is found among patients with depression diagnoses (Krittayaphong et al., 1997; Light et al., 1998), and lower vagal tone is also related to increased depressive symptoms (Kemp et al., 2010). This pattern of findings is also documented in patients with anxiety disorders, such that lower heart rate variability is found in patients with many anxiety subtypes (Pittig et al., 2013) including GAD (Thayer et al., 1996), PTSD, and PD (Blechert et al., 2007). Further, a recent study tested whether the efficiency of vagal tone in patients with generalized anxiety related to difficulties regulating emotions during a worry induction task (Levine et al., 2016). Results supported the hypothesis that PNS dysregulation, as indicated by lower vagal tone, significantly relates to the most debilitating feature of clinical anxiety: worry. Together, these results suggest that blunted PNS activity is implicated among psychiatric disorders.

Does the ANS contribute to SES disparities in mental health? One prominent model posits that this is indeed the case, specifically, that low SES might be associated with reduced efficiency of the cardiovascular system (Evans & Kim, 2007). Consistent with this idea, the general pattern of findings documented in the literature is that lower SES is associated with dysregulated ANS activity that may serve as a potential risk factor for the development of psychopathology. For example, lower SES has been consistently related to elevated baseline blood pressure (E. Chen et al., 2002), increased levels of the catecholamines epinephrine and norepinephrine (Cohen et al., 2006), and both lower heart rate variability and slower recovery of heart rate variability following stress (Boylan et al., 2018; Sloan et al., 2005). A recent meta-analysis tested the association between SES and cardiovascular responses, specifically blood pressure and heart rate reactivity, to acute stress tasks in the lab (Boylan et al., 2018). Analyses did not find that SES was associated with cardiovascular reactivity to acute laboratory stressors but did find that higher-SES individuals exhibited better cardiovascular recovery following stress. From these results, authors argue that how people recover physiologically following stress may be particularly informative for understanding the links between SES and cardiovascular risk, which is often comorbid with depression. Together these findings suggest that lower SES is associated with alterations to ANS function that may have implications for mental health.

The strongest evidence to date for the links between SES, ANS activation, and psychopathology has focused on understanding the process of intergenerational transmission of mental health problems between mother and child. Interestingly, one paper explored the vagal tone of newborn children as it related to mothers' reports of depression. In a low-income African American sample including 87 neonates, mothers' reports of past depression diagnosis and a greater number of life stressors were associated with lower heart rate variability of the baby (Jacob et al., 2009). These results indicate that stress is an important mechanism that might help explain the influence of SES and depression on ANS dysregulation very early in life. Another study exploring the influence of parent SES and psychopathology on early life ANS function examined physiological responses to stress utilizing a longitudinal design. In this study, researchers collected reports of objective and subjective stress throughout gestation and the early postpartum period. Measures of infant temperament and physiological reactivity during a stress task were collected and compared to mothers' stress reports. As expected, mothers' stress during pregnancy predicted lower emotion regulation in the infant, as well as increased heart rate reactivity to and poorer recovery from a stressor in the infants (Bush et al., 2017).

Collectively, these findings provide mechanistic evidence for how maternal psychopathology and stress can affect the offspring's physiology to potentially confer risk for the development of psychopathology in the child. Although the causal direction between SES, ANS activation, and psychiatric conditions has not been fully established, these few studies provide compelling evidence that one pathway by which SES stress may affect mental health is via intergenerational transmission of stress and concomitant ANS changes. Despite the converging evidence documenting ANS dysregulation in depression and anxiety as well as ANS dysregulation in individuals with lower SES, there is a paucity of data that directly examines the associations between SES, ANS function, and mental health. More research is needed to fully test an SES to ANS dysregulation to depression/anxiety symptoms model, which would clearly establish the relevance (or lack thereof) of the ANS in contributing to SES disparities in global mental health.

Socioeconomic Status and Inflammatory Activation

Another system that has received significant attention as a potential contributor to SES disparities in mental health outcomes is the immune system, and more specifically, inflammation. Inflammation, the innate immune system's initial, nonspecific response to a pathogen or injury and even psychological stress, can be adaptive in the short term, helping to heal wounds and fight infections. However, chronically elevated low-grade inflammation can be harmful to mental health, such that individuals with increased inflammation are at greater risk for depression (Raison et al., 2006). The most well-studied pro-inflammatory cytokines, or proteins that orchestrate the inflammatory response, are interleukin-1β (IL-1β), tumor necrosis factor-α (TNF-α), and interleukin-6 (IL-6). Another popular marker of inflammation that is examined in the literature is the acute-phase protein C-reactive protein (CRP). CRP is produced in the liver and circulating levels of CRP increase in the presence of inflammation.

A number of important models emphasize the role of elevated levels of inflammation in contributing to psychiatric symptoms (Howren et al., 2009; Nusslock & Miller, 2016). Across several disorders, increased inflammation, from prenatal exposure to adulthood, has been argued to influence risk for psychopathology (Howes & McCutcheon, 2017; A. H. Miller et al., 2017; A. H. Miller & Raison, 2016). Increased inflammation is related to anxiety and trauma-related illnesses (Michopoulos et al., 2017), as well as to depression (A. H. Miller et al., 2009) and greater depressive symptoms (Chirinos et al., 2017). In addition to differences in basal levels of inflammation, depressive symptoms have also been linked to an increased inflammatory response following an acute stressor (Fagundes et al., 2013).

The findings linking depression and inflammation have been so robust that some researchers have begun to propose that depression may be an inflammatory disease. In a 2011 paper dedicated to tackling this very question, Raison and Miller concluded that depression is not fundamentally an inflammatory disorder but that there might instead exist an inflammation-induced subtype of depression (Raison & Miller, 2011). Although the link between inflammation and depression has received much more attention than inflammation's link to other psychiatric diseases, a recent study explored levels of inflammation across hundreds of psychiatric inpatients (Osimo et al., 2018). Electronic health records from 599 patients diagnosed with psychotic, mood, neurotic, and personality disorders were included in the study. Increased inflammation was present across all disorder types and especially high for diagnoses of schizophrenia and bipolar disorder. The results from this study suggest that chronic inflammation is not necessarily specific to depression or anxiety, but is potentially a relevant feature of psychopathology more broadly. Although the association between inflammation and poor mental health has been established, what remains unclear is how these increases in inflammation arise, as well as an understanding of the factors that could be accounting for the link between inflammation and psychopathology.

One of the most consistent psychosocial factors that has been linked to elevated inflammation is socioeconomic disadvantage. Indeed, lower-SES adults and teens exhibit increased IL-6 and CRP levels at baseline (Muscatell et al., 2018; Pietras & Goodman, 2013) and show greater inflammatory reactivity to an acute stressor (Derry et al., 2013). Recent research has explored the psychological mechanisms that might underlie the association between SES and increased inflammation. One study found that lower childhood SES and greater recent negative life events predicted higher levels of CRP and IL-6 (John-Henderson et al., 2016), suggesting an "inflammatory phenotype" where low childhood SES was associated with an exaggerated inflammatory response when it was also accompanied by a context of recent negative life events. Relatedly, another study reported that lower-SES individuals exhibited greater inflammation in part due to higher levels of negative affect (Elliot & Chapman, 2016). These results provide some initial evidence supporting a link between SES, inflammation, and risk for psychopathology, particularly when lower SES is accompanied by higher life stress and greater negative affect.

Although a large body of work has examined links between SES and levels of inflammation, very few studies have explored the link between SES and psychiatric conditions as mediated by inflammation. However, a few studies have examined the link between "childhood adversity," inflammation, and depression, and included measures of SES as part of an index of "childhood adversity." One longitudinal study found that childhood adversity, with parental SES included in the measure, promoted the coupling of increased inflammation and depressive symptoms (G. E. Miller & Cole, 2012). Specifically, increases in IL-6 and CRP among those with higher early adversity preceded the development of depressive symptoms 6 months later. This co-occurrence of inflammation and depression related to child maltreatment was replicated in a longitudinal New Zealand study as well (Danese et al., 2008). Other studies have also reported that neighborhood poverty levels are associated with elevated CRP in adults and children even when adiposity, demographics, and behavioral differences are controlled for (Broyles et al., 2012). It is clear from these studies that inflammation may be an important mechanism by which SES "gets under the skin" to affect mental health.

A cultural neuroscience perspective can also provide insight into why lower SES would be linked with higher levels of inflammation. This work suggests that greater empathy and perspective taking, two common correlates of interdependence that are more prevalent among lower-SES individuals, are also associated with increased inflammation. In one study, authors set out to test whether there might be contexts in which empathy can be harmful in a sample of 143 parents and their children (Manczak et al., 2016). Analyses revealed that more empathetic parents showed greater inflammatory cytokine production to in vitro bacteria exposure if their children also reported high levels of depressive symptoms. These results suggest that parents high in empathy might be "physiologically sensitive" to their children's distress. Results from another study supported the idea that greater parental empathy was associated with psychophysiological benefits for the child but resulted in a physiological toll on the parents (Manczak, DeLongis, et al., 2016). In this study, higher parental empathy was associated with greater emotion regulation and less inflammation in the children; however, this increased empathy was also associated with greater systemic inflammation in the parents, suggesting a "physiological cost" to high empathy. Together these results propose that greater empathy, which is common among individuals from lower SES backgrounds, is associated with greater inflammation, which may put individuals at risk for developing anxiety and depression symptoms. Thus, the cultural practice of focusing on others, especially when the other is in distress, could influence mental health among lower-SES individuals. Future studies should directly test the link between SES, empathy, and physiological risk factors.

Linking Socioeconomic Status and Multisystem Dysregulation

As is evident across the physiological systems discussed previously, research has documented that individuals who mature in disadvantaged socioeconomic environments may develop a sensitivity to stress that potentially leads to dysregulated forms of affective processing and recurrent stress responses that increase risk for poor mental and physical health (Chen & Matthews, 2001; Chen et al., 2002; Taylor et al., 2004). One theory that has attempted to characterize a mechanism accounting for the relationship between SES and widespread dysregulation across physiological systems is allostatic load (McEwen, 1998). Fundamental to this theory is the idea that the body and brain are working together to maintain homeostasis or a general "set point" for effective functioning, based on inputs from the environment. As stressful experiences accumulate over time, this can alter the set point as a "price" of continually adapting to a stressful environment. Ultimately, allostatic load is a measure of cumulative threats to homeostasis brought on by repeated and costly physiological stress responses that recalibrate other biological functions to accommodate the immediate demands generated by the perceived threat (McEwen & Wingfield, 2003). Allostatic load has been conceptualized throughout the literature via measurement of dysregulation in multiple physiological systems, using subclinically relevant biomarkers to derive risk scores (McEwen & Seeman, 1999). More specifically, risk scores across several physiological systems are summed to create a global score of allostatic load. In doing so, multisystem dysregulation measures can provide more holistic information about an individual's physiological risk rather than considering a single physiological system in isolation.

To date, several papers have directly explored the links between allostatic load and mood disorders. Indeed, studies have reported that greater allostatic load is associated with increased depressive symptoms (Juster et al., 2011; Kobrosly et al., 2013; Seplaki et al., 2004). In addition to these findings, there are several theoretical papers that propose allostatic load as a mechanism that may be underlying the pathogenesis of other psychiatric disorders including bipolar disorder (Vieta et al., 2013). Interestingly, researchers have suggested that allostatic load may be a useful clinical tool for monitoring physiological dysregulations in patients with severe mental illnesses (Bizik et al., 2013).

Several studies have found that lower SES is also related to increased allostatic load scores (Gruenewald et al., 2012; McEwen & Stellar, 1993; Seeman et al., 2014), suggesting that SES may confer risk across multiple physiological systems. Not only does individual SES relate to allostatic load, but also so do neighborhood levels of SES. In some cases, neighborhood poverty is associated with greater allostatic load independent of household income, and this relationship is mediated by reports of stress and anxious arousal (Robinette et al., 2016; Schulz et al., 2012). Although a full model testing links the between SES, allostatic load, and psychiatric illnesses has not been assessed empirically, there is substantial evidence that SES is related to increases in allostatic load (Gruenewald et al., 2012; McEwen, 2003; Seeman et al., 2004, 2010). Although research in this area is currently sparse, these initial findings are exciting as they provide a mechanistic pathway linking low SES to psychiatric disease by way of physiological dysregulation across a variety of bodily systems due to chronic stress and changes in allostatic load.

Socioeconomic Status Influences on Brain Structure and Function

The final system discussed in this chapter is the central nervous system, with a focus on the brain. The brain is the primary organ that integrates stimuli from the external environment with the body's internal state and, in turn, regulates the cascades of physiological processes that help an individual respond to environmental stimuli. As such, the brain is a crucial organ to examine in efforts to understand the links between SES and mental health. Given the central role of the brain in psychological health, the National Institute of Mental Health has declared that understanding the neural risk factors implicated in mental illness is a top research priority ("Strategic Research Priorities Overview," 2017). In the following sections, we discuss both the structural and functional neural correlates of major depression and anxiety-related disorders, and the potential role SES may play in leading to neural changes that put individuals on a course toward depression and anxiety.

Brain Structure, Socioeconomic Status, and Psychopathology

Alterations in brain structure accompany most psychiatric illnesses including depression (Zhang et al., 2016) and anxiety, among others (Takagi et al., 2018). Structural magnetic resonance imaging (MRI) studies have reported alterations in cortical thickness, gray matter volume, and white matter integrity in regions within the prefrontal cortex among adults with depression (K.-M. Han et al., 2014; Zhang et al., 2016). A recent meta-analysis of 14 studies that included over 400 medication-free individuals diagnosed with MDD reported lower gray matter in the prefrontal cortex and limbic regions among individuals with depression compared to those without MDD (Zhao et al., 2014). Furthermore, a study that examined gray matter volume differences in 132 patients with MDD and 132 matched controls found that the volume of the right anterior insula and the hippocampal formation were smaller in the patient group relative to controls. Additionally, the observed findings were more pronounced based on symptom severity, such that greater symptoms and increased number of depressive episodes were related to smaller insula, hippocampi, and right amygdala volumes (Stratmann et al., 2014). Thus, depression is associated with differences in brain structure in limbic and prefrontal regions.

Structural MRI studies conducted with patients with anxiety also report alterations in brain morphology in several of the same regions noted in depression. A study that explored structural differences in individuals with social anxiety found that patients had smaller volumes in the amygdala and hippocampus and that lower hippocampal volume was associated with greater severity of symptoms (Irle et al., 2010). Another study exploring structural differences in participants with subclinical anxiety found that increased anxiety symptoms were also associated with smaller amygdala volume (Blackmon et al., 2011). A similar pattern of findings has been reported in children, such that anxiety diagnosis and symptom severity were both associated with smaller hippocampal volume (Gold et al., 2017). Finally, a study interested in exploring the structural brain overlap among patients with comorbid depression and anxiety diagnoses found that across all patients, there was less cortical thickness in the prefrontal cortex (including the medial frontal cortex and the frontal pole) and that symptom severity varied with the observed prefrontal differences (Canu et al., 2015). Thus, findings in patients with MDD and anxiety disorders suggest that smaller structural volumes in areas within the prefrontal cortex, hippocampus, and limbic system are key features of these disorders.

Despite a large literature linking brain structure to depression and anxiety, a clear understanding of the psychosocial risk factors that might be accounting for the development of these structural brain alterations is currently lacking. Given the previously reviewed evidence suggesting robust links between SES and alterations in physiological functioning, we might expect that SES would be one risk factor that could have important impacts on neural structure, with implications for psychopathology. Indeed, converging evidence highlights SES-based morphological differences in regions within the prefrontal cortex, temporal lobe, and limbic system, all of which are also implicated in depression and anxiety. Overall, socioeconomic disadvantage has been most consistently associated with differences in brain structure in regions involved in memory, executive control, and emotion, including the hippocampus, amygdala, and prefrontal cortex, such that individuals with lower SES show smaller volumes in each of these brain regions (Brito & Noble, 2014; Holz, Laucht, & Meyer-Lindenberg, 2015). Further, perceptions of social standing (i.e., subjective SES) have also been associated with smaller pregenual anterior cingulate cortex (pACC) gray matter volume, an important prefrontal region also implicated in depression (Gianaros et al., 2007). Finally, there is evidence that the effects of lower SES may be pernicious over the life course, as a recent structural MRI study documented decreased orbital frontal cortex (OFC) volume in adults aged 25 who had experienced early life poverty (Holz, Boecker, et al., 2015).

While there is substantial overlap between the brain structures affected by SES and those implicated in depression and anxiety, there are only two known studies that have examined if alterations in brain structure are a likely mechanism linking SES and psychopathology. In one study, researchers examined amygdala volume in a sample of 327 children and adolescents and explored the associations between SES, amygdala volume, and internalizing symptoms of depression and anxiety (Merz et al., 2018). Findings demonstrated that lower family income was related to smaller amygdala volume, and that lower parental education was associated with greater levels of anxiety and depression. Finally, smaller amygdala volume was associated with increased reports of internalizing symptoms. Although amygdala volume did not statistically mediate the association between parent education and internalizing symptoms in this study, results suggest a potential link between SES, brain structure, and internalizing symptoms that could be explored in future work. In the second study in this area, authors examined regional gray matter volume in the prefrontal cortex as it related to internalizing disorders among lower-SES individuals. Results showed that the observed relationship between lower family income and greater depressive symptoms was mediated by gray matter volume in the pACC extending into the dorsal anterior cingulate cortex (dACC; see Yang et al., 2016), such that greater volume in this region linked lower SES to greater depressive symptoms. This result is surprising given that most of the work in this area finds that lower SES is associated with *smaller* volume across regions. One potential explanation for this disparate finding is that the sample in this study did not exhibit wide variability in SES and depressive symptoms, as most participants were highly educated individuals with fewer depressive symptoms than found in the general population. Thus, these findings might be capturing a different phenomenon than what may be relevant for clinical depression and for individuals at the lower end of the SES spectrum. Together, these studies provide initial indication that SES-related differences in brain structure relate to psychopathology risk. More work is needed in this area to explore the potential for culture to modulate links between SES and structural differences implicated in psychopathology.

Brain Function, Socioeconomic Status, and Psychopathology

In addition to the growing literature that has examined links between SES, brain structure, and psychopathology, recent research has also examined how depression and anxiety are linked with differences in brain *functioning*, as well as the role that SES may play in shaping brain function. With regard to neural function and psychopathology, the default mode network, a set of regions that is consistently active and more connected when the brain is "at rest" (i.e., not directed toward a particular external stimulus), is especially implicated in depression, such that hyperconnectivity between regions within this network is associated with increased reports of rumination in depressed patients (Broyd et al., 2009; Nejad et al., 2013; Sheline et al., 2010). Similarly, inability to downregulate activity within the default mode network has been linked to symptoms of depression that include impaired attentional control and maladaptive rumination (Sliz & Hayley, 2012). Finally, aberrant default mode connectivity is not only linked to depressive symptoms but also to anxious states (Coutinho et al., 2016), as well as MDD (Y. Chen et al., 2015), OCD (Hou et al., 2013), and schizophrenia (Salgado-Pineda et al., 2011). Thus, aberrant activation of and connectivity within the brain's default mode network is associated with a number of negative mental health disorders.

Turning to the influences of SES on brain function, there are fewer studies suggesting that SES modulates functional neural activity (Muscatell, 2018). Complementing the structural findings reviewed earlier, one study found that SES may affect amygdala function, such that retrospective reports of lower parental social standing during childhood were related to increased amygdala activation to threatening faces in adulthood (Gianaros et al., 2008). Another study replicated this pattern of alterations in amygdala activation and found SES differences in connectivity between the amygdala and hippocampus in preschool-aged children. These observed differences in lower functional connectivity between the amygdala and hippocampus among lower-SES youth mediated the relationship between SES and depressive symptoms (Barch et al., 2016). Together, these two studies coupled with the structural findings previously demonstrate the critical role of functional connectivity between medial temporal lobe regions in linking SES and disparities in mental health.

Beyond the amygdala and hippocampus, other work has examined the modulating role of SES on activation in the mentalizing network, or a collection of neural regions activated when thinking about the thoughts and feelings of others (Frith & Frith, 2006). In both adolescent and adult samples, researchers found that activation in these regions differed by SES such that those with lower SES exhibited greater activity in the mentalizing network, and the dorsomedial prefrontal cortex (dmPFC) most robustly (Muscatell et al., 2012). Interestingly the mentalizing network shares much regional overlap with the default mode network, and, as reviewed previously, aberrant functioning in this network is implicated in several mental disorders. Another study also examined the influence of childhood SES on the connectivity within the default mode itself (Sripada et al., 2014) and reported that lower SES is associated with reduced connectivity within the network. Notably, recent work suggests that the resting default mode network might actually be critical for consolidating social information and has been studied to examine whether we are "social by default" (Meyer et al., 2018). Because the medial prefrontal cortex (mPFC) and the temporoparietal junction (TPJ) spontaneously activate during rest and are important for social inferencing, authors examined the connectivity between these regions to assess whether this communication primes an individual for social learning even at rest. Analyses revealed that connectivity between the regions increased after digesting social information and that greater connectivity also corresponded to better social memory. These findings regarding the default mode suggest that the brain might be built to practice encoding social information at rest and that activity in this network is modulated by social status to promote other-oriented activities (e.g., improved empathic accuracy, greater perspective taking, and enhanced social engagement, all key features of interdependent self-construal). A future study should simultaneously explore the relationship between magnitude of activation and measures of connectivity to provide a more complete picture of how the default mode might be implicated in the association between SES, culture, and psychiatric conditions.

Additionally, the cultural neuroscience literature documents differences in neural activation as a function of cultural orientation in circuits and regions implicated in psychopathology. Notably, Chiao and Blizinsky (2013) argue that "one of the most robust findings within cultural neuroscience is the modulation of neural response within the prefrontal regions as a function of cultural values, such as individualism and collectivism" (p. S125). Specifically, activity in the mPFC predicts how individualistic or collectivistic a person is such that individualists display greater mPFC activity when thinking about the self and collectivists show greater mPFC activity when thinking about oneself in the context of others (Chiao et al., 2009). Although low-SES context does not precisely map on to the collectivist ethnic groups explored in these studies, insights from this work can generate hypotheses about how SES might moderate neural activity in the mPFC with implications for psychopathology. Future studies should explore the conditions in which lower SES moderates activity in the mPFC, and whether this is associated with increased depression and anxiety symptoms.

Linking Socioeconomic Status, Brain Structure and Function, and Physiological Activation

As is likely now clear from the literatures reviewed previously, multilevel studies that integrate measures of SES, brain structure and function, and activation of physiological systems are critical for answering complex questions about the neural and physiological mechanisms underlying SES disparities in psychiatric disease. There are only a handful of studies to date that have utilized interdisciplinary approaches to begin shedding light on these important questions. Along these lines, given the established relationship between elevated cortisol levels and reduced hippocampal volume as markers of dysregulated HPA axis functioning, a 2013 study examined SES, HPA activity, and mothers' depressive symptoms as they relate to structural brain differences in children (Sheridan et al., 2013). The study found some mechanistic evidence that lower SES was associated with reduced levels of cortisol, and that lower subjective status of the mother was associated with lower hippocampal activation during a learning task among their offspring. These results provide initial evidence that SES-related HPA dysregulation among parents may lead to alterations in the functioning of the hippocampus among offspring. Given that the hippocampus is a brain structure critical for several cognitive and emotional processes that are important for mental well-being, this innovative study integrating across levels of analysis suggests that SES may confer risk across generations via changes in HPA axis function and hippocampus activation. More studies along these lines are warranted if we are to fully delineate the neural and physiological mechanisms linking SES to negative mental health outcomes.

Another innovative study in this area explored the relationship between SES, brain function, and inflammation, which has important implications for mental health as reviewed earlier. Peripheral inflammation has been directly linked to alterations in neural functioning relevant for psychopathology, such that inflammation is associated with decreased connectivity within the corticostriatal reward circuit in patients with depression (Felger et al., 2016). Experimentally inducing an inflammatory response has also been shown to cause mood changes via altered connectivity between the subgenual cingulate and mesolimbic regions (Harrison et al., 2009). Although the associations between peripheral inflammation and neural circuitry have been established, very little research has examined the underlying psychosocial mechanisms that can account for the patterns of observed activity. In one study, researchers sought to identify whether increased inflammatory responses to a stressful task among individuals lower in SES were mediated by activity in the dmPFC, which plays a role in mentalizing (Muscatell et al., 2016). The hypothesized mechanism was confirmed, such that those with lower subjective SES exhibited greater IL-6 responses to a stress task, and these effects were mediated by neural activity in the dmPFC in response to negative social feedback. A final noteworthy study explored the mechanisms linking SES to gene methylation of the serotonin transporter gene, amygdala reactivity to negative stimuli, and change in depressive symptoms (Swartz et al., 2017). Results from this study indicated that increases in depressive symptoms among lower-SES adolescents were mediated by a pathway from SES to epigenetic alterations in methylation of the serotonin transporter gene and greater amygdala reactivity. Together, these studies confirm the value that integration across systems has for research in this area, filling large gaps in our understanding about how disadvantage might affect psychiatric health. An important contribution to this work would be to consider how sociocultural factors might alter integration across systems to impact mental well-being.

Socioeconomic Status, Resilience, and Links Between Mental and Physical Health

Up to this point, the chapter has focused on discussing the mechanisms that may link low SES to poorer mental health. Existing evidence suggests that SES is a significant social determinant of health that has a profound impact on one's quality of life. In one provocative study, researchers exposed individuals with differing SES to a cold virus and then tracked their symptoms for 6 weeks. Findings suggest that lower-SES individuals were three times more likely to develop a cold than higher-SES individuals (Cohen et al., 2004). Interestingly, however, more than half of the lower-SES participants (55%) did not ultimately develop any cold symptoms. This finding begs the question: how do some individuals maintain good physical and psychological health despite the challenges of low-SES circumstances? Much of the work on resilience in the SES literature integrates the study of mental and physical health outcomes to generate a more complex picture of the factors promoting positive outcomes across the mental and physical domains. In what follows, we will review the primary models of resilience in the SES literature.

Common to several theories of resilience among individuals in a low-SES context is a discussion of the psychological and interpersonal resources that are beneficial for mental and physical health. Specifically, researchers maintain that personal characteristics (e.g., emotion regulation, optimism, and perceived control) as well as social support provide resources that can moderate the impact of SES on well-being. Along these lines, Taylor and Seeman (1999) discuss the role of psychosocial resources in moderating the SES–health relationship. Specifically, they argue that optimism, coping style, sense of mastery/personal control, and social support might be especially important for individuals living in contexts that limit personal control and increase chronic arousal (such as low SES), and that the absence of these psychosocial resources has been linked to depression, anxiety, suicide, and cardiovascular disease. Greater psychosocial resources are thought to reduce the stress response implicated in the etiology of mental and physical health problems because resources can influence an individual's perception of the severity of potentially stressful events. Some empirical evidence supports this theory, finding that a composite measure of psychosocial resources was associated with lower basal levels of cortisol, reduced sympathetic activation, and quicker recovery following a laboratory stressor (Taylor et al., 2003). Thus, greater psychosocial resources, including optimism, mastery, coping, and social support, may confer resilience, especially for individuals from lower-SES backgrounds.

Gallo and Matthews (2003) expanded the psychosocial resources framework by proposing that some low-SES individuals may have decreased "reserve capacity," or fewer resilient personal and interpersonal factors that can enable adaptive coping and the prevention of future stress. This model has been tested utilizing ecological momentary assessment in women with varying SES for 2 days (Gallo et al., 2005). The study found that lower-SES women had greater decreases in internal and interpersonal resources than higher-SES women, which led to increases in negative emotions and decreased positive emotions. Given the study design, authors were also able to evaluate support transactions among the women to get a better understanding of the nature and effects of social support. Interestingly, results suggested that lower-SES women experienced greater increases in positive affect following social support exchanges as compared to women in higher-SES groups. These data suggest that social support, a critical predictor of mental and physical health outcomes, may be especially important among lower-SES individuals, as high levels of support may help mitigate the risk of lower-SES environments.

Another theory of resilience, E. Chen and Miller's (2012) "shift and persist" model, focuses on the "psychological processes that mitigate perceptions of stress" to explore how these perceptions might reduce the biological cascade linked to stress in lower-SES children. In this formulation, one way to develop resilience to low-SES circumstances is to "shift," or alter one's responses to adversity by engaging in the emotion regulation strategy of reappraisal, and to "persist," or find purpose and maintain optimism about the future in spite of adversity. Role models may be critical to the development of shift-and-persist strategies as they encourage children to think positively about the future and provide an example of how to shift one's response to adversity. This theory has been tested empirically in a large, representative sample, with findings that among adults who were raised in lower-SES households, those that engaged in greater shift-and-persist strategies had the lowest allostatic load or physiological dysregulation as adults (E. Chen et al., 2012). Notably, difficulties with these strategies of emotion regulation, reappraisal, and optimism are associated with depression and anxiety (E. Chen & Miller, 2013), suggesting that the development of shift-and-persist coping strategies is one mechanism by which lower-SES individuals may thrive despite challenging life circumstances.

This body of work has identified several individual-level factors that can improve health outcomes given the context; however, there is evidence that the individual can only do so much in the face of adversity. In what they term "skin-deep resilience," Miller and colleagues (2015) find that self-control can function as a "double-edged sword" whereby it relates to better academic and psychosocial functioning but is also linked to poorer physiological health. In a sample of rural African American children under severe and persistent

SES risk, those with high levels of self-control displayed resilient behavioral and psychological outcomes and poorer physiological function years later (Brody et al., 2013). Thus, individual striving may come at a physiological cost. These results imply that while intervention efforts aimed at improving individual-level factors (e.g., self-control or "grit") may have some benefits for low-SES individuals, they may also have some costs (e.g., increased inflammation). As such, research and policy interventions must work to change societal structures that can further support individuals from lower-SES backgrounds who are upwardly mobile.

Although resilience research demonstrates how individual-level psychosocial characteristics might be fostered to improve outcomes in some domains, ultimately, these findings also speak to broader ethical considerations in studying and promoting policies targeting individual-level factors as a way to overcome SES-based disparities in mental health. The concept of medicalization widely discussed among sociologists encapsulates this very concern. Medicalization describes the process by which society shifts aspects of life or social norms toward becoming medical problems (Conrad, 2007). In her book, Becker (2013) discusses the development and tensions involved with studying stress in modern society. She argues from an anthropological and critical psychological perspective that this approach runs the risk of promoting individual blame for issues that should ultimately be resolved through social and political action. Becker contends that an individual's adaptation to adversity does not imply the adversity is no longer a problem, and she declares that "adaptation to injustice, violence, and/or poverty doesn't necessarily improve the human condition" (p. 63). Indeed, the skin-deep resilience work, documenting that individual striving comes at a physiological cost, provides support for this perspective, suggesting that ultimately reducing economic inequality (rather than helping low-SES individuals "cope" with having less) might be of paramount importance for improving health. Ongoing studies are exploring whether giving families money can attenuate the known links between poverty and brain development in children, which would point to the need for economic and policy shifts that target material resources as well as individual-level psychological resources to promote mental health equity across the SES spectrum ("Does Growing Up Poor Harm Brain Development?," 2018; Gammon, 2017).

Concluding Comments

In this chapter, we explored how SES might influence stress physiology and brain structure/function with implications for mental health. This chapter began with a discussion of how low-SES environments may foster development of an interdependent sense of self, which may in turn have relevance for mental health in this population. We discussed how interdependence within this group of individuals could potentially be costly for mental health and how an individual's cultural consonance, or degree to which an individual's life approximates the cultural prototype of success, could contribute to increased stress. With the backdrop of how cultural and psychological processes vary across the SES spectrum may confer risk for psychopathology, we next examined literature linking low

SES to alterations in physiological functioning that have implications for depression and anxiety. Generally, reviewed literature reveals that lower SES is related to dysregulation within the HPA axis, the ANS, and the immune system's pro-inflammatory response and is associated with greater multisystem dysregulation, all of which have also been associated with negative mental health outcomes. Finally, we reviewed recent neuroimaging evidence suggesting that SES can influence brain structure and function. The most conclusive findings across these different physiological and neural systems are that low SES is associated with lower cardiac vagal tone, decreased brain volume in the prefrontal cortex and limbic system, heightened functioning of the mentalizing network, and increased multisystem dysregulation. Given that these physiological and neural patterns have all been linked to major depression and clinical anxiety, a picture is beginning to emerge suggesting that lower-SES contexts can lead to changes in physiological and neural processes that put individuals on a trajectory toward psychopathology.

Although there exists strong foundational evidence for the link between SES and psychiatric conditions, there are very few studies that explore the mechanisms that might be accounting for increased depression and anxiety in this population that is most vulnerable. As reviewed earlier, literatures exploring the cultural environments of different SES strata, the physiological and neural correlates of SES, and the neurobiological bases for mental health conditions have remained largely separate to date. Thus, the time is ripe for research that integrates across social/cultural and clinical psychology, psychophysiology, neuroimaging, and epidemiology to provide a more holistic picture of the cultural, psychological, and biological pathways linking SES and mental health. Work of this nature will require team science and multidisciplinary collaboration, as well as engagement with low-SES communities via community-based participatory research, in an effort to fully explore the mechanisms that underlie SES disparities in mental health outcomes. Armed with the kind of basic science knowledge this multidisciplinary approach could generate, researchers can design more effective prevention and intervention programs that support low-SES individuals across the globe and ensure that each individual has the opportunity to thrive regardless of their income, education, or occupation.

References

Adam, E. K., Doane, L. D., Zinbarg, R. E., Mineka, S., Craske, M. G., & Griffith, J. W. (2010). Prospective prediction of major depressive disorder from cortisol awakening responses in adolescence. *Psychoneuroendocrinology*, *35*(6), 921–931. doi:10.1016/j.psyneuen.2009.12.007

Adam, E. K., Vrshek-Schallhorn, S., Kendall, A. D., Mineka, S., Zinbarg, R. E., & Craske, M. G. (2014). Prospective associations between the cortisol awakening response and first onsets of anxiety disorders over a six-year follow-up—2013 Curt Richter Award Winner. *Psychoneuroendocrinology*, *44*, 47–59. doi:10.1016/j.psyneuen.2014.02.014

Alegría, M., Canino, G., Shrout, P. E., Woo, M., Duan, N., Vila, D., Torres, M., Chen, C.-N., & Meng, X.-L. (2008). Prevalence of mental illness in immigrant and non-immigrant U.S. Latino groups. *The American Journal of Psychiatry*, *165*(3), 359–369. https://doi.org/10.1176/appi.ajp.2007.07040704

Andrade, L. H., Wang, Y.-P., Andreoni, S., Silveira, C. M., Alexandrino-Silva, C., Siu, E. R., Nishimura, R., Anthony, J. C., Gattaz, W. F., Kessler, R. C., & Viana, M. C. (2012). Mental disorders in megacities:

findings from the São Paulo megacity mental health survey, Brazil. Plos One, 7(2), e31879. https://doi.org/10.1371/journal.pone.0031879

Barch, D., Pagliaccio, D., Belden, A., Harms, M. P., Gaffrey, M., Sylvester, C. M., . . . Luby, J. (2016). Effect of hippocampal and amygdala connectivity on the relationship between preschool poverty and school-age depression. *American Journal of Psychiatry*, *173*(6), 625–634. doi:10.1176/appi.ajp.2015.15081014

Barrett, L. F. (2017). The theory of constructed emotion: An active inference account of interoception and categorization. *Social Cognitive and Affective Neuroscience*, *12*(1), 1–23. doi:10.1093/scan/nsw154

Barton, D. A., Dawood, T., Lambert, E. A., Esler, M. D., Haikerwal, D., Brenchley, C., . . . Lambert, G. W. (2007). Sympathetic activity in major depressive disorder: Identifying those at increased cardiac risk? *Journal of Hypertension*, *25*(10), 2117–2124. doi:10.1097/HJH.0b013e32829baae7

Becker, D. (2013). *One nation under stress: The trouble with stress as an idea*. Oxford University Press. doi:10.1093/acprof:osobl/9780199742912.001.0001

Belvederi Murri, M., Pariante, C., Mondelli, V., Masotti, M., Atti, A. R., Mellacqua, Z., . . . Amore, M. (2014). HPA axis and aging in depression: Systematic review and meta-analysis. *Psychoneuroendocrinology*, *41*, 46–62. doi:10.1016/j.psyneuen.2013.12.004

Berntson, G. G., Cacioppo, J. T., & Quigley, K. S. (1993). Respiratory sinus arrhythmia: Autonomic origins, physiological mechanisms, and psychophysiological implications. *Psychophysiology*, *30*(2), 183–196. doi:10.1111/j.1469-8986.1993.tb01731.x

Bizik, G., Picard, M., Nijjar, R., Tourjman, V., McEwen, B. S., Lupien, S. J., & Juster, R.-P. (2013). Allostatic load as a tool for monitoring physiological dysregulations and comorbidities in patients with severe mental illnesses. *Harvard Review of Psychiatry*, *21*(6), 296–313. doi:10.1097/HRP.0000000000000012

Blackmon, K., Barr, W. B., Carlson, C., Devinsky, O., DuBois, J., Pogash, D., . . . Thesen, T. (2011). Structural evidence for involvement of a left amygdala-orbitofrontal network in subclinical anxiety. *Psychiatry Research*, *194*(3), 296–303. doi:10.1016/j.pscychresns.2011.05.007

Blechert, J., Michael, T., Grossman, P., Lajtman, M., & Wilhelm, F. H. (2007). Autonomic and respiratory characteristics of posttraumatic stress disorder and panic disorder. *Psychosomatic Medicine*, *69*(9), 935–943. doi:10.1097/PSY.0b013e31815a8f6b

Boylan, J. M., Cundiff, J. M., & Matthews, K. A. (2018). Socioeconomic status and cardiovascular responses to standardized stressors: A systematic review and meta-analysis. *Psychosomatic Medicine*, *80*(3), 278–293. doi:10.1097/PSY.0000000000000561

Brinkmann, K., & Franzen, J. (2013). Not everyone's heart contracts to reward: Insensitivity to varying levels of reward in dysphoria. *Biological Psychology*, *94*(2), 263–271. https://doi.org/10.1016/j.biopsycho.2013.07.003

Brinkmann, K., Schüpbach, L., Joye, I. A., & Gendolla, G. H. E. (2009). Anhedonia and effort mobilization in dysphoria: reduced cardiovascular response to reward and punishment. *International Journal of Psychophysiology*, *74*(3), 250–258. https://doi.org/10.1016/j.ijpsycho.2009.09.009

Brito, N. H., & Noble, K. G. (2014). Socioeconomic status and structural brain development. *Frontiers in Neuroscience*, *8*, 276. doi:10.3389/fnins.2014.00276

Brody, G. H., Yu, T., Chen, E., Miller, G. E., Kogan, S. M., & Beach, S. R. H. (2013). Is resilience only skin deep?: Rural African Americans' socioeconomic status-related risk and competence in preadolescence and psychological adjustment and allostatic load at age 19. *Psychological Science*, *24*(7), 1285–1293. doi:10.1177/0956797612471954

Brosschot, J. F., Verkuil, B., & Thayer, J. F. (2017). Exposed to events that never happen: Generalized unsafety, the default stress response, and prolonged autonomic activity. *Neuroscience and Biobehavioral Reviews*, *74*(Pt B), 287–296. doi:10.1016/j.neubiorev.2016.07.019

Brosschot, J. F., Verkuil, B., & Thayer, J. F. (2018). Generalized unsafety theory of stress: Unsafe environments and conditions, and the default stress response. *International Journal of Environmental Research and Public Health*, *15*(3), 1–27. doi:10.3390/ijerph15030464

Broyd, S. J., Demanuele, C., Debener, S., Helps, S. K., James, C. J., & Sonuga-Barke, E. J. S. (2009). Default-mode brain dysfunction in mental disorders: A systematic review. *Neuroscience and Biobehavioral Reviews*, *33*(3), 279–296. doi:10.1016/j.neubiorev.2008.09.002

Broyles, S. T., Staiano, A. E., Drazba, K. T., Gupta, A. K., Sothern, M., & Katzmarzyk, P. T. (2012). Elevated C-reactive protein in children from risky neighborhoods: Evidence for a stress pathway linking neighborhoods and inflammation in children. *Plos One*, *7*(9), e45419. doi:10.1371/journal.pone.0045419

Burke, H. M., Davis, M. C., Otte, C., & Mohr, D. C. (2005). Depression and cortisol responses to psychological stress: A meta-analysis. *Psychoneuroendocrinology*, *30*(9), 846–856. doi:10.1016/j.psyneuen.2005.02.010

Burke, H. M., Fernald, L. C., Gertler, P. J., & Adler, N. E. (2005). Depressive symptoms are associated with blunted cortisol stress responses in very low-income women. *Psychosomatic Medicine*, *67*(2), 211–216. doi:10.1097/01.psy.0000156939.89050.28

Burmaster, K. B., Landefeld, J. C., Rehkopf, D. H., Lahiff, M., Sokal-Gutierrez, K., Adler-Milstein, S., & Fernald, L. C. H. (2015). Impact of a private sector living wage intervention on depressive symptoms among apparel workers in the Dominican Republic: A quasi-experimental study. *BMJ Open*, *5*(8), e007336. doi:10.1136/bmjopen-2014-007336

Bush, N. R., Jones-Mason, K., Coccia, M., Caron, Z., Alkon, A., Thomas, M., . . . Epel, E. S. (2017). Effects of pre- and postnatal maternal stress on infant temperament and autonomic nervous system reactivity and regulation in a diverse, low-income population. *Development and Psychopathology*, *29*(5), 1553–1571. doi:10.1017/S0954579417001237

Canu, E., Kostić, M., Agosta, F., Munjiza, A., Ferraro, P. M., Pesic, D., . . . Filippi, M. (2015). Brain structural abnormalities in patients with major depression with or without generalized anxiety disorder comorbidity. *Journal of Neurology*, *262*(5), 1255–1265. doi:10.1007/s00415-015-7701-z

Chen, E., & Matthews, K. A. (2001). Cognitive appraisal biases: an approach to understanding the relation between socioeconomic status and cardiovascular reactivity in children. *Annals of Behavioral Medicine*, *23*(2), 101–111. https://doi.org/10.1207/S15324796ABM2302_4

Chen, E., Matthews, K. A., & Boyce, W. T. (2002). Socioeconomic differences in children's health: how and why do these relationships change with age? *Psychological Bulletin*, *128*(2), 295–329.

Chen, E., & Miller, G. E. (2012). "Shift-and-persist" strategies: Why low socioeconomic status isn't always bad for health. *Perspectives on Psychological Science : A Journal of the Association for Psychological Science*, *7*(2), 135–158. doi:10.1177/1745691612436694

Chen, E., & Miller, G. E. (2013). Socioeconomic status and health: Mediating and moderating factors. *Annual Review of Clinical Psychology*, *9*, 723–749. doi:10.1146/annurev-clinpsy-050212-185634

Chen, E., Miller, G. E., Lachman, M. E., Gruenewald, T. L., & Seeman, T. E. (2012). Protective factors for adults from low-childhood socioeconomic circumstances: The benefits of shift-and-persist for allostatic load. *Psychosomatic Medicine*, *74*(2), 178–186. doi:10.1097/PSY.0b013e31824206fd

Chen, Y., Wang, C., Zhu, X., Tan, Y., & Zhong, Y. (2015). Aberrant connectivity within the default mode network in first-episode, treatment-naïve major depressive disorder. *Journal of Affective Disorders*, *183*, 49–56. doi:10.1016/j.jad.2015.04.052

Chiao, J. Y., & Blizinsky, K. D. (2013). Population disparities in mental health: Insights from cultural neuroscience. *American Journal of Public Health*, *103*(Suppl 1), S122–S132. doi:10.2105/AJPH.2013.301440

Chiao, J. Y., Harada, T., Komeda, H., Li, Z., Mano, Y., Saito, D., . . . Iidaka, T. (2009). Neural basis of individualistic and collectivistic views of self. *Human Brain Mapping*, *30*(9), 2813–2820. doi:10.1002/hbm.20707

Chiavegatto Filho, A. D. P., Kawachi, I., Wang, Y. P., Viana, M. C., & Andrade, L. H. S. G. (2013). Does income inequality get under the skin? A multilevel analysis of depression, anxiety and mental disorders in Sao Paulo, Brazil. *Journal of Epidemiology and Community Health*, *67*(11), 966–972. doi:10.1136/jech-2013-202626

Chirinos, D. A., Murdock, K. W., LeRoy, A. S., & Fagundes, C. (2017). Depressive symptom profiles, cardiometabolic risk and inflammation: Results from the MIDUS study. *Psychoneuroendocrinology*, *82*, 17–25. doi:10.1016/j.psyneuen.2017.04.011

Cohen, S., Doyle, W. J., & Baum, A. (2006). Socioeconomic status is associated with stress hormones. *Psychosomatic Medicine*, *68*(3), 414–420. doi:10.1097/01.psy.0000221236.37158.b9

Cohen, S., Doyle, W. J., Turner, R. B., Alper, C. M., & Skoner, D. P. (2004). Childhood socioeconomic status and host resistance to infectious illness in adulthood. *Psychosomatic Medicine*, *66*(4), 553–558. doi:10.1097/01.psy.0000126200.05189.d3

Conrad, P. (2007). *The medicalization of society: On the transformation of human conditions into treatable disorders.* Johns Hopkins University Press.

Coutinho, J. F., Fernandesl, S. V., Soares, J. M., Maia, L., Gonçalves, Ó. F., & Sampaio, A. (2016). Default mode network dissociation in depressive and anxiety states. *Brain Imaging and Behavior*, *10*(1), 147–157. doi:10.1007/s11682-015-9375-7

Critchley, H. D., & Garfinkel, S. N. (2017). Interoception and emotion. *Current Opinion in Psychology*, *17*, 7–14. doi:10.1016/j.copsyc.2017.04.020

Danese, A., Moffitt, T. E., Pariante, C. M., Ambler, A., Poulton, R., & Caspi, A. (2008). Elevated inflammation levels in depressed adults with a history of childhood maltreatment. *Archives of General Psychiatry*, *65*(4), 409–415. doi:10.1001/archpsyc.65.4.409

Derry, H. M., Fagundes, C. P., Andridge, R., Glaser, R., Malarkey, W. B., & Kiecolt-Glaser, J. K. (2013). Lower subjective social status exaggerates interleukin-6 responses to a laboratory stressor. *Psychoneuroendocrinology*, *38*(11), 2676–2685. doi:10.1016/j.psyneuen.2013.06.026

Dittmann, A. G., & Stephens, N. M. (2017). Interventions aimed at closing the social class achievement gap: Changing individuals, structures, and construals. *Current Opinion in Psychology*, *18*, 111–116. doi:10.1016/j.copsyc.2017.07.044

Does growing up poor harm brain development? (2018, May 3). *The Economist*.

Dressler, W. W. (2007). Cultural consonance. In D. Bhugra & K. Bhui (Eds.), *Textbook of cultural psychiatry* (pp. 179–190). Cambridge University Press. doi:10.1017/CBO9780511543609.016

Dressler, W. W., Balieiro, M. C., & dos Santos, J. E. (2017). Cultural consonance in life goals and depressive symptoms in urban Brazil. *Journal of Anthropological Research*, *73*(1), 43–65. doi:10.1086/690610

Dressler, W. W., Balieiro, M. C., Ribeiro, R. P., & dos Santos, J. E. (2007). A prospective study of cultural consonance and depressive symptoms in urban Brazil. *Social Science & Medicine*, *65*(10), 2058–2069. doi:10.1016/j.socscimed.2007.06.020

Elliot, A. J., & Chapman, B. P. (2016). Socioeconomic status, psychological resources, and inflammatory markers: Results from the MIDUS study. *Health Psychology*, *35*(11), 1205–1213. doi:10.1037/hea0000392

Evans, G. W., & Kim, P. (2007). Childhood poverty and health: Cumulative risk exposure and stress dysregulation. *Psychological Science*, *18*(11), 953–957. doi:10.1111/j.1467-9280.2007.02008.x

Fagundes, C. P., Glaser, R., Hwang, B. S., Malarkey, W. B., & Kiecolt-Glaser, J. K. (2013). Depressive symptoms enhance stress-induced inflammatory responses. *Brain, Behavior, and Immunity*, *31*, 172–176. doi:10.1016/j.bbi.2012.05.006

Faravelli, C., Lo Sauro, C., Godini, L., Lelli, L., Benni, L., Pietrini, F., . . . Ricca, V. (2012). Childhood stressful events, HPA axis and anxiety disorders. *World Journal of Psychiatry*, *2*(1), 13–25. doi:10.5498/wjp.v2.i1.13

Felger, J. C., Li, Z., Haroon, E., Woolwine, B. J., Jung, M. Y., Hu, X., & Miller, A. H. (2016). Inflammation is associated with decreased functional connectivity within corticostriatal reward circuitry in depression. *Molecular Psychiatry*, *21*(10), 1358–1365. doi:10.1038/mp.2015.168

Fernald, L. C. H., Burke, H. M., & Gunnar, M. R. (2008). Salivary cortisol levels in children of low-income women with high depressive symptomatology. *Development and Psychopathology*, *20*(2), 423–436. doi:10.1017/S0954579408000205

Franzen, J., & Brinkmann, K. (2015). Blunted cardiovascular reactivity in dysphoria during reward and punishment anticipation. *International Journal of Psychophysiology*, *95*(3), 270–277. https://doi.org/10.1016/j.ijpsycho.2014.11.007

Frith, C. D., & Frith, U. (2006). The neural basis of mentalizing. *Neuron*, *50*(4), 531–534. doi:10.1016/j.neuron.2006.05.001

Gallo, L. C., Bogart, L. M., Vranceanu, A.-M., & Matthews, K. A. (2005). Socioeconomic status, resources, psychological experiences, and emotional responses: A test of the reserve capacity model. *Journal of Personality and Social Psychology*, *88*(2), 386–399. doi:10.1037/0022-3514.88.2.386

Gallo, L. C., & Matthews, K. A. (2003). Understanding the association between socioeconomic status and physical health: Do negative emotions play a role? *Psychological Bulletin*, *129*(1), 10–51. doi:10.1037/0033-2909.129.1.10

Gammon, K. (2017, September 22). Could giving families cash help children's brain development? https://www.centerforhealthjournalism.org/2017/09/20/could-giving-families-cash-help-children%E2%80%99s-brain-development

Gianaros, P. J., Horenstein, J. A., Cohen, S., Matthews, K. A., Brown, S. M., Flory, J. D., . . . Hariri, A. R. (2007). Perigenual anterior cingulate morphology covaries with perceived social standing. *Social Cognitive and Affective Neuroscience*, *2*(3), 161–173. doi:10.1093/scan/nsm013

Gianaros, P. J., Horenstein, J. A., Hariri, A. R., Sheu, L. K., Manuck, S. B., Matthews, K. A., & Cohen, S. (2008). Potential neural embedding of parental social standing. *Social Cognitive and Affective Neuroscience*, *3*(2), 91–96. doi:10.1093/scan/nsn003

Gold, A. L., Steuber, E. R., White, L. K., Pacheco, J., Sachs, J. F., Pagliaccio, D., . . . Pine, D. S. (2017). Cortical thickness and subcortical gray matter volume in pediatric anxiety disorders. *Neuropsychopharmacology*, *42*(12), 2423–2433. doi:10.1038/npp.2017.83

Gone, J. P., & Trimble, J. E. (2012). American Indian and Alaska Native mental health: Diverse perspectives on enduring disparities. *Annual Review of Clinical Psychology*, 8, 131–160. doi:10.1146/annurev-clinpsy-032511-143127

Grossmann, I., & Varnum, M. E. W. (2011). Social class, culture, and cognition. *Social Psychological and Personality Science*, 2(1), 81–89. doi:10.1177/1948550610377119

Gruenewald, T. L., Karlamangla, A. S., Hu, P., Stein-Merkin, S., Crandall, C., Koretz, B., & Seeman, T. E. (2012). History of socioeconomic disadvantage and allostatic load in later life. *Social Science & Medicine*, 74(1), 75–83. doi:10.1016/j.socscimed.2011.09.037

Han, K.-M., Choi, S., Jung, J., Na, K.-S., Yoon, H.-K., Lee, M.-S., & Ham, B.-J. (2014). Cortical thickness, cortical and subcortical volume, and white matter integrity in patients with their first episode of major depression. *Journal of Affective Disorders*, 155, 42–48. doi:10.1016/j.jad.2013.10.021

Han, S., Northoff, G., Vogeley, K., Wexler, B. E., Kitayama, S., & Varnum, M. E. W. (2013). A cultural neuroscience approach to the biosocial nature of the human brain. *Annual Review of Psychology*, 64, 335–359. doi:10.1146/annurev-psych-071112-054629

Harrison, N. A., Brydon, L., Walker, C., Gray, M. A., Steptoe, A., & Critchley, H. D. (2009). Inflammation causes mood changes through alterations in subgenual cingulate activity and mesolimbic connectivity. *Biological Psychiatry*, 66(5), 407–414. doi:10.1016/j.biopsych.2009.03.015

Heim, C., & Binder, E. B. (2012). Current research trends in early life stress and depression: Review of human studies on sensitive periods, gene-environment interactions, and epigenetics. *Experimental Neurology*, 233(1), 102–111. doi:10.1016/j.expneurol.2011.10.032

Hek, K., Direk, N., Newson, R. S., Hofman, A., Hoogendijk, W. J. G., Mulder, C. L., & Tiemeier, H. (2013). Anxiety disorders and salivary cortisol levels in older adults: A population-based study. *Psychoneuroendocrinology*, 38(2), 300–305. doi:10.1016/j.psyneuen.2012.06.006

Herbert, J., Goodyer, I. M., Grossman, A. B., Hastings, M. H., de Kloet, E. R., Lightman, S. L., . . . Seckl, J. R. (2006). Do corticosteroids damage the brain? *Journal of Neuroendocrinology*, 18(6), 393–411. doi:10.1111/j.1365-2826.2006.01429.x

Hezel, D. M., & McNally, R. J. (2014). Theory of mind impairments in social anxiety disorder. *Behavior Therapy*, 45(4), 530–540. doi:10.1016/j.beth.2014.02.010

Holz, N. E., Boecker, R., Hohm, E., Zohsel, K., Buchmann, A. F., Blomeyer, D., . . . Laucht, M. (2015). The long-term impact of early life poverty on orbitofrontal cortex volume in adulthood: Results from a prospective study over 25 years. *Neuropsychopharmacology*, 40(4), 996–1004. doi:10.1038/npp.2014.277

Holz, N. E., Laucht, M., & Meyer-Lindenberg, A. (2015). Recent advances in understanding the neurobiology of childhood socioeconomic disadvantage. *Current Opinion in Psychiatry*, 28(5), 365–370. doi:10.1097/YCO.0000000000000178

Hou, J., Song, L., Zhang, W., Wu, W., Wang, J., Zhou, D., . . . Li, H. (2013). Morphologic and functional connectivity alterations of corticostriatal and default mode network in treatment-naïve patients with obsessive-compulsive disorder. *Plos One*, 8(12), e83931. doi:10.1371/journal.pone.0083931

Howes, O. D., & McCutcheon, R. (2017). Inflammation and the neural diathesis-stress hypothesis of schizophrenia: A reconceptualization. *Translational Psychiatry*, 7(2), e1024. doi:10.1038/tp.2016.278

Howren, M. B., Lamkin, D. M., & Suls, J. (2009). Associations of depression with C-reactive protein, IL-1, and IL-6: A meta-analysis. *Psychosomatic Medicine*, 71(2), 171–186. doi:10.1097/PSY.0b013e3181907c1b

Hughes, J. W., Watkins, L., Blumenthal, J. A., Kuhn, C., & Sherwood, A. (2004). Depression and anxiety symptoms are related to increased 24-hour urinary norepinephrine excretion among healthy middle-aged women. *Journal of Psychosomatic Research*, 57(4), 353–358. doi:10.1016/j.jpsychores.2004.02.016

Irle, E., Ruhleder, M., Lange, C., Seidler-Brandler, U., Salzer, S., Dechent, P., . . . Leichsenring, F. (2010). Reduced amygdalar and hippocampal size in adults with generalized social phobia. *Journal of Psychiatry & Neuroscience*, 35(2), 126–131.

Jacob, S., Byrne, M., & Keenan, K. (2009). Neonatal physiological regulation is associated with perinatal factors: A study of neonates born to healthy African American women living in poverty. *Infant Mental Health Journal*, 30(1), 82–94. doi:10.1002/imhj.20204

John-Henderson, N. A., Marsland, A. L., Kamarck, T. W., Muldoon, M. F., & Manuck, S. B. (2016). Childhood socioeconomic status and the occurrence of recent negative life events as predictors of circulating and stimulated levels of interleukin-6. *Psychosomatic Medicine*, 78(1), 91–101. doi:10.1097/PSY.0000000000000262

Jones, A. D. (2017). Food insecurity and mental health status: A global analysis of 149 countries. *American Journal of Preventive Medicine*, 53(2), 264–273. doi:10.1016/j.amepre.2017.04.008

Juruena, M. F. (2014). Early-life stress and HPA axis trigger recurrent adulthood depression. *Epilepsy & Behavior, 38*, 148–159. doi:10.1016/j.yebeh.2013.10.020

Juster, R.-P., Marin, M.-F., Sindi, S., Nair, N. P. V., Ng, Y. K., Pruessner, J. C., & Lupien, S. J. (2011). Allostatic load associations to acute, 3-year and 6-year prospective depressive symptoms in healthy older adults. *Physiology & Behavior, 104*(2), 360–364. doi:10.1016/j.physbeh.2011.02.027

Kemp, A. H., Quintana, D. S., Gray, M. A., Felmingham, K. L., Brown, K., & Gatt, J. M. (2010). Impact of depression and antidepressant treatment on heart rate variability: A review and meta-analysis. *Biological Psychiatry, 67*(11), 1067–1074. doi:10.1016/j.biopsych.2009.12.012

Kessler, R. C. (1994). Lifetime and 12-month prevalence of DSM-III-R psychiatric disorders in the United States. *Archives of General Psychiatry, 51*(1), 8. doi:10.1001/archpsyc.1994.03950010008002

Kim, H. S., Sherman, D. K., & Taylor, S. E. (2008). Culture and social support. *American Psychologist, 63*(6), 518–526.

Kobrosly, R. W., Seplaki, C. L., Cory-Slechta, D. A., Moynihan, J., & van Wijngaarden, E. (2013). Multisystem physiological dysfunction is associated with depressive symptoms in a population-based sample of older adults. *International Journal of Geriatric Psychiatry, 28*(7), 718–727. doi:10.1002/gps.3878

Kraus, M. W., Côté, S., & Keltner, D. (2010). Social class, contextualism, and empathic accuracy. *Psychological Science, 21*(11), 1716–1723. doi:10.1177/0956797610387613

Kraus, M. W., & Keltner, D. (2009). Signs of socioeconomic status: A thin-slicing approach. *Psychological Science, 20*(1), 99–106. doi:10.1111/j.1467-9280.2008.02251.x

Kraus, M. W., Piff, P. K., & Keltner, D. (2011). Social class as culture: The convergence of resources and rank in the social realm. *Current Directions in Psychological Science, 20*(4), 246–250. doi:10.1177/0963721411414654

Kreibig, S. D. (2010). Autonomic nervous system activity in emotion: A review. *Biological Psychology, 84*(3), 394–421. doi:10.1016/j.biopsycho.2010.03.010

Krittayaphong, R., Cascio, W. E., Light, K. C., Sheffield, D., Golden, R. N., Finkel, J. B., . . . Sheps, D. S. (1997). Heart rate variability in patients with coronary artery disease: Differences in patients with higher and lower depression scores. *Psychosomatic Medicine, 59*(3), 231–235.

Ladin, K. (2008). Risk of late-life depression across 10 European Union countries: Deconstructing the education effect. *Journal of Aging and Health, 20*(6), 653–670. doi:10.1177/0898264308321002

Levine, J. C., Fleming, R., Piedmont, J. I., Cain, S. M., & Chen, W.-J. (2016). Heart rate variability and generalized anxiety disorder during laboratory-induced worry and aversive imagery. *Journal of Affective Disorders, 205*, 207–215. doi:10.1016/j.jad.2016.07.019

Light, K. C., Kothandapani, R. V., & Allen, M. T. (1998). Enhanced cardiovascular and catecholamine responses in women with depressive symptoms. *International Journal of Psychophysiology, 28*(2), 157–166. doi:10.1016/S0167-8760(97)00093-7

Lupien, S. J., King, S., Meaney, M. J., & McEwen, B. S. (2000). Child's stress hormone levels correlate with mother's socioeconomic status and depressive state. *Biological Psychiatry, 48*(10), 976–980.

MacCormack, J. K., & Lindquist, K. A. (2017). Bodily contributions to emotion: Schachter's legacy for a psychological constructionist view on emotion. *Emotion Review, 9*(1), 36–45. doi:10.1177/1754073916639664

Manczak, E. M., Basu, D., & Chen, E. (2016). The price of perspective taking: Child depressive symptoms interact with parental empathy to predict immune functioning in parents. *Clinical Psychological Science: A Journal of the Association for Psychological Science, 4*(3), 485–492. doi:10.1177/2167702615595001

Manczak, E. M., DeLongis, A., & Chen, E. (2016). Does empathy have a cost? Diverging psychological and physiological effects within families. *Health Psychology, 35*(3), 211–218. doi:10.1037/hea0000281

Markus, H. R., & Kitayama, S. (1991). Culture and the self: Implications for cognition, emotion, and motivation. *Psychological Review, 98*(2), 224–253. doi:10.1037/0033-295X.98.2.224

Marmot, M. G. (2004). Status syndrome: How your social standing directly affects your health and life expectancy. London: Bloomsbury Pub.

Marmot, M., Allen, J., Bell, R., & Goldblatt, P. (2012). Building of the global movement for health equity: From Santiago to Rio and beyond. *The Lancet, 379*(9811), 181–188. doi:10.1016/S0140-6736(11)61506-7

Maselko, J., Bates, L., Bhalotra, S., Gallis, J. A., O'Donnell, K., Sikander, S., & Turner, E. L. (2018). Socioeconomic status indicators and common mental disorders: Evidence from a study of prenatal depression in Pakistan. *SSM - Population Health, 4*, 1–9. doi:10.1016/j.ssmph.2017.10.004

McEwen, B S. (1998). Stress, adaptation, and disease: Allostasis and allostatic load. *Annals of the New York Academy of Sciences, 840*, 33–44.

McEwen, B. S. (2003). Mood disorders and allostatic load. *Biological Psychiatry*, *54*(3), 200–207. doi:10.1016/S0006-3223(03)00177-X

McEwen, B. S., & Seeman, T. (1999). Protective and damaging effects of mediators of stress: Elaborating and testing the concepts of allostasis and allostatic load. *Annals of the New York Academy of Sciences*, *896*, 30–47.

McEwen, B. S., & Stellar, E. (1993). Stress and the individual. Mechanisms leading to disease. *Archives of Internal Medicine*, *153*(18), 2093–2101. https://doi.org/10.1001/archinte.153.18.2093

McEwen, B. S., & Wingfield, J. C. (2003). The concept of allostasis in biology and biomedicine. *Hormones and Behavior*, *43*(1), 2–15. doi:10.1016/S0018-506X(02)00024-7

Merz, E. C., Tottenham, N., & Noble, K. G. (2018). Socioeconomic status, amygdala volume, and internalizing symptoms in children and adolescents. *Journal of Clinical Child and Adolescent Psychology*, *47*(2), 312–323. doi:10.1080/15374416.2017.1326122

Meyer, M. L., Davachi, L., Ochsner, K. N., & Lieberman, M. D. (2019). Evidence That Default Network Connectivity During Rest Consolidates Social Information. *Cerebral cortex*, *29*(5), 1910–1920. https://doi.org/10.1093/cercor/bhy071

Michopoulos, V., Powers, A., Gillespie, C. F., Ressler, K. J., & Jovanovic, T. (2017). Inflammation in fear- and anxiety-based disorders: PTSD, GAD, and beyond. *Neuropsychopharmacology*, *42*(1), 254–270. doi:10.1038/npp.2016.146

Miller, A. H., Haroon, E., & Felger, J. C. (2017). The immunology of behavior-exploring the role of the immune system in brain health and illness. *Neuropsychopharmacology*, *42*(1), 1–4. doi:10.1038/npp.2016.229

Miller, A. H., Maletic, V., & Raison, C. L. (2009). Inflammation and its discontents: The role of cytokines in the pathophysiology of major depression. *Biological Psychiatry*, *65*(9), 732–741. doi:10.1016/j.biopsych.2008.11.029

Miller, A. H., & Raison, C. L. (2016). The role of inflammation in depression: From evolutionary imperative to modern treatment target. *Nature Reviews. Immunology*, *16*(1), 22–34. doi:10.1038/nri.2015.5

Miller, G. E., & Cole, S. W. (2012). Clustering of depression and inflammation in adolescents previously exposed to childhood adversity. *Biological Psychiatry*, *72*(1), 34–40. doi:10.1016/j.biopsych.2012.02.034

Miller, G. E., Yu, T., Chen, E., & Brody, G. H. (2015). Self-control forecasts better psychosocial outcomes but faster epigenetic aging in low-SES youth. *Proceedings of the National Academy of Sciences of the United States of America*, *112*(33), 10325–10330. doi:10.1073/pnas.1505063112

Muscatell, K. A. (2018). Socioeconomic influences on brain function: Implications for health. *Annals of the New York Academy of Sciences*, *1428*(1), 14–32. doi:10.1111/nyas.13862

Muscatell, K. A., Brosso, S. N. & Humphreys, K. L. Socioeconomic status and inflammation: a meta-analysis. *Mol Psychiatry*, 25, 2189–2199 (2020). https://doi.org/10.1038/s41380-018-0259-2

Muscatell, K. A., Dedovic, K., Slavich, G. M., Jarcho, M. R., Breen, E. C., Bower, J. E., . . . Eisenberger, N. I. (2016). Neural mechanisms linking social status and inflammatory responses to social stress. *Social Cognitive and Affective Neuroscience*, *11*(6), 915–922. doi:10.1093/scan/nsw025

Muscatell, K. A., Morelli, S. A., Falk, E. B., Way, B. M., Pfeifer, J. H., Galinsky, A. D., . . . Eisenberger, N. I. (2012). Social status modulates neural activity in the mentalizing network. *Neuroimage*, *60*(3), 1771–1777. doi:10.1016/j.neuroimage.2012.01.080

Nejad, A. B., Fossati, P., & Lemogne, C. (2013). Self-referential processing, rumination, and cortical midline structures in major depression. *Frontiers in Human Neuroscience*, *7*, 666. doi:10.3389/fnhum.2013.00666

Nusslock, R., & Miller, G. E. (2016). Early-life adversity and physical and emotional health across the lifespan: A neuroimmune network hypothesis. *Biological Psychiatry*, *80*(1), 23–32. doi:10.1016/j.biopsych.2015.05.017

Osimo, E. F., Cardinal, R. N., Jones, P. B., & Khandaker, G. M. (2018). Prevalence and correlates of low-grade systemic inflammation in adult psychiatric inpatients: An electronic health record-based study. *Psychoneuroendocrinology*, *91*, 226–234. doi:10.1016/j.psyneuen.2018.02.031

Pariante, C. M., & Lightman, S. L. (2008). The HPA axis in major depression: Classical theories and new developments. *Trends in Neurosciences*, *31*(9), 464–468. doi:10.1016/j.tins.2008.06.006

Pietras, S. A., & Goodman, E. (2013). Socioeconomic status gradients in inflammation in adolescence. *Psychosomatic Medicine*, *75*(5), 442–448. doi:10.1097/PSY.0b013e31828b871a

Piff, P. K., Stancato, D. M., Martinez, A. G., Kraus, M. W., & Keltner, D. (2012). Class, chaos, and the construction of community. *Journal of Personality and Social Psychology*, *103*(6), 949–962. doi:10.1037/a0029673

Pittig, A., Arch, J. J., Lam, C. W. R., & Craske, M. G. (2013). Heart rate and heart rate variability in panic, social anxiety, obsessive-compulsive, and generalized anxiety disorders at baseline and in response to relaxation and hyperventilation. *International Journal of Psychophysiology, 87*(1), 19–27. doi:10.1016/j.ijpsycho.2012.10.012

Raison, C. L., Capuron, L., & Miller, A. H. (2006). Cytokines sing the blues: Inflammation and the pathogenesis of depression. *Trends in Immunology, 27*(1), 24–31. doi:10.1016/j.it.2005.11.006

Raison, C. L., & Miller, A. H. (2011). Is depression an inflammatory disorder? *Current Psychiatry Reports, 13*(6), 467–475. doi:10.1007/s11920-011-0232-0

Robinette, J. W., Charles, S. T., Almeida, D. M., & Gruenewald, T. L. (2016). Neighborhood features and physiological risk: An examination of allostatic load. *Health & Place, 41*, 110–118. doi:10.1016/j.healthplace.2016.08.003

Salgado-Pineda, P., Fakra, E., Delaveau, P., McKenna, P. J., Pomarol-Clotet, E., & Blin, O. (2011). Correlated structural and functional brain abnormalities in the default mode network in schizophrenia patients. *Schizophrenia Research, 125*(2–3), 101–109. doi:10.1016/j.schres.2010.10.027

Sapolsky, R. M. (2004). *Why zebras don't get ulcers: The acclaimed guide to stress, stress-related diseases, and coping.* Henry Holt and Company.

Schulz, A. J., Mentz, G., Lachance, L., Johnson, J., Gaines, C., & Israel, B. A. (2012). Associations between socioeconomic status and allostatic load: Effects of neighborhood poverty and tests of mediating pathways. *American Journal of Public Health, 102*(9), 1706–1714. doi:10.2105/AJPH.2011.300412

Seeman, T., Epel, E., Gruenewald, T., Karlamangla, A., & McEwen, B. S. (2010). Socio-economic differentials in peripheral biology: Cumulative allostatic load. *Annals of the New York Academy of Sciences, 1186*, 223–239. doi:10.1111/j.1749-6632.2009.05341.x

Seeman, T. E., Crimmins, E., Huang, M.-H., Singer, B., Bucur, A., Gruenewald, T., . . . Reuben, D. B. (2004). Cumulative biological risk and socio-economic differences in mortality: MacArthur studies of successful aging. *Social Science & Medicine, 58*(10), 1985–1997. doi:10.1016/S0277-9536(03)00402-7

Seplaki, C. L., Goldman, N., Weinstein, M., & Lin, Y.-H. (2004). How are biomarkers related to physical and mental well-being? *Journals of Gerontology. Series A, Biological Sciences and Medical Sciences, 59*(3), 201–217.

Sheline, Y. I., Price, J. L., Yan, Z., & Mintun, M. A. (2010). Resting-state functional MRI in depression unmasks increased connectivity between networks via the dorsal nexus. *Proceedings of the National Academy of Sciences of the United States of America, 107*(24), 11020–11025. doi:10.1073/pnas.1000446107

Sheridan, M. A., How, J., Araujo, M., Schamberg, M. A., & Nelson, C. A. (2013). What are the links between maternal social status, hippocampal function, and HPA axis function in children? *Developmental Science, 16*(5), 665–675. doi:10.1111/desc.12087

Sliz, D., & Hayley, S. (2012). Major depressive disorder and alterations in insular cortical activity: A review of current functional magnetic imaging research. *Frontiers in Human Neuroscience, 6*, 323. doi:10.3389/fnhum.2012.00323

Sloan, R. P., Huang, M.-H., Sidney, S., Liu, K., Williams, O. D., & Seeman, T. (2005). Socioeconomic status and health: Is parasympathetic nervous system activity an intervening mechanism? *International Journal of Epidemiology, 34*(2), 309–315. doi:10.1093/ije/dyh381

Snibbe, A. C., & Markus, H. R. (2005). You can't always get what you want: Educational attainment, agency, and choice. *Journal of Personality and Social Psychology, 88*(4), 703–720. doi:10.1037/0022-3514.88.4.703

Sripada, R. K., Swain, J. E., Evans, G. W., Welsh, R. C., & Liberzon, I. (2014). Childhood poverty and stress reactivity are associated with aberrant functional connectivity in default mode network. *Neuropsychopharmacology, 39*(9), 2244–2251. doi:10.1038/npp.2014.75

Stellar, J. E., Manzo, V. M., Kraus, M. W., & Keltner, D. (2012). Class and compassion: Socioeconomic factors predict responses to suffering. *Emotion, 12*(3), 449–459. doi:10.1037/a0026508

Stephens, N. M., Fryberg, S. A., Markus, H. R., Johnson, C. S., & Covarrubias, R. (2012). Unseen disadvantage: How American universities' focus on independence undermines the academic performance of first-generation college students. *Journal of Personality and Social Psychology, 102*(6), 1178–1197. doi:10.1037/a0027143

Stephens, N. M., Markus, H. R., & Fryberg, S. A. (2012). Social class disparities in health and education: Reducing inequality by applying a sociocultural self model of behavior. *Psychological Review, 119*(4), 723–744. doi:10.1037/a0029028

Stephens, N. M., Townsend, S. S. M., & Dittmann, A. G. (2019). Social-Class Disparities in Higher Education and Professional Workplaces: The Role of Cultural Mismatch. Current Directions in Psychological Science, 28(1), 67–73. https://doi.org/10.1177/0963721418806506

Strategic Research Priorities Overview. (2017). https://www.nimh.nih.gov/about/strategic-planning-reports/strategic-research-priorities/index.shtml

Stratmann, M., Konrad, C., Kugel, H., Krug, A., Schöning, S., Ohrmann, P., . . . Dannlowski, U. (2014). Insular and hippocampal gray matter volume reductions in patients with major depressive disorder. *Plos One*, *9*(7), e102692. doi:10.1371/journal.pone.0102692

Swartz, J. R., Hariri, A. R., & Williamson, D. E. (2017). An epigenetic mechanism links socioeconomic status to changes in depression-related brain function in high-risk adolescents. *Molecular Psychiatry*, *22*(2), 209–214. doi:10.1038/mp.2016.82

Takagi, Y., Sakai, Y., Abe, Y., Nishida, S., Harrison, B. J., Martínez-Zalacaín, I., . . . Tanaka, S. C. (2018). A common brain network among state, trait, and pathological anxiety from whole-brain functional connectivity. *Neuroimage*, *172*, 506–516. doi:10.1016/j.neuroimage.2018.01.080

Taylor, S. E., Lerner, J. S., Sage, R. M., Lehman, B. J., & Seeman, T. E. (2004). Early environment, emotions, responses to stress, and health. *Journal of Personality*, *72*(6), 1365–1393. doi:10.1111/j.1467-6494.2004.00300.x

Taylor, S. E., Lerner, J. S., Sherman, D. K., Sage, R. M., & McDowell, N. K. (2003). Are self-enhancing cognitions associated with healthy or unhealthy biological profiles? *Journal of Personality and Social Psychology*, *85*(4), 605–615. doi:10.1037/0022-3514.85.4.605

Taylor, S. E., & Seeman, T. E. (1999). Psychosocial resources and the SES-health relationship. *Annals of the New York Academy of Sciences*, *896*, 210–225. doi:10.1111/j.1749-6632.1999.tb08117.x

Thayer, J. F., Friedman, B. H., & Borkovec, T. D. (1996). Autonomic characteristics of generalized anxiety disorder and worry. *Biological Psychiatry*, *39*(4), 255–266. doi:10.1016/0006-3223(95)00136-0

Tibi-Elhanany, Y., & Shamay-Tsoory, S. G. (2011). Social cognition in social anxiety: First evidence for increased empathic abilities. *Israel Journal of Psychiatry and Related Sciences*, *48*(2), 98–106.

Ursache, A., Merz, E. C., Melvin, S., Meyer, J., & Noble, K. G. (2017). Socioeconomic status, hair cortisol and internalizing symptoms in parents and children. *Psychoneuroendocrinology*, *78*, 142–150. doi:10.1016/j.psyneuen.2017.01.020

Varghese, F. P., & Brown, E. S. (2001). The Hypothalamic-Pituitary-Adrenal Axis in Major Depressive Disorder: A Brief Primer for Primary Care Physicians. Primary care companion to the Journal of clinical psychiatry, 3(4), 151–155. https://doi.org/10.4088/pcc.v03n0401

Vellakkal, S., Subramanian, S. V., Millett, C., Basu, S., Stuckler, D., & Ebrahim, S. (2013). Socioeconomic inequalities in non-communicable diseases prevalence in India: Disparities between self-reported diagnoses and standardized measures. *Plos One*, *8*(7), e68219. doi:10.1371/journal.pone.0068219

Vieta, E., Popovic, D., Rosa, A. R., Solé, B., Grande, I., Frey, B. N., . . . Kapczinski, F. (2013). The clinical implications of cognitive impairment and allostatic load in bipolar disorder. *European Psychiatry*, *28*(1), 21–29. doi:10.1016/j.eurpsy.2011.11.007

Vos, T., Flaxman, A. D., Naghavi, M., Lozano, R., Michaud, C., Ezzati, M., et al. (2012). Years lived with disability (YLDs) for 1160 sequelae of 289 diseases and injuries 1990-2010: A systematic analysis for the Global Burden of Disease Study 2010. *The Lancet*, *380*(9859), 2163–2196. doi:10.1016/S0140-6736(12)61729-2

Walters, K. L., & Simoni, J. M. (2002). Reconceptualizing native women's health: An "indigenist" stress-coping model. *American Journal of Public Health*, *92*(4), 520–524. doi:10.2105/AJPH.92.4.520

Williams, D. R. (1999). Race, socioeconomic status, and health: The added effects of racism and discrimination. *Annals of the New York Academy of Sciences*, *896*, 173–188. doi:10.1111/j.1749-6632.1999.tb08114.x

Yang, J., Liu, H., Wei, D., Liu, W., Meng, J., Wang, K., . . . Qiu, J. (2016). Regional gray matter volume mediates the relationship between family socioeconomic status and depression-related trait in a young healthy sample. *Cognitive, Affective & Behavioral Neuroscience*, *16*(1), 51–62. doi:10.3758/s13415-015-0371-6

Zainal, N. H., & Newman, M. G. (2018). Worry amplifies theory-of-mind reasoning for negatively valenced social stimuli in generalized anxiety disorder. *Journal of Affective Disorders*, *227*, 824–833. doi:10.1016/j.jad.2017.11.084

Zhang, K., Zhu, Y., Zhu, Y., Wu, S., Liu, H., Zhang, W., . . . Tian, M. (2016). Molecular, functional, and structural imaging of major depressive disorder. *Neuroscience Bulletin*, *32*(3), 273–285. doi:10.1007/s12264-016-0030-0

Zhao, Y. J., Du, M. Y., Huang, X. Q., Lui, S., Chen, Z. Q., Liu, J., . . . Gong, Q. Y. (2014). Brain grey matter abnormalities in medication-free patients with major depressive disorder: A meta-analysis. *Psychological Medicine*, *44*(14), 2927–2937. doi:10.1017/S0033291714000518

Autobiographical Memory and Culture

Yoojin Chae *and* Qi Wang

Abstract

Research has demonstrated the crucial role of culture in shaping how the self is represented and how autobiographical event information is organized, retained, and retrieved. Specifically, the style, accuracy, content, emergence, and general accessibility of autobiographical memories in children and adults have been found to vary across cultures, which reflects the cultured self. This chapter provides an overview of research that has identified language, family narrative practices, and emotion knowledge as potent mechanisms responsible for cultural effects on self-views and autobiographical memory. It further discusses cross-cultural differences in the simulation of future events based on neuropsychological research findings and also within-culture variations in socioeconomic status in relation to the development of self and autobiographical memory. This line of research has important applied implications for clinical and educational professionals given the significant contributions of autobiographical memory to human functioning and psychological well-being in cultural contexts.

Key Words: autobiographical memory; self; culture; well-being; neuropsychology; cross-cultural difference

Autobiographical memory, that is, memory for event information pertaining to the self, can be shaped by our concept of self. The fundamental significance of the self for the development of autobiographical remembering has long been underscored by a number of theorists (e.g., Conway & Pleydell-Pearce, 2000; Howe, Courage, & Edison, 2003). For instance, according to the personalization theory of autobiographical memory delineated by Howe and Courage (1993, 1997), the acquisition of the cognitive self at about 18 to 24 months of age, indexed by mirror self-recognition, is a prerequisite to the emergence of autobiographical memory. With the cognitive self in place, life events can take on personal meaning, and such personal experiences can be organized and retained in memory related to "me." Indeed, empirical studies have shown that the onset of the cognitive self is followed shortly by the emergence of autobiographical memory (e.g., Howe, Courage, & Peterson, 1994).

The emergence and development of self and autobiographical memory encompass the contributions of sociolinguistic and cultural factors (Nelson & Fivush, 2004; Wang, 2013). In particular, a growing body of research has demonstrated systematic differences in autobiographical memories between European American and East Asian children, which may reflect the influence of different cultural norms, beliefs, traditions, languages, and socialization practices on how the self is represented and how autobiographical event information is organized, retained, and retrieved (for reviews, see Wang, 2014; Wang & Senzaki, 2019). In this chapter, we provide a selective review of research that has documented the crucial contributions of sociocultural environment, language, family narrative practices, and emotion knowledge to the development of self and autobiographical memory. Cross-cultural differences in the simulation of future events are also discussed given the neuropsychological research findings that have revealed a striking neural overlap in past and future episodic thinking. Next, we turn to adults' autobiographical memories that have also been shown to differ across cultures. We then describe how autobiographical memory can in turn contribute to human functioning and psychological well-being in cultural contexts. Finally, we consider within-culture variations in socioeconomic status in relation to the development of self and autobiographical memory.

The Cultured Self and Autobiographical Memory

How we process, organize, and represent information about the self is influenced by our sociocultural environment. There is considerable evidence that individuals in different cultures have different conceptions of selfhood (e.g., Markus & Kitayama, 1991; Miyamoto et al., 2018; Wang, 2001a, 2004, 2006a). In Western, especially European American, cultures that value individuality, personal distinctiveness, and self-sufficiency, an autonomous self-concept is promoted. European Americans are encouraged to refer to their unique inner qualities, attributes, and opinions, independent of others or of social contexts, in defining themselves. In contrast, in East Asian cultures that emphasize interdependence, collective solidarity, and relational hierarchy, a relational self-concept is promoted. Asian people are motivated to focus on their social roles, group memberships, and ongoing relationships with significant others and the community in defining themselves.

These different self-concepts across cultures emerge early in life and, in turn, influence whether children put a premium on remembering personal experiences and how they attend to, process, and retain information from significant personal events (Wang, 2004, 2013). In European American cultures, remembering significant personal experiences is perceived as a crucial way to distinguish oneself from others and as a necessary part of a unique individual identity (Nelson, 2003; Wang, 2013). This cultural context may motivate individuals to remember specific, one-moment-in-time events and to focus on their own roles and perspectives. Accordingly, European Americans may process and encode event information highlighting their uniqueness and autonomy and elaborately represent such information in their memory system. They may further produce elaborate and lengthy accounts of personal experiences and center on their own roles, feelings, and perspectives. In contrast, in East Asian cultures that emphasize group solidarity and interconnectedness, the retention of social knowledge, rather than development of a structured personal event memory system, may be valued to a greater extent. Accordingly, Asian people's memories may focus on the role of others and often concern generic events, which help to reaffirm interpersonal relations and social conventions. They are also likely to provide relatively brief and skeleton accounts and to focus their memories on group activities and interactions. In addition, given that autobiographical memory is considered important in constructing a unique individual self and identity, which is prioritized in Western (e.g., European American) cultures, detailed and elaborate encoding of personal event information may be promoted in Western cultures.

Cross-Cultural Differences in Early Autobiographical Memory

In line with the theoretical analysis, a number of empirical studies have shown that the style, accuracy, content, emergence, and general accessibility of children's autobiographical memories vary as a function of culture (Wang, 2013). With regard to memory style, European American children tend to remember their life experiences in richer episodic details and to recall more unique, one-time (as opposed to generic, repeated) events, compared with East Asian children. In a study by Han, Leichtman, and Wang (1998), European American, Korean, and Chinese 4- and 6-year-old children were interviewed about recent personal experiences. It was found that in comparison with Korean and Chinese children, European American children produced more complex, elaborate, specific, and detailed narratives, speaking a greater number of words per proposition, using more descriptive terms, temporal markers, and causal language, and giving more accounts of specific, one-point-in-time episodes. In another study, children of ages 8, 11, and 14 from European Canadian and Chinese cultures were asked to recall in a 4-minute period as many early memories as possible from before they went to school (Peterson, Wang, & Hou, 2009). Results indicated that European Canadian children recalled more specific, one-time episodes from their early childhood than did Chinese children. Furthermore, both when recalling past personal events and when constructing future personal events, European American 7- to 10-year-old children generated more distinct information details about the events than did their Chinese counterparts (Wang, Capous, Koh, & Hou, 2014).

European American culture's emphasis on more detailed and elaborate narratives, however, may negatively influence another important aspect of children's memory, namely, memory accuracy. Researchers have recently begun to examine cross-cultural differences in children's memory accuracy. In a study by Klemfuss and Wang (2017), European American and Chinese American 6-year-old children experienced a staged event. A researcher played with individual children in the laboratory a "zookeeper game" adapted from McGuigan and Salmon (2004), with various distinct episodes (e.g., to find a lost baby elephant, to clean up a giraffe). Children were interviewed about the event 6 months later to assess their memory accuracy. Chinese American children were more accurate in their responses to recall prompts (e.g., "Tell me what happened when you got ready to be the zookeeper"), compared with European American children, who provided more inaccurate details. Similarly, Wang and Song (2018) found that 6-year-old European American children produced stories that differed to a greater extent from their mothers' reports of the same events, compared with their Chinese American counterparts. This may suggest that European American children were less accurate in their event memories than were Chinese children. Together, these cultural differences in memory accuracy may reflect a greater appreciation for good storytelling, as opposed to accurate remembering, in European American than in East Asian cultures (Wang, Leichtman, & Davies, 2000).

In terms of the content of children's memories, studies have consistently shown that children from European American cultures elaborated more on their subjective views (i.e., personal meaning or reactions) and referred more frequently to their internal states (e.g., emotions, cognitions, preferences) than East Asian children (Han et al., 1998; Wang & Song, 2018). For instance, in Peterson et al.'s (2009) study of grade school children's early childhood memories, European Canadian children were twice as likely as Chinese children to recall memories that focused on themselves (e.g., "playing alone at home"), whereas Chinese children were more likely to recall memory events involving group activities and other people (e.g., "telling stories with friends"). In fact, European Canadian children most frequently recalled events of solitary play, whereas Chinese children most frequently recalled events concerning family interactions.

Although these cross-cultural differences in children's autobiographical memory reports have been thought to reflect different cultural traditions and norms, an alternative interpretation is also plausible. Rather than implying actual differences in children's memories, such findings may simply stem from the differences in children's daily life experiences. Perhaps compared with European American children, Asian children simply spend more time with significant others and more frequently engage in socially oriented activities, which may explain why they remember more about social interactions and other people. European American children, in contrast, may more frequently participate in self-initiated activities and therefore remember more self-focused event details. To examine whether children from different cultures would still demonstrate stylistic and content differences in their memory reports when interviewed about the same event, Chae, Kulkofsky, and Wang (2006) tested memory for the same staged classroom event in European American and Korean immigrant preschoolers. Consistent with the cultural differences observed in children's personal event memories, American children produced more voluminous and cohesive reports and made more objective descriptions of the factual details about the staged event than did Koreans. Cultural differences were found in the content of children's memories as well, such that American children produced more details about objects and actions and more autonomous phrases (e.g., "I like pizza"), whereas Korean children talked more about other people. Thus, even when children recounted the same event, remarkable cultural differences were observed.

Pertaining to the emergence and general accessibility of autobiographical memory, the study by Peterson and colleagues (2009) demonstrated that, when asked what their earliest childhood memory was, European Canadian children (ages 8, 11, and 14) recalled earlier first memories than did their Chinese peers, whereby the average age of Canadian children's earliest memory was more than a year earlier than that of Chinese children (28 vs. 41 months). Furthermore, although Canadian children of different age groups did not differ in the age of earliest memory, Chinese 8- and 11-year-olds had significantly earlier first memories than did Chinese 14-year-olds. Across all age groups, the ages of earliest memory of Canadian children were significantly earlier than the average age of earliest memory in North American adults. However, whereas the ages of earliest memory provided by Chinese 8- and 11-year-olds were also earlier than the average age of earliest memory in Chinese adults, the earliest memory of 14-year-old Chinese children, dated at 50 months, was comparable to that of Chinese adults. These findings suggest that while Canadian children still have earlier access to childhood memories than do North American adults, Chinese children by age 14 already exhibit adult-like childhood amnesia. In this study, cultural differences were found in the number of early memories as well, such that Canadian children recalled a greater number of early childhood events than did Chinese children. Additionally, in the Canadian sample, 11- and 14-year-olds recalled more memories than did 8-year-olds, reflecting that the memory task might be more cognitively demanding for younger children. In contrast, in the Chinese sample, 8- and 11-year-olds produced more memories than did 14-year-olds, which also implies that by the time Chinese children are 14 years of age the degree of childhood amnesia already resembles the Chinese adult pattern.

There is empirical evidence that these cultural differences in children's autobiographical remembering are due in part to the cultured self. In a study by Wang (2006b), the mediating role of child self-concept in the relations between culture and autobiographical memory abilities was directly tested in 3-year-olds from Chinese families in China, first-generation Chinese immigrant families in the United States, and European American families. The children were asked to recall two specific, one-time events and to describe themselves. Compared with both Chinese groups, European American children focused more on their personal qualities, attributes, beliefs, or behaviors in describing themselves (e.g., "I'm happy," "I have a teddy bear") rather than making collective or public self-descriptions (e.g., "I am a boy," "I love my mommy"), and they also recalled more details about past events. Mediation analyses further demonstrated that child self-concept accounted for cultural differences in autobiographical memory.

Mechanisms Underlying Cultural Effects on Autobiographical Memory Development

In addition to the cultured self, other cultural elements may also contribute to cultural differences in autobiographical memory that emerge early in development.

Language

A critical mechanism that underlies the cultural differences in self-concept and, in turn, autobiographical memory is language. Research has revealed the important role of language in the development and maintenance of cultured self and autobiographical memory. In a study by Wang, Shao, and Li (2010), for instance, English-Chinese bilingual children ages 8–14 from Hong Kong were interviewed in either English or Chinese. They were asked to recount personal experiences and to provide self-descriptions, and then to indicate their agreement with Chinese interdependent values (e.g., interpersonal harmony, group solidarity, social compliance, humility) versus Western independent values (e.g., individual autonomy, personal sufficiency, pride). Regardless of age, children interviewed in English provided lengthier accounts about themselves and their autobiographical memories, and they focused more on unique personal attributes and qualities in their self-descriptions and talked more about their own roles and perspectives in their autobiographical memories, when compared with children interviewed in Chinese, who produced less elaborate and more socially oriented self-descriptions and memory accounts. In addition, across all age groups, children interviewed in Chinese reported higher agreement with interdependent values and lower agreement with independent values than did children interviewed in English. Hence, linguistic usage (i.e., Chinese vs. English) seems to shape the endorsement of cultural belief systems (i.e., interdependence vs. independence), which in turn contributes to the degrees of autonomous self and memory self-focus. These findings imply that language is a crucial mechanism that activates and reinforces cultural beliefs and culturally promoted self-concepts, which can, in turn, motivate children to retain and retrieve autobiographical information in culture-specific ways.

Family Narrative Practices

According to social-interactionist theories, discussions of personal experiences with significant others help children develop coherently organized memories that remain accessible and verbalized over time (Nelson & Fivush, 2004; Pillemer, 1998; Wang, 2013). Particularly, the role of parent-child reminiscing in autobiographical memory development has been highlighted. Joint parent-child memory sharing begins early in the child's life as the parent helps to reconstruct the stories of the child's life even before the child is able to participate in recalling the events. Families converse about the past in different ways and the parent's reminiscing styles influence the child's autobiographical memory skills (for a review, see Nelson, 2007). Specifically, parental styles vary in the amount of detail and in the richness of discourse when parents discuss the past with their children

(Fivush, Reese, & Haden, 2006). Elaborative parents tend to provide rich background details about the event being discussed and ask novel, complex, and typically open-ended questions to the child. In contrast, parents who are characterized as repetitive (non-elaborative) tend not to add much background to the event discussed and instead ask many repetitive questions. Parental reminiscing styles predict children's early ability to recall the past, such that children of elaborative parents have more detailed memories of their past experiences than children of repetitive parents (e.g., Harley & Reese, 1999; Leichtman, Pillemer, Wang, Koreishi, & Han, 2000).

Notably, research has demonstrated cross-cultural differences in the style and content of parental reminiscing. Compared with East Asian parents, European American parents tend to more frequently engage in memory sharing with their children and also use more elaborative reminiscing styles (e.g., Kulkofsky, Wang, & Koh, 2009; Wang, 2006b, 2007; Wang, Leichtman, & Davies, 2000). For example, in a study by Wang and Fivush (2005), European American and Chinese mother-child dyads talked about two shared past events. One event was extremely positive to the child, and the other was extremely stressful. American mothers initiated more interactive and elaborative conversations focusing on the child's roles and preferences, and they used a "cognitive approach" to emotional regulation by providing explanations for the cause of children's emotional states. In comparison, Chinese mothers assumed a leading role in the conversation, posting and repeating memory questions and focusing on social interaction. They further used a "behavioral approach" to emotional regulation by emphasizing behavioral expectation and discipline to their children.

These cross-cultural variations in the ways that parents reminisce with their children may stem from different underlying values, socialization goals, and beliefs about the functions of sharing memoires. In European American cultures, highly elaborative reminiscing about shared experiences is believed to be an effective means to strengthen emotional bonding and to create a sense of togetherness between parents and children (Fivush, Berlin, Sales, Mennuti-Washburn, & Cassidy, 2003; Fivush & Vasudeva, 2002). In contrast, in Asian cultures, a low-elaboration style may help emphasize social hierarchy by placing the parent at the center of the conversation and requiring the child to provide "right" answers through directive questioning (Wang, 2006b). The relation between parental cultural value orientations and parental reminiscing styles was directly tested in a study by Wang (2007). Mothers and children from Chinese families in China, first-generation Chinese immigrant families in the United States, and European American families talked about past events in which they both participated at three time points: when children were 3, 3.5, and 4.5 years old. Mothers' agreement with independent (e.g., "I do my own thing, regardless of what others think") and interdependent self-values (e.g., "I will sacrifice my self-interest for the benefit of the group I am in") was also measured. European American mothers scored higher on independence and lower on interdependence than did both Chinese and Chinese immigrant mothers. Furthermore, maternal elaborative reminiscing was positively related to mothers' endorsement of independence and negatively to their orientation toward interdependence.

Kulkofsky and colleagues (2009) further examined parental beliefs regarding the purposes of sharing memories with children and the links between these beliefs and parent-child reminiscing behaviors in a cross-cultural context. European American and Chinese mothers were asked when and why they reminisce with their children. They also talked with their children about two specific one-time events. Findings revealed cultural differences in maternal beliefs about the purpose of reminiscing. Compared with Chinese mothers, European American mothers were more likely to emphasize social functions, such as having a conversation and relationship maintenance (e.g., "to give us something to talk about"; "as a way of bonding"). Mothers' beliefs about the goals of memory sharing further predicted their reminiscing behaviors. Mothers who focused on the social functions of memory conversations were more elaborative during reminiscing with their children, independent of culture. These findings suggest that parents' reminiscing styles are influenced by their cultural value orientations and beliefs about memory sharing, which further contribute to children's autobiographical memory. European American children often recall more event details with their parents than do Chinese children, but regardless of culture, parents' use of elaborations is positively associated with the amount of event details that children recall (Wang, 2006b; Wang & Fivush, 2005; Wang et al., 2000). A recent meta-analytic review conducted by Wu and Jobson (2019) showed that maternal elaborative reminiscing was positively related to children's ability to recall more detailed autobiographical memory concurrently and longitudinally, regardless of culture.

In Wang's (2006b) study of autobiographical memories in native Chinese, Chinese immigrant, and European American 3-year-olds, the potential mediating role of parental reminiscing styles in the relation between cultural contexts and children's memory abilities was examined. Results indicated that parental reminiscing style significantly mediated cultural effects on children's shared and independent autobiographical memory. Furthermore, in a longitudinal study, Wang (2007) explored the long-term contributions of parental elaborative reminiscing to children's shared autobiographical memory skills in cultural contexts. Across all time points, European American mothers were more elaborative than Chinese mothers, and European American children contributed more information to the memory conversations than did Chinese children. Furthermore, mothers' use of elaborations uniquely predicted children's memory responding both concurrently and over the long term, independent of culture. Through family reminiscing practices, children learn culture-specific ways of personal remembering.

Emotion Knowledge

Children's emotional knowledge is an additional important mechanism accounting for cultural variations in autobiographical memory. Given that significant personal events typically involve emotional reactions, knowledge of emotion can help children process, organize, interpret, and retain the event information, thereby enhancing their autobiographical remembering. Cross-cultural research has shown that European American children have overall better understanding of emotion situations than East Asian children. For instance, compared with Chinese children, American children better identified the appropriate emotions of story protagonists in various situations and also better described situations likely to provoke happy, sad, fearful, or angry emotions (e.g., Wang, 2003; Wang, 2008; Wang, Hutt, Kulkofsky, McDermott, & Wei, 2006). Such cultural differences in children's emotion understanding may stem from different beliefs and practices of emotion socialization in Western and East Asian families (Chao, 1995; Wang, 2001b; Wang & Fivush, 2005). In Western cultures where self-expression and individuality are valued, children often have many opportunities to participate in emotional conversations with their parents, which then promote their understanding of emotions. In comparison, in East Asian cultures where mutual dependence and social conformity are highlighted, emotions are considered potentially disruptive to interpersonal harmony and thus children are not encouraged to talk about emotions (Chao, 1995; Chen, 2000). These varied beliefs and practices contribute to cultural differences in children's emotion knowledge (Doan & Wang, 2010).

Empirical studies have demonstrated that emotion knowledge serves as a significant mediator that leads to cultural variations in children's autobiographical memory. In a longitudinal investigation by Wang (2008), European American children demonstrated greater emotion understanding and also provided more elaborations and specific details in their memory narratives of autobiographical events, when compared with native Chinese children and Chinese immigrant children. Furthermore, children's emotion knowledge was found to mediate culture effects on their autobiographical memory.

Remembering the Past and Imagining the Future

Cultural differences have been further examined with regard to the imagination of potential future personal events. For instance, Wang, Capous, Koh, and Hou (2014) compared European American and Chinese children's memories for past events and simulation of future events. Children were asked to recall two specific past events and to imagine two specific future events. Of the past events, one happened to children recently and one happened when they were little. Of the future events, one could happen to children soon and one when they grow up. Compared with Chinese children, European American children produced more specific details about what, where, and when for both past and future events, with the difference particularly pronounced for temporally near events. At the individual level, children who remembered the past in greater episodic details also imagined the future in richer details, and children who produced more general details about their past events produced more general details about the future events as well, regardless of culture.

Findings from neuroimaging studies have consistently demonstrated remarkable similarities in cognitive and neural processes between remembering previous experiences and simulating possible future scenarios (Addis, Wong, & Schacter, 2007; Addis, Wong, & Schacter, 2008; Schacter & Addis, 2007; Szpunar, 2010; Szpunar, Watson, & McDermott, 2007). In particular, the left hippocampus has been found to be engaged in the construction of both past and future episodes, along with posterior visuospatial regions. According to the constructive-episodic-simulation hypothesis, imagination of possible future events involves recombining episodic information from the past into novel scenarios (Schacter & Addis, 2007). That is, autobiographical information can be utilized to imagine future events. Individuals can extract, recombine, and reassemble the episodic details of the past to construct potential future events (Addis et al., 2007, 2008). Thus, European Americans who tend to produce more specific and more elaborate memories than do Asians might be able to envision more detailed future episodes by using the rich details stored in their memories.

Culture and Autobiographical Memory in Adults

Cultural differences revealed in various dimensions (e.g., style, content, emergence, general accessibility) of children's autobiographical memories have also been reflected in adults' memories. For example, compared with Asian adults, European American adults more often described their own thoughts and feelings when recalling their autobiographical memories (Wang & Conway, 2004). European American adults also produced more specific event details in remembering the past and envisioning the future than did Chinese adults (Wang, Hou, Tang, & Wiprovnick, 2011).

A study by Jobson and O'Kearney (2008) further indicated that cultural variations in autobiographical memories are moderated by the memories' themes. When European Australians and Asians were asked to provide autobiographical memories of events that shaped who they were as individuals (i.e., self-defining memories), Australians recalled more autonomy-themed self-defining events (e.g., academic achievement, sporting endeavors) than Asians, and Asians recalled more relatedness-themed events (e.g., collective activities of family, workplace, or other social groups) than Australians, which reflects different self-goals prioritized in respective cultures. Of note, there was a significant interaction between culture and theme for elaboration, such that Australians elaborated on autonomy-themed memories more than relatedness-themed memories, whereas Asians elaborated on relatedness-themed memories more than autonomy-themed memories.

Self-views that vary across cultures may further result in differences in memory accuracy or distortion between European Americans and East Asians. In a meta-analysis of cross-cultural studies, Heine and Hamamura (2007) reported that Westerners emphasize self-enhancing motivations, whereas Asians emphasize self-improving motivations. That is, Westerners have a stronger self-serving bias and are more likely to view themselves in a positive light than Asians. For instance, significant discrepancies in self-appraisals were found between Canadian and Japanese participants, whereby Canadians reported a greater number of favorable than unfavorable self-appraisals in their self-descriptions, whereas Japanese were generally evenhanded in their self-descriptions without being self-critical or self-enhancing (Ross, Heine, Wilson, & Sugimori, 2005). Self-enhancing motivations emphasized by Westerners may in turn encourage them to reconstruct their memories to maintain favorable self-views. In contrast, self-improving motivations emphasized by Asians may encourage them to retain their personal memories more objectively for genuine improvement.

Research findings obtained by Oishi (2002) provided support for such expectations. European Americans and Asian Americans completed a life satisfaction form every day for 7 consecutive days. The form included items on daily satisfaction (i.e., "How good or bad was today?") on 6-point scales, as well as domain-specific satisfaction items. At the end of the week, participants rated their satisfaction for the week on the same 6-point scales (e.g., "How good or bad was the week?"). Findings showed that although there was no cultural difference in actual daily satisfaction over the 7-day period, in retrospection, European Americans rated the week as a whole significantly more favorably than did Asians. Furthermore, while Asians did not differ in their average daily satisfaction and their retrospective judgment of the week, European Americans' retrospective judgment was significantly more positive than their average daily satisfaction. Hence, Western individuals reconstruct their memories to be more positive than they actually were, whereas Asians do not exhibit such memory distortion.

Self-enhancing motivations of Westerners are also revealed in people's estimates of the subjective temporal distance of positive and negative life events and their reports of the ease with which they recall such events. In the study by Ross et al. (2005), Canadians reported that they felt closer in time to proud events than to embarrassing events, and that embarrassing events were more difficult to recall than similarly distant proud events. Japanese, however, reported no difference in the ease of recalling proud and embarrassing events, and they stated that proud and embarrassing events felt equally far away and were equally memorable. These cross-cultural differences in the valence of personal memories are in line with the self-goals in respective cultural contexts. In a similar vein, American participants viewed their own future health more favorably than others' future health, whereas Koreans considered their own and others' future health to be similar (Jeon, Wang, Burrow, & Ratner, 2020).

Cross-cultural differences have also been found in perceived functions and usages of autobiographical memory (Alea & Wang, 2015). In general, there appears to be a greater appreciation for autobiographical memories of specific events in Western cultures than in East Asian cultures. Although the three major functions of autobiographical memory identified among Western populations—directing behavior, social bonding, and self-continuity—have also been observed in other populations, Chinese young adults (Kulkofsky, Wang, & Hou, 2010) and mothers (Kulkofsky et al., 2009) and Japanese adults (Maki, Kawasaki, Demiray, & Janssen, 2015) recognize to a lesser degree the various functions of autobiographical memory than their European American peers. Furthermore, in many Western cultures, autobiographical memory is viewed as defining elements of the self and as a therapeutic tool. In contrast, in many East Asian cultures, autobiographical memory is valued for its intellectual and moral functions to provide insight about life (Wang, 2013). Wang, Koh, Song, and Hou (2015) examined memory function knowledge in European American and Asian adults and children. Compared with Asians, European American children were more likely to use autobiographical memories for maintaining a sense of self or for regulating negative affect. Compared with European Americans, Asian adults were more likely to use autobiographical memories for learning lessons, solving problems, and future preparation. These findings suggest cultural variations in perceived values of autobiographical memory.

Culture, Autobiographical Memory, and Psychological Well-Being

Autobiographical memories that vary across cultures can, in turn, contribute in different ways to individuals' mental health and psychological well-being (Jobson, Moradi, Rahimi-Movaghar, Conway, & Dalgleish, 2014; Valentino, 2011; Williams et al., 2007; Wang, 2021). For instance, among Western individuals, detailed and specific memory can be beneficial for emotion regulation and coping with stressors (Jing, Madore, & Schacter, 2016), whereas impaired retrieval of specific events from autobiographical memory has been associated with depressive symptoms and post-traumatic stress (Hitchcock, Nixon, & Weber, 2014). Yet researchers have suggested the need to understand the functions of autobiographical memory in cultural contexts (Alea & Wang, 2015; Wang, 2013). Autobiographical memory may have different implications for psychological outcomes across cultures. In Western cultures, where individuality and autonomy are emphasized, detailed remembering of specific, one-moment-in-time episodes is valued as it is thought to consolidate an individual's unique identity. In East Asian cultures, however, remembering specific events with idiosyncratic details may not fit well with the cultural emphasis on downplaying personal uniqueness. According to the person-culture-fit framework, psychological adjustment is associated with the congruence between individual characteristics and cultural norms (Caldwell-Harris & Ayçiçegi, 2006; Chen, 2018; Lerner, 2002; Wang, 2021).

In a study by Wang, Hou, Koh, Song, and Yang (2018), the effects of cultural fit in remembering autobiographical events on psychological well-being were examined among adults and children from European American and East Asian cultures. The findings showed that culture moderated the associations between autobiographical memory specificity and various aspects of psychological well-being. Specifically, whereas increased memory specificity was associated with decreased use of avoidant coping among European Americans, it

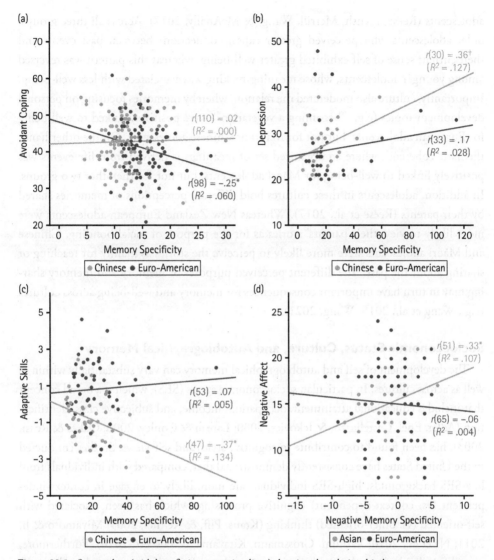

Figure 29.1. Scatterplots (with best fitting regression lines) showing the relationship between memory specificity and (a) avoidant coping (Study 1), (b) depressive symptoms (Study 2), (c) adaptive skills (Study 3), and (d) negative affect (Study 4) for each culture. † p =.053; * p <.05.

Figure reprinted with permission from Wang, Q., Hou, Y., Koh, J. B. K., Song, Q., & Yang, Y. (2018). Culturally motivated remembering: The moderating role of culture for the relation of episodic memory to well-being. *Clinical Psychological Science*, 6(6), 860–871. doi:10.1177/2167702618784012.

predicted elevated depressive symptoms, decreased adaptive skills, and increased negative emotions among East Asians (see Figure 29.1). Hence, as the person-culture-fit framework suggests, the link between autobiographical memory and psychological well-being may vary across cultures.

In the same vein, Reese and colleagues examined the relation of memory meaning-making to psychological well-being in New Zealand Māori, European, and Chinese adolescents (Reese, Fivush, Merrill, Wang, & McAnally, 2017). Across all three groups, older adolescents who perceived greater causal connections between past events and their current sense of self exhibited greater well-being, whereas this pattern was reversed among younger adolescents, whose meaning-making was associated with less well-being. Importantly, culture also moderated the relation, whereby memories focusing on personal development topics (e.g., "becoming a vegetarian") were positively linked to well-being for European adolescents, but not for Māori or Chinese adolescents. On the other hand, thematic coherence where an organized set of meanings is derived from life events was positively linked to well-being for Māori adolescents, but not for the other two groups. In addition, adolescents in these cultures hold different perceptions of memories shared by their parents (Reese et al., 2017). Whereas New Zealand European adolescents were more likely to view their parents' stories as for the purpose of social bonding, Chinese and Māori adolescents were more likely to perceive the stories as mainly for teaching or sharing about the past. The different perceived purposes of memory and memory sharing may in turn have important consequences for memory and well-being across cultures (e.g., Wang et al., 2015; Wang, 2021).

Socioeconomic Status, Culture, and Autobiographical Memory

The development of self and autobiographical memory can vary substantially within as well as across cultures. In particular, socioeconomic status (SES), which is a broad concept that includes educational attainment, occupation, income, and subjective class identification (Adler, Epel, Castellazzo, & Ickovics, 2000; Lareau & Conley, 2008; Oakes & Rossi, 2003), has been found to contribute to cognitive styles and self-views. Studies conducted in the United States have consistently demonstrated that, compared with individuals from low-SES backgrounds, high-SES individuals are more likely to engage in context-independent (vs. context-dependent) cognitive processing, which has been associated with self-oriented (vs. other-oriented) thinking (Kraus, Piff, & Keltner, 2009; Miyamoto & Ji, 2011; Na et al., 2010; Varnum, Grossmann, Kitayama, & Nisbett, 2010). Furthermore, low-SES individuals tend to endorse more interdependent self-views and show less self-inflation than those from high-SES backgrounds (Grossmann & Varnum, 2011). In addition, people from low-SES backgrounds were more likely to make choices that put them in a similar situation with others, whereas people from high-SES backgrounds were more likely to make choices that make them stand out from others (Stephens, Markus, & Townsend, 2007). Drawing on all these findings that demonstrate significant associations between higher social status and greater independence, one would expect high-SES individuals to produce more elaborate, specific, and detailed narratives of autobiographical events, to focus more on their own subjective views, and to have greater access to personal events more generally, when compared with their low-SES counterparts.

In a study on parent-child reminiscing, Wiley, Rose, Burger, and Miller (1998) observed differences between working-class and middle-class mothers in European American communities. Specifically, although mothers in both communities encouraged their children to develop autonomous selves, the versions of autonomy that they tried to promote varied such that middle-class mothers gave the children more latitude to express their own views than working-class mothers did. Oppositions to children were typically mitigated in middle-class communities. When children provided incorrect information, middle-class mothers conveyed their opposition by taking the children's claims as "different" rather than "wrong" (e.g., "*Santa Claus? Does Santa Claus come at Easter?*"). In contrast, working-class mothers often contradicted the children's statements in a direct and matter-of-fact manner (e.g., "*No, we didn't buy Batman*"). Such within-culture variations in parent-child reminiscing may further influence the way children remember and recount their personal life events.

Of note, however, several studies have shown that cultural contexts moderate the influence of SES on psychological attributes and socialization values. In European American culture and in Western cultures in general, high-SES individuals tend to engage in tasks emphasizing the self and self-set goals (i.e., self-orientation) that support independence of the self. In comparison, in East Asian cultures where Confucian teaching has promoted interdependent views of the self, high-SES individuals are likely to engage in tasks focusing on the relationships or others' benefits (i.e., other-orientation) that reinforce interdependence of the self. In a study by Miyamoto and Wilken (2010), American participants who were assigned to be a leader (vs. follower) exhibited more context-independent cognitive styles. In contrast, Japanese participants who were assigned to be a leader showed context-dependent cognitive styles, the same as those assigned to be a follower. Similarly, Miyamoto et al. (2018) demonstrated that Japanese from higher SES backgrounds had higher levels of other-orientation than Japanese from lower SES backgrounds, whereas such links were weaker or even reversed among Americans. The positive relation between SES and other-orientation observed among Japanese further extends to other cultures with Confucian influences, whereas the negative association between SES and other-orientation in Americans can be generalized to other Western cultures. Hence, high-SES individuals are more likely than their low-SES peers to exhibit psychological tendencies that are prevalent in their culture. These patterns of findings concerning SES in interaction with culture may translate to ways of autobiographical remembering as well, which will be an important topic for future research.

Conclusion

In this chapter, we have focused on autobiographical memory and its development in cultural contexts. The concept of self, which is a cognitive requirement for remembering personal life events, is conditioned by cultural values, beliefs, and practices, which, in turn, motivates individuals to develop culture-specific ways of remembering the past and also envisioning the future. Research in this area over the past two decades has revealed potent mechanisms, such as language, family narrative practices, and emotion knowledge, that account for the striking cross-cultural differences in self-views and autobiographical memories and that suggest differences within cultures as well. In addition, recent investigations using neurophysiological measures have further deepened our knowledge about past and future episodic thinking. A complete understanding of autobiographical memory and its development must be situated in cultural contexts. We call for more research to examine how individuals in different cultures and subcultures organize, retain, and retrieve autobiographical information. Such research has important applied implications for clinical and educational professionals as well, given the significant contributions of autobiographical remembering to mental health and psychological well-being.

References

Addis, D. R., Wong, A. T., & Schacter, D. L. (2007). Remembering the past and imagining the future: Common and distinct neural substrates during event construction and elaboration. *Neuropsychologia, 45*, 1363–1377.

Addis, D. R., Wong, A. T., & Schacter, D. L. (2008). Age-related changes in the episodic simulation of future events. *Psychological Science, 19*, 33–41.

Adler, N. E., Epel, E. S., Castellazzo, G., & Ickovics, J. R. (2000). Relationship of subjective and objective social status with psychological and physiological functioning: Preliminary data in healthy white women. *Health Psychology, 19*, 586–592.

Alea, N., & Wang, Q. (2015). Going global: The functions of autobiographical memory in cultural context. *Memory, 23*, 1–10.

Caldwell-Harris, C., & Ayçiçegi, A. (2006). When personality and culture crash: The psychological distress of allocentrics in an individualistic culture and idiocentrics in a collectivistic culture. *Transpersonal Psychiatry, 43*, 331–361.

Chae, Y., Kulkofsky, S., & Wang, Q. (2006). What happened in our pizza game? Memory of a staged event in Korean and European American preschoolers. In M. A. Vanchevsky (Ed.), *Frontiers in cognitive psychology* (pp. 71–89). Hauppauge, NY: Nova Science.

Chao, R. K. (1995). Chinese and European American cultural models of the self reflected in mothers' child-drearing beliefs. *Ethos, 23*, 328–354.

Chen, X. (2000). Growing up in a collectivist culture: Socialization and socioemotional development in Chinese children. In H. Comunion & V. Gielen (Eds.), *International perspectives on human development* (pp. 331–353). Padua, Italy: Cadam.

Chen, X. (2018). Culture, temperament, and social and psychological adjustment. *Developmental Review, 50*, 42–53.

Conway, M., & Pleydell-Pearce, C. W. (2000). The construction of autobiographical memories in the self-memory system. *Psychological Review, 107*, 261–288.

Doan, S. N., & Wang, Q. (2010). Maternal discussions of mental states and behaviors: Relations to emotion situation knowledge in European American and immigrant Chinese children. *Child Development, 81*, 1490–1503. doi:10.1111/j.1467-8624.2010.01487.x

Fivush, R., Berlin, L., Sales, J. D., Mennuti-Washburn, J., & Cassidy, J. (2003). Functions of parent-child reminiscing about emotionally negative events. *Memory, 11*, 179–192.

Fivush, R., Reese, E., & Haden, C. A. (2006). Elaborating on elaborations: The role of maternal reminiscing style in cognitive and socioemotional development. *Child Development, 77*, 1568–1588.

Fivush, R., & Vasudeva, A. (2002). Reminiscing and relating: Correlations among maternal reminiscing style, attachment and emotional warmth. *Journal of Cognition and Development, 3*, 73–90.

Grossmann, I., & Varnum, M. W. (2011). Social class, culture, and cognition. *Social and Psychological & Personality Science, 2*, 81–89.

Han, J. J., Leichtman, M. D., & Wang, Q. (1998). Autobiographical memory in Korean, Chinese, and American children. *Developmental Psychology, 34*, 701–713.

Harley, K., & Reese, E. (1999). Origins of autobiographical memory. *Developmental Psychology, 35*, 1338–1348.

Heine, S. J., & Hamamura, T. (2007). In search of East Asian self-enhancement. *Personality and Social Psychology Review, 11*, 4–27.

Hitchcock, C., Nixon, R. D., & Weber, N. (2014). A review of overgeneral memory in child psychopathology. *British Journal of Clinical Psychology, 53*, 170–193.

Howe, M. L., & Courage, M. L. (1993). On resolving the enigma of infantile amnesia. *Psychological Bulletin, 113*, 305–326.

Howe, M. L., & Courage, M. L. (1997). The emergency and early development of autobiographical memory. *Psychological Review, 104*, 499–523.

Howe, M. L., Courage, M. L., & Edison, S. C. (2003). When autobiographical memory begins. *Developmental Review, 23*, 471–494.

Howe, M. L., Courage, M. L., & Peterson, C. (1994). How can I remember when "I" wasn't there: Long-term retention of traumatic experiences and emergence of the cognitive self. *Consciousness and Cognition, 3*, 327–355.

Jeon, H. J., Wang, Q., Burrow, A. L., & Ratner, K. (2020). Perspectives of future health in self and others: The moderating role of culture. *Journal of Health Psychology, 25*(5), 703–712.

Jing, H. G., Madore, K. P., & Schacter, D. L. (2016). Worry about the future: An episodic specificity induction impacts problem solving, reappraisal, and well-being. *Journal of Experimental Psychology: General, 145*, 402–418.

Jobson, L., Moradi, A. R., Rahimi-Movaghar, V., Conway, M. A., & Dalgleish, T. (2014). Culture and the remembering of trauma. *Clinical Psychological Science, 2*, 696–713.

Jobson, L., & O'Kearney, R. (2008). Cultural differences in retrieval of self-defining memories. *Journal of Cross-Cultural Psychology, 39*, 75–80.

Klemfuss, J. Z., & Wang, Q. (2017). Narrative skills, gender, culture, and children's long-term memory accuracy of a staged event. *Journal of Cognition and Development, 18*, 577–594.

Kraus, M. W., Piff, P. K., & Keltner, D. (2009). Social class, sense of control, and social explanation. *Journal of Personality and Social Psychology, 97*, 992–1004.

Kulkofsky, S., Wang, Q., & Hou, Y. (2010). Why I remember that: The influence of contextual factors on beliefs about everyday memory. *Memory & Cognition, 38*, 461–473.

Kulkofsky, S., Wang, Q., & Koh, J. B. K. (2009). Functions of memory sharing and mother-child reminiscing behaviors: Individual and cultural variations. *Journal of Cognition and Development, 10*, 92–114.

Lareau, A., & Conley, D. (2008). *Social class: How does it work?* New York, NY: Russell Sage Foundation.

Leichtman, M. D., Pillemer, D. B., Wang, Q., Koreishi, A., & Han, J. J. (2000). When Bay Maisy came to school: Mothers' interview styles and preschoolers' event memories. *Cognitive Development, 15*, 99–114.

Lerner, R. (2002). *Concepts and theories of human development* (3rd ed.). Mahwah, NJ: Lawrence Erlbaum.

Maki, Y., Kawasaki, Y., Demiray, B., & Janssen, S. M. J. (2015). Autobiographical memory functions in young Japanese men and women. *Memory, 23*(1), 11–24. doi:10.1080/09658211.2014.930153.

Markus, H., & Kitayama, S. (1991). Culture and the self: Implications for cognition, emotion, and Motivation. *Psychological Review, 98*, 224–253.

McGuigan, F., & Salmon, K. (2004). The time to talk: The influence of the timing of adult–child talk on children's event memory. *Child Development, 75*, 669–686. doi:10.1111/j.1467-8624.2004.00700.x.

Miyamoto, Y., & Ji, L. J. (2011). Power fosters context-independent analytic cognition. *Personality and Social Psychology Bulletin, 37*, 1449–1458.

Miyamoto, Y., Yoo, J., Levine, C. S., Park, J., Boylan, J. M., Sims, T.,... Ryff, C. D. (2018). Culture and social hierarchy: Self- and other-oriented correlates of socioeconomic status across cultures. *Journal of Personality and Social Psychology, 115*, 427–445.

Miyamoto, Y., & Wilken, B. (2010). Culturally contingent situated cognition: Influencing other people fosters analytic perception in the United States but not in Japan. *Psychological Science, 21*, 1616–1622.

Na, J., Grossmann, I., Varnum, M. E. W., Kitayama., S., Gonzalez, R., & Nisbett, R. E. (2010). Cultural differences are not always reducible to individual differences. *Proceedings of the National Academy of Sciences of the United States of America, 107*, 6192–6197.

Nelson, K. (2003). Self and social functions: Individual autobiographical memory and collective narrative. *Memory, 11*, 125–136.

Nelson, K. (2007). *Young minds in social worlds: Experience, meaning, and memory.* Cambridge, MA: Harvard University Press.

Nelson, K., & Fivush, R. (2004). The emergence of autobiographical memory: A social cultural developmental theory. *Psychological Review, 111,* 486–511.

Oakes, J. M., & Rossi, P. H. (2003). The measurement of SES in health research: Current practice and steps toward a new approach. *Social Science & Medicine, 56,* 769–784.

Oishi, S. (2002). Experiencing and remembering of well-being: A cross-cultural analysis. *Personality and Social Psychology Bulletin, 28,* 1398–1406.

Peterson, C., Wang, Q., & Hou, Y. (2009). "When I was little": Childhood recollections in Chinese and European Canadian grade school children. *Child Development, 80,* 506–518.

Pillemer, D. B. (1998). *Momentous events, vivid memories.* Cambridge, MA: Harvard University Press.

Reese, E., Fivush, R., Merrill, N., Wang, Q., & McAnally, H. (2017). Adolescents' intergenerational narratives across cultures. *Developmental Psychology, 53,* 1142–1153. http://dx.doi.org/10.1037/dev0000309.

Reese, E., Myftari, E., McAnally, H. M., Chen, Y., Neha, T., Wang, Q., Jack, F., & Robertson, S. (2017). Telling the tale and living well: Adolescent narrative identity, personality traits, and well-being across cultures. *Child Development, 88,* 612–628. doi:10.1111/cdev.12618.

Ross, M., Heine, S. J., Wilson, A. E., & Sugimori, S. (2005). Cross-cultural discrepancies in self-appraisals. *Personality and Social Psychology Bulletin, 31,* 1175–1188.

Schacter, D. L. & Addis, D. R. (2007). The cognitive neuroscience of constructive memory: Remembering the past and imagining the future. *Philosophical Transactions of the Royal Society B: Biological Sciences, 362,* 773–786.

Szpunar, K. K. (2010). Episodic future thought: An emerging concept. *Perspectives on Psychological Science, 5,* 142–162.

Szpunar, K. K., Watson, J. M., & McDermott, K. B. (2007). Neural substrates of envisioning the future. *Proceedings of the National Academy of Sciences, USA, 104,* 642–647.

Stephens, N. M., Markus, H. R., & Townsend, S. S. (2007). Choice as an act of meaning: The case of social class. *Journal of Personality and Social Psychology, 93,* 814–830.

Valentino, K. (2011). A developmental psychopathology model of overgeneral autobiographical memory. *Developmental Review, 31,* 32–54.

Varnum, M. E. W., Grossmann, I., Kitayama., S., & Nisbett, R. E. (2010). The origin of cultural differences in cognition: The social orientation hypothesis. *Current Directions in Psychological Science, 19,* 9–13.

Wang, Q. (2001a). Cultural effects on adults' earliest childhood recollection and self-description: Implications for the relation between memory and the self. *Journal of Personality and Social Psychology, 81,* 220–233.

Wang, Q. (2001b). "Did you have fun?" American and Chinese mother-child conversations about shared emotional experiences. *Cognitive Development, 16,* 693–715.

Wang, Q. (2003). Emotion situation knowledge in American and Chinese preschool children and adults. *Cognition & Emotion, 17,* 725–746.

Wang, Q. (2004). The emergence of cultural self-constructs: Autobiographical memory and self-description in European American and Chinese children. *Development Psychology, 40,* 3–15.

Wang, Q. (2006a). Culture and the development of self-knowledge. *Current Directions in Psychological Science, 15,* 182–187.

Wang, Q. (2006b). Relations of maternal style and child self-concept to autobiographical memories in Chinese, Chinese immigrant, and European American 3-year-olds. *Child Development, 77,* 1794–1809.

Wang, Q. (2007). "Remember when you got the big, big bulldozers?" Mother-child reminiscing over time and across cultures. *Social Cognition, 25,* 455–471.

Wang, Q. (2008). Emotion knowledge and autobiographical memory across the preschool years: A cross-cultural longitudinal investigation. *Cognition, 108,* 117–135.

Wang, Q. (2013). *The autobiographical self in time and culture.* New York, NY: Oxford University Press.

Wang, Q. (2014). The cultured self and remembering. In P. J. Bauer & R. Fivush (Eds.), *The Wiley handbook on the development of children's memory* (pp. 605–625). West Sussex, UK: John Wiley & Sons.

Wang, Q. (2021). Cultural pathways and outcomes of autobiographical memory development. *Child Development Perspectives, 15(3),* 196-202.

Wang, Q., Capous, D., Koh, J. B. K., & Hou, Y. (2014). Past and future episodic thinking in middle childhood. *Journal of Cognition and Development, 15,* 625–643.

Wang, Q., & Conway, M. A. (2004). The stories we keep: Autobiographical memory in American and Chinese middle-aged adults. *Journal of Personality, 72*, 911-938.

Wang, Q., & Fivush, R. (2005). Mother-child conversations of emotionally salient events: Exploring the functions of emotional reminiscing in European American and Chinese families. *Social Development, 14*, 473–495.

Wang, Q., Hou, Y., Koh, J. B. K., Song, Q., & Yang, Y. (2018). Culturally motivated remembering: The moderating role of culture for the relation of episodic memory to well-being. *Clinical Psychological Science, 6*, 860–871.

Wang, Q., Hou, Y., Tang, H., & Wiprovnick, A. (2011). Traveling backward and forward in time: Culture and gender in the episodic specificity of past and future events. *Memory, 19*, 103–109.

Wang, Q., Hutt, R., Kulkofsky, S., McDermott, M., & Wei, R. (2006). Emotion situation knowledge and autobiographical memory in Chinese, immigrant Chinese, and European American 3-year-olds. *Journal of Cognition and Development, 7*, 95–118.

Wang, Q., Koh, J. B. K., Song, Q., & Hou, Y. (2015). Knowledge of memory functions in European and Asian American adults and children: The relation to autobiographical memory. *Memory, 23*, 25–38.

Wang, Q., Leichtman, M. D., & Davies, K. I. (2000). Sharing memories and telling stories: American and Chinese mothers and their 3-year-olds. *Memory, 8*, 159–177.

Wang, Q., & Senzaki, S. (2019). Culture and cognition. In D. Matsumoto & H. C. Hwang (Eds.), *Oxford handbook of culture and psychology* (2nd ed., pp. 318–360). New York, NY: Oxford University Press.

Wang, Q., Shao, Y., & Li, Y. J. (2010). "My way or Mom's way?" The bilingual and bicultural self in Hong Kong Chinese children and adolescents. *Child Development, 81*, 555–567.

Wang, Q., & Song, Q. (2018). He says, she says: Mothers and children remembering the same events. *Child Development, 89*, 2215–2229.

Wiley, A. R., Rose, A. J., Burger, L. K., & Miller, P. J. (1998). Constructing autonomous selves through narrative practices: A comparative study of working-class and middle-class families. *Child Development, 69*, 833–847.

Williams, J. M. G., Barnhofer, T., Crane, C., Herman, D., Raes, F., Watkins, E., & Dalgleish, T. (2007). Autobiographical specificity and emotional disorder. *Psychological Bulletin, 133*, 122–148.

Wu, Y., & Jobson, L. (2019). Maternal reminiscing and child autobiographical memory elaboration: A meta-analysis review. *Developmental Psychology, 55*, 2505–2521.

Conclusion

Joan Y. Chiao, Shu-Chen Li, Robert Turner, Su Yeon Lee-Tauler, *and* Beverly A. Pringle

Mental disorders are a major contributor to the global burden of disease. Mental, neurological, and substance abuse (MNS) disorders contribute to morbidity and mortality across geographic regions. The prevalence of mental disorders is an unmet societal and economic burden. Across nations, investment in research in the discovery and delivery science of cures for, preventions of, and interventions for mental disorders is lower than the disease burden. Global concerns that threaten protections for mental health are a considerable source of environmental threat. Stigma and human rights violations further challenge the conditions of mental health of vulnerable populations. Effective protection from threats and empowerment of individuals and communities are essential to overall mental health and well-being. The alleviation of mental disorders is necessary for quality of life and fulfillment of human potential.

The *Oxford Handbook of Cultural Neuroscience and Global Mental Health* provides an in-depth, comprehensive overview of foundations in cultural neuroscience and global mental health. Research in cultural neuroscience and global mental health is essential to the identification of cures for, preventions of, and interventions for mental disorders. Research approaches in the field consist of scientific processes for the discovery of root causes of mental disorders. The generation of novel scientific knowledge is necessary for the translation of research into evidence-based practice and policy. Research approaches that advance the development and implementation of preventions of and interventions for mental disorders are necessary for mental health promotion.

Scientific processes in the field postulate theoretical approaches to explain causal relations between culture and mental health. In particular, theoretical models seek to identify root causes of mental disorders across cultures. Methodological approaches facilitate the observation and measurement of biomarkers of mental disorders across cultural contexts. Methodological tools measure the dynamical relations of cultural processes within multilevel mechanisms that vary across spatiotemporal scales. Empirical approaches consist of programs of research that systematically investigate cultural processes within the structure and function of the organization of the nervous system. Research that builds on foundations in the field contributes to the generation and sharing of novel scientific knowledge that is necessary for addressing grand challenges in global mental health.

Summary of the Handbook

Part I examines theoretical foundations in cultural neuroscience and global mental health. Chapters 1 through 9 present reviews of theoretical approaches in cultural neuroscience in the study of the root causes of, prevention for, and interventions for mental disorders. Scientific frameworks for the investigation of the etiology of mental health disorders across cultures are introduced. Conceptual models that postulate causal patterns of influences in cultural and neurobiological systems contribute to the identification of biomarkers underlying mental disorders across cultural contexts.

The importance of culture in mental health is paramount to understanding the meaning and significance of human experience. Global concerns as environmental influences affect societal exposure to the risk and resilience factors that contribute to mental disorders. Lack of protection from threats to security compromise environmental conditions that are necessary for mental health. Cross-national variation in the prevalence of mental disorders illustrates the importance of understanding the etiology of mental disorders across cultural contexts.

Scott (Chapter 1) shows that cross-national prevalence of mental disorders illustrates variation in the manifestation and assessment of mental disorders across cultural contexts. Culture plays a fundamental role in the malleability of risk and protective factors for mental disorders. Cultural factors contribute to the maintenance and regulation of the well-being of individuals, societies, and nations.

Uchiyama and Muthukrishna (Chapter 2) introduce theories of cultural evolutionary neuroscience. The cultural evolutionary framework postulates that cumulative cultural and genetic evolution shape the evolutionary history of the adaptive brain. Causal models of brain adaptation consist of relations among characteristics of cultural and neural systems, including brain size, group size, adaptive knowledge, and social learning. Cultural processes that are cumulative in knowledge and transmittable through social learning contribute to greater complexity in functional specialization of brain adaptation.

Matsumoto and Hwang (Chapter 3) review basic models of how human culture affects psychological processes and behaviors. Human cultures regulate the psychological processes that influence subjective elements of behavior. Culture influences affective, cognitive, and social processes underlying the etiology of mental disorders. Cultural variation in the content and function of psychological processes affects mental health and well-being.

Northoff (Chapter 4) introduces scientific concepts fundamental to the study of culture and neurophilosophy. Cultural and neural systems consist of fundamental mechanisms of mental health. The concepts of embrainment and enculturation reflect the influence of culture on mechanisms of neuronal activity. Embrainment refers to the encoding of neuronal activity that occurs within cultural contexts. Enculturation reflects the neural mechanisms of cognitive and affective functions that manifest cultural contexts. Concepts of embrainment and enculturation constitute neuroidentity relations that describe functional associations of the mind and the brain. The centrality of the self to the encoding and generation of culture in neuronal activity illustrates a standard paradigm for embrainment and enculturation.

Chiao, Mano, Li, Bebko, Blizinsky, and Turner (Chapter 5) review theoretical, methodological, and empirical foundations in cultural neuroscience. Research priorities in cultural neuroscience include the study of cultural influence on neurobiological systems of behavior. Methodological tools that vary in spatial and temporal dimensions facilitate the observation and measurement of the structure and function of the nervous system. Empirical approaches in cultural neuroscience consist of research programs that systematically investigate cultural processes in multilevel mechanisms of the nervous system. The scientific study of culture and the nervous system is essential to the discovery of fundamental laws and principles of cultural processes and their physical instantiation in the natural world.

Chiao and Sadato (Chapter 6) review psychophysiological approaches in cultural neuroscience and global mental health. Brain dynamics of the nervous system illustrate the temporal and sequential properties of mental constructs and multilevel mechanisms. Psychophysiological approaches investigate the spatiotemporal properties of psychophysiological components and their relation to mental functions of cultural contexts. Conceptual models that postulate cultural processes as sequences of mental functions in neural mechanisms provide a theoretical basis for the study of psychophysiological components of culture. Spatiotemporal properties of cultural processes contribute to the identification of biomarkers affecting mental health.

Chiao, Li, and Sadato (Chapter 7) review cultural variation in the human genome. The population structure of the human genome characterizes sources of geographic and cultural variations of populations. Geographic and cultural variations contribute to the epidemiology of disease and disorder. Cross-national prevalence of mental disorders is explained in patterns of cultural and genetic variations. Understanding the sources of variation in the human genome is essential to the discovery and delivery of cures for, preventions of, and interventions for mental disorders.

Vasquez-Salgado and Greenfield (Chapter 8) introduce theoretical frameworks in sociocultural developmental neuroscience. Sociocultural factors play an important role in brain development. Cultural acquisition depends on functional brain maturation during development periods. Cultural resources affect the socialization and functional brain maturation of youth. Research in sociocultural developmental neuroscience systematically investigates the influence of sociocultural factors on neurodevelopmental trajectories of behavior.

Li (Chapter 9) reviews global aging and its implications for cultural neuroscience and global mental health. Growth in the aging population presents several challenges in global mental health. Discovery of cures, preventions, and interventions that bolster mental functioning in the aging brain is necessary to address the needs of the aging population. The aging brain consists of brain plasticity illustrating the malleability of risk and protective factors to mental disorders in older age. Cultural resources that buffer cognitive decline and enhance social and emotional functioning are an important protective factor in older age. Cultural changes that produce technological developments for behavioral intervention have the potential to provide considerable benefits to aging societies.

Part II reviews empirical approaches to the study of the etiology of mental disorders across cultural contexts. Chapters 10 through 18 present programs of research that systematically investigate cultural processes in multilevel mechanisms of mental functions. Cultural processes are generated and regulated within a range of mental constructs and neurobiological mechanisms. Understanding molecular and cellular mechanisms of brain functioning across cultural contexts is essential to discovery and delivery science that contributes to the alleviation of mental disorders.

Chiao, Mano, Stein, and Sadato (Chapter 10) review cultural processes in neurobiological mechanisms of emotion. Culture influences the generation, experience, and regulation of emotion. Research on cultural variation in emotion shows distinct processes of negative and positive affect across cultural contexts. Cultural variation in negative and positive affect is observed within neurotransmitter systems and patterns of functional activity within the nervous system. The regulation of emotion across cultural contexts modulates patterns of brain dynamics. Cultural processes that are fundamental to emotion contribute to mental health and well-being.

Nomura, Tsuda, and Rappleye (Chapter 11) discuss cultural differences in positive emotion and its implications for global mental health. Culture affects the experience of positive emotions. The experience of positive emotion in the cultural context plays an important protective role in sociocultural and psychological adaptation. Cultural variation in positive emotion may serve an adaptive function in response to and recovery from humanitarian settings. The study of cultural variation in positive emotion is important for understanding how protective factors reduce vulnerabilities and enhance resilience in the mental health and well-being of populations.

Masuda, Lee, and Russell (Chapter 12) review empirical approaches in the study of culture and perception. Cultural orientations influence the cognitive processes and neural mechanisms of perception. Analytic and holistic systems of thought are composed of cultural variation in fundamental cognitive processes of attention and perception. Cultural systems of perception show variation in attentional focus either on objects or on the surrounding context. Cultural variation in perception illustrates the importance of shared meaning systems as a bidirectional influence on mental and neural patterns of perception. Cultural variation in perception contributes to the protective factors that bolster mental health and well-being.

Tang and Tang (Chapter 13) review cultural differences in numerical cognition. The representation and processing of numerical cognition differ across cultures. Cultural factors affect the acquisition of numerical cognition. Cultural variation is observed in distinct functional patterns in the neural mechanisms of numerical processing. Cultural differences in motivational style may influence the ease of acquisition in numerical cognition.

Gutchess, Mukadam, Zhang, and Zhang (Chapter 14) review memory and aging across cultures. Structural and functional components of the aging brain affect memory. Cultural factors affect the processes of memory across the lifespan. Cultural influences on encoding reflect variation in memory representation and function. Cultural differences are observed in age-related patterns of neural function within the ventral visual pathway. Systematic investigation of aging and memory across cultures contributes to the identification of root causes of, preventions of, and interventions for mental disorders in global mental health.

Goto, Lewis, and Grayzel-Ward (Chapter 15) review cultural differences in self-construal. Cultural variation in self-construal affects cognitive, affective, and motivational processes of behavior. Independent and interdependent self-construal characterize distinct sets of mental processes that define the self. Cultural influences on self-construal describe behavioral and neural patterns of independent and interdependent mental functions. Cultural differences in self-construal characterize situational factors that affect the generation and regulation of mental and neural functioning.

Blais and Caldara (Chapter 16) discuss cultural differences in visual perception. Culture affects the cognitive processes of social perception. The social processing of faces and emotion in multilevel mechanisms shows cultural variation. Cultural variation in top-down and bottom-up processing of social cues illustrates distinct patterns of mental function in perceptual systems.

Gianola and Reynolds Losin (Chapter 17) review theoretical, methodological, and empirical foundations of cultural learning in the imitative neural system. Imitation is a core cognitive process to cultural learning. Cultural variation in the imitative neural system illustrates distinct patterns of neural and behavioral function within mechanisms of cultural learning. Research on the imitative neural system across cultural contexts contributes to the identification of root causes of, preventions of, and interventions for mental disorders.

Sands and Harris (Chapter 18) review intergroup theories of dehumanization and its implications for global mental health. Dehumanization presents a considerable threat to social equality. Patterns of social cognitive practices that ease the arbitrary moral distinction of self and others in intergroup contexts illustrate the antecedents and consequences of bias. Dehumanization of others is a societal risk factor that contributes to prejudice and discrimination. The development and implementation of preventions and interventions that ameliorate the processes of dehumanization enhance resilience and reduce vulnerabilities of populations.

Part III explores the cultural factors that contribute to the design of prevention and early intervention in global mental health. Understanding mental disorders in the context of cultures is informative for the design of preventions and early interventions in mental health that are widely accepted. Cultural factors demonstrate the malleability of risk and protective factors of mental disorders. Culture is a potent resource for the bolstering of mental capital and underlying multilevel mechanisms that are vital to mental health and well-being.

Varnum and Hampton (Chapter 19) articulate a framework for the study of cultural change in the structure and function of the human brain. Cultural change occurs as patterns of change in thought and behavior. Cultural change in thought and behavior manifests in dynamic patterns of attitudes and values. The structure and function of the human brain undergoes dynamic change across situational and cultural contexts. Fundamental principles of learning describe neural mechanisms that support the acquisition of novel knowledge. Cultural change may be particularly adaptive in response to ecological and technological conditions that protect mental health and well-being.

Goh (Chapter 20) reviews the theoretical foundations of culture and neuroplasticity as fundamental principles of the human brain. Culture affects the structure and function of the organization of the human brain. Neuroplasticity contributes to the patterns of neuronal activity that encode cultural information. Neural processing of prediction error facilitates processing of information that is congruent with social norms within the cultural context. Learning principles that maintain and strengthen skill acquisition improve understanding of cellular mechanisms that reduce vulnerability and improve resilience to disorders. The development and implementation of behavioral training paradigms advance prevention and early intervention in global mental health.

Chiao, Mano, and Sadato (Chapter 21) review the importance of culture in technological innovations for global mental health. Technology provides essential tools for the discovery and delivery science of health equity across nations. Technology that improves capability across cultural contexts ensures access to and use of information necessary for the achievement of health equity. Technological innovation that improves cultural competence is beneficial to the development and implementation of preventions and early interventions in global mental health.

Chiao, Mano, and Sadato (Chapter 22) review the role of culture in the maintenance and regulation of risk and protective factors in the social and physical environment. Cultural dimensions serve a protective role in adaptive response to conditions of environmental threat. Cultural dimensions consist of patterns of thought and behavior that reduce societal exposure to risk factors of environmental threat. Cultural dimensions characterize protective factors that strengthen resilience and support social and physical well-being. Culture that strengthens the perception of protection and empowerment in the social and physical environment is an effective strategy for prevention of and early intervention for disorders in global mental health.

Jensen (Chapter 23) discusses the role of globalization in culture. Globalization enhances opportunities for cultural contact among diverse populations. Globalization is one of the most efficient strategies for the popularization of culture. Globalization affects the processes of acculturation and cultural identity. Globalization is a potent influence on the human development of individuals, societies, and nations. Understanding the influence of globalization on mental health and well-being is important to human fulfillment and the achievement of human potential.

Part IV discusses societal conditions that affect the improvement of treatments and access to care in global mental health.

Iidaka (Chapter 24) reviews the societal factors that affect premature mortality worldwide. The cross-national prevalence of premature mortality from suicide is affected by social and economic conditions. The cross-national prevalence of premature mortality from suicide has been in steady decline in the past 15 years. Religion and economic growth are protective factors that contribute to the reduction of premature mortality.

Tang and Tang (Chapter 25) discuss cultural differences that affect mental health promotion. The integrated health model (IHM) addresses mental health promotion and prevention in global mental health. The IHM of mental health promotion involves the development of culturally adapted preventions and interventions for mental health promotion.

Part V discusses ways of raising awareness of the global burden of mental health disorders. Cultural factors affect mental health disparities in access to and use of health services. Cultural strategies are beneficial for the amelioration of the stigma, discrimination, and social exclusion associated with mental disorders. The manifestation and prevalence of mental disorders vary across ethnic groups within and across nations. Understanding how cultural factors affect the prevalence of mental disorders across ethnic groups is essential to the amelioration of mental disorders.

Chiao and Blizinsky (Chapter 26) review research in cultural neuroscience that contributes to closing the gap in population disparities in mental health. Population disparities in mental health refer to the variation in the prevalence of mental disorders due to unequal conditions across racial and ethnic groups. Population variation in mental health disparities suggests the importance of cultural factors in the etiology of mental disorders. Understanding the root causes of mental disorders across racial and ethnic groups contributes to the amelioration of population disparities in mental health. Evidence-based approaches in cultural neuroscience inform policymaking to achieve health equity for all.

Bart-Plange and Trawalter (Chapter 27) review the role of stigma in health disparities. Stigma contributes to the social construction of mental and physical health disparities. Stigma occurs not only among individuals but also within societal contexts that contribute to health disparities. Structural stigma refers to the institutional and cultural resources that contribute to health and well-being. Favorable environmental conditions that promote social equality and eliminate racial prejudice and discrimination are necessary to ameliorate stigma and health disparities.

Alvarez and Muscatell (Chapter 28) review the root causes of socioeconomic health disparities. Socioeconomic factors contribute to neural and physiological mechanisms of health behavior. Cultural factors affect the social processes underlying socioeconomic status. Culture influences the perception of self and others across varying levels of socioeconomic status. Cultural differences in socioeconomic status contribute to variations in neural and physiological responding that contribute to health disparities. Understanding the role of cultural factors in socioeconomic status and underlying multilevel mechanisms is essential to the elimination of health disparities.

Chae and Wang (Chapter 29) review cultural differences in autobiographic memory, with a focus on the effects of language, family narrative practices, and emotional knowledge in affecting an individual's memory of personal experiences. Differences in these mechanisms between European-American and Asian cultures contribute to global diversities in the emergence and maintenance of autobiographic memory during childhood and across adult life, respectively. Having a stable self-identity is essential for an individual's psychological well-being. Disturbances or disruptions of autobiographical memory affect the stability of self-identity, which is associated with many common mental health problems including depression and dementia. Thus, understanding cultural differences in mechanisms underlying autobiographic memory is important for improving interventions for mental disorders of the self and its memory.

Implications

Research in cultural neuroscience and global mental health is a necessary resource for the amelioration of mental disorders and the achievement of health equity. Evidence-based approaches in cultural neuroscience generate novel knowledge of the root causes of, preventions for, and interventions for mental disorders in global mental health. The identification of biomarkers of mental disorders differs across cultural contexts. Culture influences neurobiological mechanisms of behavior. Understanding the root causes of mental disorders across cultural contexts is fundamental to the discovery of cures, preventions, and interventions in global mental health.

Cultural factors affect the malleability of risk and protective factors that contribute to mental disorders. Cultural processes affect societal exposure to risk and protective factors of ethnocultural groups. Culture strengthens resilience and reduces vulnerabilities to mental disorders. Culture influences the perception of protection and empowerment that is necessary for human development.

Future Directions

Future directions in the field include systematic, large-scale efforts to generate novel scientific knowledge and translate research into practice and policy. Social and financial investment to build research capacity is essential to the development and implementation of targeted development initiatives that address key priorities in the field. The goal to advance novel scientific knowledge in the field may lead to substantial societal and economic benefits for health equity.

Research and policy interventions are beneficial to the design of effective strategies that improve mental health and quality of life around the world. Mental health and well-being are necessary to human development across nations. The transformation of health systems and policies through evidence-based approaches is a fundamental goal of the development agenda for the achievement of health equity for all.

INDEX

Tables, figures and boxes are indicated by *t*, *f* and *b* following the page number. Numbers followed by n. indicate footnotes.